W. Domschke S.J. Konturek (Eds.)

The Stomach

Physiology, Pathophysiology and Treatment

With 155 Figures

Springer-Verlag
Berlin Heidelberg New York
London Paris Tokyo
Hong Kong Barcelona
Budapest

Professor W. Domschke, MD MD(hon) FACG
Chairman of the Department of Medicine B
University of Münster
Albert-Schweitzer-Str. 33
D-48149 Münster
Germany

Professor S.J. Konturek, MD
Chairman of the
Institute of Physiology
University of Kraków
ul. Grzegórzecka 16
PL-31531 Kraków
Poland

ISBN-13:978-3-540-56613-7 e-ISBN-13:978-3-642-78176-6
DOI: 10.1007/978-3-642-78176-6

Library of Congress Cataloging-in-Publication Data. The stomach/[edited by] W. Domschke, S.J. Konturek. p. cm. Based on the International Symposium on the Stomach in Münster in Sept. 1992. Includes bibliographical references and index. ISBN-13:978-3-540-56613-7
1. Stomach—Diseases—Congresses. 2. Stomach—Pathophysiology—Congresses. 3. Stomach—Physiology—Congresses. I. Domschke, Wolfram. II. Konturek, Stanislaw J. III. International Symposium on the Stomach (1992: Münster in Westfalen, Germany) [DNLM: 1. Stomach—physiology—congresses. 2. Stomach—physiopathology—congresses. 3. Stomach Diseases—therapy—congresses. WI 300 S876 1992] RC816.S833 1993 616.3'3—dc20
DNLM/DLC for library of Congress 93-21900

Typesetting: Macmillan India Ltd., Bangalore 25
23/3145/SPS-5 4 3 2 1 0-Printed on acid-free paper

Preface

Members of the European Gastro Club, which celebrates its 25th anniversary this year, wrote this book, together with friends and colleagues from all over the world. Their purpose was to make available to a wider audience the information assembled at the International Symposium on the Stomach in Münster in September 1992.

Their contributions approach the theme "The Stomach and Its Diseases" from a variety of different angles at different levels of biological organization, covering current topics of clinical, morphological, pharmacological, physiological, biochemical, and cell and molecular biological interest. What unites the authors – accepted experts in their field – is their desire to achieve a better understanding of the stomach and its diseases, a broadening and deepening of our knowledge from which the patients entrusted to our care may benefit in the end.

Working with our colleagues, the ladies and gentlemen of Springer-Verlag and of EuMeCom, Medizin Information Fortbildung GmbH, Hamburg, has been a pleasure. Our thanks are due to all those who have helped make possible the publication of this book in its present form.

Münster and Krakow,
March 1993

WOLFRAM DOMSCHKE
STANISLAW J. KONTUREK

Preface

Contents

List of Contributors

BERSTAD, A., Prof. Dr., Section of Gastroenterology, Medical Department, University of Bergen, Haukeland Hospital, N-Bergen, Norway

BIANCHI PORRO, G., Prof. Dr., Gastrointestinal Unit, Ospedale "L. Sacco", Via G.B. Grassi, 74, 1-20157 Milano, Italy

DOMSCHKE, W., Prof. Dr. Dr.h.c., Dept. of Medicine B, University of Münster, Albert-Schweitzer-Str. 33, D-48149 Münster, Germany

FOERSTER, E., Priv.-Doz. Dr. Dr., Dept. of Medicine B, University of Münster, Albert-Schweitzer-Str. 33, D-48149 Münster, Germany

FORTE, J.G., Prof. Dr., Dept. of Molecular and Cell Biology, 241 LSA, University of California, Berkeley, CA 94720, USA

GALMICHE, J.P., Prof. Dr., Centre Hospitalier Régional et Universitaire de Nantes, Hôpital Guillaume et René Laennec, B.P. 1005, F-44035 Nantes, Cedex 01, France

GARNER, A., Prof. Dr. Dr., Dept. of Biochemistry, The University College of Wales, GB-Aberystwyth, Dyfed SY23 3DD, Great Britain

HALTER, F., Prof. Dr., Dept. of Gastroenterology, University Hospital Inselspital, CH-3010 Bern, Switzerland

HELANDER, H.F., Prof. Dr., Astra Hässle, Kärragatan 5, S-43183 Mölndal, Sweden

HÖGEMANN, B., Prof. Dr., Dept. of Medicine B, University of Münster, Albert-Schweitzer-Str. 33, D-48149 Münster, Germany

KITAJIMA, M., Prof. Dr., Dept. of Surgery, Keio University, 35 Shinanomachi, Shinjuku-ku, Tokyo, Japan

KONTUREK, S.J., Prof. Dr., Institute of Physiology, University School of Medicine, Grzegórzecka 16, PL-31531 Kraków, Poland

LAMERS, C.B.H.W., Prof. Dr., Dept. of Gastroenterology and Hepatology, Academisch Ziekenhuis Leiden, Building 1, C4-PO15, Rijnsburgerweg 10, NL-2300 Leiden, Netherlands

LEWIN, M.J.M., Prof. Dr., Hôpital Bichat, 170, Boulevard Ney, F-75877 Paris, Cedex 18, France

LOH, C.S., Prof. Dr., National Medical Laser Centre, The Rayne Institute, 5 University Street, GB-London WC 1E 6JJ, Great Britain

MATON, P.N., Prof. Dr., Oklahoma Foundation for Digestive Research, 711 Stanton L. Young Blvd., Suite 501, OK 73104, USA

OGURO, Y., Dr., National Cancer Center, Division of Endoscopy, 5-1-1 Tsukiji, Chuo-ku, Tokyo, Japan

PIASECKI, Ch., Prof. Dr., Dept. of Anatomy, Royal Free Hospital School of Medicine, Rowland Hill St., GB-London NW 32 PF, Great Britain

PREUSSER, P., Prof. Dr., Dept. of General Surgery, University of Münster, Jungeblodtplatz 1, D-48149 Münster, Germany

RACHMILEWITZ, D., Prof. Dr., Dept. of Gastroenterology, Hadassah University Hospital, P.O. Box 24035, Jerusalem 91240, Israel

REERS, B., Prof. Dr., Dept. of General Surgery, University of Münster, Jungeblodtplatz 1, D-48149 Münster, Germany

RUTGEERTS, P., Prof. Dr., Universitaire Ziekenhuizen Leuven, U.Z. Gasthuisberg, Herestraat 49, B-3000 Leuven, Belgium

SLOMIANY, A., Prof. Dr., UMDJ, Dental Research Center, 110 Bergen Street, Newark, NJ 07103-2425, USA

SLOMIANY, B.L., Prof. Dr., UMDJ, Dental Research Center, 110 Bergen Street, Newark, NJ 07103-2425, USA

SONNENBERG, A., Prof. Dr., Gastroenterology Service, Veterans Administration, Medical Center, 5000 West National Av., Milwaukee, WI 53295, USA

SZABO, S., Prof. Dr. Dr., Division of Chemical Pathology, Brigham and Women's Hospital, Harvard University School of Medicine, 75 Francis Street, Boston, MA 02115, USA

TARNAWSKI, A.S., Prof. Dr., Dept. of Medicine, California College of Medicine, UCI-Long Beach Medical Program, Veterans Administration Medical Center, 5901 E. Seventh Street, Long Beach, CA 90822, USA

TIO, T.L., Prof. Dr., Division of Gastroenterology, Georgetown University Medical Center, 3800 Reservoir Road NW, Washington, DC 20007-2197, USA

WHITTLE, B.J.R., Dr., Dept. of Pharmacology, Wellcome Research Labs., Langley Court, GB-Beckenham, Kent BR3 3BS, Great Britain

WYLE, F.A., Prof. Dr., Dept. of Medicine, Veterans Administration Medical Center, 5901 E. Seventh Street, Long Beach, CA 90822, USA

Gastric Physiology and Pathophysiology

Parietal Cell Receptors of Acid Secretion

M.J.M. Lewin

Introduction

The gastric parietal cell is a highly differentiated cell whose main and almost sole biological role is to secrete hydrochloric acid. In contrast to this narrow specialization, the functional regulation of the parietal cell involves a large span of physiological mediators of various chemical nature: ions (including H^+ itself), biogenic monoamines such as histamine and acetylcholine, peptides (i.e. the so-called gastrointestinal "hormones"), and fatty acid derivatives such as prostagladins and platelet-activating factor (PAF). Some of these mediators are locally released from nerves or "endocrine" cells and act through neurocrine or paracrine pathways. This is notably the case for histamine and somatostatin. Others are released at a distance from the parietal cell, and for their action to occur they need to be transported by the blood, i.e. they act as true endocrine mediators, as gastrin does for instance. In addition, autocrine regulatory pathways may also occur with membrane-diffusible lipidic mediators. A further complication is the fact that many of the acid secretion mediators do not act directly on the parietal cell but require the intervention of one or several relay cell(s) which generate several feed-back effects and regulatory loops (Fig. 1).

Because of this complex pattern, a specific approach to parietal cell receptors is extremely difficult to carry out in vivo, and this is why most of our present knowledge in this area comes from in vitro studies on isolated glands, cells or membranes. Such studies have already made it possible to characterize several parietal cell receptors in terms of binding kinetics and intracellular signalling pathways. Moreover, for some of them, the primary structure has been elucidated by genetic cloning.

Stimulatory Receptors

Three main stimulatory receptors are present on the parietal cell, namely, the histamine, gastrin and muscarinic receptors. For a long time, our knowledge of these receptors has been restricted to their pharmacological features. However, during the last few years there has been a dramatic acceleration in the approach to their biochemistry, their mechanistics and their molecular structure. Furthermore, additional stimulatory receptors have been recently suggested on the

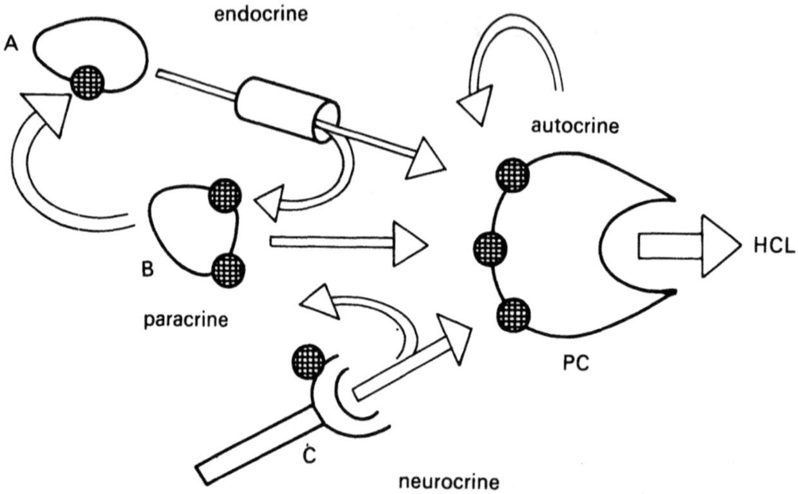

Fig. 1. Regulatory pathways of acid secretion. The gastric parietal cell is controlled by a set of receptors (*dark balls*) located on the parietal cell itself (*PC*) or on various relay cells (*A*, *B*, *C*). These are "endocrine cells" or neurons. Several endocrine, paracrine, neurocrine and autocrine feedback loops are operating (*arrows*)

parietal cell whose physiological role is still unclear. These particularly include the GLP-1 and PAF receptors.

Histamine Receptor

This receptor is by far the best documented among the parietal cell receptors. Early identified as a H_2 subtype, it was the subject of extensive pharmacological investigations which led to the development of the well-known series of specific antagonists as antiulcer drugs [1]. In addition to their importance for therapy, these pharmacological investigations shed some light on the chemical requirement at the receptor level. They indicated that binding of histamine or structurally related molecules to the receptor should be conditional on the recognition of a pentagonal nucleus containing at least one nitrogen atom (not necessarily an imidazole ring, as believed at first), while receptor activation should be triggered by the positively charged nitrogen of the aliphatic side chain. Furthermore, for this activation to occur, they suggested the requirement of a tautomeric equilibrium between two free pairs of electrons in the chemical nucleus [2, 3]. This empirical model proved to be consistent with the receptor molecular structure as recently characterized by cDNA recombinant techniques in canine [4] and human [5] parietal cells as well as in rat brain [6]. The H_2 receptor is a 70-kDa glycoprotein [7] whose primary structure is typical of that of the so-called seven-transmembrane-domain receptors (Fig. 2). The members of this family are known to interact with GTP-binding regulatory "G" proteins to produce their intracellular effects. Such a feature is consistent with the current

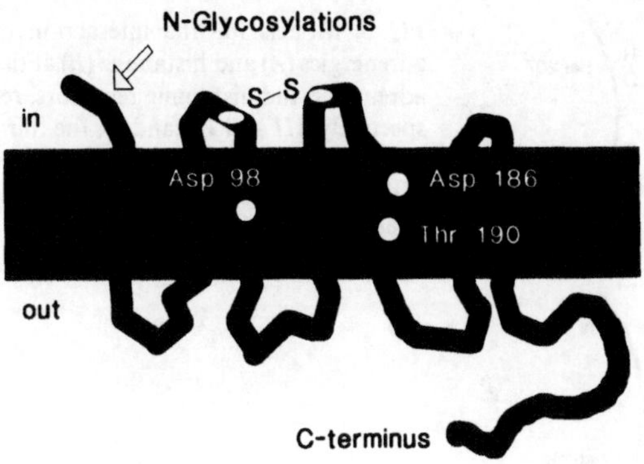

Fig. 2. Molecular structure of the parietal cell histamine H_2-receptor. This structure is characterized by seven hydrophobic domains which span the plasma membrane. The amino acids Asp 98, Asp 186 and Thr 190 are believed to play a crucial role for receptor activation

knowledge on signal transduction at the H_2 parietal cell receptor, i.e. a Gs-mediated activation of adenylate cyclase [8]. An interesting piece of information revealed by the H_2-receptor primary structure is the structural homologies of this receptor with the other monoamine receptors, particularly the widely studied β_2-adrenergic receptor [9]. In this latter receptor, an aspartate residue located in the third transmembrane domain (Asp 113) and two serine residues located in the fifth transmembrane domain (Ser 207 and Ser 204) are believed to play a critical role in the binding to and activation of the receptor by epinephrine [10]. The H_2-receptor also contains an aspartic residue in the third transmembrane domain (Asp 98), but the two serine residues in the fifth transmembrane domain are replaced by an aspartate and a threonine residue (Asp 186 and Thr 190). By analogy with the β_2-adrenergic receptor, it has been postulated that Asp 98 interacts with the protonated nitrogen of the histamine side chain, whereas Asp 186 and Thr 190 interact with the nitrogen atoms of the imidazole ring [11, 12] (Fig. 3). Recent mutagenesis studies are consistent with this view: replacement of Asp 186 by Ala 186 and of Gly 187 by Ser 187 was found to result in a "bifunctional" H_2/β_2-adrenergic receptor [13]. On the other hand, the aspartate and threonine residues that are suggested to be critical for the H_2-receptor's functioning are lacking in the H_1-receptor and replaced by threonine and asparagine, respectively [14]. This finding could provide a molecular basis for the specificity of H_2- vs H_1-agonists. The H_1-agonists are characterized by a hetero-aromatic nucleus containing one nitrogen atom with a free pair of electrons on the position next to an ethylamine side chain (position π). This π nitrogen atom is suggested to bind to the above-mentioned threonine or asparagine residues. Thus, the activation of the H_1-receptor would involve one critical hydrogen bond instead of two for the H_2-receptor. Furthermore, the requirement of imidazole ring tautomerism for histamine activation of the H_2-receptor suggests that a hydrogen exchange could be involved [15] (Fig. 4). In the furane and thiazole nucleus of the highly potent and specific H_2-receptor inhibitors ranitidine and famotidine (respectively) there is indeed no tautomerism and no possibility for such an exchange to occur [16].

Although a substantial amount of information is now available on the H_2-receptor protein and molecular functioning, much remains to be elucidated

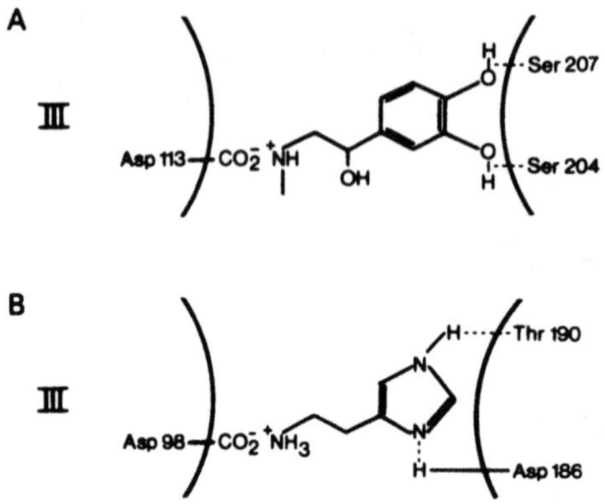

Fig. 3. Models for the interaction of adrenergics (*A*) and histamine (*B*) at the adrenergic and histamine receptors, respectively. *III* and *V* stand for the third and fifth receptor transmembrane domains. (From Birdsall [11] and Gantz et al. [12])

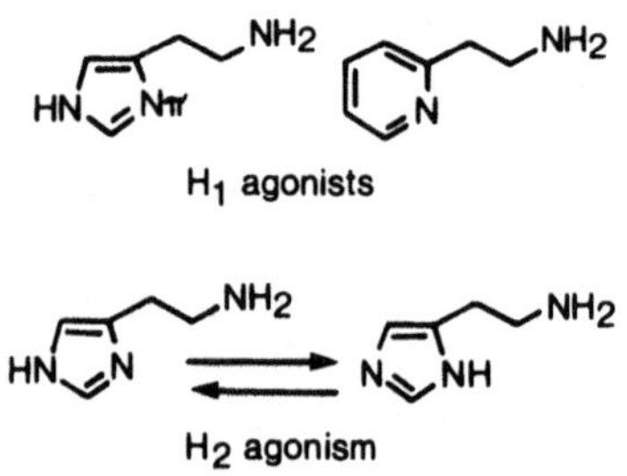

Fig. 4. Model of H_1 vs H_2 agonisms at the parietal histamine receptor. (Redrawn from Timmerman [15])

regarding the post-receptor events triggered by its activation. As already mentioned, adenylate cyclase stimulation and subsequent elevation of cAMP levels by the H_2-receptor have been extensively documented. However, there are observations suggesting that the H_2-receptor could also trigger a cAMP-independent transient increase in intracellular Ca^{2+} concentration in (some ?) parietal cells [17]. Furthermore, evidence has recently been provided for a cAMP- and Ca^{2+}-independent inhibition of phospholipase-A_2 activity and arachidonate release by the H_2-(brain)-receptor [18]. To date, these alternative signalling pathways remain unexplained. On the other hand, it is a matter of a current knowledge that the intracellular cAMP produced as a consequence of H_2-receptor occupation by histamine results in cAMP-dependent protein kinase(s)-mediated protein phosphorylations [19] (Fig. 5). A great deal of effort has been devoted to the characterization of histamine- or cAMP-phosphorylated proteins in the parietal cell. Several candidates have been suggested with various molecular masses and subcellular locations [20–23]. Some of these could operate as regulators of ionic channels, especially of the apical chloride channel [24]. Others could stand for those cytoskeleton proteins that are believed to be involved in the morphological rearrangement of the parietal cell which accompanies the onset of acid secretion (e.g. ezrin) [25]. However, further investigations are required to better characterize the role of these phosphoproteins in stimulus-secretion coupling.

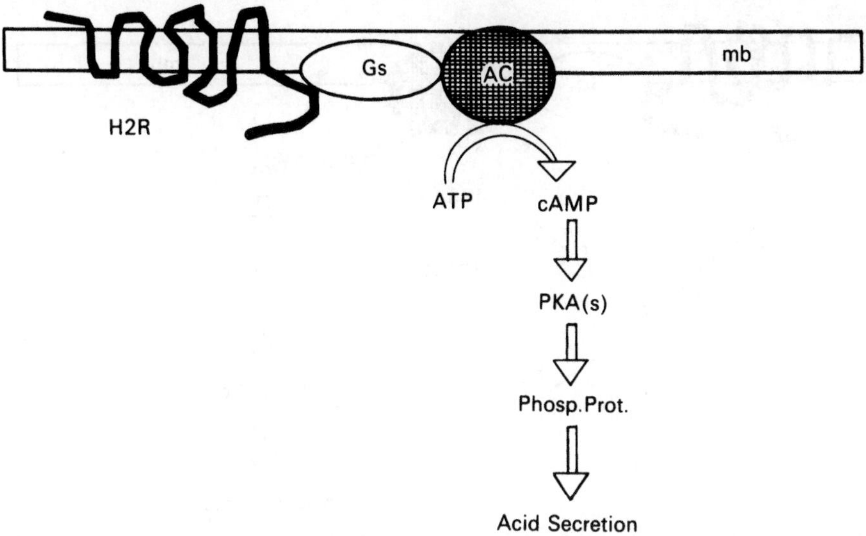

Fig. 5. The intracellular signalling pathway at the parietal H_2-receptor. *H2R*, histamine H_2-receptor; *Gs*, stimulatory coupling G-protein; *AC*, adenylate cyclase; *mb*, plasma membrane

Gastrin Receptor

The importance of gastrin as a physiological and pathophysiological regulator of acid secretion has been recognized for a long time, but there have been, and still are, a lot of controversies as to the exact place of this peptide in the regulatory pathway. Central to this issue is the question of whether or not a gastrin receptor is present on the parietal cell. Evidence for binding of tritiated [26] or iodinated [27] gastrin to isolated and highly purified rat and canine parietal cells was provided early by our laboratory and others. However, this evidence has for several years been obscured by the growing attention payed to histamine as a putative final common mediator. The crucial role of histamine in the stimulation of gastric acid secretion is now well documented and widely recognized, and this role is consistent with the remarkable efficacy of the histamine H_2-antagonists as inhibitory drugs. It is generally agreed that a primary stimulus event in physiological gastric acid secretion is histamine release from mucosal storage cells, identified as enterochromaffin-like (ECL) cells [28, 29]. Gastrin (as well as cholinergic) stimulation of mucosal histamine release has been indeed reported [29, 30]. Although this finding supports the presence of a gastrin (and a cholinergic) receptor on the ECL cells, it does not, however, preclude the possibility of the parietal cell's having its own gastrin (and cholinergic) receptor. As a matter of fact, a new line of evidence has emerged from recent studies which strengthens the hypothesis of a gastrin receptor on the parietal cell: (a) gastrin stimulation of [^{14}C] aminopyrine uptake (as an index of acid secretion) has been demonstrated in isolated and purified canine [31], rabbit [32–35] and rat [36] parietal cells, under conditions where the contribution of histamine was eliminated by the presence of H_2-blockers; (b) this

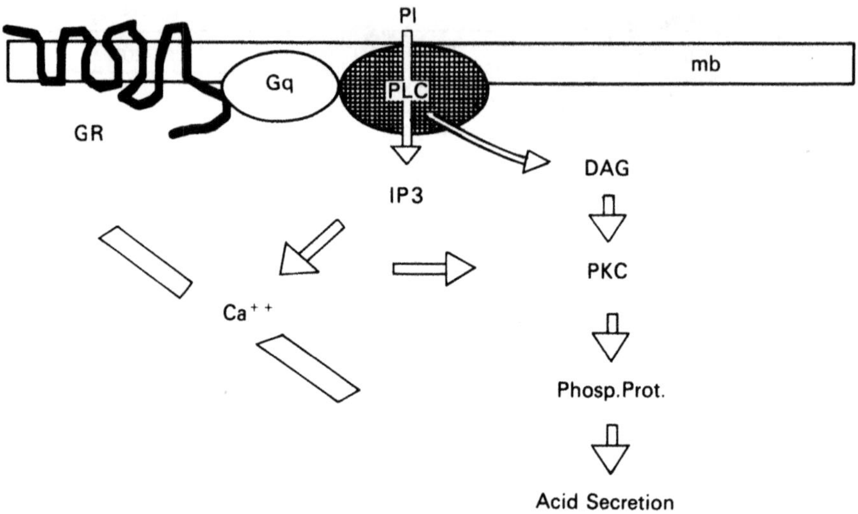

Fig. 6. The intracellular signalling pathway at the parietal cell gastrin receptor. *GR*, Gastrin receptor; *Gq*, coupling G-protein; *PLC*, phospholipase C (β isoform); *mb*, secretory membrane; IP_3 inositol triphosphate; *DAG*, diacylglycerol; *PKC*, calcium protein kinase

stimulation was found to coincide with membrane phosphatidylinositide turnover activation and subsequent increase in intracellular Ca^{2+} as monitored by the fluorescent dye Fura-2 AM [32, 37, 38]; (c) a gastrin-dependent Ca^{2+} increase in single canine [17] and rat [39] parietal cells was demonstrated by microfluorimetry; and (d) genetic cloning of the gastrin receptor has been recently achieved from a canine parietal cell cDNA expression library [40].

As is the case with the H_2-receptor, the primary structure of the gastrin receptor is consistent with a G-protein-coupled-seven-transmembrane-domain model of receptor. However, compared to the H_2-receptor, the gastrin receptor displays a larger third cytoplasmic loop and a shorter carboxyl terminal. This feature, which is also found in the H_1-histamine, the m_1-muscarinic and the D_2-dopamine receptors, is thought to be characteristic of Ca^{2+} mobilizing receptors [14] (Fig. 6). Expression of the cloned parietal cell gastrin receptor in the COS cell has confirmed its capacity to increase intracellular Ca^{2+} as the native receptor does. Moreover, these genetic cloning and in vitro expression studies have allowed the relationship between the gastrin receptor and the CCK receptor subtypes to be elucidated. It is now recognized that the parietal cell cloned gastrin receptor has the pharmacological features of a CCK_B receptor [41]. It is molecularly similar to the brain CCK_B receptor and distinct from the CCK_A type, which occurs in other peripheral targets such as the pancreatic cell [42]. That the gastrin receptor of the parietal cell does not clearly discriminate between gastrin and CCK makes it unlikely that it will be possible to design gastrin receptor antagonists devoid of CCK-like side effects.

Muscarinic Receptor

As is the case for gastrin stimulation, the characterization of cholinergic stimulation of acid secretion has long been hampered by the existence of indirect actions such as gastrin [43] and histamine [44] release. It is only recently that studies on isolated gastric glands or isolated and purified parietal cells have provided unambiguous evidence of a parietal cell muscarinic receptor [45]. The IC_{50} values for inhibition of this receptor by cholinergic antagonists were found to be in the following order of potency: HHSID (M_3-antagonist) $\gg$ 4-DAMP (M_1/M_3-antagonist) = atropine (nonspecific antagonist) $\gg$ pirenzepine (M_1-antagonist) $\gg$ AF-DX 116 (M_2-antagonist) [46]. This finding characterizes the receptor as an M_3-subtype. In accord with this pharmacological evidence, the polymerase chain reaction (PCR) amplification of the mRNAs with oligonucleotidic primers designed for the detection of all known muscarinic receptor subtypes confirmed the exclusive presence of M_3-subtype transcripts in the parietal cell [47]. The primary sequences of the five muscarinic receptors so far identified indicate that they belong to the seven-transmembrane-domain receptor family, and hence should involve G-proteins for their cellular effects. While the M_2- and M_4-subtypes couple to adenylate cyclase inhibition via G_i or G_o, the M_3- as well as the M_1- and M_5-subtypes are known to couple to phosphatidyl inositol via several possible G-proteins [48]. The molecular evidence for an M_3-subtype on the parietal cell is therefore in good accord with the increase in intracellular Ca^{2+} observed in this cell during cholinergic stimulation of acid secretion. However, it has been further suggested that this Ca^{2+} increase could also result from Ca^{2+} entry through a receptor-activated plasma membrane channel. An attractive hypothesis is that the receptor activates both pathways by coupling to two different G-proteins [45]. More experiments are required to clarify this point. However, since the M_3-receptor subtype is not specific to the parietal cell, it appears not to be a pharmacological target of interest for the design of antisecretory drugs.

GLP-1 Receptor

The GLP-1s are molecular variants of glucagon (1–37) that are produced by transactional processing of the precursor peptide in the intestinal L cell. Three main forms have been identified, i.e. GLP-1 (7–37), GLP-1 (1–36) and GLP-1 (7–36) and the two latter have been shown to be released into the circulation during the digestive phase. Besides their insulinotropic properties (stimulation of insulin secretion, biosynthesis and genomic transcription) the GLP-1s have been suggested to participate in the intestinal regulation of acid secretion, but this enterogastrone role is still controversial. Evidence has been recently provided that all three forms stimulated [^{14}C] aminopyrine uptake by isolated and purified rat parietal cells. Furthermore, this stimulatory effect was found to be mediated through activation of adenylate cyclase via a pertussis toxin-sensitive Gs-type subunit, as in the case of the H_2-receptor [49]. Clearly, these in vitro findings support the existence of a stimulatory GLP-1 receptor on the parietal cell, at least in the rat. Whether such a receptor could account for the physiological effects, if any, of the GLP-1s in human remains, however, to be investigated.

PAF Receptor

The platelet activating factor (PAF) is a phospholipid mediator involved in a variety of pathophysiological events. In the rat, intracerebral administration of PAF was shown to inhibit gastric acid secretion [50]. Furthermore, in this species PAF was suggested to partially mediate inhibition of pentagastrin acid secretion by endotoxic shock [51] and to inhibit vagal reflex stimulation of acid secretion as induced by pylorus ligation [52]. In the human digestive tract, PAF has been implicated in inflammatory processes associated with gastritis, RCH and Crohn's disease [53, 54]. However, the putative physiological role of PAF is still unknown. A stimulatory effect of PAF on [^{14}C] aminopyrine uptake by isolated guinea pig parietal cells has been reported [55]. Furthermore, evidence has been recently obtained in our laboratory for a stimulatory effect of PAF on [^{14}C] aminopyrine uptake by isolated rabbit gastric glands. This effect was insensitive to H_2-receptor blockade by ranitidine, whereas it was competitively inhibited by the specific antagonist BN50727 as well as the calcium channel inhibitor verapamil or intracellular calcium chelators (unpublished observations). Such findings strongly suggest that a PAF receptor has a role in the physiological control of acid secretion. Since it has been shown to be secreted in the gastric juice [53], PAF could act as an autocrine factor. Our preliminary findings indicate that the putative PAF receptor could be located on the parietal cell (its effect is H_2-receptor-independent) and that it could involve intracellular calcium as second messenger [56]. This signalling pathway would be consistent with the molecular structure of the PAF receptor (i.e. a seventh-transmembrane-domaine type) as recently characterized from guinea pig lung [57, 58]. However, future studies are required to ascertain the location on the parietal cell of this proposed new acid secretion stimulatory receptor and to further examine its physiological relevance in vivo.

Inhibitory Receptors

The inhibitory receptors of the parietal cell play an essential role in the control of acid secretion by modulating the effects of the stimulatory receptors. They lower the "physiological baseline" for stimulation and graduate the parietal cell response by allowing negative feedbacks to operate from other gastric cells. Two such inhibitory receptors are relatively well documented, i.e. the somatostatin and the prostaglandin receptors. Other candidate receptors have recently been suggested which deserve further investigations as to their biological nature and actual role in human physiology. These include (not exhaustively) transforming growth factor α/epidermal growth factor and the histamine H_3-receptor.

Somatostatin Receptor

That somatostatin is a physiological inhibitor of gastric acid secretion is supported by a line of evidence [59]. The existence of specific receptor sites for somatostatin on the isolated and purified rat parietal cell was first reported by our group [60, 61]. We and others further reported somatostatin inhibition of adenylate cyclase stimulation by the H_2-receptor. Since this effect was sensitive to pertussis toxin we suggested that somatostatin inhibition of gastric acid secretion could be explained by negative control of the H_2-receptor via a G_i-protein-coupled somatostatin receptor [62]. Similar findings and conclusions have been reported and proposed in subsequent studies by others on isolated canine [63] and rat [64] parietal cells as well as on the isolated mouse stomach [65].

To date, no less than three somatostatin receptor subtypes have been characterized by genetic cloning. The so-called $SSTR_1$ and $SSTR_2$ receptors have been obtained by PCR from mRNAs from human pancreatic islets. They differ slightly in size (391 and 369 amino acids, respectively) but there is 46% identity and 70% homology in their primary structures. Northern blot analysis of their distribution in human tissue indicates that they are expressed at the highest level in jejunum and stomach [66]. A third subtype has been identified by expression in the COS-7 of PCR extended fragments from a cDNA rat brain library. This subtype is 391 amino acids long and has 97.5% structural identity to $SSTR_1$ but less than 45% identity to $SSTR_2$. It is expressed in brain (hippocampus and cerebral cortex) but is apparently lacking in the peripheral tissue, including stomach [67].

Could $SSTR_1$ and/or $SSTR_2$ account for the parietal cell somatostatin receptor(s)? Both subtypes display a primary structure with seven potential transmembrane domains, hence consistent with their coupling to an adenylate cyclase inhibitory G_i-protein. However, as suggested from these reports, there seems to be a whole family of somatostatin receptor genes with tissue-specific expression. It is, therefore, possible that the parietal cell receptor pertains to another, still unidentified subtype. On the other hand, G_i-mediated adenylate cyclase inhibition might not be the only transduction pathway for somatostatin inhibition of acid secretion. Indeed, somatostatin was suggested to inhibit Ca^{2+} influx in a number of cells [68, 69], and we recently reported somatostatin inhibition of formation of inositol triphosphate in the rat pancreatic acini [70]. We also demonstrated, several years ago, a somatostatin-dependent protein dephosphorylation in isolated rat parietal and pancreatic cells [71–73], and we proposed that the somatostatin receptor could couple a phosphoprotein phosphatase [74]. Such a dephosphorylating effect could well account for the general inhibitory action of somatostatin on the various cellular functions, particularly acid secretion. The hypothesis of somatostatin receptor coupling to a phosphoprotein phosphatase has been recently re-emitted by three other groups. In addition, evidence was provided that somatostatin could dephosphorylate tyrosine as well as serine and threonine residues, but this effect would be more specifically related to cell growth regulation [75–78]. In an attempt to gain a deeper insight into the nature of the parietal cell somatostatin receptor(s), studies in progress in our laboratory are directed at the molecular characterization of an 87-kDa somatostatin-binding protein immunopurified from the HGT1 cell [68, 79]. Several somatostatin analogues have been synthesized which have proved to be useful as inhibitors of endocrine secretions (especially gastrinoma secretions) and are full of promise as inhibitors of tumoral cell growth [59, 80]. These can also produce inhibition of acid secretion, but this inhibition has a limited efficacy (because of the balance between G_s- and G_i-proteins in the parietal cell) and it is largely unspecific. Thus, unless a particular somatostatin receptor is discovered in the parietal cell, the somatostatin inhibitory pathway of the parietal cell appears of limited interest for the design of new acid secretion inhibitors.

Prostaglandin Receptor

Several observations support the assumption that the prostaglandins from the E and I series (PGE and PGI) are physiological inhibitors of gastric acid secretion. Furthermore, their inhibitory effect is more pronounced on histaminic stimulation, which suggests that they exert a direct effect via a parietal cell receptor(s) [81]. This view is consistent with early in vitro observations showing that PGE and PGI inhibited adenylate cyclase activity in isolated canine parietal cells (whereas they stimulated it in the nonparietal cells) [82] and the evidence for PGE binding sites on pig parietal cells [83]. Additional supports come from more recent studies on isolated canine [84], rat [85] and rabbit [86] parietal cells. These demonstrated that prostaglandin inhibition of cAMP adenylate cyclase was mediated through a pertussis toxin-sensitive G_i-protein, i.e. similarly to somatostatin inhibition. Such findings are consistent with the recent report on cloning and CHO cell expression of the lung PGE_3-receptor [87]. PGE_3-receptor mRNA has been detected in mouse stomach [87]. Furthermore, pharmacological evidence supports the theory that the parietal cell receptor is an E_3 subtype [88]. However, to date prostaglandin northern blot analysis has not been carried out on purified parietal cells.

In contrast to their inhibitory effect on acid secretion, the prostaglandins stimulate gastric secretion of mucus and bicarbonate. Furthermore, they are currently suggested to have a mitogenic effect. These interesting properties have prompted pharmaceutical firms to develop synthetic analogues as putative "cytoprotective" drugs (e.g. enprostil and misoprostol). The use of such analogues as acid secretion inhibitors would be theoretically possible using higher dosages. However, for the same reasons as mentioned above for somatostatin, prostaglandin inhibition of parietal cells is of limited efficacy and specificity.

TGFα/EGF Receptor

Epidermal growth factor (EGF) and transforming growth factor (TGFα) are currently suggested to play a gastroprotective role through various mechanisms including stimulation of mitogenesis [89], stimulation of gastrin gene transcription [90] and perhaps prostaglandin-mediated proto-oncogene (c-*myc*) expression [91, 92]. Both of these growth factors also exert an inhibitory effect on gastric acid secretion in vivo as well as in vitro [93–95]. Furthermore, EGF-receptor-binding sites have been demonstrated in isolated guinea pig gastric glands [96] and isolated porcine parietal cells [97]. The inhibitory effect has been suggested to be mediated in a similar way to that of somatostatin and the PGEs, i.e. via a pertussis toxin-sensitive inhibition of adenylate cyclase [64, 98, 99]. However, such a signalling pathway is somewhat unexpected from the molecular structure of the EGF receptor. Indeed, this differs from that of G-protein-coupled receptors by the presence of only one membrane-spanning domain. Furthermore, the only known membrane event triggered by the EGF-receptor is activation of phospholipase C(γ) by tyrosine phosphorylation, resulting in elevation of intracellular Ca^{2+} concentration [100]. Should such an activation occur in the parietal cell, it would result in a stimulatory rather than an inhibitory effect on acid secretion. Therefore, the intracellular pathway(s) mediating EGF-receptor inhibition of acid secretion remain to be elucidated. Interestingly enough, TGFα and EGF share the same receptor. Furthermore, coexpression of TGFα and EGF-receptor has been suggested by some authors to occur in normal as well as pathological gastric mucosal cells [101–103], including the parietal cell [104]. This would argue for an autocrine regulatory role of TGFα. It is possible that TGFα could participate in this way in the control of acid secretion, although it appears more likely that its major role would be dealing with the regulation of cell renewal and growth [89, 105]. On the other hand, there are still controversies about the expression of EGF-receptors in the adult normal gastrointestinal mucosa and their cellular and subcellular location [106–108].

Histamine H_3-receptor

The novel "H_3" type of histamine receptor was first demonstrated in the brain, where it is suggested to act as an autoreceptor mediating histamine inhibition of histamine synthesis and release from histaminergic nerves. This receptor is pharmacologically characterized by a poor sensitivity to the current H_1- and H_2-agonists and antagonists, whereas it is specifically activated and inhibited by the histamine derivatives R(α)-methylhistamine and thioperamide, respectively [109, 110].

Because of the crucial role played by histamine in the stimulation of acid secretion, the hypothesis of a gastric H_3-receptor was explored in our laboratory. In a first series of in vivo experiments carried out on the cat we found that R(α)-methylhistamine inhibited pentagastrin as well as meal-stimulated gastric acid secretion and that these effects were concentration-dependently prevented by thioperamide [111, 112]. In subsequent in vitro studies carried out on isolated gastric rabbit glands we obtained evidence for a R(α)-methylhistamine-sensitive thioperamide stimulation of [^{14}C]aminopyrine uptake by the parietal cells. Interestingly, this stimulation was parallelled by a significant release of histamine in the suspension medium. These findings do support the existence of a histamine H_3-receptor on the ECL cells (Fig. 7). However, thioperamide stimulation of [^{14}C]aminopyrine uptake was not inhibited by ranitidine. Furthermore, R(α)-methylhistamine inhibited histamine as well as carbachol stimulation of this uptake. This supports the existence of additional H_3-receptors on other cell types including the parietal cell itself [113] (Fig. 8). We have recently been able to affinity purify human H_3-receptor protein from the HGT1 cell [111, 114]. This would allow us to achieve its genetic cloning and to specify its cellular

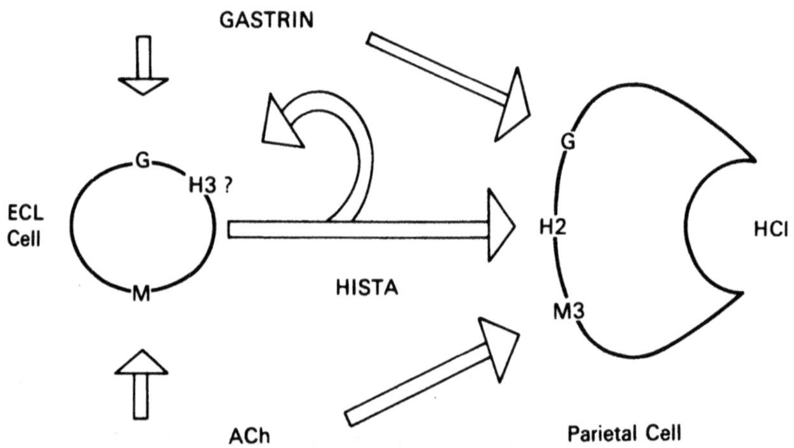

Fig. 7. The putative enterochromaffin-like (ECL) cell histamine H_3-receptor. This receptor would modulate histaminergic stimulation of acid secretion by exerting negative control on histamine synthesis and release. *G*, Gastrin receptor; M_3, muscarinic M_3-receptor; H_2, histamine H_2 receptor

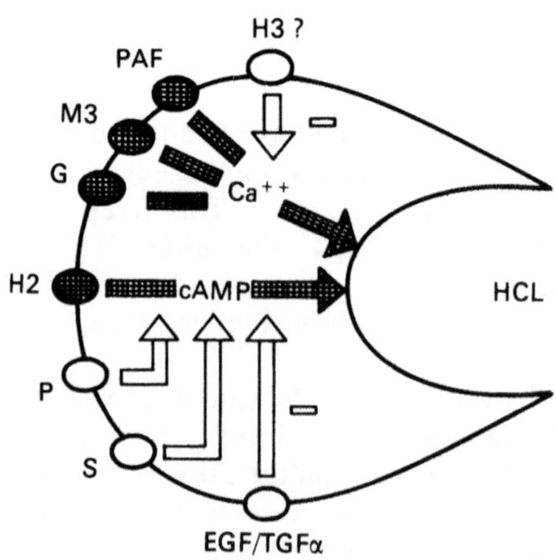

Fig. 8. The parietal cell receptors. The histaminic H_2 receptor (H_2) stimulates acid secretion via an increase in intracellular cAMP concentration. The gastrin (*G*), muscarinic (M_3) and putative PAF receptors stimulate acid secretion via an increase in intracellular calcium concentration. The prostaglandin (*P*), somatostatin (*S*) and EGF/TGFα receptors inhibit acid secretion via inhibition of cAMP formation. The putative histamine H_3-receptor is suggested to inhibit acid secretion via inhibition of intracellular calcium mobilization

expression. We have recently obtained evidence that the signalling pathway at this receptor should rely on G-protein-mediated inhibition of membrane phosphatidylinositide turnover [113]. Thus, the putative H_3-receptor could exert a negative control on intracellular Ca^{2+}-mobilizing receptors in a manner mirroring the negative control exerted by the prostaglandin, the somatostin and the EGF-receptors on cAMP-producing receptors.

Conclusion and Projections to the Future

This brief review shows that outstanding progress has been achieved in our knowledge of parietal cell receptors. In particular, the recent elucidation of the molecular structures of the histamine H_2- and gastrin receptors represents a major step towards the understanding of the initial events of acid secretion stimulation. Furthermore, the characterization of new receptors may provide important clues for a deeper and more comprehensive approach to gastric physiology and pathophysiology.

For the sake of clarity we have restricted our focus to the major biochemical pathways. This simplification should not mislead the reader into believing that all is known about receptor regulation of acid secretion. In fact, many aspects of this area remain obscure and need a great deal of further investigation. Among the important issues to be addressed in the future is the question of how the receptor proteins themselves are regulated. Desensitization of the β-adrenergic and the EGF-receptors has been shown to occur as a result of receptor phosphorylation, whereas tyrosine phosphorylation is known to be a prerequisite for EGF-receptor activation. Such mechanisms of phosphorylation-mediated receptor regulation could also operate in the parietal cell. Furthermore, as has been suggested for other G-protein-coupled receptors, it is possible that the parietal cell receptors pertaining to this family could auto- or cross-regulate their mRNA levels and their gene transcription through cAMP- or Ca^{2+}-mediated phosphorylations of a set of specific proteins (e.g. cyclic AMP responsible element binding proteins).

Another important issue is concerned with the multiplicity of the cellular events triggered by a given receptor as a consequence of its interaction with several types of G-proteins. This multiplicity provides a further intricacy in attempts to clarify the various postreceptor interactions between different stimuli. In addition, very little is still known about the nature of the phosphoproteins linking the activation of the secretory pathways to the turning on of the secretory machinery.

On the other hand, it is important to compare the in vitro findings from animal preparations to those obtained from human material [115, 116] and to evaluate the relevance of these finding in human physiology and pathophysiology. One may hope that new antisecretory drugs will emerge from the future advances in this field. However, with the single exception of the H_2-receptor, most of the parietal cell receptors so far identified appear to be of little interest as putative antisecretory targets. With regard to all these aspects, therefore, it appears essential to learn still more about the structure (particularly the three-dimensional conformation) and the biochemical nature of the parietal cell receptors.

References

1. Lewin MJM (1992) Cell physiology and pharmacology of gastric acid secretion. Therapie 47:93–96
2. Weinstein H, Chou D, Johnson CL, Kang S, Green JP (1976) Tautomerism and the receptor action of histamine: a mechanistic model. Mol Pharmacol 12:738–745
3. Gannelin CR (1982) Chemistry and structure-activity relationships of drugs acting at histamine receptors. In: Gannelin CR & Parsons ME (eds) Pharmacology of histamine receptors. Wright PSG, Bristol, p. 10–102
4. Gantz I, Schaffer M, DelValle J, Logsdon C, Campbell V, Uhler M, Yamada T (1991) Molecular cloning of a gene encoding the histamine H_2 receptor. Proc Natl Acad Sci USA 88:429–433
5. Gantz I, Munzert G, Tashiro T, Schaffer M, Wang L, DelValle J, Yamada T (1991) Molecular cloning of the human histamine H_2 receptor. Biochem Biophys Res Commun 178:1386–1392
6. Ruat M, Traiffort E, Arrang JM, Leurs R, Schwartz JC (1991) Cloning and tissue expression of a rat histamine H_2 receptor gene. Biochem Biophys Res Commun 179:1470–1478
7. Reyl-Desmars F, Cherifi Y, Le Romancer M, Pigeon C, Le Roux S, Lewin MJM (1991) Solubilisation, purification et caractérisation moléculaire du récepteur histaminique H_2 ă partir des cellules tumorales gastriques humaines HGT1. CR Acad Sci III 312:221–224
8. Cheret AM, Pignal F, Lewin MJM (1981) Effect of H_2-receptor antagonists cimetidine, ranitidine, and ICI 125, 211 on histamine-stimulated adenylate cyclase activity in guinea pig gastric mucosa. Mol Pharmacol 20:326–330
9. Dohlman HG, Bouvier M, Benovic JL, Caron MG, Lefkowitz RJ (1987) The multiple membrane spanning topography of the β_2-adrenergic receptor. Localization of the sites of binding, glycosylation, and regulatory phosphorylation by limited proteolysis. J Biol Chem 262:14282–14288
10. Strader CD, Sigal IS, Candelore MR, Rands E, Hill WS, Dixon RA (1988) Conserved aspartic acid residues 79 and 113 of the β-adrenergic receptor have different roles in receptor function. J Biol Chem 263:10267–10271
11. Birdsall NJM (1991) Cloning and structure-function of the H_2 histamine receptor. Trends Pharmacol Sci 12:9–10
12. Gantz I, DelValle J, Wang L, Tashiro T, Munzert G, Guo YJ, Konda Y, Yamada T (1992) Molecular basis for the interaction of histamine with the histamine H_2 receptor. J Biol Chem 267:20840–20843
13. DelValle J, Wang L, Gantz I, Guo Y, Yamada T (1992) Construction of a novel bifunctional receptor via mutagenesis of the fifth transmembrane domain of the histamine H_2 receptor. Regul Pept 40:132 (abst)
14. Yamashita M, Fukui H, Sugama K, Horio Y, Ito S, Mizuguchi H, Wada H (1991) Expression cloning of a cDNA encoding the bovine histamine H_1 receptor. Proc Natl Acad Sci USA 88:15515–15519
15. Timmerman H (1992) Cloning of the H_1 histamine receptor. Trends Pharmacol Sci 13:6–7
16. Cheret AM, Scarpignato C, Lewin MJM, Bertaccini G (1984) Inhibition of the histamine-stimulated adenylate cyclase activity of guinea pig gastric cells by the H_2-receptor antagonists cimetidine, oxmetidine and SKF 93479; Pharmacology 28:268–274
17. DelValle J, Tsunoda Y, Williams JA, Yamada T (1992) Regulation of (Ca^{2+}) by secretagogue stimulation of canine gastric parietal cells. Am J Physiol 262:G420–G426
18. Traiffort E, Ruat M, Arrang JM, Leurs R, Piomelli D, Schwartz JC (1992) Expression of a cloned rat histamine H_2 receptor mediating inhibition of arachidonate release and activatiton of cAMP accumulation. Proc Natl Acad Sci USA 89:2649–2653

19. Mangeat P, Marchis-Mouren G, Cheret AM, Lewin MJM (1980) Specific activation of cyclic AMP-dependent protein kinase(s) by H_2-receptor agonists in isolated gastric mucosal cells from guinea-pig. Biochim Biophys Acta 629:604–608
20. Chew CS, Brown MR (1987) Histamine increases phosphorylation of 27- and 40-kDa parietal cell proteins. Am J Physiol 253:G823–G829
21. Malinowska DH, Sachs G, Cuppoletti J (1988) Gastric H^+ secretion: histamine (cAMP-mediated) activation of protein phosphorylation. Biochim Biophys Acta 972:95–109
22. Urushidani T, Hanzel DK, Forte JG (1989) Characterization of an 80-kDa phosphoprotein involved in parietal cell stimulation. Am J Physiol 256:G1070–G1081
23. Modlin IM, Oddsdottir M, Adrian TE, Zdon MJ, Zucker KA, Goldenring JR (1987) A specific histamine-stimulated phosphoprotein in isolated parietal cells. J Surg Res 42:348–353
24. Soumarmon A, Abastado M, Bonfils S, Lewin MJM (1980) Cl^- transport in gastric microsomes. An ATP-dependent influx sensitive to membrane potential and to protein kinase inhibitor. J Biol Chem 255:11682–11687
25. Hanzel D, Reggio H, Bretscher A, Forte JG, Mangeat P (1991) The secretion-stimulated 80K phosphoprotein of parietal cells is ezrin, and has properties of a membrane cytoskeletal linker in the induced apical microvilli. EMBO J 10:2363–2373
26. Soumarmon A, Cheret AM, Lewin MJM (1977) Localization of gastrin receptors in intact isolated and separated rat fundic cells. Gastroenterology 73:900–903
27. Soll AH, Amirian DA, Thomas LP, Reedy TJ, Elashoff JD (1984) Gastrin receptors on isolated canine parietal cells. J Clin Invest 73:1434–1447
28. Rangachari PK (1992) Histamine: mercurial messenger in the gut. Am J Physiol 262:G1–G13
29. Hakanson R, Sundler F (1991). Do histamine-storing cells in the gastric mucosa mediate the acid-stimulating action of gastrin? In: Uvnas B (Ed.) Histamine and histamine antagonists. Handbook of experimental pharmacology. Vol 97. Springer, Berlin, p. 325–346
30. Berqvist E, Obrink KJ (1979). Gastrin-histamine as a normal sequence in gastric acid stimulation in the rabbit. Uppsala J Med Sci 84:145–154
31. Soll AH (1980) Secretagogue stimulation of [^{14}C]aminopyrine accumulation by isolated canine parietal cells. Am J Physiol 238:G366–G375
32. Muallem S, Fimmel CJ, Pandol SJ, Sachs G (1986). Regulation of free cytosolic Ca^{2+} in the peptic and parietal cells of the rabbit gastric gland. J Biol Chem 261:2660–2666
33. Roche S, Bali JP, Magous R (1990) Involvement of a pertussis toxin-sensitive G protein in the action of gastrin on gastric parietal cells. Biochim Biophys Acta 1055:287–294
34. Chew CS, Ljungstrom M, Smolka A, Brown MR (1989) Primary culture of secretagogue-responsive parietal cells from rabbit gastric mucosa. Am J Physiol 256:G254–G263
35. Chew CS, Hersey SJ (1982) Gastrin stimulation of isolated gastric glands. Am J Physiol 242:G504–G512
36. Cabero JL, Li Z, Mardh S (1991) Gastrin potentiates histamine-stimulated aminopyrine accumulation in isolated rat parietal cells. Am J Physiol 261:G621–G627
37. Roche S, Magous S (1989) Gastrin and CCK-8 induce inositol 1, 45-triphosphate formation in rabbit gastric parietal cells. Biochim Biophys Acta 1014:313–318
38. Chew CS, Brown MR (1986) Release of intracellular Ca^{2+} and elevation of inositol triphosphate by secretagogues in parietal and chief cells isolated from rabbit gastric mucosa. Biochim Biophys Acta 888:116–125
39. Cabero JL, Grapengiesser E, Gylfe E, Li Z, Mardh S (1992) Effects of gastrin on cytosolic free Ca^{2+} in individual acid-secreting rat parietal cells. Biochem Biophys Res Commun 183:1097–1102
40. Kopin AS, Lee YM, McBride EW, Miller LJ, Lu M, Lin HY, Kolakowski LF (1992) Expression cloning and characterization of the canine parietal cell gastrin receptor. Proc Natl Acad Sci USA 89:3605–3609
41. Wank SA, Harkins R, Jensen RT, Shapira H, DE Weerth A, Slattery T (1992) Purification, molecular cloning, and functional expression of the cholecystokinin receptor from rat pancreas. Proc Natl Acad Sci USA 89:3125–3129
42. Wank SA, Pisegna JR, de Weerth A (1992) Brain and gastrointestinal cholecystokinin receptor family: structure and functional expression. Proc Natl Acad Sci USA 89:8691–8695
43. Schubert ML, Bitar KN, Makhlouf GM (1982) Regulation of gastrin and somatostatin secretion by cholinergic and non-cholinergic intramural neurons. Am J Physiol 243:G442–G447
44. Hirschowitz BI, Molina E (1983) Effects of four H_2 histamine antagonists on bethanechol stimulated acid and pepsin secretion in the dog. J Pharmacol Exp Ther 224:341–345

45. Wilkes JM, Kajimura M, Scott DR, Hersey SJ, Sachs G (1991) Muscarinic responses of gastric parietal cells. J Membr Biol 122:97–110
46. Pfeiffer A, Hanack C, Kopp R, Tacke R, Moser U, Mutschler E, Lambrecht G, Herawi M (1990) Human gastric mucosa expressed glandular M_3 subtype of muscarinic receptors. Dig Dis Sci 35:1468–1472
47. Kajimura M, Reuben MA, Sachs G (1992) The muscarinic receptor gene expressed in rabbit parietal cells is the M_3 subtype. Gastroenterology 102:870–875
48. Pfeiffer A, Rochlitz H, Herz A, Paumgartner G (1988) Stimulation of acid secretion and phosphoinositol production by rat parietal cell muscarinic M2 receptors. Am J Physiol 254:G622–G629
49. Schepp W, Schmidtler J, Dehne K, Schusdziarra V, Classen M (1992) Pertussis toxin-sensitive and pertussis toxin-insensitive inhibition of parietal cell response to GLP-1 and histamine. Am J Physiol 262:G660–G668
50. Cucala M, Wallace JL, Salas A, Guarner F, Rodriguez R, Malagelada JR (1989) Central regulation of gastric acid secretion by platelet-activating factor in anesthesized rats. Prostaglandins 37:275–285
51. Martinez-Cuesta MA, Esplugues JV, Barrachina MD, Pique JM, Wittle BJR (1992) PAF and nitric oxide mediate the inhibition by endotoxin of pentagastrin-stimulated gastric acid secretion. Gastroenterology 102:A119
52. Defaux JP, Thonier F, Etienne A, Braquet P (1992) Platelet-activating factor (PAF) inhibits the secretion of gastric acid in rats: possible involvement of prostaglandins. First United European Gastroenterology Week (XIV Int Congress of Gastroenterology and VII Eur Congress of Digestive Endoscopy), Athens, 25–30 September 1992. Abstract book p. 58
53. Sobhani I, Denizot Y, Vissuzaine C, Vatier J, Benveniste J, Lewin MJM, Mignon M (1992) Significance and regulation of gastric secretion of platelet-activating factor (PAF-acether) in man. Dig Dis Sci 37:1583–1592
54. Sobhani I, Hochlaf S, Denizot Y, Vissuzaine C, René E, Benveniste J, Lewin MJM, Mignon M (1992) Raised concentrations of platelet activating factor in colonic mucosa of Crohn's disease patients. Gut 33:1220–1225
55. Nogami M, Suko M, Miyamoto T (1990) The effect of platelet-activating factor on [^{14}C] aminopyrine uptake by isolated guinea pig parietal cells. Biochem Biophys Res Commun 168:1047–1052
56. Sobhani I, Denizot Y, Laboisse C, Bourgeois M, Sainte Beuve AM, Benveniste J, Lewin MJM (1993) Production of PAF-acether (PAF) by a human gastric cell line: effects of neuromediators. Gastroenterology (in press)
57. Honda Z, Nakamura M, Miki I, Minami M, Watanabe T, Seyma Y, Okado H, Toh H, Ito K, Miyamato T, Shimizu T (1991) Cloning by functional expression of platelet-activating factor receptor from guinea-pig lung. Nature 349:342–346
58. Shukla SD (1992) Platelet-activating factor receptor and signal transduction mechanisms. FASEB J 6:2296–2301
59. Lewin MJM (1992) The somatostatin receptor in the GI tract. Annual Rev Physiol 54:455–468
60. Reyl F, Silve C, Lewin MJM (1979) Somatostatin receptors on isolated gastric cells. In: Rosselin G, Fromageot P, Bonfils S (eds) Hormone receptors in digestion and nutrition. Elsevier, Amsterdam, pp 391–399
61. Lewin MJM (1986) Somatostatin receptors. Scand J Gastroenterol (suppl. 119) :42–46
62. Reyl-Desmars F, Laboisse C, Lewin MJM (1986) A somatostatin receptor negatively coupled to adenylate cyclase in the human gastric cell line HGT-1. Regul Pept 16:207–215
63. Park J, Chiba T, Yamada T (1987) Mechanisms for direct inhibition of canine gastric parietal cells by somatostatin. J Biol Chem 262:14190–14196
64. Schmidtler J, Rosenthal W, Offermanns S, Schusdziarra V, Classen M, Schepp W (1992) Pertussis toxin reverses prostaglandin-E(2)- and somatostatin-induced inhibition of rat parietal cell H^+-production. Cell Signal 4:321–329
65. Schubert ML, Hightower J, Makhlouf GM (1989) Linkage between somatostatin and acid secretion: evidence from use of pertussis toxin. Am J Physiol 256:G418–G422
66. Yamada Y, Post SR, Wang K, Tager HS, Bell GI, Seino S (1992) Cloning and functional characterization of a family of human and mouse somatostatin receptors expressed in brain, gastrointestinal tract, and kidney. Proc Natl Acad Sci USA 89:251–255

67. Li XJ, Forte M, North RA, Ross CA, Snyder SH (1992) Cloning and expression of a rat somatostatin receptor enriched in brain. J Biol Chem 267:21307–21312
68. Lewin MJM, Reyl-Desmars F (1990) Molecular characterization of a purified human gastric somatostatin receptor. Metabolism 39:74–78
69. Yamada T, Chiba T (1989) Somatostatin. In: Schultz ST, Makhlouf GM (eds) Handbook of physiology. The gastrointestinal system II. Oxford University Press, Oxford, pp 431–453
70. Linard C, Reyl-Desmars F, Lewin MJM (1992) Somatostatin inhibition of phosphoinositides turnover in isolated rat acinar pancreatic cells: interaction with bombesin. Regul Pept 41:219–226
71. Reyl F, Lewin MJM (1981) Somatostatin is a potent activator of phosphoprotein phosphatases in the digestive tract. Biochim Biophys Acta 675:297–300
72. Reyl F, Lewin MJM (1982) Intracellular receptor for somatostatin in gastric mucosal cells: decomposition and reconstitution of somatostatin-stimulated phosphoprotein phosphatases. Proc Natl Acad Sci USA 79:978–982
73. Reyl-Desmars F, Zeytin F (1985) Somatostatin inhibits growth hormone-releasing factor-stimulated adenylate cyclase activity in GH3 cells. Biochem Biophys Res Commun 127: 986–991
74. Reyl F, Lewin MJM (1984) Cellular mechanism of action of somatostatin in the gastric mucosa: an hypothesis. In: Raptis S, Rosenthal J, Gerich J (eds) 2nd International symposium on Somatostatin, Athens, June 1981. Attempto, Tubingen, pp 293–295
75. White RE, Schonbrunn A, Armstrong DL (1991) Somatostatin stimulates Ca^{2+}-activated K^+ channels through protein dephosphorylatin. Nature 351:570–573
76. Tahiri-Jouti N, Cambillau C, Viguerie N, Vidal C, Buscail L, Saint Laurent N, Vaysse N, Susini C (1992) Characterization of a membrane tyrosine phosphatase in AR43J cells: regulation by somatostatin. Am J Physiol 262:G1007–G1014
77. Liebow C, Reilly C, Serrano M (1989) Somatostatin analogues inhibit growth of pancreatic cancer by stimulating tyrosine phosphatase. Proc Natl Acad Sci USA 86:2003–2007
78. Hierowsky MT, Liebow C, Du Sapin K (1985) Stimulation by somatostatin of dephosphorylation of membrane proteins in pancreatic cancer MIA PaCa-2 cell line. FEBS Lett 179:252–256
79. Reyl-Desmars F, Le Roux S, Linard C, Benkouka F, Lewin MJM (1989) Solubilization and immunopurification of a somatostatin receptor from the human gastric tumoral cell line HGT-1. J Biol Chem 264:18787–18795
80. Ruszniewski P, Lehy T, Reyl-Desmars F, Le Roux F, Lewin MJM (1993) Octreotide (SMS 201–995) inhibits the growth of colon peritoneal carcinomatosis in BDIX rats. Regul Pept 43:141–147
81. Whittle BJR, Vane JR (1987) Prostanoids as regulators of gastrointestinal function. In: Johnson LR (ed) Physiology of the gastrointestinal tract, 2nd edn. Raven, New York, pp 143–180
82. Major JS, Scholes P (1983) The localization of a histamine H_2-receptor adenylate cyclase system in canine parietal cells and its inhibition by prostaglandins. Agents Actions 8:324–331
83. Tepperman B, Soper B (1981) Prostaglandin E2-binding sites and cAMP production in porcine fundic mucosa. Am J Physiol 241:313–320
84. Chen MCY, Amirian DA, Toomey M, Sanders MJ, Soll AH (1988) Prostanoid inhibition of canine parietal cells: mediation by the inhibitory guanosine-triphosphate-binding protein of adenylate cyclase. Gastroenterology 94:1221–1229
85. Schepp W, Kath D, Tatge C, Zimmerhackl B, Schusdziarra V, Classen M (1989) Leukotrienes C_4 and D_4 potentiate acid production by isolated rat parietal cells. Gastroenterology 97:420–429
86. Choquet A, Leonard A, Magous R, Bali JP (1990) Intracellular coupling of prostaglandin inhibition of acid secretion in isolated rabbit gastric parietal cells. Biochem Pharmacol 39:1905–1911
87. Sugimoto Y, Namba T, Honda A, Hayashi Y, Negishi M, Ichikawa A, Narumiya S (1992) Cloning and expression of a cDNA for mouse prostaglandin E receptor EP3 subtype. J Biol Chem 267:6463–6466

88. Beinborn M, Degen V, Unruh E, Netz S, Sewing K (1992) Expression of prostaglandin E2 receptor subtypes in porcine parietal and chief cells. Gastroenterology 102:A40 (abst)
89. Konturek SJ, Brzozowski T, Majka J, Dembinski A, Slomiany A, Slomiany BL (1992) Transforming growth factor alpha and epidermal growth factor in protection and healing of gastric mucosal injury. Scand J Gastroenterol 27:649–655
90. Merchant JL, DelValle J, Wilson E (1992) EGF regulates gastrin gene expression in canine primary G cells. Regul Pept 40:A208
91. Handler JA, Danilowicz RM, Eling TE (1990) Mitogenic signaling by epidermal growth factor (EGF), but not platelet-derived growth factor, requires arachidonic acid metabolism in BALB/c 3T3 cells. Modulation of EGF-dependent c-myc expression by prostaglandins. J Biol Chem 265:3669–3673
92. Skouteris GG, McMenamin M (1992) Transforming growth factor α induced DNA synthesis and c-myc expression in primary rat hepatocyte cultures is modulated by indomethacin. Biochem J 281:729–733
93. Konturek SJ, Cieszkowski M, Jaworek J, Konturek J, Brzozowski T, Gregory H (1984) Effects of epidermal growth factor on gastrointestinal secretions. Am J Physiol 246:G580–G586
94. Rackoff PJ, Zdon MJ, Tyshkov M, Modlin IM (1988) Epidermal growth factor (EGF) inhibits both intrinsic factor secretion and acid secretion in histamine-stimulated isolated gastric glands. Regul Pept 21:279–287
95. Dembinski A, Drozdowicz D, Gregory H, Konturek SJ, Warzecha Z (1988) Inhibition of acid formation by epidermal growth factor in the isolated rabbit gastric glands. J Physiol 378:347–357
96. Forgue-Lafitte ME, Kobari L, Gespach C, Chamblier MC, Rosselin G (1984) Characterization and repartition of epidermal growth factor-urogastrone receptors in gastric glands isolated from young and adult guinea pigs. Biochim Biophys Acta 798:192–198
97. Sjodin L, Dahlen HG, Vittanen E (1992) Binding of epidermal growth factor to receptors in preparation of enriched porcine parietal cells and inhibition of aminopyrine uptake. Scand J Gastroenterology 27:495–500
98. Lewis JJ, Goldenring JR, Asher VA, Modlin IM (1990) Effects of epidermal growth factor on signal transduction in rabbit parietal cells. Am J Physiol 258:G476–G483
99. Yakabi K, Masaoka I, Nakamura T (1990) The mechanism for direct inhibition of canine gastric parietal cells by epidermal growth factor. Gastroenterology 98:A150
100. Pandiella A, Beguinot L, Vicentini LM, Meldolesi J (1989) Transmembrane signalling at the epidermal growth factor receptor. Trends Pharmacol Sci 20:411–414
101. Bennett C, Paterson IM, Corbishley CM, Luqmani YA (1989) Expression of growth factor and epidermal growth factor receptor encoded transcripts in human gastric tissues. Cancer Res 49:2104–2111
102. Cartlidge SA, Elder JB (1989) Transforming growth factor α and epidermal growth factor levels in normal human gastrointestinal mucosa. Br J Cancer 60:657–660
103. Yoshida K, Kyo E, Tsujino T, Sano T, Niimoto M, Tahara E (1990) Expression of epidermal growth factor, transforming growth factors and their receptor genes in human gastric carcinomas; implication for autocrine growth. Jpn J Cancer Res 81:43–51
104. Beauchamp RD, Barnard JA, McCutchen CM, Cherner JA, Coffey RJ Jr. (1989) Localization of transforming growth factor α and its receptor in gastric mucosal cells. J Clin Invest 84:1017–1023
105. Polk WH, Dempsey PJ, Russell WE, Brown PI, Beauchamp RD, Barnard JA, Coffey Jr RJ (1992) Increased production of transforming growth factor α following acute gastric injury. Gastroenterology 102:1467–1474
106. Thomas DM, Nasim MM, Gullick WJ, Alison MR (1992) Immunoreactivity of transforming growth factor alpha in the normal adult gastrointestinal tract. Gut 33:628–631
107. Slomiany BL, Lin J, Yao P (1990) Characterization of the epidermal growth factor receptor in gastric mucosa. Digestion 47:181–190
108. Polk WH, Saroka CJ, Goldenring J, Modlin IM, Bundz S, Dempsey PJ, Coffey RI (1991) Immunolocalization of transforming growth factor alpha (TGFα) and its receptor to the parietal cell in normal gastric mucosa. Gastroenterology 100:A660
109. Arrang JM, Garbarg M, Schwartz JC (1983) Auto-inhibition of brain histamine release by a novel class (H3) of histamine receptor. Nature 302:832–837

110. Arrang JM, Garbarg M, Lancelot JC, Lecomte JM, Pollard H, Robba M, Schunack W, Schwartz JC (1987) Highly potent and selective ligands for histamine H3-receptors. Nature 327:177–123
111. Lewin MJM, Bado A, Cherifi Y, Reyl-Desmars F (1993) Gastric H_3 receptors: a review. Yale J Biol Med 65 (in press)
112. Bado A, Hervatin F, Lewin MJM (1991) Pharmacological evidence for histamine H3 receptors in the control of gastric acid secretion in the cat. Am J Physiol 260:G631–G635
113. Bado A, Moizo L, Laigneau JP, Lewin MJM (1992) Pharmacological characterization of histamine H3-receptors in isolated rabbit gastric glands. Am J Physiol 262:G56–G61
114. Cherifi Y, Pigeon C, Le Romancer M, Bado A, Reyl-Desmars F, Lewin MJM (1992) Purification of a H_3 receptor negatively coupled to phosphoinositide turnover in the human gastric cell line HGT1. J Biol Chem 267:25315–25320
115. Haglund U, Elander B, Fellenius E, Leth R, Rehnberg O, Olbe L (1982) The effects of secretagogues on isolated human gastric glands. Scand J Gastroenterol 17:455–460
116. Leth R, Lundell L, Olbe L (1991) Effects of some gastrointestinal peptides on human and rabbit gastric glands. Scand J Gastroenterol 26:89–96

Structural and Functional Significance of the Gastric H^+, K^+-ATPase

J.G. FORTE and D.C. CHOW

Introduction

The apical plasma membrane of gastric parietal cells is highly adapted to perform its major physiological role in the secretion of concentrated HCl and at the same time maintain a resistance against the caustic degeneration from its very acidic secretory product. The predominant protein in the apical membrane of the secreting parietal cell is the proton pump protein, the H^+, K^+-ATPase. This membrane protein not only functions as the primary force for generation of HCl secretion, but must also be endowed with special properties that make it insensitive to pepsinolysis and H^+ degradation.

H^+, K^+-ATPase is a member of the family of cation pump proteins called P-type ATPases, which include the ubiquitous Na^+, K^+-ATPase and the Ca^{++}-ATPases of sarcoplasmic reticulum and plasma membrane [12, 14]. Unifying features in this family of pump proteins include the ability to form a phosphoenzyme intermediate, or E·P, in their catalytic cycle, and the relatively high degree of amino acid sequence homology, especially in the region of ATP binding and phosphorylation. Indeed, the sequence homology within the ATP binding domain was strategically used by Shull and Lingrel (1986) to design a nucleic acid probe to screen, and clone, the gene for the gastric H^+, K^+-ATPase. In a comparison of amino acid sequences among the various P-type ATPases it was pointed out that the H^+, K^+-ATPase shares the highest degree of homology with the Na^+, K^+-ATPase (~60% identity) and probably represents a fairly recent evolutionary modification that was functionally retained by the stomach [14].

In addition to sequence homology, Na^+, K^+-ATPase and H^+, K^+-ATPase share at least two additional features: they are both cation exchangers, including the cellular uptake of K^+ in exchange for exported Na^+ or H^+, respectively; and both pumps consist of $\alpha\beta$-subunit heterodimers. Generally, the α-subunit, with a M_r of about 110 kDa, is considered to be the catalytic subunit of the enzyme, containing sites for ATP binding and phosphoenzyme formation. For the Na^+, K^+-ATPase the α-subunit contains the ouabain binding site topologically localized to the extracellular domain [20]. H^+, K^+-ATPase does not have a ouabain binding site; however, its α-subunit does contain the site of omeprazole binding, which also appears to be in the extracellular domain [25]. For both the Na^+, K^+-ATPase and H^+, K^+-ATPase the α-subunits are thought to have eight transmembrane segments with intervening loops of peptide extending from the membrane; at least 70% of the α-subunit peptide mass is distributed within the cytoplasmic domain where interactions with ATP occur. Further information on the structural and functional activities of the α-subunit of the H^+, K^+-ATPase can be found in several reviews on the cell biology and biochemistry of gastric acid secretion [9, 25].

The purpose of this presentation is to review some of the structural and functional features of the much less studied β-subunit of the H^+, K^+-ATPase. In fact, it was only recently that a β-subunit for the H^+, K^+-ATPase had been suggested and demonstrated [23], and within months of this discovery five different laboratories published amino acid sequences for the subunit [4, 21, 24, 27, 28]. A comparison of sequence homology for the gastric β-subunit for six species, including human and an unpublished partial bovine sequence, is shown in Fig. 1.

Primary Structure of the Gastric β-Subunit

Unlike the α-subunit, the β-subunit of the H^+, K^+-ATPase is a glycoprotein with a single transmembrane segment, and over 70% of the 34-kDa peptide mass is positioned on the extracellular side of the plasma membrane. The β-subunit is heavily *N*-glycosylated, thus contributing to the apparently much higher molecular mass and its broad band of staining in the 60- to 80-kDa region on SDS-polyacrylamide gel electrophoresis (SDS-PAGE). Considering that all of the oligosaccharides are on the outer membrane surface, this suggests that more than 90% of the β-subunit mass is extracellular. From the available sequence data there are seven potential sites for *N*-linked glycosylation in the extracellular domain of the β-subunits from all species except the pig, for which there are only six such sites predicted (Fig. 1).

Among the many other homologous features for the β-subunits from these various species is location of nine cysteine residues. We were particularly struck by the extended homology when we compared β-subunits from the H^+, K^+-ATPase with various β-subunit isoforms of the Na^+, K^+-ATPase, finding that the six cysteine residues in the extracellular domain of all β-subunits examined were in identical locations [4]. Such a high degree of conservation in functionally divergent enzymes was consistent with an assumption of some fundamental role for these cysteine residues, possibly stabilizing tertiary structure through disulfide cross-linking.

Functional Activity of Disulfide Bonds in H^+, K^+-ATPase

Studies on the Na^+, K^+-ATPase suggested that cysteine residues in the extracellular domain of the β-subunit normally exist in the oxidized state as three disulfide bonds [15, 17], and that enzyme activity of the Na^+, K^+-ATPase

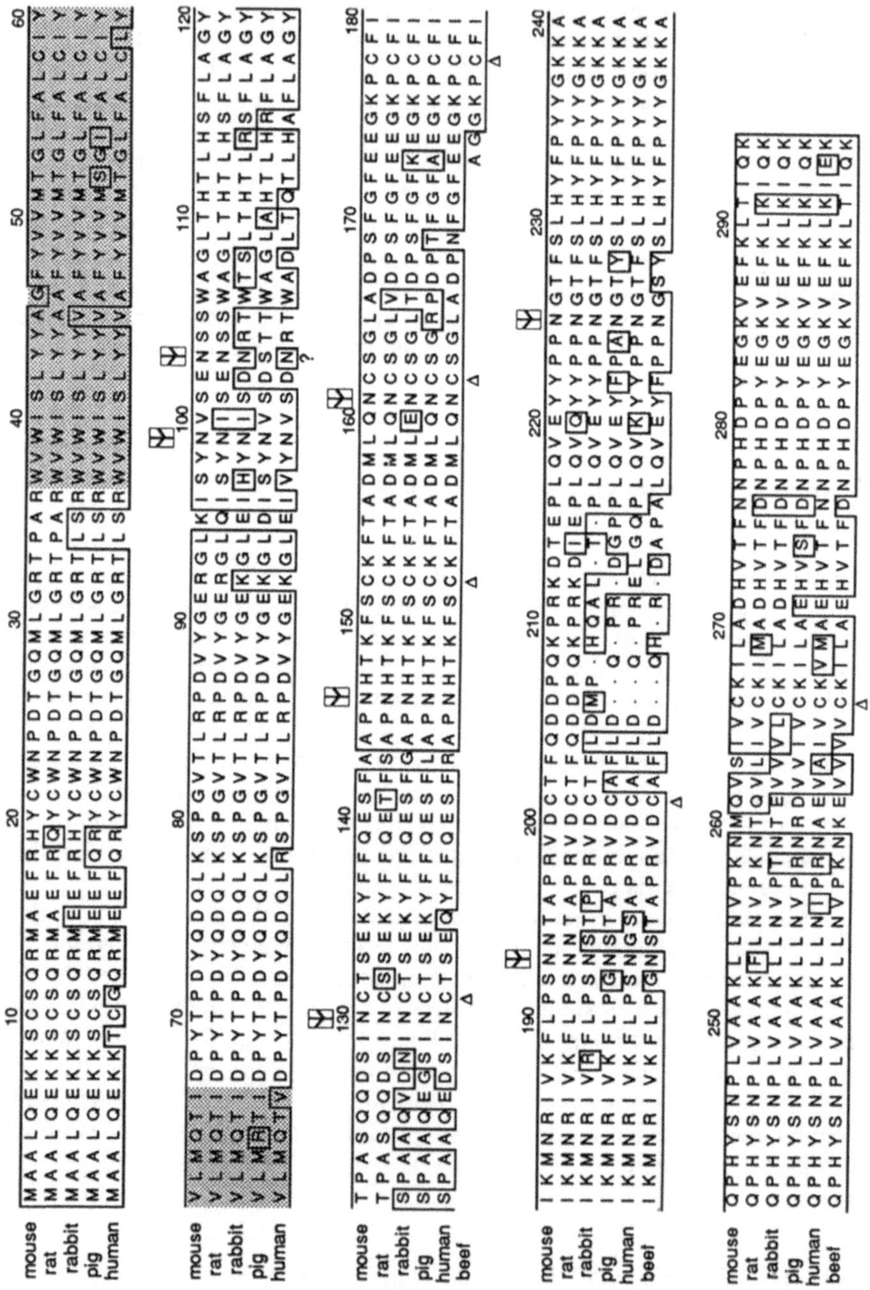

was inhibited under reducing conditions where the disulfides were at least partially reduced [15–18]. Because of the homologies with respect to the extracellular cysteine residues in the β-subunits of the cation-transporting ATPases, we tested the sensitivity of gastric H^+, K^+-ATPase activity to reducing conditions.

Strong reducing conditions, using relatively high concentrations of 2-mercaptoethanol or dithiothreitol at elevated temperatures, produced a time-dependent loss of either ATPase or K^+-stimulated pNPPase activities, as shown in Fig. 2. Interestingly, the degree of inhibition was attenuated in the presence of K^+, as had been shown for Na^+, K^+-ATPase [15, 18], indicating that the K^+-bound form of the enzyme was more resistant to reduction of disulfide bonds. Congeners of K^+, including Tl^+ and Rb^+, were shown to provide analogous protection of H^+, K^+-ATPase activity from disulfide reduction (Fig. 3). Also shown in Fig. 3 are the calculated ED_{50} values for the protection afforded by each of the three alkali cations and their effectiveness in stimulating the hydrolysis of pNPP (K_a values from [8]). The close correspondence between the ED_{50} and K_a values for Tl^+, K^+, and Rb^+ indicates that the protective effect was not some nonspecific ionic interaction, but rather related to the E_2 conformational state of the enzyme promoted by K^+ congeners. Furthermore, high concentrations of Na^+ antagonized the protective effects of 10 m*M* KCl, just as high concentrations of Na^+ antagonize the ability of K^+ to activate the phosphatase activity of the H^+, K^+-ATPase [5].

Separate experiments were carried out to quantitate the number of disulfide bonds in the β-subunit and to correlate their reduction, from -SS- to 2SH, with the loss of enzyme activity. Using sulfhydryl group-specific fluorescent labeling, as exemplified in Fig. 4, we estimated that about 70% of cysteine residues in the β-subunit are normally present in the oxidized state. Since there are nine cysteine residues in the β-subunit, we concluded that six of them are stabilized in the oxidized state and cross-linked as three disulfide bonds. On the other hand, for the α-subunit, our data suggest that less than 10% of cysteine residues in the α-subunit are in the oxidized state. Even this small extent of apparent oxidized α-subunit cysteines may be an overstimate due to nonspecific labeling and backgound noise; thus, there may be no disulfide bonds in the α-subunit. Recent experiments have shown that the β-subunit of the H^+, K^+-ATPase can act as a

---

Fig. 1. Comparison of amino acid sequences for the β-subunits of the H^+, K^+-ATPase of several species. The deduced amino acid sequence for the β-subunit of the mouse H^+, K^+-ATPase [3] was aligned with those of the rat [4, 27], the rabbit [24], the pig [28], and the human H^+, K^+-ATPase [21]. A partial sequence of the β-subunit of bovine H^+, K^+-ATPase (Canfield et al., unpublished data) is also shown. Lapses in the sequence allow optimal alignment for amino acid insertions/deletions. Identical residues are enclosed. The β-subunit of the mouse H^+, K^+-ATPase is numbered above. The β-subunit consists of a relatively short, amino-terminal, cytoplasmic segment; a single transmembrane segment, as indicated by the shading; and a long extracellular portion including sites for glycosylation and containing critical cyteine residues. The *triton symbols* indicate potential *N*-linked glycosylation sites (the *question mark* indicates a possible difference in glycosylation for the pig β-subunit). The *triangles* indicate the locations of the extracellular cysteine residues, which are highly conserved with those of the Na^+, K^+-ATPase

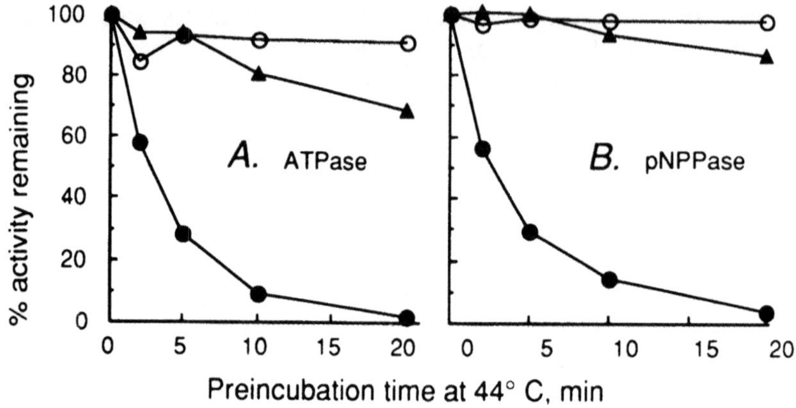

Fig. 2. Kinetics of inactivation of H^+, K^+-ATPase by 2-mercaptoethanol (2-ME) and the protective effect of K^+. Enzyme was preincubated with or without 0.46 *M* 2-ME at 44°C, in the presence or absence of 10 m*M* KCl, for the indicated times, and then diluted for assay of both K^+-stimulated ATPase (*panel A*) and K^+-stimulated pNPPase activities (*panel B*). Preincubation conditions were as follows: control enzyme with no 2-ME, ○; enzyme with 0.46 *M* 2-ME, ●; enzyme with 0.46 *M* 2-ME and 10 m*M* KCl, ▲. (From Chow et al. [5])

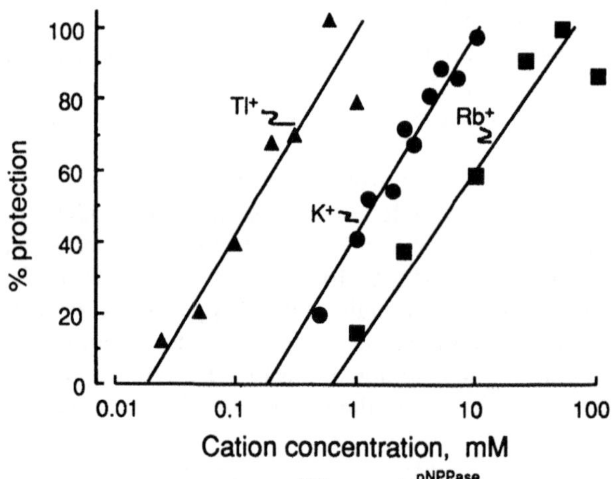

	ED_{50}	$K_a^{pNPPase}$
Tl^+	0.16	0.2
K^+	1.7	2.5
Rb^+	4.5	4.0

Fig. 3. Comparison of K^+, Tl^+, and Rb^+ in their effectiveness at protecting the H^+, K^+-ATPase against inactivation by 2-ME. Enzyme was treated with 0.48 *M* 2-ME and various concentrations of monovalent cation for 20 min at 44°C, then diluted for assay of K^+-stimulated pNPPase as our marker of H^+, K^+-ATPase activity. All data are expressed as the percentage of activity compared to samples that had not been inactivated by 2-ME (adapted from Chow et al. [5]). Below the graph are shown values for the estimated ED_{50} for protection by the three cations calculated from the present data, and K_a values for activation of pNPPase stimulated by the three cations from Forte et al. [8]

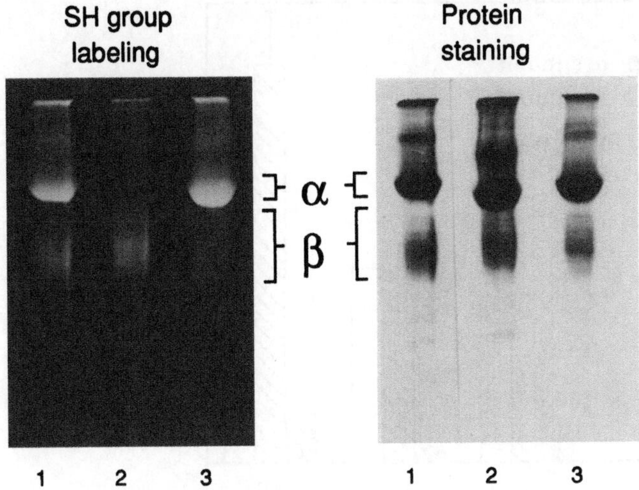

Fig. 4. Selective labeling of free and total cysteine sulfhydryl groups and cysteine disulfide groups in the α- and β-subunits of the H^+, K^+-ATPase. Results are shown for SDS-PAGE for (*left*) the fluorescence image of H^+, K^+-ATPase labeled with fluorescein maleimide (F-M) under various treatments, and (*right*) the corresponding protein pattern stained with Coomassie blue. *Lane* 1, Total cysteine labeling: treated with F-M after solubilization and full reduction by DTT. *Lane* 2, Disulfide cysteine labeling: samples were first blocked with *N*-ethyl maleimide, reduced with DTT, and then labeled with F-M. *Lane* 3, Free sulfhydryl cysteine labeling: samples were treated with F-M without any prior reduction. Quantitative assay of the bands revealed that 68% of the cysteine residues in the β-subunit were present in the oxidized disulfide form, indicating a total of three -SS- bonds. On the other hand, more than 88% of the cysteine residues in the α-subunit are in the reduced -SH form. (From Chow et al. [5])

surrogate β-subunit for the Na^+, K^+-ATPase [7, 11]; and since functional stability of the holoenzyme depends on the β-subunit, we conclude that the disulfide bond configuration within these two homologous β-subunits is most likely the same.

In order to examine the relationship between the oxidation state of cysteine residues and enzyme activity, these functions were measured at various times after the enzyme was treated with reducing agents. Microsomal membranes were exposed to 2-mercaptoethanol in the presence and absence of KCl, and parallel assays were carried out for both disulfide bonds and enzymatic activity. Figure 5 shows that the number of disulfide bonds in the β-subunit correlated with the remaining enzyme activity, and that there was no change in the state of cysteine residues within the α-subunit over the time course of the treatment. One additional point to be made, as indicated in the legend to Fig. 5, is that KCl protects the H^+, K^+-ATPase from inactivation as well as preventing the reduction of disulfide bonds within the β-subunit. This strongly suggests that the disulfide bonds in the β-subunit are important for establishing a functional conformation of the H^+, K^+-ATPase, and, conversely, that the stability of disulfide bonds is related to the conformational state of the H^+, K^+-ATPase,

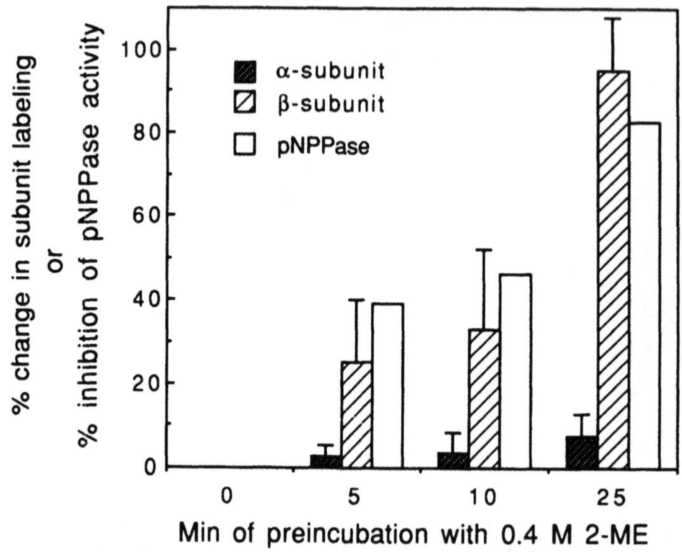

Fig. 5. Correlation between the loss of enzyme activity and increase in sulfhydryl group labeling in the β-subunit of the H^+,K^+-ATPase. Enzyme was treated at 44°C with 0.4 *M* 2-ME for 0, 5, 10, and 25 min, then stopped by a 20-fold dilution. After dilution, samples were taken for assay of enzyme activity and for labeling of reduced sulfhydryl groups. Details for labeling and quantitating sulfhydryl groups are described elsewhere [5]. The percentage change is defined as the percentage change at any given incubation time with respect to the control (time 0). The data clearly show that there is a good correlation between increase in -SH labeling (loss of disulfide bonds) and decrease in enzyme activity. Additional tests run with samples that included 10 m*M* KCl and treated with 0.4 *M* 2-ME at 44°C for 25 min showed no difference from the control. Therefore, K^+ protected both from loss of enzyme and loss of disulfide bonds

i.e., the disulfide bonds are more stable in the E_2 state of the enzyme that is promoted by K^+.

Stability of the H^+, K^+-ATPase to Alcohols and Denaturants

Another important issue in the functional stability of the H^+, K^+-ATPase is its resistance against denaturants, such as organic solvents and detergents. For example, the sensitivity of the gastric epithelium to alcohols is of immediate clinical significance. To address this problem at the membrane level, we measured the dose-dependent inactivation of the H^+, K^+-ATPase induced by various alcohols in the presence and absence of 10 m*M* KCl. Dose-response curves for ethanol and 1-propanol are shown in Fig. 6. The measured IC_{50} values for a series of alcohols are shown in Table 1, along with published values of the respective oil/water partition coefficients. There are several instructive features in these inhibitory data. First, K^+ stabilized the enzyme, providing protection against inhibition by alcohol, as it did for reducing agents. Secondly,

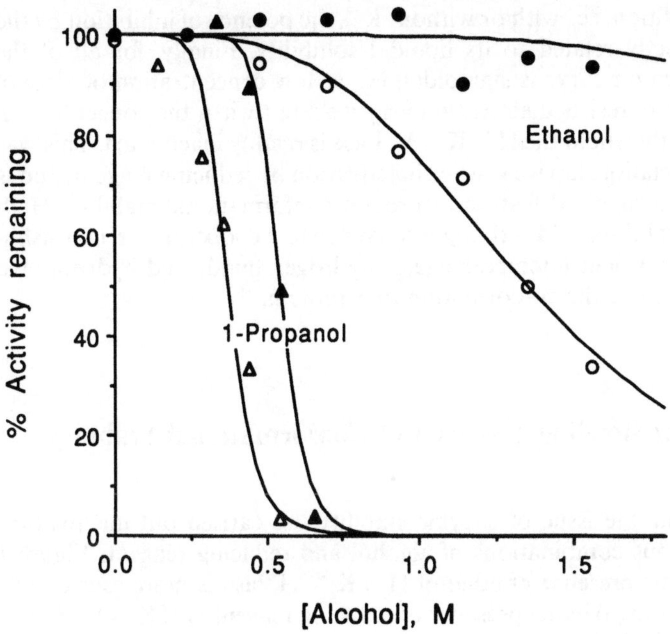

Fig. 6. Dose-dependent inhibition of H^+, K^+-ATPase by 1-propanol and ethanol in the presence or absence of KCl. Enzyme was preincubated with the designated concentration of alcohol in the presence or absence of 10 m*M* KCl for 20 min at 44°C, then diluted for assay of K^+-stimulated pNPPase activity. The data are expressed as the percentage of enzyme activity measured at zero concentration of alcohol. The alcohols are represented by ethanol (○, ●) and 1-propanol (△, ▲), with the *open symbols* representing absence of KCl and the *solid symbols* representing presence of 10 m*M* KCl

Table 1. Comparison of the partition coefficient for various alcohols with their ability to inhibit H, K-ATPase activity

Alcohol	Partition coefficient (PC)	1/PC	IC_{50} (*M*) (No K^+)	IC_{50} (*M*) (10 m*M* K^+)
Methanol	0.20	5.1	≫ 2.5	≫ 2.5
Ethanol	0.48	2.1	1.2	~2.5
2-Propanol	1	1	0.67	1.0
1-Propanol	2.22	0.45	0.38	0.56
n-Butanol	7.69	0.13	0.07	0.19

Partition coefficients and the reciprocal of the partition coefficients (1/PC) are indicated. Also shown are the measured IC_{50} values for inhibition of enzyme activity in the absence of K^+ and in the presence of 10 m*M* K^+. The data show a direct correlation between the lipoidal solubility of the alcohol and its inhibitory potency in the absence of K^+. An analogous correlation exists in the presence of K^+, but inhibition requires about twice as much alcohol. For methanol, with its low partition coefficient, the concentrations required for inhibition were far above the highest tested

for any given condition, i.e., with or without K^+, the potency of inhibition by the alcohols was directly related to its lipoidal solubility. Finally, for all of the alcohols the inhibition curve is sigmoidal, i.e., at low concentration of alcohol the H^+, K^+-ATPase resists inactivation very well, but when the concentration achieves a critical threshold the H^+, K^+-ATPase is readily inactivated. This was the same kind of relationship we saw for inactivation by reducing reagent, and is one ubiquitously recognized feature of protein conformational stability. High sensitivity at critical threshold is thought to be due to a cooperative relationship among weak noncovalent interactions (e.g., hydrogen bonds and hydrophobic interaction) to stabilize the conformation of a protein.

Cooperativity of Bonding Forces and Conformational Stability

To further examine the issue of enzyme stability, we carried out inactivation studies using various combinations of alcohol and reducing reagent. Figure 7 shows that (i) in the presence of ethanol H^+, K^+-ATPase is more sensitive to reducing reagent, and (ii) in the presence of reducing reagent H^+, K^+-ATPase is more sensitive to alcohol. An extensive series of this kind of experiment showed

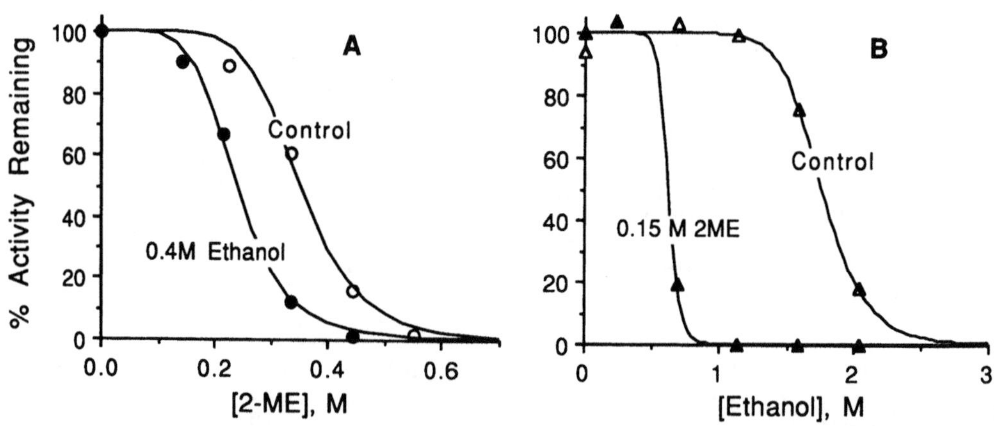

Fig. 7A, B. Cooperative inhibition of H^+,K^+-ATPase activity by combining reducing reagents and denaturants. Ethanol decreases the IC_{50} of 2-ME and 2-ME decreases the IC_{50} of ethanol. **A** Dose-dependent inhibition of H^+,K^+-ATPase by 2-ME in the presence (●) or absence (○) of 0.4 *M* ethanol. **B** Dose-dependent inhibition of H^+, K^+-ATPase by ethanol in the presence (▲) or absence (△) of 0.15 *M* 2-ME. Enzyme was preincubated with the designated combinated concentration of ethanol and 2-ME for 20 min at 44°C, then diluted for assay of K^+-stimulated pNPPase activity. The data are expressed as the percentage of enzyme activity measured at zero concentration of the titrating reagent

that the H^+, K^+-ATPase is sensitive to the additive effect of both reducing reagent and alcohol. These data indicate that the stability of the H^+, K^+-ATPase is contributed by noncovalent interactions within holoenzyme and disulfide bonds interactions specifically within the β-subunit.

From available primary sequence data and from topological and structural considerations, it can be reasoned that the α-subunit of the H^+, K^+-ATPase has over 70% of its mass distributed within the cytoplasmic domain. It is this cytoplasmic region of the α-subunit that contains functionally important sites for binding ATP, phosphorylation, hydrolysis of pNPP, and, possibly, the K^+ binding site [25]. As pointed out above, over 70% of the peptide mass of the β-subunit projects into the extracellular domain, just opposite to the α-subunit. We have shown that reduction of disulfide bonds within the extracellular domain of the β-subunit leads to inactivation of the holoenzyme, including those steps which are known to be associated with the cytoplasmic domain of the α-subunit [5]. On the other hand, binding of K^+ to the enzyme, which has also been suggested to be localized to the cytoplasmic domain of the α-subunit, not only alters the conformational state of the α-subunit, but also changes the stability of the disulfide bonds within the β-subunit. Thus, the extracellular domain of the β-subunit is linked conformationally with the cytoplasmic domain of the α-subunit, by some allosteric noncovalent interactions between the two subunits. The existence of such an association between the two subunits is further confirmed by present data showing the cooperative effects of reducing reagents and organic solvents in destabilizing enzyme function.

Extensive studies in very simple soluble enzyme systems have established that the stability of disulfied bonds within the protomer is quantitatively related to the functional stability of the enzyme and that the stabilities are related to conformation of the protein. Such intramolecular interactions to stabilize structural and functional activity of proteins has been termed "cooperativity" (for further discussion of cooperativity see [6]). The gastric H^+, K^+-ATPase is a much more complex molecule; it is a membrane protein and it is an oligomer made up of two distinct subunits. Organic solvents destabilize the holoenzymatic activity, probably by interfering with noncovalent interactions within the protein structure or at the protein/lipid interface, and they also destabilize disulfide bonds in the β-subunit. Conversely, reducing reagents that break disulfide bonds of the β-subunit destabilize the holoenzyme by making it more susceptible to denaturants. Therefore, the stability of the disulfide bonds in the β-subunit and the stability of the H^+, K^+-ATPase are linked with each other cooperatively. Such a close association between the two subunits not only indicates that the β-subunit is a structural part of the holoenzyme, but also suggests that the β-subunit is a functional component of the enzyme. Several reports have suggested a possible functional role for the β-subunit in the operation of the Na^+, K^+-ATPase [7, 11, 13]. We have extended this suggestion to the H^+, K^+-ATPase through the present studies and through our recent demonstration that functional activity of the gastric enzyme was altered by a monoclonal antibody that specifically bound to the cytoplasmic domain of the β-subunit.

Carbohydrate Structure and Function Within the β-Subunit

General Carbohydrate Properties

The studies presented above demonstrate that conformational stability of the β-subunit confers a stability and activity to the H^+, K^+-ATPase holoenzyme. Furthermore, the conformation of the holoenzyme induced by ligands (and substrates) influences the stability of the β-subunit. In the secreting parietal cell, over 70% of the mass of the β-subunit resides in the highly acidic and possibly pepsin-active extracellular environment. We would like to propose that the β-subunit plays a primary role in stabilizing the H^+, K^+-ATPase from acid and proteolytic damage and maintaining functional activity of the stomach. At the present time such an hypothesis is difficult to substantiate directly and is largely based on the inferences from the studies on enzyme stability; however, we might examine another specialized feature of the extracellular domain of the β-subunit, that is, the associated oligosaccharides.

The gastric β-subunit is rich in carbohydrate. Analyses reveal that a large part of the total gastric β glycoprotein mass is carbohydrate [23]; the bulk of the sugar consists of *N*-acetylglucosamine (glcNAc), galactose (gal), and mannose (man). Unlike β-subunit isoforms from Na^+, K^+-ATPase, gastric β contains no sialic acid [1, 19]. By virtue of its affinity to various lectins, and its sensitivity to selected glycosidases, we can make some general conclusions regarding the nature of the glycosylations on the β-subunit. Gastric β does not bind to concanavalin A, but binds avidly to a several other lectins, including ricinus communis agglutinin, wheat germ agglutinin, helix pomatia agglutinin [22, 23], and tomato and potato lectins [2]. The mature form of gastric β is completely insensitive to endoglycosidase H, but it is rapidly deglycosylated by peptide: *N*-glycosidase F (PNGase). From these data on glycosidase sensitivity, as well as those on lectin binding, we conclude that oligosaccharides of gastric β are not of the high-mannose or hybrid types, but of the complex type, most likely in a tri- or tetra-antennary structure. Furthermore, the reported strong affinity for tomato and potato lectins suggests [2] that gastric β-subunit oligosaccharides are rich in poly-*N*-acetyllactosamine sequences (i.e., repeating glcNAc-gal sequences). The poly-*N*-acetyllactosamine structure is also a characteristic for binding to wheat germ agglutinin [10].

Seven Sites of *N*-Glycosylation on the β-Subunit

In recent experiments we used an antibody for the 60- to 80-kDa β-subunit to identify a 52-kDa glycopeptide present in gastric membrane fractions rich in rough ER. The 52-kDa glycopeptide not only reacted with β-subunit antibody, but was also bound by *Galanthus nivalis* lectin (GNA; specific for high mannose) and was deglycosylated by endoglycosidase H to the immunoreactive 34-kDa core peptide of the β-subunit. Thus, we concluded that the 52-kDa glycopeptide from the rough ER-enriched membranes is a high-mannose precursor form of

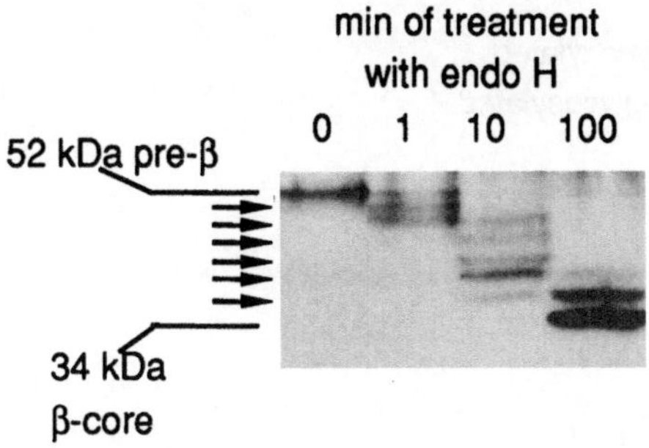

Fig. 8. Western blot analysis of progressive deglycosylation of the 52-kDa precursor β-subunit by endoglycosidase H. The rough ER-enriched fraction was treated with endoglycosidase H at pH 8.0 for 0 min, 1 min, 10 min, and 100 min. Samples were run on SDS-PAGE and blotted to nitrocellulose. The blots were probed with antibody against the β-subunit. In addition to the 52-kDa pre-β band seen at zero time, and the 34-kDa β-subunit core peptide seen after 100 min, one can discern six intermediates, partially deglycosylated, forms of the β-subunit (*arrows*), demonstrating that there are a total of seven oligosaccharides that are removed during the deglycosylation

the β-subunit (pre-β). Because the 52-kDa glycopeptide was so well focused on SDS-PAGE, it was amenable to a deglycosylation study seeking to determine the number of *N*-linked glycosylations on the β-subunit. Figure 8 shows the results of time-dependent deglycosylation of pre-β by endoglycosidase H. Six transient intermediates and the final β-subunit core peptide were all identified by the same antibody on western blots. The molecular weight differences between successive bands were similar ($\sim$2.6 kDa), indicating that the carbohydrate side chains of the 52-M_r pre-β are relatively homogenous and that successive bands reflect removal of single oligosaccharide groups. Thus, there are seven *N*-linked oligosaccharides in the β-subunit of the rabbit gastric H^+, K^+-ATPase. Because of the slight differences in primary sequence noted above, it will be of interest to subject the β-subunit of the pig stomach to the same analyses.

Glycosylation of β-Subunit Confers Resistance to Pepsinolysis

It is difficult to test the total functional significance of the oligosaccharides in the gastric β-subunit, but it is clear that they reside on the extracellular molecular mass that is exposed to conditions of low pH and pepsin, so we considered the hypothesis that the β-subunit might contribute to resistance of the holoenzyme to pepsin attack. To study the possible protective role of carbohydrate side chains, we subjected mature glycosylated and deglycosylated β-subunit to pepsinolysis at low pH, and analyzed a series of timed samples by western blot. The kinetics of digestion for both the glycosylated and deglycosylated forms were dependent on pepsin concentration, pH, and temperature, but for any set of conditions, hydrolysis was significantly slower for the glycosylated than for the deglycosylated β-subunit. For example, as shown by the results plotted in

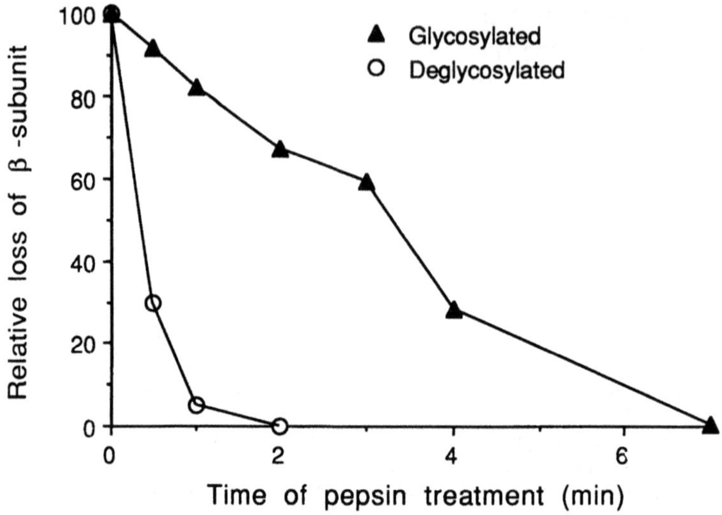

Fig. 9. Comparison of the peptic breakdown for the glycosylated and deglycosylated forms of the β-subunit. Samples of gastric H^+,K^+-ATPase were solubilized in NP-40 and either treated with PNGase F to produce the fully deglycosylated β-subunit, or left untreated to obtain the glycosylated form of the β-subunit. The samples were brought to pH 2 and pure pepsin was added. Samples were withdrawn at various times and taken for SDS-PAGE and western blots. The density volumes of the 60- to 80-kDa fully glycosylated β-subunit band and the 34-kDa core β-subunit band were assayed by densitometry, and plotted as a function of time of treatment with pepsin. The zero time of treatment was taken as 100% of the respective β-subunit. The estimated half times for the pepsinolysis of the glycosylated and deglycosylated β-subunit forms were 3.5 min and 0.4 min, respectively

Fig. 9, the measured half-time for degradation of the glycosylated β-subunit was decreased eight-fold after deglycosylation. It must be underscored that these data were obtained in a completely unphysiological state with β-subunit suspended in detergent solution. Because of the requirements for deglycosylation by PNGase, membranes containing β-subunit had to be solubilized in detergent (NP-40). However, the marked increase in susceptibility to pepsin after deglycosylation suggests a protective role for the carbohydrate side chains, even if this only represents a steric factor.

Summary

Highly complex structural interactions are essential for the operation of the H^+, K^+-ATPase as the primary source of gastric hydrochloric acid, as well as for its ability to protect itself from autolysis. The H^+, K^+-ATPase is a proteic dimer of α-subunit and the β-subunit peptides forming the functional holoenzyme with an asymmetric distribution of subunit mass to opposite sides of the secretory membrane. We have shown that stability of disulfide bonds within the β-subunit is cooperatively linked to conformational stability within the peptides and between peptide and phospholipid annulus, which, in turn, are all related to the conformational and functional state of the holoenzyme. The observed cooperativity between the structural stability of the β-subunit and enzymatic activity provides evidence for the involvement of the β-subunit in the function of the H^+, K^+-ATPase. The high degree of homology between the β-subunit of the

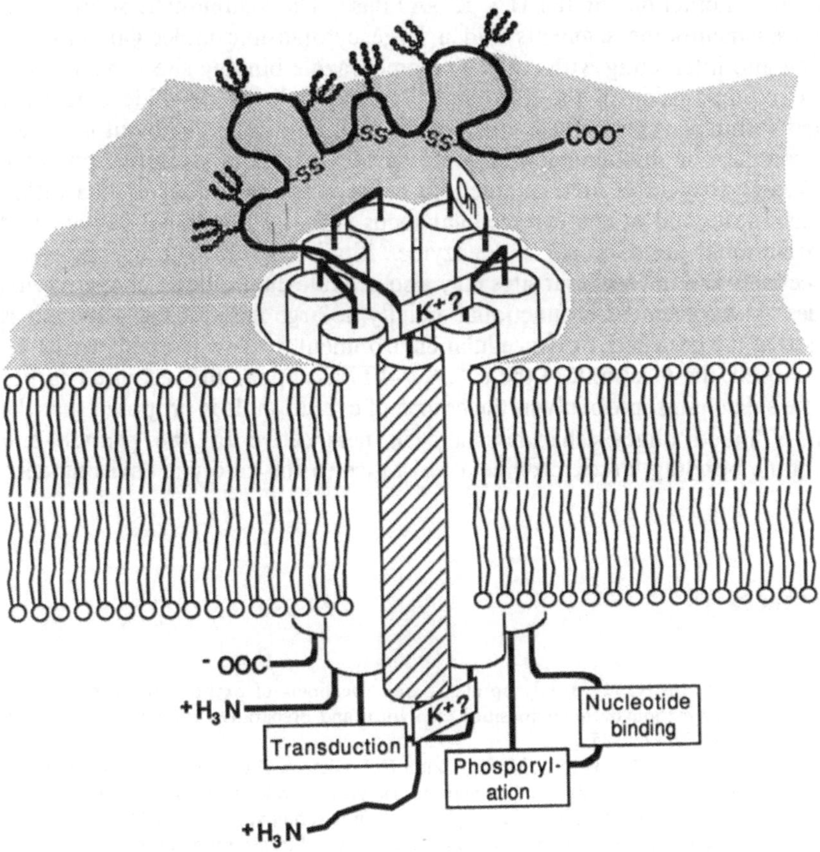

Fig. 10. Schematic representation of the organization of the α- and β-subunits of the H^+,K^+-ATPase within a membrane. The α-subunit is shown with eight transmembrane segments, a large cytoplasmic molecular mass for binding and interacting with ATP, and includes the omeprazole binding site (*Om*) within the extracellular domain. The β-subunit, indicated by the single *shaded* transmembrane segment, includes a relatively short, amino-terminal, cytoplasmic segment and a longer extracellular portion including sites for glycosylation and containing three stabilizing disulfide bonds. Interactions between the α- and β-subunits occur within the membrane and at the extracellular locus to stabilize functional activity and conformational state of the holoenzyme. Binding of K^+ at its respective extracellular and intracellular sites is known to influence subunit interaction and protein conformation, but precise location of the sites is tentative. The extensive glycosylation through seven *N*-linked oligosaccharides may serve an important function in protecting the enzyme from the destructive extracellular environment

H^+, K^+-ATPase and that of the Na^+, K^+-ATPase, and the observed exchangeability between the two β-subunits in conveying functional activity, provide a basis for postulating that the disulfide bonding configuration is the same for both subunits. Borrowing the fact that the region of interaction for the αβ subunits of the Na^+, K^+-ATPase has been localized to the extracellular or transmembrane domains, the interactive region for the αβ subunits of the H^+, K^+-ATPase is also likely to be localized to the extracellular domain.

The model presented in Fig. 10 displays projected sites of intra- and intermolecular interaction for the H^+, K^+-ATPase. The α-subunit is shown with eight transmembrane segments and a large cytoplasmic molecular mass for binding and interacting with ATP. The omeprazole binding site is depicted at the extracellular side of the α-subunit. Three stabilizing disulfide bonds are located within the extracellular mass of the β-subunit. The β-subunit is replete with complex, multiantennary oligosaccharides at all of its seven potential *N*-linked glycosylation sites. Interactions between the α- and β-subunits within the membrane and at the extracellular locus stabilize functional activity and conformational state of the holoenzyme. Binding of K^+ at its respective extracellular and intracellular sites may also provide dual subunit cooperativity. Besides its involvement in functional activity, a large mass of the β-subunit is exposed to the destructive extracellular environment, i.e., low pH and pepsin. To protect itself, the β-subunit of the H^+, K^+-ATPase apparently acquired carbohydrate side chains, probably in the course of evolution. It is proposed that the seven *N*-linked oligosaccharides, held in perspective by the peptide and membrane bonding forces, provide a resistance to the autolytic environment.

References

1. Beesley RC, Forte JG (1973) Glycoproteins and glycolipids of oxyntic cell microsomes. I. Glycoproteins: carbohydrate composition, analytical and preparative fractionation. Biochem Biophys Acta 307:372–385
2. Callaghan JM, Toh BH, Pettitt JM, Humphris DC, Gleeson PA (1990) Poly-*N*-acetyllactosamine-specific tomato lectin interacts with gastric parietal cells. Identification of a tomato-lectin binding 60–90 × 10^3 M_r membrane glycoprotein of tubulovesicles. J Cell Sci 95:563–576
3. Canfield VA, Levenson R (1991) Structural organization and transcription of the mouse gastric H^+, K^+-ATPase beta subunit gene. Proc Natl Acad Sci USA 88:8247–8251
4. Canfield VA, Okamoto CT, Chow D, Dorfman J, Gros P, Forte JG, Levenson R (1990) Cloning of the H, K-ATPase β-subunit: tissue-specific expression, chromosomal assignment, and relationship to Na, K-ATPase β-subunits. J Biol Chem 265:19878–19884
5. Chow DC, Browning CM, Forte JG (1992) Gastric H, K-ATPase activity is inhibited by reduction of disulfide bonds in the β-subunit. Am J Physiol (Cell Physiol 32) 263:C39–C46
6. Creighton TE (1990) Protein folding. Biochem J 270:1–16
7. Eakle KA, Kim KS, Kabalin MA, Farley RA (1992) High-affinity ouabain binding by yeast cells expressing Na^+, K^+-ATPase alpha subunits and the gastric H^+, K^+-ATPase beta subunit. Proc Natl Acad Sci USA 89:2834–2838
8. Forte JG, Ganser AL, Ray TK (1976) The K^+-stimulated ATPase from oxyntic glands of gastric mucosa. In: Kasbekar DK, Sachs G, Rehm W (eds) Gastric hydrogen ion secretion. Dekker, New York, pp 302–330

9. Forte JG, Soll A (1989) Cell biology of hydrochloric acid secretion. In: Forte JG, Schultz SG (eds) Handbook of physiology, sect 6: The gastrointestinal system, Vol 3. American Physiological Society, Bethesda, pp 207–228
10. Gallagher JT, Morris A, Dexter TM (1985) Identification of two binding sites for wheat-germ agglutinin on polyactosamine-type oligosaccharides. Biochem J 231:115–122
11. Horisberger JD, Jaunin P, Reuben MA, Lasater LS, Chow DC, Forte JG, Sachs G, Rossier, BC, Geering K (1991) The H, K-ATPase β-subunit can act as a surrogate for the β-subunit of the Na, K pump. J Biol Chem 26:19131–19134
12. Inesi G, Kirtley MR (1992) Structural Features of Cation Transport ATPase. J Bioenerg Biomembr 24:271–284
13. Jaisser F, Canessa CM, Horisberger JD, Rossier BC (1992) Primary sequence and functional expression of a novel ouabain-resistant Na, K-ATPase. The beta subunit modulates potassium activation of the Na, K-pump. J Biol Chem 267:16895–16903
14. Jørgensen PL, Andersen JP (1988) Structural basis for E1–E2 conformational transitions in Na, K-ATPase and Ca-ATPase. J Membrane Biol 103:95–120
15. Kawamura M, Nagano K (1984) Evidence for essential disulfide bonds in the β-subunit of (Na^+ + K^+)-ATPase. Biochem Biophys Acta 774:188–192
16. Kawamura M, Ohmizo K, Morohashi M, Nagano K (1985) Protective effect of Na^+ and K^+ against inactivation of (Na^+ + K^+)-ATPase by high concentrations of 2-mercaptoethanol at high temperatures. Biochem Biophys Acta 821:115–120
17. Kirley TL (1989) Determination of three disulfide bonds and one free sulfhydryl in the β-subunit of (Na, K)-ATPase. J Biol Chem 264:7185–7192
18. Kirley TL (1990) Inactivation of (Na^+, K^+)-ATPase by β-mercaptoethanol. J Biol Chem 265:4227–4232
19. Kyte J (1972) Properties of 2 polypeptides of sodium-dependent and potassium-dependent adenosine-triphosphatase. J Biol Chem 247:7642–7649
20. Lingrel JB (1992) Na, K-ATPase: isoform structure, function, and expression. J Bioenerg Biomembr 24:263–270
21. Ma JY, Song YH, Sjostrand SE, Rask L, Mardh S (1991) cDNA cloning of the beta-subunit of the human gastric H^+, K^+-ATPase. Biochem Biophys Res Commun 180(1) :39–45
22. Okamoto CT, Forte JG (1988) Distribution of lectin-binding sites in oxyntic and chief cells of isolated rabbit gastric glands. Gastroenterology 95:334–342
23 Okamoto CT, Karpilow JM, Smolka A, Forte JG (1990) Isolation and characterization of gastric microsomal glycoproteins. Evidence for a glycosylated β-subunit of the H^+, K^+-ATPase. Biochim Biophys Acta 1037:360–372
24. Reuben MA, Lasater LS, Sachs G (1990) Characterization of a beta subunit of the gastric H^+/K^+-transporting ATPase. Proc Natl Acad Sci USA 87:6767–6771
25. Sachs G, Kaunitz J, Mendlein J, Wallmark B (1989) Biochemistry of gastric acid secretion. In: Forte JG, Schultz SG (eds) Handbook of physiology, sect 6: The gastrointestinal system, Vol. 3. American Physiological Society, Bethesda, pp 229–254
26. Shull GE, Lingrel JB (1986) Molecular cloning of the rat stomach (H^+ + K^+)-ATPase. J Biol Chem 231:16788–16791
27. Shull GE (1990) cDNA cloning of the β-subunit of the rat gastric H, K-ATPase. J Biol Chem 265:12123–12126
28. Toh BH, Gleeson PA, Simpson RJ, Moritz RL, Callaghan JM, Goldkorn I, Jones CM, Martinelli TM, Mu FT, Humphris DC (1990) The 60- to 90-kDa parietal cell autoantigen associated with autoimmune gastritis is a beta subunit of the gastric H^+/K^+-ATPase (proton pump). Proc Natl Acad Sci USA 87: 6418–6422

New Insights into the Regulation of Gastric Secretion in Duodenal Ulcer Patients*

C.B.H.W. Lamers

Introduction

Duodenal ulcer is believed to result from an imbalance between aggressive and defensive factors [1, 2]. Hypersecretion of gastric acid and pepsinogen is accepted as playing a key role in the pathogenesis of the ulcer diathesis [1–3]. However, this crucial role of acid has only been proven in a small subgroup of patients with hypergastrinemia or increased histamine secretion [3, 4]. On the other hand, the impressive efficacy of acid-reducing drugs in the healing of duodenal ulcer supports the assumption of the significance of acid in the pathogenesis of duodenal ulcer [5]. Numerous studies on the regulation of gastric secretion have been performed in order to unravel the mystery of the pathogenesis of duodenal ulcer. These studies, comprising investigations into the regulation of gastric acid, pepsinogens, and gastrin, have pointed to the presence of hypersecretion in many duodenal ulcer patients. However, in more than half of the patients secretion levels are well within the normal range [3]. Partly on the basis of these heterogeneous abnormalities of gastric secretion, it has been suggested that duodenal ulcer is a heterogeneous disorder in which various genetic and environmental factors lead to the same end result, i.e. the ulcer in the duodenal bulb [6]. Increased serum levels of pepsinogen A, previously called pepsinogen I and an exaggerated serum gastrin response to meals have been considered as genetic markers for duodenal ulcer disease [7–11].

Gastric Secretory Abnormalities in Duodenal Ulcer

The mechanism of the increased acid load to the duodenal bulb in duodenal ulcer is multifactorial and includes abnormalities of the parietal cells, the gastrin-producing G-cells in the antrum, and the gastric emptying mechanism (Table 1). The predominant feature of these abnormalities is the impaired feedback regulation between gastric acid and serum gastrin secretion [3, 4]. Several reports have pointed to abnormalities of gastrin in the antral mucosa

* The author is indebted to Ms J.W. van Spronsen for excellent secretarial assistance.

Table 1. Gastric secretory abnormalities in duodenal ulcer

- Parietal cell abnormalities:
  - Increased parietal cell mass
  - Parietal cell dysfunctions:
    - increased basal acid output
    - increased nocturnal acid output
    - increased response to cephalic stimulation
    - increased sensitivity to gastrin stimulation
    - failure to decrease acid secretion in the presence of low pH
    - increased meal-stimulated acid output
- Chief cell abnormalities:
  - Increased chief cell mass
  - Increased sensitivity to stimuli
- G-cell abnormalities:
  - Increased G-cell mass
  - G-cell dysfunction:
    - increased secretion after stimuli
    - reduced suppression by acid

and plasma of duodenal ulcer patients. Numerous studies have shown that in duodenal ulcer disease, basal plasma gastrin levels are not appropriately reduced by the high gastric acid secretion, pointing to a deficient negative feedback mechanism between gastric acid and gastrin secretion [2–4]. The impairment of this feedback mechanism is further corroborated by the finding that, compared with normal control subjects, patients with duodenal ulcer show enhanced gastrin secretion in the presence of increased gastric acid secretion after feeding [2–4]. This abnormal autoregulation of meal-stimulated gastrin secretion is still apparent when patients with duodenal ulcer disease are divided into those with normal and those with increased gastric acid secretion [12, 13]. Thus, duodenal ulcer patients with normal gastric acid secretion have an increased gastrin response to feeding, while those with gastric acid hypersecretion have postprandial serum gastrin concentrations in the normal range [12, 13]. An impaired feedback mechanism between gastric acid and postprandial gastrin secretion is also suggested by the finding that, compared with normal subjects, duodenal ulcer patients show a reduced inhibition of postprandial gastrin secretion after acidification of the meal [14].

The mechanism of the impaired autoregulation of gastrin in duodenal ulcer disease is not completely understood. However, recent animal and in vitro experiments have greatly enhanced our insight into the regulation of gastrin secretion [15, 16]. These studies have shown that somatostatin, in close interaction with the cholinergic, adrenergic, and peptidergic (gastrin-releasing peptide) nervous system, plays a key role in the regulation of gastrin secretion [15, 16]. It has been shown that secretion of antral somatostatin is stimulated by lowering the intragastric pH [15, 16]. Furthermore, the finding that immunoneutralization of somatostatin by a somatostatin antiserum enhances gastrin release from the antrum suggests that the gastrin-secreting G-cells are under constant restraint by the somatostatin-secreting D-cells in the antral mucosa

[17]. In the presence of high gastric acid concentrations this restraint will be increased, resulting in reduced gastrin secretion, whereas in the presence of low gastric acid secretion this restraint will be reduced, resulting in enhanced gastrin secretion. It has therefore been claimed that somatostatin is the major mediator of the inhibition of gastrin secretion by gastric acid [18]. In contrast to the important role of antral somatostatin acting in a local, paracrine manner, it is unlikely that postprandial circulatory somatostatin concentrations affect gastrin secretion [19]. In duodenal ulcer patients basal and postprandial plasma somatostatin concentrations are normal [17, 18], and on the basis of infusion studies with somatostatin, they are considered to be too low to inhibit gastrin secretion [19].

Whether a somatostatin deficiency in the antrum is involved in the impaired gastric acid-serum gastrin feedback mechanism in duodenal ulcer disease is a matter of controversy. However, several groups have found evidence of such a somatostatin deficiency in peptic ulcer disease. Chayvialle et al. [20] were the first to demonstrate significantly reduced somatostatin concentrations in the antrum of duodenal ulcer patients. This finding was supported by a study from Japan showing significantly reduced antral somatostatin concentrations in duodenal ulcer patients [21]. Since the antral gastrin content was within normal limits, as in most other studies, the calculated gastrin to somatostatin ratio was increased in the peptic ulcer patients. These authors further found that the correlation between antral gastrin and antral somatostatin and that between gastric acid secretion and antral somatostatin, present in normal subjects, is absent in duodenal ulcer patients. In other words, in duodenal ulcer patients antral somatostatin is reduced irrespective of antral gastrin content or gastric acid secretion. The aforementioned findings have been confirmed in another Japanese study [18]. That study also showed that the antral somatostatin deficiency was most pronounced in those duodenal ulcer patients who have a high rate of gastric acid secretion. Recently, decreased somatostatin concentrations in the antrum of duodenal ulcer patients were also found in a study from Spain [22].

The study by Arnold et al. [23], showing a normal number of somatostatin producing D-cells and a normal G-cell to D-cell ratio in the antral mucosa, is in contrast with the above-mentioned studies. This discrepancy cannot be simply attributed to differences in analytical techniques – that is, counting of peptide-producing cells versus determination of peptide concentrations – since a reduced number of D-cells in the antral mucosa have been found by others [18, 24]. An additional interesting observation pointing to antral somatostatin deficiency in duodenal ulcer patients is the finding of a decreased release of somatostatin accompanied by an enhanced release of gastrin from antral mucosal explants from such patients [25]. It has been hypothesized that the enhanced gastrin secretion due to the antral somatostatin deficiency is the primary, possibly genetic, abnormality in duodenal ulcer disease, and that the other pathophysiologic abnormalities, such as the increased number of parietal cells, the increased gastric acid secretion, and the increased pepsinogen secretion, are secondary to the trophic actions of gastrin on the gastric mucosa [18]. However, it is possible that the somatostatin deficiency of the antral mucosa is not genetically determined, but is secondary to other factors, such as vagal drive [16, 26], gastritis or previous therapy with antisecretory drugs [27].

Gastric acid hypersecretion in duodenal ulcer may also be due to impaired acid inhibition irrespective of the defective gastrin regulation. In fact, it has been shown in the isolated, luminally perfused mouse stomach that acid in the gastric lumen stimulates somatostatin secretion from D-cells in the gastric body [28]. On the basis of these findings it was proposed that acid-induced release of somatostatin in proximity to parietal cells serves as a negative feedback mechanism, restraining acid secretion. This inhibitory effect of somatostatin may directly affect the parietal cells, but may also act by inhibiting gastrin-induced histamine release [29].

In addition, several circulating hormones with inhibitory actions on gastric acid secretion have been suggested to act as physiologic inhibitors of gastric acid secretion, such as secretin, cholecystokinin (CCK), Peptide YY (PYY), gastric inhibitory polypeptide (GIP), and somatostatin. However, secretin and GIP, when administered in physiologic doses, do not reduce gastric acid secretion in man. On the other hand, when postprandial plasma somatostatin concentrations are mimicked by infusion of somatostatin, gastric acid secretion is significantly reduced [19].

Recent studies employing CCK-receptor antagonists have shown that CCK does act as an enterogastrone. Pretreatment of normal subjects with type A CCK-receptor antagonists, such as loxiglumide and L-364, 718, increased not only basal gastric acid secretion but also the acid response to a meal and to infusion of CCK or bombesin [30–34]. Somatostatin produced locally by gastric D-cells may play a crucial role in acid inhibition by cholecystokinin. In fact, it has been shown that somatostatin release from gastric D-cells is stimulated by CCK [35]. Furthermore, pretreatment with the CCK-receptor antagonist loxiglumide inhibited somatostatin secretion into the gastric lumen during CCK stimulation in normal subjects [31]. However, so far no studies employing CCK-receptor antagonists have been performed to demonstrate or rule out that inhibition of gastric acid by CCK is impaired in duodenal ulcer patients.

Role of *H. pylori*

The discovery of *Helicobacter pylori* and its accompanying chronic active gastritis in practically all duodenal ulcer patients has raised the question as to whether the abnormalities in gastric secretion in duodenal ulcer are primary or secondary to the gastric infection with this microorganism. Recent studies have shown that several of the gastric secretory abnormalities of duodenal ulcer patients may be secondary to the chronic infection with *Helicobacter pylori*. Levi et al. [36] found that basal and pentagastrin-stimulated gastric acid secretion was higher in *Helicobacter pylori*-positive duodenal ulcer patients than in patients without infection with this organism. The authors further demonstrated that basal and meal-stimulated serum gastrin levels were also higher in the patients with gastric *Helicobacter pylori* infection. These increased serum gastrin values appeared not to be restricted to duodenal ulcer patients, since Smith et al. [37] found serum gastrin levels, measured hourly for 24 h, to be higher in *Helicobacter pylori*-positive asymptomatic subjects than in asymptomatic subjects without this infection. However, there was no significant difference in median integrated 24 h intragastric acidity between the *Helicobacter pylori*-positive and *Helicobacter pylori*-negative subjects. Serum pepsinogen A and C levels were also found to be increased in an asymptomatic *Helicobacter pylori*-positive Japanese population, while the pepsinogen A, C ratio was decreased [38]. Eradication of the microorganism by antibiotic therapy reduced basal and meal- and bombesin-stimulated serum gastrin concentrations in duodenal ulcer patients and asymptomatic *Helicobacter pylori*-positive subjects, [39–43]. In addition, serum pepsinogen A and C concentrations were significantly decreased after *Helicobacter pylori* eradication to levels comparable to those found in *Helicobacter pylori*-negative subjects, while no change was found in patients in whom eradication was not achieved, [40, 44].

Interestingly, eradication of the microorganism did not alter nocturnal gastric acid secretion and daytime intragastric pH in duodenal ulcer patients [41]. However, Moss and Calam [43] found in duodenal ulcer patients that basal gastric acid secretion did decrease after *Helicobacter* eradication, whereas pentagastrin-stimulated gastric acid secretion was unchanged [41, 43]. This finding suggests that the increased basal acid secretion in *Helicobacter*-positive ulcer patients is due to the increased basal serum gastrin secretion, while the maximum capacity of the stomach to secrete acid in response to (penta)gastrin is not affected by the infection. In this respect it is interesting to analyze whether the gastric acid secretion capacity of the stomach in *Helicobacter pylori*-positive subjects is dependent on the presence of the microorganism in the gastric body, which is the case in about 70% of *Helicobacter pylori*-infected persons while the antrum is infected in practically all *Helicobacter pylori*-positive subjects. Haruma et al. [45] tested the hypothesis that the increased serum gastrin secretion was due to a low antral somatostatin content of the antral mucosa in the *Helicobacter pylori*-positive subjects, and indeed, *Helicobacter pylori*-positive patients who also had increased basal and postprandial serum gastrin concentrations had a markedly reduced antral somatostatin content. Similarly, Murthy et al. [46] found that the number of somatostatin-producing D-cells in the antral mucosa was decreased in *Helicobacter pylori*-positive subjects, while the number of G-cells was similar to that in the noninfected controls. These findings suggest that somatostatin deficiency due to reduction of the number of D-cells is responsible for the increased gastrin secretion from the antral mucosa in *Helicobacter pylori*-infected subjects. This suggestion was substantiated by Moss et al. [47], who showed in duodenal ulcer patients that eradication of *Helicobacter pylori* led to an increase in somatostatin mRNA but did not alter gastrin mRNA.

Conclusion

Recent studies suggest that the abnormal gastrin and pepsinogen secretion in duodenal ulcer patients cannot be considered to be primary genetic defects, as previously suggested, but rather appear to be due to gastric infection with *Helicobacter pylori*. These abnormalities may be due to the *Helicobacter pylori* infection itself or to the associated chronic active gastritis. The increased serum gastrin secretion has been shown to be secondary to deficiency of somatostatin-producing D-cells in the antral mucosa of *Helicobacter pylori*-infected subjects. The increased basal and postprandial gastric acid secretion is probably due to increased serum gastrin levels in *Helicobacter pylori*-infected subjects. The finding that eradication of the microorganism does not change pentagastrin-stimulated gastric acid secretion suggests that the high maximum acid secretion in duodenal ulcer patients is not directly due to the infection. It may, however, be possible that the high pentagastrin-stimulated gastric acid secretion is due to the large number of parietal cells in duodenal ulcer patients, possibly due to the chronic hypergastrinemia secondary to *Helicobacter pylori* infection. If this hypothesis is correct, long-term follow-up after eradication would have to reveal a progressive reduction of pentagastrin-stimulated gastric acid secretion, pointing to a reduction of the parietal cell mass.

In conclusion, *Helicobacter pylori* infection is responsible for several of the abnormalities of gastric secretion in duodenal ulcer patients, which have previously been considered as primary genetically determined features. This finding has dramatically changed our understanding of the pathogenesis of duodenal ulcer. However, we should make clear to ourselves that *Helicobacter pylori* infection is a major factor in but not the cause of duodenal ulcer disease, because the majority of *Helicobacter pylori*-infected subjects do not suffer from duodenal ulcer disease.

References

1. Kovacs TOG, Soll AH (1992) Pathophysiology of peptic ulcer disease. In: Gustavsson S, Kumar D, Graham DY (eds) The stomach. Churchill Livingstone, London, pp 230–245
2. Pounder RE, Prewett EJ (1992) Gastric secretion of health and disease. In: Gustavsson S, Kumar D, Graham DY (eds) The stomach. Churchill Livingstone, London, pp 53–80
3. Lam SK (1985) Heterogeneous origin of hyperacidity in duodenal ulcer. Progr Clin Biol Res 173:255–271
4. Lamers CBHW (1988) Hormonal regulation of gastric acid in peptic ulcer. Scand J Gastroenterol 23 (Suppl 146):5–10
5. Bianchi Porro G, Lazzaroni M (1992) Medical treatment of peptic ulcer disease. In: Gustavsson S, Kumar D, Graham DY (eds) The stomach. Churchill Livingstone, London, pp 246–265
6. Rotter JI (1980) Genetic approaches to ulcer heterogeneity. In: Rotter JI, Samloff IM, Rimoin DL (eds) The genetics and heterogeneity of common gastrointestinal disorders. Academic, New York, pp 111–128
7. Rotter JI, Perersen GM, Samloff IM (1985) Pepsinogens and other physiologic markers in genetic studies of peptic ulcer and related disorders. Progr Clin Biol Res 173:227–244

8. Rotter JI, Sones JQ, Samloff IM, Richardson CT, Gursky JG, Walsh JH, Rimoin DL (1979) Duodenal ulcer disease associated with elevated serum pepsinogen I, an inherited autosomal dominant disorder. N Engl J Med 300:63–66
9. Rotter JI, Petersen GM, Samloff IM, McConnell RB, Ellis A, Spence MA, Rimoin DL (1979) Genetic heterogeneity of familial hyperpepsinogenemic I and normopepsinogemic I duodenal ulcer disease. Ann intern Med 91:372–377
10. Taylor IL, Calam J, Rotter JI et al. (1981) Family studies of hypergastrinemic hyperpepsinogenemic I duodenal ulcer. Ann intern Med (1985) 95:421–424
11. Lamers CBHW, Jansen JBMJ, Rotter JI, Samloff IM (1985) Serum pepsinogen I in hereditary hypergastrinemic peptic ulcer syndromes. Progr Clin Biol Res 173:273–281.
12. Byrnes DJ, Lam SK, Sircus W (1976) The relation between functioning parietal cell and gastric cell masses in two groups of duodenal patients. Clin Sci Mol Med 50:375–383
13. Fritsch WP, Hausamen TU, Rick W (1976) Gastric and extragastric gastrin release in normal subjects, in duodenal ulcer patients and patients with partial gastrectomy (Billroth I). Gastroenterology 71:552–557
14. Walsh JH, Richardson T, Fordtran J (1975) pH dependence of acid secretion and gastrin release in normal and ulcer subjects. J Clin Invest 55:462–468
15. Saffouri B, Weir CG, Bitar KN, Makhlouf G (1980) Gastrin and somatostatin secretion by perfused rat stomach: functional linkage of antral peptides. Am J Physiol 238:495–501
16. Schubert ML, Makhlouf G (1982) Regulation of gastrin and somatostatin by intramural neurons; effect of nicotinic receptor stimulation with dimethyl-phenylpiperazinium. Gastroenterology 82:626–632
17. Saffouri B, Weir G, Makhlouf G (1979) Stimulation of gastrin secretion by perfused rat stomach by somatostatin antiserum. Life Sci 25:1749–1754
18. Kishimoto S, Takaba N, Ogawa M et al. (1985) Gastrin and somatostatin in patients with hyperchlorhydric duodenal ulcer. Hiroshima J Med Sci 34:441–449
19. Colturi TJ, Unger R, Feldman M (1984) Role of circulatory somatostatin in regulation of gastric secretion, gastrin release, and islet cell function: studies in healthy subjects and duodenal ulcer patients. J Clin invest 74:417–423
20. Chayvialle JAP, Descos P, Bernard C, Martin A, Barbe C, Partensky C (1978) Somatostatin in mucosa of stomach and duodenum in gastroduodenal disease. Gastroenterology 75:13–19
21. Sumii K, Fukushima T, Hirata T et al. (1981) Antral gastrin and somatostatin concentrations in peptic ulcer patients. Peptides 2 (Suppl 2):281–283
22. Torres AJ, Fernandez-Durango R, Suarez A et al. (1987) Gastric mucosal somatostatin-like immunoreactivity in peptic ulcer. Surg Gynaecol Obstet 164:313–318
23. Arnold R, Koop H, Schwarting H, Tuch K, Willemer B (1986) Effect of acid inhibition on gastric endocrine cells. Scand J Gastroenterol 21 (Suppl 125):14–19
24. Polak JH, Bloom SR, Bishop HF, McGrossan MV (1978) D-cell pathology in duodenal ulcers and achlorydria. Metabolism 27 (Suppl 1):1239–1242
25. Harty RF, Malco DG, McGuigan JE (1986) Antral release of gastrin and somatostatin in duodenal ulcer and control subjects. Gut 27:652–658
26. Uvnas-Moberg K, Anderson B, Posloncec B (1981) Initial fall in peripheral plasma somatostatin-like immunoreactivity levels following feeding in humans indicating a vagal inhibitory control of somatostatin levels. Acta Physiol Scand 113:411–413
27. Allen JM, Bishop AE, Daly MG, Larsson H, Carlsson E, Polak JM, Bloom SR (1986) Effect of inhibition of acid secretion on the regulatory peptides in rat stomach. Gastroenterology 90:970–977
28. Schubert ML, Edwards NF, Makhlouf GM (1988) Regulation of gastric somatostatin secretion in the mouse by luminal acidity: a local feedback mechanism. Gastroenterology 94:317–322
29. Sandvik AK, Waldum HL (1988) The effect of somatostatin on baseline and stimulated acid secretion and vascular histamine release from the totally isolated vascularly perfused rat stomach. Regul Peptides 20:233–239
30. Jebbink MCW, Lamers CBHW, Mooy DH, Rovati LC, Jansen JBMJ (1992) Effect of loxiglumide on basal and gastrin- and bombesin-stimulated gastric acid and serum gastrin levels. Gastroenterology 103:1215–1220
31. Verhulst ML, Gielkens HAJ, Hopman WPM, Tangerman A, Lamers CBHW, Jansen JBMJ (1992) Cholecystokinin both stimulates and inhibits gastric acid secretion in man. Regul Peptides 40:271

32. Konturek JW, Konturek SJ, Maczka M, Domschke W (1992) Cholecystokinin in the control of gastric acid secretion in humans. Regul Peptides 40:185
33. Schmidt WE, Schenk S, Otto J, Nustede R, Rovati LC, Fölsch UR, Creutzfeld W (1992) Cholecystokinin (CCK) inhibits gastric acid secretion in humans via a CCK-A receptor mediated mechanism. Regul Peptides 40:246
34. Burckhardt B, Delco F, Aufderhaar U, Ketterer S, Beglinger C (1992) Effects of CCK-A receptor antagonist on gastric acid secretion in man. Regul Peptides 40:178
35. Soll AH, Amirian DA, Park JL, Elashoff JD, Yamada T (1985) Cholecystokinin potently releases somatostatin from canine fundic mucosal cells in short-term culture. Am J Physiol 248:G569–573
36. Levi S, Beardshall K, Haddad G, Playford R, Ghosh P, Calam J (1989) Campylobacter pylori and duodenal ulcers; the gastrin link. Lancet I:1167–1168
37. Smith JTL, Pounder RE, Nwokolo CU, Lanzon-Miller S, Evans DG, Graham DY, Evans DJ (1990) Inappropriate hypergastrinaemia in asymptomatic healthy subjects infected with Helicobacter pylori. Gut 31:522–525
38. Asaka M, Kimura T, Kudo M et al. (1992) Relationship of Helicobacter pylori to serum pepsinogens in an asymptomatic Japanese population. Gastroenterology 102:760–766
39. Prewett EJ, Smith JTL, Nwokolo CU, Hudson M, Sawyerr AM, Pounder RE (1991) Eradication of Helicobacter pylori abolishes 24-hour hypergastrinaemia: a prospective study in healthy subjects. Aliment Pharmacol Ther 5:283–290
40. Chittajallu RS, Dorrian CA, Ardill JES, McColl KEL (1992) Effect of Helicobacter pylori on serum pepsinogen I and plasma gastrin in duodenal ulcer patients. Scand J Gastroenterol 27:20–24
41. McColl KEL, Fullarton GM, Chittajallu R, El Nujumi AM, MacDonald AMI, Dahill SW, Hilditch TE (1991) Plasma gastrin, daytime intragastric pH, and nocturnal acid output before and at 1 and 7 months after eradication of Helicobacter pylori in duodenal ulcer patients. Scand J Gastroenterol 26:339–346
42. Graham DY, Opekun A, Lew GM, Klein PD, Walsh JH (1991) Helocibacter pylori-associated exaggerated gastrin release in duodenal ulcer patients. Gastroenterology 100:1571–1575
43. Moss SF, Calam J (1992) Changes in acid secretion and parietal cell sensitivity to gastrin in duodenal ulcer patients after eradication of Helicobacter pylori. Gut 32:S 28
44. Fraser AG, Prewett EJ, Pounder RE, Samloff IM (1992) Twenty-four-hour hyperpepsinogenaemia in Helicobacter pylori-positive subjects is abolished by eradication of the infection. Aliment Pharmacol Ther 6:389–394
45. Haruma K, Sumii K, Okamoto S et al. (1992) Helicobacter pylori infection causes low antral somatostatin content: pathogenesis of inappropriate hypergastrinemia. Gastroenterology 102: A 80
46. Murthy UK, Linscheer R, Cho C (1992) The hypergastrinemia in Helicobacter pylori gastritis is due to a decrease in antral D cell density and D: G cell ratio. Gastroenterology 102:A 130
47. Moss SF, Legon S, Calam J (1992) Helicobacter pylori infection decreases gastric somatostatin mRNA in duodenal ulcer patients. Gut 33:S 27

Kinetics of the Gastric Epithelial Cells

H. F. HELANDER

Introduction

In the study of gastrointestinal physiology and pathophysiology, much attention is focused on the formation of new cells, their survival, migration and ultimate death. Particularly in the small intestine, various types of treatment or disease are known to bring about significant changes in the thickness of the mucosa, which reflect modifications to the kinetics of the mucosal cells. These may be due to an altered rate of formation of new cells, a change in the life span of the cells, or a combination of both.

This review will summarize some of the methods used in the study of cell kinetics, and will then focus on the kinetics of the various types of gastric epithelial cells under normal conditions. In addition, a few examples of pathological disturbances will be discussed. For further results and opinions the reader should consult previous reviews on this topic (e.g. Lipkin 1973; Willems 1981; Wright and Alison 1984).

Methods

The first tool to be used in quantitative studies of cell kinetics was *counting mitoses*; the results were usually presented as the mitotic index, which is the percentage of mitotic cell nuclei in relation to the total number of cell nuclei. Since the M (mitotic) phase only lasts for less than 1 h, and the proportion of mitotic cells is often quite small (Fig. 1), various agents such as colchicine were sometimes used to block the mitosis in metaphase. Thus, the proportion of cell nuclei recognized in the M phase was increased. The disadvantage was the toxicity of the compounds.

Using these methods in the rat, Stevens and Leblond (1953) pioneered the research concerning cell renewal in the gastric mucosa. Hunt (1957) described an increase in the mitotic rate after refeeding starved rats, and he also observed markedly increased mitotic activity in the area immediately surrounding experimental gastric ulcers (Hunt 1958).

The introduction of radioactive isotopes in biomedical research resulted in new and far more sensitive methods for studying cellular kinetics. ^{3}H-Thymidine was utilized, since this synthetic nucleotide is incorporated into nuclear

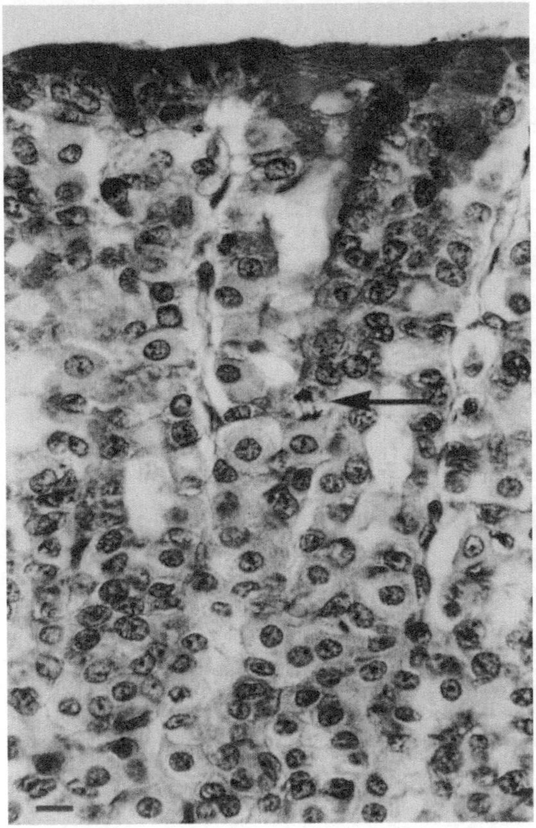

Fig. 1. Superficial layers of rat oxyntic mucosa showing a mitotic figure (*arrow*). Periodic acid-Schiff stain; × 500; bar = 10 μm

DNA during the S (synthetic) phase of the mitotic cycle. It remains there as a marker throughout the entire life span of the cell. Autoradiography can be used to calculate the number of *labelled nuclei*; the relation between labelled nuclei and the total number of nuclei is referred to as the labelling index. In addition, any movement of the labelled cells from their supposed origin can be recorded.

Messier and Leblond (1960) utilized ^{3}H-Thymidine labelling to study cell proliferation and migration in a large number of organs, including the gastric mucosa, and more detailed studies on the oxyntic mucosa were published soon afterwards by Hunt and Hunt (1962).

In recent years, bromodeoxyuridine (BrdU) has emerged as a non-radioactive alternative to ^{3}H-Thymidine, which can be detected by immunohistochemical methods (Fig. 2); some investigators also have used this compound in patients (Danova et al. 1988). Such procedures, as well as the injection of ^{3}H-Thymidine into patients (MacDonald et al. 1964, Lipkin 1972), will require comprehensive discussions with ethical committees before they are repeated.

The chain of events that leads to a complete cell division involves the expression of a series of specific proteins, some of which may be used as markers for the mitotic process (e.g. DNA polymerase α, proliferating cell nuclear

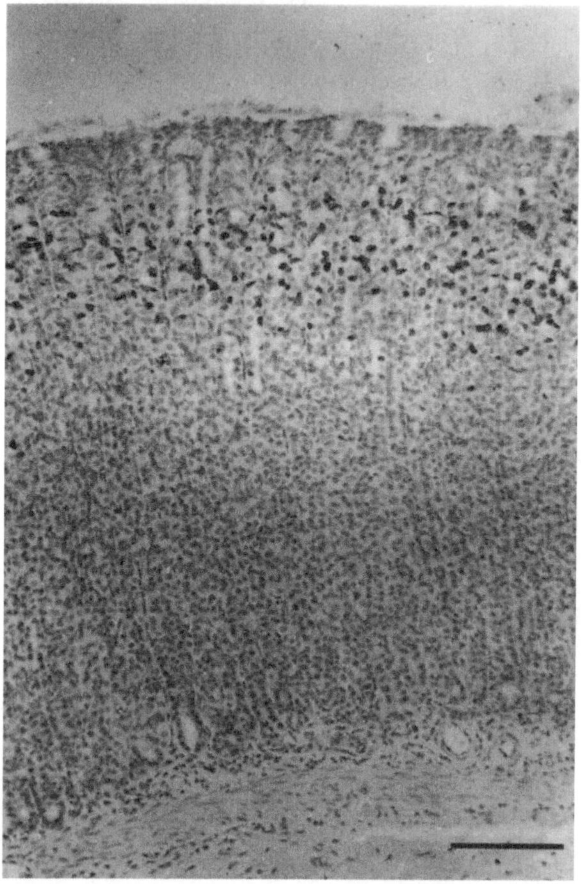

Fig. 2. Oxyntic mucosa from rat given bromodeoxyuridine (BrdU) 1 h before death. The dark-stained cell nuclei in the isthmus-neck region have incorporated BrdU into their nuclear DNA, indicating that the cells have entered S phase. Peroxidase antibody stain; ×150; bar = 100 μm

antigen). These products can be readily detected by immunohistochemical methods.

A comprehensive study of the theory of renewing cell populations has been published by Wright and Alison (1984).

Proliferating Cells of the Gastric Epithelium

The great majority of the dividing cells are found in the "progenitor zone" in the isthmus and neck regions of the gastric glands (Figs. 1, 2; additional mitoses are seen in endocrine cells – see the section on endocrine cells below). The position of the progenitor zone in the gastric mucosa contrasts to that of the intestine, where cell proliferation takes place mainly in the bottom part of the intestinal glands. It should be noted that, during perinatal development, the dividing cells are distibuted throughout all levels of the gastric mucosa. As the various epithelial cells mature, a progenitor zone is established in the neck-isthmus region (Yeomans and Trier 1976; Kataoka et al. 1984).

The progenitor zone is also spread out during the healing of gastric ulcers, and mitoses can be observed at all levels of the glands in the ulcer margin (Helander 1983, Helpap et al. 1981). Although most investigators have referred to the dividing cells as "immature mucous neck cells" or "stem cells", the identity of these cells has been much debated. In a couple of articles, Kataoka and coworkers (Kataoka 1970; Kataoka et al. 1986) investigated the cell renewal in the mouse gastric mucosa. They observed mitoses in the undifferentiated cells (devoid of secretory granules), in immature mucous neck cells (containing secretory granules), and in immature surface mucous cells (also containing secretory granules). Similarly, in the hamster gastric mucosa, Tamura and Fujita (1983) described uptake of ^{3}H-Thymidine in immature surface mucous cells and mucous neck cells within a few hours of injection.

In a recent study of the mouse oxyntic mucosa, Karam (1990) confirmed and extended these observations. The three types of dividing cells included the non-granulated stem cell (Fig. 3), the pre-mucous neck cell, which contained

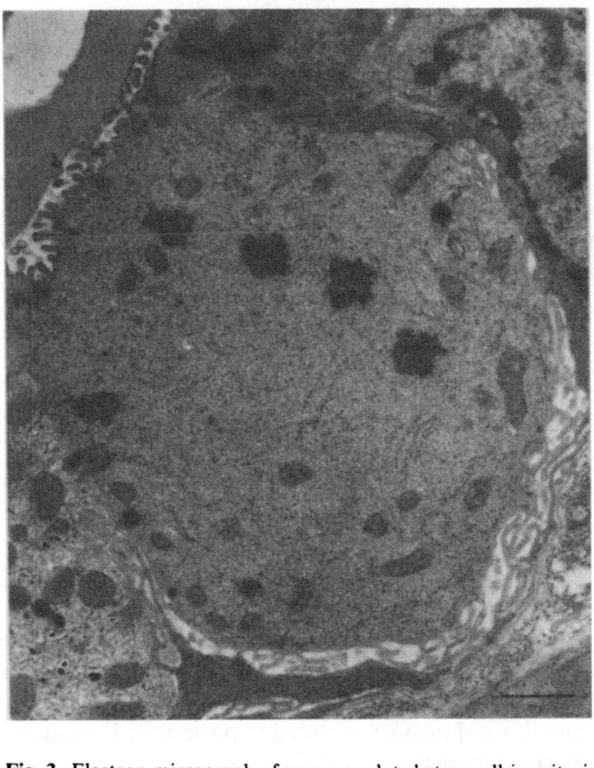

Fig. 3. Electron micrograph of non-granulated stem cell in mitosis. ×11 000; bar = 1 μm

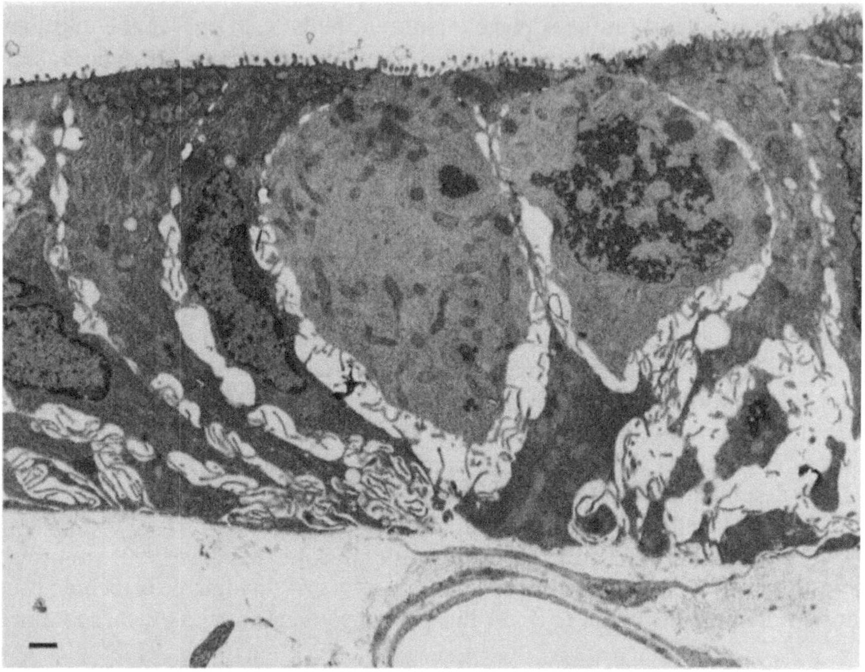

Fig. 4. Electron micrograph of dividing pre-mucous neck cells from rat oxyntic mucosa. Specimen was taken from ridge surrounding an experimental ulcer. × 3600; bar = 1 μm

secretory granules similar to those of the mature mucous neck cells (Fig. 4), and the pre-pit cells with granules similar to those found in the mature surface mucous cells. All these three types of cell were labelled 30 min after an injection of ^{3}H-Thymidine, and their turnover time, i.e. the time required to replace all cells of a certain type, was about 3 days.

Physiological Variations

Perhaps the most important physiological variation is the diurnal variation. This has been studied in other parts of the digestive tract (Scheving et al. 1980), and there is every reason to believe that in the gastric mucosa, too, the rate of cell proliferation changes as a result of diurnal influence (see Wegener et al. 1971).

Feeding is known to raise the mitotic rate considerably (Hunt 1957; Willems 1981). In the canine oxyntic mucosa DNA synthesis started to increase 8 h after food ingestion, peaked at 16 h, and could still be observed after 20 h (Willems et al. 1971). The mitotic index was increased between 20 and 24 h after food ingestion (however, in vitro studies of human gastric biopsies from three healthy volunteers failed to show any diurnal or post-prandial variations in the mitotic index or the labelling index (Hart-Hansen et al. 1976)).

The reasons for the post-prandial increase in cell proliferation are complex. Willems (1981) has emphasized the role of desquamation of the surface epithelium during a meal, and he also pointed out the obvious connection with the elevated levels of several gastrointestinal hormones, most notably gastrin. In dogs, a 4-h intravenous infusion of gastrin caused a four-fold increase in the mitotic index of the oxyntic mucosa 16 h after the start of the infusion. The mitotic index rose from the 20th h (Willems et al. 1972b). In gastric biopsies from healthy volunteers who were given a 2-h intravenous infusion of pentagastrin, Hart-Hansen et al. (1976) observed a doubling of the labelling index in the foveolar epithelium of the corpus. No change was recorded in the antrum.

In hypergastrinaemia—produced in rats by continuous infusion of gastrin-17 for 12 days—there was a significant increase in the labelling index in the progenitor zone of the oxyntic mucosa, but not of the antral mucosa. A similar effect was evoked when endogenous gastrin secretion was stimulated by the inhibition of gastric acid secretion (Ryberg et al. 1990).

It is obvious that other hormones, as well as growth factors, may play an important role in regulating cell proliferation in the gastric mucosa.

Pathological Variations

Acute stress appears to inhibit epithelial cell proliferation in the rat oxyntic mucosa, but has no effect on the antral mucosa. Chronic indomethacin administration stimulates the proliferation in the oxyntic mucosa, but not in the antral mucosa (Kuwayama and Eastwood 1985).

Several investigators have utilized endoscopic biopsies from the gastric mucosa in patients; the biopsies have been incubated with ^{3}H-Thymidine for a few hours and then used for autoradiography. These studies indicated an accelerated rate of mitosis in atrophic gastritics. Since the gastric mucosa was much thinner than normal, it was concluded that the turnover time of the epithelial cells was probably reduced (Hart Hansen et al. 1977). Assad and Eastwood (1980) found increased epithelial proliferation in biopsies from the oxyntic mucosa in patients subjected to antrectomy and vagotomy. This effect was attributed mainly to the development of gastritis, but other factors could also play a role.

These studies were followed by several others, in which the effects of various drugs were tested on endoscopic biopsies. Fich et al. (1985) found a decreased turnover of the gastric epithelial cells in biopsies from patients given misoprostol; in contrast, cimetidine caused increased gastric cell turnover.

Where ^{3}H-Thymidine labelling was used in the studies mentioned above, Levi et al. (1990) employed microdissected glands from endoscopic biopsy specimens instead. Using a modified Feulgen stain, they were able to recognize dividing cells and to obtain a proliferative activity index, defined as the number of cells in mitosis per gland. In the ulcer edge area the number of mitoses per gland averaged 11.6 ± 1.37, vs 3.75 ± 0.37 in the adjacent mucosa.

Non-steroidal anti-inflammatory drugs inhibited cell proliferation, an effect which was reversed by misoprostol.

Surface Mucous Cells

Upon their transition to the gastric pits, the pre-pit cells differentiate into mature surface mucous cells, which then migrate to the surface of the gastric mucosa. The turnover time from the mitosis to the shedding of the these cells into the gastric cavity amounts to about 3 days in the mouse (Karam 1990). In an early study by MacDonald et al. (1964), ^{3}H-Thymidine was given intravenously to two cancer patients, and the migration of the labelled cells was followed in repeated gastric biopsies up to 14 days after the injection. The transit time from the gastric pits to the surface was estimated to be about 4–6 days. In vitro studies of the human foveolar cells in antral biopsies from healthy volunteers have shown a turnover time of 65 h, and 63 h in corpus biopsies. In cases with gastritis, the turnover times were significantly shorter (Hart-Hansen et al. 1979).

The death and desquamation of the surface mucous cells have been studied by several authors (Kataoka et al. 1985, Tatsumi and Fujita 1988, Grosse et al. 1991). In gastric biopsies from healthy volunteers, Mackercher et al. (1978) observed that, on average, 2.4% of the surface mucous cells were damaged or dead. An interesting detail in the process leading to desquamation is the capacity of the surface mucous cells to repair wounds in their apical plasma membrane and thus postpone the ultimate death of the cell (McNeil and Ito 1989).

Special conditions seem to exist for the repair of superficial injuries of the gastric mucosa. The damaged cells are lifted off like a piece of foil from the viable part of the mucosa to form a protective layer together with mucus, fibrin and other cell debris. In a study in rats, the viable epithelial cells underlying this layer started to form long lamellipodia within 7 min of the injury. These projections of cytoplasm rapidly covered the bare basement membrane (Lacy 1988).

Wegener et al. (1971) compared mucous cell kinetics in rat oxyntic and pyloric mucosa and found shorter generation times in the pyloric mucosa. Experimental uraemia reduced the generation times of the mucous cells in both the corpus and the antrum.

Mucous Neck Cells and Zymogenic (Chief) Cells

The pre-mucous neck cells have a turnover time of about 3 days in the mouse, and after this time they have acquired the characteristics of the mature mucous neck cells (Karam 1990). These cells then migrate towards the bottom of the glands, but in the process their morphological characteristics gradually change. The rough endoplasmic reticulum grows, and the secretory granules become more similar to those of the zymogenic cells (Fig. 5; Suzuki et al. 1983).

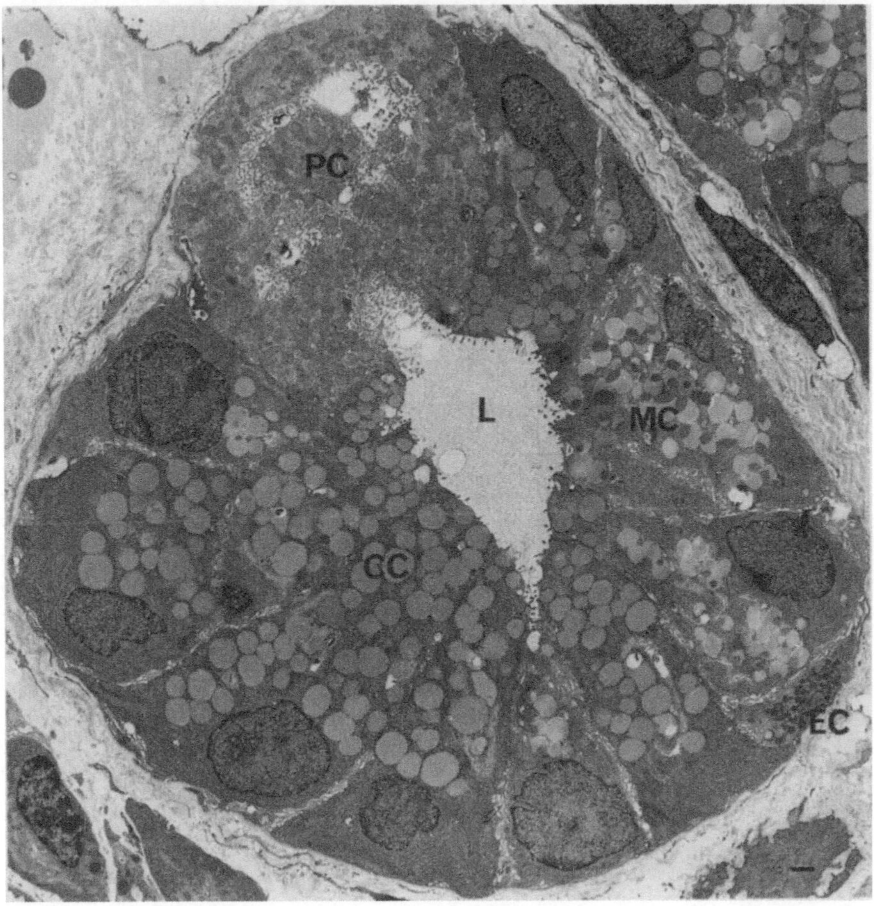

Fig. 5. Electron micrograph of cross-sectioned oxyntic gland from rat. Typical mucous neck cells (*MC*) and typical chief cells (*CC*) are seen, as well as transitional forms. *EC*, endocrine cell; *L*, gland lumen; *PC*, parietal cell. ×3300; bar = 1 μm

The origin of the zymogenic cells of the oxyntic glands has been debated (see Kataoka 1970, Hattori and Fujita 1976, Willems 1981, Karam 1990). Some investigators have claimed to observe mitoses in mature zymogenic cells; this "self-replication" would account for the formation of new zymogenic cells under normal circumstances. However, most authors have described a transition from mucous neck cells to zymogenic cells, also referred to as *the muco-zymogenic cell* (Karam 1990). It cannot be ruled out that there are species differences, but much of this uncertainty has been due to the use of relatively thick paraffin sections, in which cell identification can sometimes be difficult. The introduciton of thinner plastic sections has largely resolved this problem.

In the mouse, the turnover time of the muco-zymogenic cells has been estimated to be 78 days, and at the end of this period they have developed into

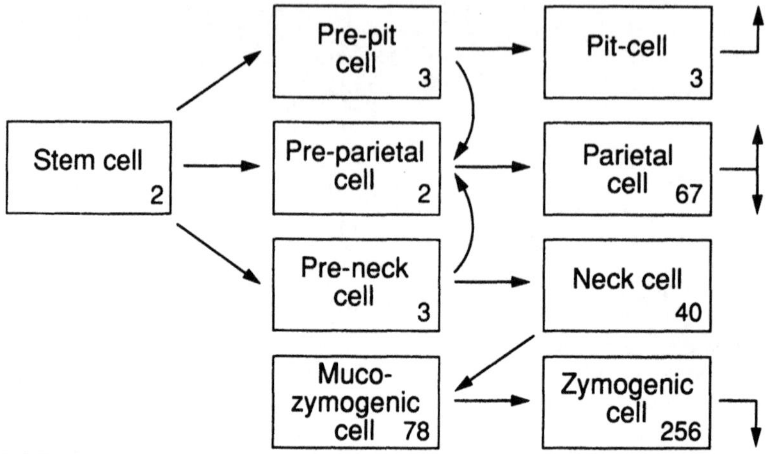

Fig. 6. Development of the epithelial cells in the mouse oxyntic mucosa. The numbers indicate the calculated turnover times in days. The *vertical arrows* to the right show the migration towards the mucosal surface or the bottom of the glands. (Adapted from Karam [18])

mature zymogenic cells with an additional turnover time calculated to be 256 days (Fig. 6; Karam 1990). In the golden hamster, Hattori and Fujita (1976) estimated the life span of the zymogen cells to be 200 ± 100 days.

Parietal Cells

The most primitive type of parietal cell is found in the isthmus-neck region of the oxyntic glands. It is characterized by small secretory canaliculi, many free ribosomes, a relatively large nucleus and small mitochondria (Karam and Leblond 1992). In some species a few mucous secretory granules have been observed (Helander 1988) in these cells. Shortly (30 min to a few hours) after an injection of ^{3}H-thymidine these cells – as all other parietal cells – remain unlabelled, and it must therefore be concluded that parietal cells do not divide under normal circumstances. A couple of days later, however, the parietal cells of the isthmus-neck region become labelled, indicating that they are derived from the proliferating cells in this region (Hunt and Hunt 1962, Ragins et al. 1968, Kataoka 1970, Willems 1981, Karam 1990).

During the following weeks and months, the majority of the parietal cells migrate towards the bottom of the glands, where they finally die. A few of them move towards the mucosal surface instead (Karam 1990). Ragins et al. (1968) estimated the half-life of the parietal cells in the mouse to be roughly 23 days and the survival to be about 90 days. In the golden hamster, the life span was calculated to be 200 ± 100 days (Hattori and Fujita 1976). More recent studies in the mouse by Karam (1990) indicate a turnover time of 67 days. Lipkin (1972) studied the proliferation of gastric epithelial cells from patients given a single injection of ^{3}H-thymidine. His results suggested replacement of the parietal and zymogen cell populations within one to several years.

Under stimulated conditions in man, the secretory surface (i.e. the apical plus the canalicular plasma membrane) of the parietal cells in the isthmus-neck region is about twice as large as in the parietal cells of the gland base, but under non-stimulated conditions, no such difference is observed (Helander et al. 1986). Similar observations have been made in the rat (Helander 1976; Jacobs and Sturtevant 1982) and have led to the speculation that the older parietal cells found in the bottom of the glands secrete acid at a lower rate than the younger parietal cells in the superfical layers of the mucosa.

In man, 4% of the parietal cells and 1% of the zymogenic cells display two nuclei (Helander et al. 1986). The significance of the binucleate cells is unknown, but it should be noted that they are twice as large as the corresponding mononucleate cells.

Endocrine Cells

In the gastric mucosa a minute fraction (about 1% of the volume) is taken up by various types of endocrine cells. In the oxyntic mucosa the most common type is the enterochromaffin-like (ECL) cell, and in the antral mucosa the gastrin (G) cells dominate.

The proliferation of the ECL cell has been studied in the rat by Tielemans et al. (Tielemans et al. 1989, Ryberg et al. 1990), using antibodies to histamine to identify the cells. One hour after an injection of ^{3}H-thymidine some labelled ECL cells were observed, mainly in the bottom half of the oxyntic mucosa. The turnover time of the ECL cells has not been determined. The first study on the kinetics of the G cells was published by Lehy and Willems (1976), who calculated a turnover time of 2–4 months in the mouse. The majority of the gastrin cells appeared to be renewed through replication of other gastrin cells.

In contrast, Fujimoto et al. (1980), who investigated the hamster, concluded that the large majority of the antral G cells originated from immature precursor cells at the isthmus of the pyloric glands and then migrated downwards towards the bottom of the glands. Only a small number of G cells appeared to undergo mitosis. It took 5 days for the immature generative cell to develop into a mature gastrin cell. The half-life of the hamster G cells was estimated to be 10–15 days.

The identification of the various endocrine cells is carried out by immunological methods using antibodies against their secretory products. Koop et al. (1987) pointed out that some antral G cells of the rat were "empty", i.e. their cytoplasm contained so little gastrin that the cells were not stained by antibodies against gastrin; only upon stimulation was it possible to identify these cells. Because of this uncertainty in the identification, data on endocrine cell kinetics should be interpreted with some caution.

References

1. Assad RT, Eastwood GL (1980) Epithelial proliferation in human fundic mucosa after antrectomy and vagotomy. Gastroenterology 79:807–811
2. Danova M, Riccardi A, Brugnatelli S, Fiocca R, Girino M, Villani L, Giordano P, Dionigi P, Giordano M, Buttini R, Ucci G, Mazzini G (1988) In vivo bromodeoxyuridine incorporation in human gastric cancer: a study on formalin-fixed and paraffin-embedded sections. Histochem J 20:125–130
3. Grosse G, Manthey N, Merker HJ, Niedobitek F (1991) Elektronenmikroskopische Untersuchungen am Oberflächenepitel der Magenschleimhaut des Menschen unter Berücksichtigung sekretorischer Vorgänge und der Zelldesquamation. Pathologe 12:239–245
4. Fich A, Arber N, Sestieri M, Zajicek G, Rachmilewitz D (1985) Effects of misoprostol and cimetidine on gastric cell labelling. Gastroenterology 89:57–61.
5. Fujimoto S, Hattori T, Kimoto K, Yamashita S, Fujita S, Kawai K (1980) Tritiated thymidine autoradiographic study on origin and renewal of gastrin cells in antral area of hamsters. Gastroenterology 79:785–791
6. Hart-Hansen O, Johansen AA, Larsen JK, Svendsen LB (1979) Cell proliferation in normal and diseased gastric mucosa. Acta Pathol Microbiol Scand Sect A87:217–222.
7. Hart-Hansen O, Pedersen T, Larsen JK (1976) Cell proliferation kinetics in normal human gastric mucosa. Studies on diurnal fluctuations and effect of food ingestion. Gastroenterology 70:1051–1054
8. Hart-Hansen O, Pedersen T, Larsen JK, Rehfeld JF (1976) Effect of gastrin on gastric mucosal cell proliferation in man. Gut 17:536–541
9. Hattori T (1974) On cell proliferation and differentiation of the fundic mucosa in the golden hamster. Cell Tiss Res 148:213–226
10. Hattori T, Fujita S (1976) Tritiated thymidine autoradiographic study on cellular migration in the gastric gland of the golden hamster. Cell Tiss Res. 172:171–184
11. Helander HF (1976) Stereological changes in rat parietal cells after vagotomy and antrectomy. Gastroenterology 71:1010–1018

12a. Helander HF (1983) Morphological studies on the margin of gastric corpus wounds in the rat. J Submicrosc Cytol 15:627–643

12b. Helander HF (1988) Parietal cells are not equal. In: Davison JS, Shaffer EA (eds) Gastrointestinal and hepatic secretions: mechanism and control. University of Calgary Press, Calgary, pp 107–110

13a. Helander HF, Leth R, Olbe L (1986) Stereological investigations on human gastric mucosa: II. Normal oxyntic mucosa. Anat Rec 216:373–380

13b. Helpap B, Hattori T, Gedigk P (1981) Repair of gastric ulcer. A cell kinetic study. Virch. Arch. Pathol Anat 392:159–170

14. Hunt TE (1957) Mitotic activity in the gastric mucosa of the rat after fasting and refeeding. Anat Rec 127:539–550
15. Hunt TE (1958) Regeneration of the gastric mucosa in the rat. Anat Rec 131:193–211
16. Hunt TE, Hunt EA (1962) Radioautographic study of proliferation in the stomach of the rat using thymidine-H^3 and compound 48/80. Anat Rec 142:505–517
17. Jacobs DM, Sturtevant RP (1982) Circadian ultrastructural changes in rat gastric parietal cells under altered feeding regimens: a morphometric study. Anat Rec 203:101–113
18. Karam SM (1990) Cell dynamics in the body (corpus) of the mouse stomach. PhD Thesis, McGill University, Montreal
19. Karam SM, Leblond CP (1992) Identifying and counting epithelial cell types in the "corpus" of the mouse stomach. Anat Rec 232:231–246
20. Kataoka K (1970) Electron microscopic observations on cell proliferation and differentiation in the gastric mucosa of the mouse. Arch Histol Jpn 32:251–273
21. Kataoka K, Sakano Y, Miura J (1984) Histogenesis of the mouse gastric mucosa, with special reference to type and distribution of proliferative cells. Arch Histol Jpn 47:459–474
22. Kataoka K, Takeoka Y, Hirano S (1985) Electron microscopic observations of surface mucous cells in the mouse gastric mucosa during physiological denegeration and extrusion. Arch Histol Jpn 48:327–339
23. Kataoka K, Takeoka Y, Maesako J (1986) Electron microscopic observations on immature chief and parietal cells in the mouse gastric mucosa. Arch Histol Jpn 49:321–331

24. Koop H, Schubert B, Schwarting H, Schikierka D, Eissele R, Willemer S, Arnold R (1987) Increased visualization of antral gastrin-producing G-cells after acute stimulation of gastrin in the rat. Eur J Clin Invest 17: 111–116
25. Kuwayama H, Eastwood GL (1985) Effects of water immersion restraint stress and chronic indomethacin ingestion on gastric antral and fundic epithelial proliferation. Gastroenterology 88:362–365
26. Lacy ER (1988) Epithelial restitution in the gastrointestinal tract. J Clin Gastroenterol 10, suppl. 1:S72–S77
27. Lehy T, Willems G (1976) Population kinetics of antral gastric cells in the mouse. Gastroenterology 71:614–619
28. Lipkin M (1972) Proliferation and differentiation of mucus containing cells in normal and diseased mucosa. Digestive mucous secretions. Biol Gastroenterol 61:500c
29. Lipkin M (1973) Proliferation and differentiation of gastrointestinal cells. Physiol Rev 53:891–915
30. MacDonald WC, Trier JS, Everett NB (1964) Cell proliferation and migration in the stomach, duodenum, and rectum of man: radioautographic studies. Gastroenterology 46:405–417
31. Mackercher PA, Ivey KJ, Baskin WN, Krause WJ (1978) A scanning electron microscopic study of normal human oxyntic mucosa using blunt dissection and freeze fracture. Dig Dis 23:449–459
32. McNeil PL, Ito S (1989) Gastrointestinal cell plasma membrane wounding and resealing in vivo. Gastroenterology 96:1238–1248
33. Messier B, Leblond CP (1960) Cell proliferation and migration as revealed by radioautography after injection of thymidine-H^3 into rats and mice. Am J Anat 106:247–285
34. Ragins H, Wincze F, Liu SM, Dittbrenner M (1968) The origin and survival of gastric parietal cells in the mouse. Anat Rec 162:99–110
35. Ryberg B, Tielemans Y, Axelson J, Carlsson E, Håkanson R, Mattsson H, Sundler F, Willems G (1990) Gastrin stimulates the self-replication rate of enterochromaffinlike cells in the rat stomach. Effects of omeprazole, ranitidine and gastrin-17 in intact and antrectomized rats. Gastroenterology 99:935–942
36. Scheving LA, Yaeh YC, Tsai TH, Scheving LE (1980) Circadian phase dependent stimulatory effects of epidermal growth factor on desoxyribonucleic acid synthesis in the duodenum, jejunum, ileum, caecum, colon and rectum of the adult mouse. Endocrinology 106:1498–1503
37. Stevens CE, Leblond CP (1953) Renewal of the mucous cells in the gastric mucosa of the rat Anat Rec 115:231–245
38. Suzuki S, Tsuyama S, Murata F (1983) Cells intermediate between mucous neck cells and chief cells in rat stomach. Cell Tiss Res 233:475–484
39. Tamura S, Fujita H (1983) Fine structural aspects on the renewal and development of surface mucous cells and glandular cells of the gastric body of the adult hamster. Arch Jpn Histol 46:501–521
40. Tatsumi H, Fujita H (1988) Ultrastructural aspects of the turnover of stomach mucosal epithelium. In: Motta PM, Fujita H, Correr S (eds) Ultrastructure of the digestive tract. Nijhoff, Boston, pp 53–66
41. Tielemans Y, Willems G (1990) Cellular kinetics in the oxyntic mucosa of the rat with special reference to the enterochromaffin-like (ECL) cells: influence of circulating gastrin. Res Clin Forums 12:81–92
42. Wegener K, Börner M, Krempien B, Wanke M, Rotz E (1971) Urämie und Proliferation an der Magenschleimhaut. Autoradiographische Untersuchungen über Teilphasen des Zellcyclus und der Generationszeiten des Magenschleimhautepithelien urämischer Ratten. Virch Arch B 8:186–195
43. Willems G (1981) Cellular kinetics and gastric mucosal disease. In: Domscke W and Wormsley KG (eds) Magen und Magenkrankheiten. Thieme, Stuttgart, pp 195–204
44. Willems G, Galand P, Vansteenkiste Y, Zeitoun P (1972a) Cell population kinetics of the zymogen and parietal cells in the stomach of mice. Z Zellforsch 134:505–518
45. Willems G, Vansteenkiste Y, Limbosch JM. (1972b) Stimulating effect of gastrin on cell proliferation kinetics in canine fundic mucosa. Gastroenterology 62:583–589
46. Willems G, Vansteenkiste Y, Smets P (1971) Effects of food ingestion on the cell proliferation kinetics in the canine fundic mucosa. Gastroenterology 61:323–329
47. Wright N, Alison M (1984) The biology of epithelial cell populations. Clarendon, Oxford
48. Yeomans ND, Trier JS (1976) Epithelial cell proliferation and migration in the developing rat gastric mucosa. Develop Biol 53:206–216

Trophic Effects of Gastrin: Therapeutic and Pathophysiological Implications

F. HALTER and A. SCHMASSMANN

Introduction

Gastrin is an important regulator of gastric acid secretion. In addition, it exerts well-defined trophic effects on the gastrointestinal tract which have long been linked to the pathogenesis of peptic ulcer disease [1, 2]. Moreover, hypergastrinaemia occuring during ulcer treatment with acid inhibitors is considered by many to be a risk factor fostering early ulcer relapse and development of malignant gastric tumours [for references see [3]]. Conversely, it has been postulated that as a growth factor gastrin could, in a manner analogous to epidermal growth factor, enhance reepithelialization of ulcers and possibly act as a mucosal protective factor [3].

Gastrin as a Potential Risk Factor in Peptic Ulcer Disease

Findings Based on Clinical Observations

Gastrin represents a direct pathogenic factor only in rare subgroups of ulcer patients, such as in those with the Zollinger-Ellison syndrome, the antral G-cell hyperplasia syndrome, and those in whom the gastric antrum was erroneously retained following partial gastrectomy. These three conditions can be cured through resection of the source of excessive gastrin production, e.g. a gastrinoma or the hyperplastic antrum or antral stump.

In most patients suffering from simple duodenal ulcer disease, fasting plasma gastrin is normal but the postprandial gastrin release is disproportionately enhanced [2]. This has been linked hypothetically to the overall increase in maximum acid secretory capacity of duodenal ulcer patients [4], which indirectly represents an increase in the parietal cell mass [5]. In addition, the increased sensitivity of the parietal cell to gastrin [6] has been linked to a possibly gastrin mediated up-regulation of the parietal cell [7].

The theory that gastrin could play a pivotal role in simple peptic ulcer disease has been reactivated following the discovery that colonization by *Helicobacter pylori* may be responsible for the disproportionate postprandial gastrin release [8], since this is reversible once *H. pylori* is eradicated [9–10]. In this theory the *H. pylori* infection acts as the trigger mechanism for the development of hypergastrinaemia and subsequent increase of the parietal cell mass, and possibly also an increase in the sensitivity of the parietal cell to gastrin. This hypothesis is weakened, however, by the observation that maximum acid secretory capacity and gastrin sensitivity do not return to normal once gastrin levels are normalized following eradication of *H. pylori* [11].

Findings Based on Animal Experiments

Some of the circumstantial evidence for a causative role of gastrin in the pathogenesis of gastrin stems from early animal experiments on the trophic effects of gastrin. The parietal cell was the first established target of the trophic effects of gastrin in the rat. More than two decades ago it was shown that gastrin can enhance cell proliferation within the gastric corpus mucosa. This in part results from an increase in parietal cell density resulting from a disproportionate maturation of parietal cells from stem cells [12]. Such an increase can be induced in the rat by repeated application of gastrin [13], by surgically induced mild hypergastrinaemia [14], and has also been observed following phasic increase of gastrin as induced by competitive histamine receptor antagonists [15].

By contrast, the trophic effect induced by surgical models inducing sustained hypergastrinaemia [16] or by prolonged acid inhibition with H^+/K^+-ATPase inhibitor [17] appears to be specifically targeted towards the enterochromaffin-like (ECL) cell type, and ECL cell density can increase up to fivefold whilst that of the parietal cell appears not to be affected [18]. This discrepancy was recently confirmed by Brenna et al. [19]. Since prolonged acid inhibition with an insurmountable histamine-H_2 antagonist also failed to enlarge parietal cell density, it is possible that a secretory product of the ECL cell induces an antitrophic effect on the acid-producing cell. In the rat, histamine would be a possible candidate. In the latter species, the ECL cell density increases proportionately to the degree of drug-induced hypergastrinaemia and can eventually lead to formation of carcinoid-like tumours provided prolonged acid suppression is extended through the whole life cycle of the animal [20]. Subtotal abolition of the pool of gastrin-producing G cells by antrectomy largely prevents this increase in ECL cells in rats treated with omeprazole [21].

Studies in Man

In man it is tempting to attribute both acid rebound and tolerance, as observed following acid inhibition with histamine H_2 receptor antagonists, to trophic effects of gastrin.

Acid Rebound

Several investigators have reported a rebound increase in gastric acid secretion after withdrawal of H_2-receptor antagonists [22–24]. Since prolonged acid inhibition almost inevitably leads to slight hypergastrinaemia, it is difficult to rule out definitely a possible causal relation between enhanced acid secretion and the trophic effects of gastrin. The same phenomenon could also supply a plausible explanation of the observation that the failure of acid secretory responses to fall following duodenal ulcer healing could be responsible for early ulcer recurrences [25–27]. Acid rebound and early recurrence can, however, also occur in the absence of hypergastrinaemia [23, 28], and the cause of acid rebound and early ulcer recurrence is presently not fully understood. One possible mechanism concerns "up-regulation" of the gastrin or histamine H_2-receptor of the parietal cell [29]. Up-regulation of either of the two receptors can be confirmed only by demonstrating an increase in the numbers or density of receptors in tissue binding studies, and such studies have not been performed. The availability of antibodies against the cloned parent receptors would facilitate such studies.

Tolerance to Histamine H_2-Receptor Antagonists

A number of studies in healthy volunteers have shown a decrease in the effect of histamine H_2-receptor antagonists on intragastric acidity after 7–14 days administration, especially if higher and/or more frequent doses than normal were used [30–36]. This phenomenon was not regularly associated with a progressive rise in plasma gastrin levels [32, 34], but in all studies gastrin failed to fall with the relative increase in intragastric acidity. An argument against gastrin as a causative factor in the phenomenon of tolerance stems from recent observations that tolerance occurs as early as 1 day after onset of acid inhibition [37].

Formation of Carcinoid-Like Gastric Tumours

Carcinoid-like gastric tumours have occasionally been observed in man in patients suffering from Zollinger-Ellison syndrome or in patients with pernicious anaemia [38–40]. Such neoplastic lesions have, however, not been observed to date in man. Following prolonged acid inhibition, despite experience with very large patient groups [41]. In man, by contrast to the rat, the degree of induced hypergastrinaemia is relatively small, much lower than observed in patients suffering from pernicious anaemia [42].

All these data suggest that gastrin is unlikely to be a major risk factor in peptic ulcer disease, except in very particular conditions such as in the presence of a gastrinoma [Zollinger-Ellison-Syndrome] or when the gastric antrum was retained during partial gastrectomy.

Gastrin as a Possible Beneficial Factor in Peptic Ulcer Disease

Hypotheses Based on Clinical Observations

There are theoretical grounds for believing that gastrin could influence ulcer formation and, less probably, also ulcer healing, either by enhancing mucosal protection or, directly, by its mitogenic property. The only suggestive evidence that gastrin could enhance healing of peptic ulcers comes from the apparently direct relationship between the degree of acid inhibition and the induced hypergastrinaemia, and the fact that more potent acid inhibitors result in more rapid ulcer healing than moderate acid suppressors [3].

Support From Animal Experiments

Effect of Gastrin on Healing of Experimental Ulcers

Support for this hypothesis comes from studies by Tarnawski and his associates [43], who compared the healing of acetic acid-induced ulcers in the rat during omeprazole treatment in intact and antrectomized rats. Removal of the antrum, the main source of gastrin production, delayed healing, but since this operation modifies gastric emptying it is not possible to attribute this delay unequivocally to gastrin. Okabe and coworkers [44] suppressed gastrin during omeprazole therapy in rats with an intact antrum with concomitant somatostatin therapy, but this failed to delay healing. Again, these results have to be interpreted with caution, since somatostatin in addition to gastrin suppresses many other known and unknown hormones. There is thus a great need to study healing of experimental ulcers during suppression of gastrin activity with a potent and specific gastrin receptor antagonist displaying prolonged action. We planned such a study but the limited supply of currently available gastrin receptor antagonists precluded realization of this project and we had to restrict ourselves to acute experiments on the effect of gastrin on mucosal protection.

Effect of Gastrin on Mucosal Protection

The presently available data on whether gastrin can protect the gastric mucosa are conflicting. Using rats depleted of gastrin by a liquid diet, Takeuchi and Johnson [45] found a marked decrease in DNA synthesis in the oxyntic mucosa, which by itself did not lead to ulcer formation, but greatly increased the ulcerogenity of restraint stress. Injection of pentagastrin reversed the decrease in DNA synthesis caused by a liquid diet and significantly protected against stress ulcers, suggesting that regeneration might be an important protective factor. This was indirectly supported by stress ulcer studies performed by Sakamoto et al. [46], but pentagastrin prevention of stress ulcers was attributed to the release of endogenous somatostatin.

Pentagastrin has also been reported to reduce gastric ulceration induced by acetylsalicylic acid in a dose-dependent manner in the gastrin-depleted model described above [47]. A significant positive correlation was observed between ulcer index and the ratio of DNA loss to DNA synthesis. The damage caused by acetylsalicylic acid could be partly reduced by pentagastrin infusion. Konturek et al. [48], however, were unable to confirm the protective effect of gastrin against acetylsalicylic acid challenge in normally fed rats.

We used a more direct approach and pretreated rats with a new and potent gastrin receptor antagonist [PD-136, 450]. This new, "dipeptoid" gastrin receptor antagonist, has been reported to display a very high affinity for the gastrin receptor in guinea-pig gastric mucosa [$IC_{50} = 0.6$ n*M*], is equally powerful in competing for the binding of 125_1-CCK in cerebral cortex [CCK_B site, $IC_{50} = 0.7$ n*M*], and is 1000-fold selective at this site over the CCK_A site in rat pancreas, with an ED_{50} of 0.8 *M* [49]. It has been reported that PD-136, 450 blocks the acid secretory response to pentagastrin in the in situ-perfused rat stomach preparation [Ghosh & Schild] with an ED_{50} of 0.03 mg/kg [50]. In addition, PD-136, 450 antagonized, at high doses, trophic changes inclusive ECL cell hyperplasia in the oxyntic mucosa of the rat as found after prolonged hypergastrinaemia induced by a potent proton pump blocker [51].

Male Wistar rats [6–12/group] were divided into nine groups and received vehicle, dimethyl-prostaglandin E_2, gastrin-17, PD-136, 450, omeprazole or combinations of these drugs, prior to intragastric administration of 1 ml 70% ethanol. The dose given, the time schedule, and the number of rats per group are shown in Table 1. Animals were killed after 15 min and the stomach was excised and opened along the greater curvature, rinsed with 0.9% NaCl and photographed. Coded colour slides were evaluated and the areas of gross haemorrhagic necrosis were measured planimetricaly using a semi-automatic image analysis system. The results were expressed as a percentage of damage to the total glandular mucosal area [mean ± SEM]. Dimethyl-prostaglandin E_2 was donated by the Upjohn Company, Kalamazoo, Mich., omeprazole by AB Hässle, Mölndal, Sweden.

The significance of differences was determined by unpaired *t*-test. Probability values of less than 0.05 were regarded as significant. Results were expressed as mean ± SEM.

Table 1. Gastric mucosal protection induced by gastrin and PD-136,450

Group	Dose (per kg, s.c.)	Time (min.)	Number of rats	Lesion index
Vehicle	0.3 ml	30	12	14.6 ± 3.3 *
Omeprazole	40 μmol	240	12	33.4 ± 4.3
Dimethyl-PGE_2	100 μg i.g.(!)	30	6	0.2 ± 0.2 **
Gastrin	8 μg	30	6	4.0 ± 2.4 *
Gastrin	128 μg	30	6	0.2 ± 0.2 **
Gastrin + PD-136,450	128 μg/18mg	30/45	6	0.5 ± 0.3 **
Gastrin + omeprazole	128 μg/40 μmol	30/240	6	17.0 ± 5.3 *
PD-136,450	18 mg	30	12	1.0 ± 0.5 **
PD-136,450 + omeprazole	18 mg/40 μmol	30/240	6	2.0 ± 1.4 *

Significant difference ($p < 0.05$; unpaired *t*-test) to omeprazole * or vehicle **

Gastrin strongly stimulated acid secretion to 360 μmol/kg H^+/h. Omeprazole [40 μmol/kg s.c.] virtually abolished basal, gastrin-, and PD-136, 450-induced acid secretion, reducing it to less than 1 μmol/kg H^+/h [pH of acid juice > 6] (Fig. 1). Gastrin enhanced dose-dependent gastroprotection (Table 1). It significantly reduced the macroscopic necrotic lesions induced by 70% ethanol. In agreement with results obtained with the prostanoid, both gastrin and PD-136, 450 almost completely prevented damage induced by 70% ethanol (Fig. 2). By contrast, intraperitoneal injection of omeprazole significantly augmented the ethanol damage. Pretreatment with omeprazole significantly [$p < 0.05$] reduced the gastroprotective effect of gastrin, but not that induced by PD-136, 450 (Table 1, Fig. 3).

These results are difficult to interpret, since both gastrin and its receptor antagonist were gastroprotective. A more detailed analysis of the receptor

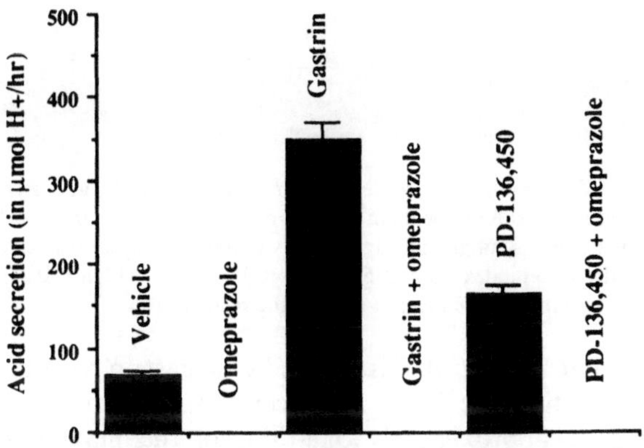

Fig. 1. Effect of omeprazole on gastrin- and PD-136, 450-induced acid secretion. Gastrin (128 μg/kg s.c.) increased acid secretion to 320 ± 21 (mean ± SEM, $n = 6$) and PD-136,450 (18 mg/kg s.c.) increased it to 170 ± 10 μmol/kg H^+ h. Omeprazole (40 μmol/kg s.c.) virtually abolished basal, gastrin- and PD-136,450-induced acid secretion, reducing it to less than 1 μmol/kg H^+ h (pH of acid juice > 6)

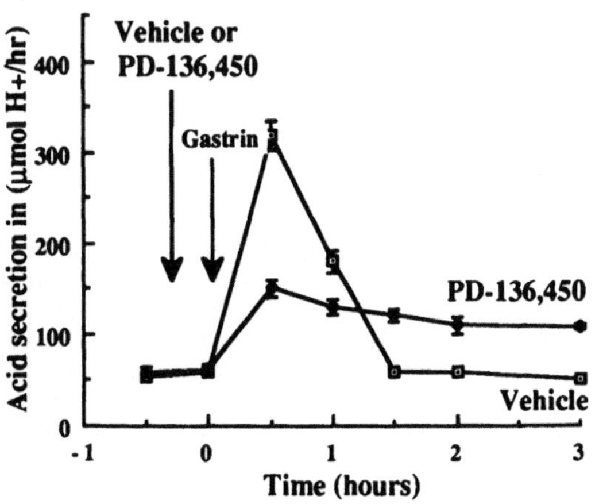

Fig. 2. Antagonist effect of PD-136,450 on gastrin-stimulated acid secretion in conscious rats. After subcutaneous pretreatment with 4.5 mg PD-136,450, gastrin-stimulated (32 mg/kg s.c.) acid secretion was reduced by $60 \pm 5\%$ (mean ± SEM)

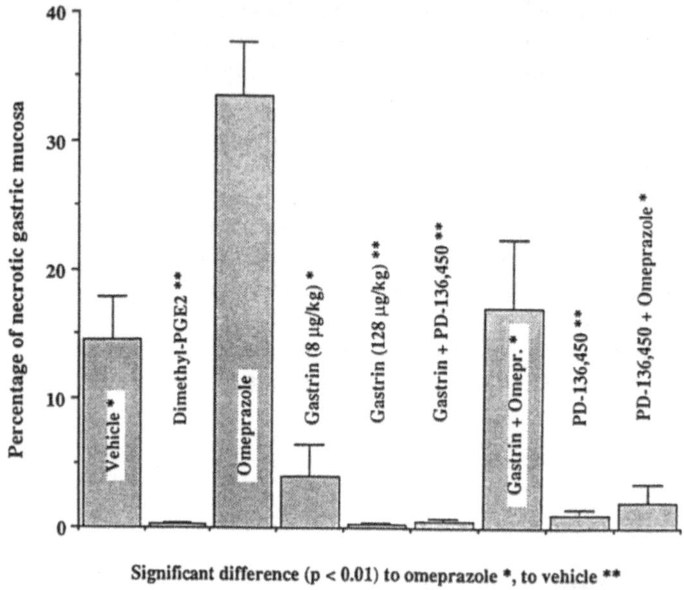

Fig. 3. Gastric mucosal protection of dimethyl-prostaglandin E_2, omeprazole, gastrin and PD-136,450. Gastrin reduced the lesion index in a dose-dependent manner from 14.6 ± 3.3 to 0.2 ± 0.2 (mean ± SEM, $n = 12$, $p < 0.01$). Omeprazole strongly and significantly reduced the cytoprotective effect of gastrin. PD-136,450 reduced the lesion index from 14.6 ± 3.3 to 1.0 ± 0.5 ($n = 12$, $p < 0.01$). Complete inhibition of acid secretion by omeprazole did not change the results

antagonist revealed, however, that PD-136, 450 is a mixed type gastrin receptor antagonist which can partially stimulate basal acid secretion, its maximum stimulatory effect amounting to approximately one-third of the maximum gastrin response (Figs. 2, 4). It is thus likely that acid secretion, possibly by diluting the 70% ethanol load, contributed to the "protective" effect induced by both the receptor antagonist and pharmacological doses of gastrin. This is indirectly supported by the observation that omeprazole, which at the chosen dose completely abolishes gastric acid secretion, potentiated the damaging effect of ethanol. The acid-dilutory effect seems, however, not to be the only mech-

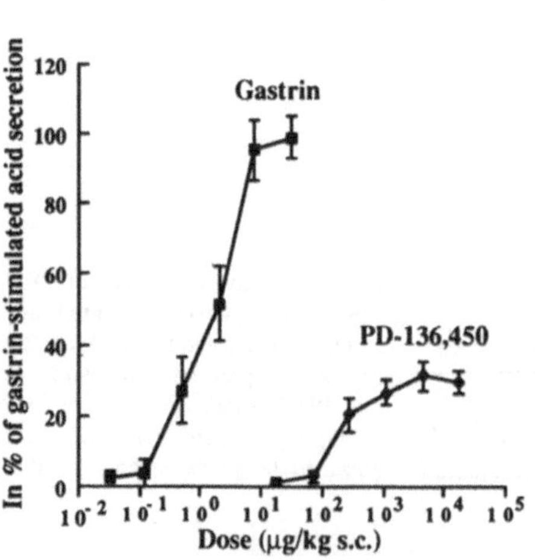

Fig. 4. The agonist effect of PD-136,450 on acid secretion is shown in comparison to gastrin in conscious gastric fistula rats. PD-136,450 displayed a partial agonist effect of 30 ± 5% of the maximal gastrin-induced acid output. ED_{50} of PD-136,450 was 0.2 mg/kg and the response was greatest at 4.5 mg/kg

anism through which the gastrin receptor antagonist PD-136, 450 enhances mucosal protection, since it counteracted the negative impact omeprazole induced on mucosal integrity without interfering with its acid-inhibitory effect. A stimulatory effect of mucosal microcirculation would yield a plausible explanation, since acid secretion is in general parallelled by a corresponding increase in blood flow. Moreover, gastrin has been shown to enhance gastric mucosal blood flow by different techniques [52, 53].

Further characterization of PD-136, 450 revealed that PD-136, 450 is not only active as mixed-type receptor antagonist at the CCK_B receptors but also as full agonist at the CCK_A receptors [54]. Activation of CCK_A receptors via vagal capsaicin-sensitive fibres protects the gastric mucosa against ethanol [55]. Thus in omeprazole pretreated rats PD-136, 450 but not gastrin may exert mucosal gastroprotective activity by interaction at the CCK_A receptors of vagal capsaicin-sensitive fibres.

The results of our studies do not completely clarify the role of gastrin on mucosal protection and underline the need for more specific full gastrin receptor antagonists. They also demonstrate the difficulty in separating the trophic action of gastrin from its stimulatory effect on acid secretion.

Summary and Conclusion

The trophic effects of gastrin in the pathogenesis of peptic ulcer disease are still not fully elucidated, but substantial progress may be expected once potent and specific gastrin receptor antagonists and receptor antibodies are available for use in man. Present data do not, however, support the notion that this hormone plays a central role in peptic ulcer disease outside rare conditions such as Zollinger-Ellison syndrome and retained antrum.

References

1. Johnson LR (1976) The trophic action of gastrointestinal hormone. Gastroenterology 70:278–288
2. Walsh JH (1979) Pathogenic role for the gastrins. In: Rehfeld JF, Amdrup E (eds) Gastrins and the vagus. Academic, London, pp 181–198
3. Pounder R, Smith J (1990) Drug-induced changes of plasma gastrin concentration. In: Hunt RH (ed) Gastroenterology clinics of north america: peptic ulcer disease. Saunders, London, Vol 19, No. 1 pp 141–154
4. Wormsley KG, Grossman MI (1965) Maximal histology test in control subjects and patients with peptic ulcer. Gut 6:427–435
5. Card WI, Marks IN (1960) The relationship between the acid output of the stomach following "maximal" histamine stimulation and parietal cell mass. Clin Sci 19:147–163
6. Isenberg JI, Grossman MI, Maxwell V, Walsh JH (1975) Increased sensitivity to stimulation of acid secretion by pentagastrin in duodenal ulcer. J Clin Invest 55:330–337
7. Betrachini G (1988) Receptors involved in the regulation of gastric acid secretion. SAMJ Suppl 74:3–4
8. Smith JTL, Pounder RE, Nwokolo CU, Lanzon-Miller S, Evans DG, Graham DY, Evans DJ (1990] Inappropriate hypergastrinaemia in asymptomatic healthy subjects infected with *Helicobacter pylori*. Gut 311:522–525

9. Graham DY, Apekum A, Ginger PA-C, Lew PA, Doyle PA, Evans J et al (1990) Ablation of exaggerated meal-stimulated gastrin release in duodenal ulcer patients after clearance of *Helicobacter* (*Campylobacter*) *pylori* infection. Am J Gastroent 85:394–398
10. Levi S, Beardshall K, Swift I, Foulkes W, Playford R, Ghosh P, Calam J (1989) Antral *Helicobacter pylori*, hypergastrinaemia, and duodenal ulcers: effect of eradicating the organism. BMJ 29:1504
11. Chittajallu RS, Harwood J, Dorrian CA, MCKoll KEL (1991) Is *Helicobacter pylori* related hypergastrinaemia due to the bacterium inhibiting parietal cell function? Gut 31:A 1206
12. Willems G, Lehy T (1975) Radioautographic and quantitative studies on parietal and peptic cell kinetics in the mouse: a selective effect of gastrin on parietal cell proliferation. Gastroenterology 69:416– 425
13. Crean GP, Marshall MW, Rumsey RDE (1969) Parietal cell hyperplasia induced by the administration of pentagastrin (ICI 50, 123) to rats. Gastroenterology 57:147–155
14. Lehy T, Bonnefond A, Dubrasquet M, Nasca S, Lewin M, Bonfils S (1973) Comparative effects of antrocolic transposition and antrectomy on fundic mucosa and acid secretion of the rat. Gastroenterology 64:421– 428
15. Witzel L, Halter F, Olah AJ, Häcki WH (1977) Effects of prolonged metiamide medication on the fundic mucosa. A secretory and histomorphometric study in the rat. Gastroenterology 73:797–803
16. Alumets J, EL Munshid HA, Hakanson R, Liedberg G, Oscarson J, Rehfeld JF, Sundler F (1979) Effect of antrum exclusion on endocrine cells of rat stomach. J Physiol 286:145–155
17. Hakanson R, Blom H, Carlsson E, Larsson H, Ryberg B, Sundler F (1986) Hypergastrinemia produces trophic effects in stomach but not in pancreas and intestines. Regulatory Peptides 13:225–233
18. Inauen W, Eigenmann F, Varga L, Koelz HR, Halter F (1990) Effects of gastric acid inhibition on plasma gastrin and oxyntic mucosal growth in the rat. Eur J Gastroenterol Hepatol 2:297–303
19. Brenna E, Waldum HL, Sandwik AK, Schultze Sognen B, Kristensen (1992) Effects on the rat oxyntic mucosa of the histamine H_2-antagonist loxtidine and the H^+K^+ATPase inhibitor omeprazole. Aliment Pharmacol Ther 6:335–349
20. Ekman L, Hansson E, Havu N, Lundberg C (1985) Toxicological studies on omeprazole. Scand J Gastroenterol 20 (suppl 108):53 – 69
21. Larsson H, Carlsson E, Mattsson H, Lundell L, Sundler F, Sundell G, Wallmark B, Watanabe T, Hankanson R (1986) Plasma gastrin and gastric enterochomaffinlike cell activation and proliferation. Studies with omeprazole and ranitidine in intact and antrectomized rats. Gastroenterology 90:391–399
22. Chiverton SG, Hunt RH (1989] Initial therapy and relapse of duodenal ulcer: possible acid secretory mechanisms. Gastroenterology 96:632–639
23. Fullarton GM, McLaughlan G, MacDonald A, Crean GP, McColl KEL (1989) Rebound nocturnal hypersecretion after four weeks treatment with an H_2 antagonist. Gut 30:449– 454
24. Marks IN, Johnston DA, Young GO (1991) Acid secretory changes and early relapse following duodenal ulcer healing with sucralfate, ranitidine, antacids or omeprazole. In: Halter F, Garner A, Tytgat CNJ (eds) Mechanisms of peptic ulcer healing. Kluwer, Dordrecht, pp 273–282
25. Yanaka A, Muto H (1988) Increased parietal cell responsiveness to tetragastrin in patients with recurrent duodenal ulcer. Dig Dis Sci 33:1459–1465
26. Marks IN (1991) Sucralfate: efficacy and basis for therapy. In: Swabb EA, Szabo S (eds), Ulcer disease-investigation and basis for therapy. Dekker, New York, pp 263–285
27. Bardhan K, Cole DS, Hawkins BW, Franks CR (1982) Does treatment with cimetidine extended beyond initial healing of duodenal ulcer reduce the subsequent relapse rate? Br Med J 284:621– 623
28. Prewett EJ, Hudson M, Nwokolo CU, Sawyer AFM, Pounder RE (1991) Nocturnal intragastric acidity during and after a period of dosing with either ranitidine or omeprazole. Gastroenterology 100:873–877
29. Jones DB, Howden CW, Burget DW, Silletti C, Hunt RH (1988) Alteration of H_2 receptor sensitivity in duodenal ulcer patients after maintenance treatment with an H_2 receptor antagonist. Gut 29:890– 893
30. Halter F (1990) H_2-receptor antagonsits: intragastric acidity after repeated doses. Aliment Pharmacol Therap 4 (Suppl. 1):1–6

31. Wilder-Smith CH, Halter F, Ernst T, Gennoni M, Zeyen B, Varga L, Roehmel JJ, Merki HS (1990) Loss of acid suppression during dosing with H_2 receptor antagonists. Aliment Pharmacol Therap 4 (Suppl 1):15–27
32. Nwokolo CU, Smith JTL, Gavey C, Sawyerr A, Pounder RE (1990) Tolerance during 29 days of conventional dosing with cimetidine, nizatidine, famotidine or ranitidine. Aliment Pharmacol Therap 4 (Suppl 1):29– 45
33. Wilder-Smith CH, Ernst T, Gennoni M, Zeyen B, Halter F, Merki HS (1990) Tolerance to oral H_2-receptor antagonists. Dig Dis Sci 35:976–983
34. Misiewicz JJ (1990) Clinical relevance to peptic ulcer healing and relapse. Aliment Pharmacol Therap 4 (Suppl 1):85–96
35. Smith JTL, Gavey C, Nwokolo CU, Pounder RE (1990) Tolerance during 8 days of high dose H_2 blockade: placebo-controlled studies of 24-hr acidity and gastrin. Aliment Pharmacol Therap 4 (Suppl 1):47– 63
36. Rogers MJ, Holmfield JHM, Primrose JN, Johnston D (1990) The effects of 15 days of dosing with placebo, sufotidine 600 mg nocte or 600 mg twice daily upon 24-hour intragastric acidity and 24-hour gastrin. Aliment Pharmacol Therap 4 (Suppl 1):65–74
37. Hürliman S et al. unpublished data
38. Harvey RF, Bradshaw MJ, Davidson CM, et al. (1985) Multifocal gastric carcinoid tumours, achlorhydria, and hypergastrinaemia. Lancet i:951–953
39. Borch K, Renvall H, Liedberg G (1985) Gastric endocrine cell hyperplasia and carcinoid tumours in pernicious anemia. Gastroenterology 88:638–648
40. Bardram L, Thomsen P, Stadil F (1986) Gastric endocrine cells in omeprazole treated and untreated patients with the Zollinger-Ellison syndrome. Digestion 35 [Suppl 1):116 –122
41. Berlin RG [1991) Omeprazole. Gastrin and gastric endocrine cell data from clinical studies. Dig Dis Sci 36:129–136
42. Lanzon-Miller S, Pounder RE, Hamilton MR et al. (1987) Twenty-four hour intragastric acidity and plasma gastrin concentration in healthy subjects and patients with duodenal or gastric ulcer, or pernicious anaemia. Aliment Pharmacol Ther 1:225–237
43. Tarnawski, personal communication
44. Okabe S, personal communication
45. Takeuchi K, Johnson LR (1979) Pentagastrin protects against stress ulceration in rats. Gastroenterology 76:327–334
46. Sakamoto T, Swierczek JS, Odgen D et al. (1985) Cytoprotective effect of pentagastrin and epidermal growth factor. Ann Surg 201:290–295
47. Takeuchi K, Johnson LR (1982) Effect of cell proliferation and loss in aspirin-induced gastric damage in the rat. Am J Physiol 243:G463–G468
48. Konturek SJ, Brzozowski T, Radecki I, et al. (1982) Cytoprotective effects of gastrointestinal hormones. In: Gut Peptides and Hormones. Biomedical Research Foundation, Tokyo, p 411
49. Horwell DC, Hughes J, Hunter JC, Pritchard MC, Richardson RS, Roberts E, Woodruff GN (1991) Rationally designed "dipeptoid" analogues of CCK. α-Methyl-tryptophan derivatives as highly selective and orally active gastrin and CCK-B antagonists with potent anxiolygic properties. J Med Chem 34:404–414
50. Lotti VJ, Chang RSL (1989) A new potent and selective non-peptide gastrin antagonist and brain cholecystokinin receptor (CCK-B) ligand: L-365,260. Eur J Pharmacol 162:273–280
51. Eissele R, Koop H, Patberg H, Rosskopf B, Frank M, Lorenz W, Arnold R (1991) The new gastric receptor antagonist Cam 1189 prevents ECL-cell hpyerplasia induced by the propton pump inhibitor BY 308 in the rat stomach. Europ J Gastroenterol Hepatol 3. Suppl, S34
52. Jacobson ED, Lindorf RH and Grossman MI (1966) Gastric secretion in relation to mucosal blood flow studied by a clearance technique. J Clin Invest 45:1–13
53. Ivarson IE, Darle N, Hulten L, Lindhagen J, Lundgren O (1982) Gastric blood flow and distribution: Effect of pentagastrin in anesthetized cat and man studied by an inert gas elimination technique. Scand J Gastroentol 17:1037–1048
54. Schmassmann A, Varga L, Flogerzi B, Sanner M, Garner A, Halter F (1992) The gastrin receptor antagonist Cam-1189 is a partial secretory agonist in the stomach and pancreas of the rat. Gastroenterology 102 Suppl A160
55. Evangalista S, Maggi CA (1991) Protection induced by cholecystokin-8 (CCK-8) in ethanol-induced gastric lesions in mediated via vagal capsaicin-sensitive fibres and CCK_A receptors. Br J Pharmacol 102: 119–122

Gastric Mucosal Damage and Protection: Involvement of Novel Endothelium-Derived Mediators

B.J.R. WHITTLE and J. LOPEZ-BELMONTE

Introduction

The vascular endothelium synthesizes and releases a number of potent biologically active mediators that can exert both protective and injurious actions on the gastric mucosa. Such endogenous mediators may be involved in the regulation of gastric mucosal integrity and in the pathogenesis of peptic ulceration.

Prostacyclin

The labile cyclo-oxygenase product prostacyclin (PGI_2) can be synthesized from the fatty acid precursor arachidonic acid by endothelial cells (Moncada and Vane 1978). Its formation can be detected in gastric mucosal tissue using bioassay or radioimmunoassay techniques and is inhibited by non-steroid anti-inflammatory drugs such as aspirin and indomethacin (Whittle et al. 1980; Whittle and Vane 1987).

Prostacyclin, like the other major prostanoid synthesized in the gastric mucosa, prostaglandin E_2 (PGE_2), is a potent vasodilator in the gastric microcirculation (Whittle et al. 1978; Gerkins et al. 1978; Walus et al. 1980; Kauffman and Whittle 1982). Furthermore, like PGE_2, prostacyclin can inhibit gastric acid secretion in a number of experimental preparations (Whittle et al. 1978; Gerkins et al. 1978; Kauffman et al. 1979; Konturek et al. 1980; Whittle, 1981; Shea-Donohue et al. 1982) and can stimulate the secretion of bicarbonate, a luminal protective factor (Whittle et al. 1984). Such a profile of properties has been suggested to contribute to the protective actions of PGE_2 (Robert et al. 1979; Whittle and Vane 1987) and may likewise underlie the protective properties of prostacyclin and its more stable analogues against mucosal damage observed in a number of experimental models (Whittle et al. 1978; Whittle and Boughton-Smith, 1979; Konturek et al. 1981, 1984).

The involvement of such endogenous prostanoids in the modulation of mucosal integrity is suggested by the enhanced susceptibility of the gastric mucosa to challenge following cyclo-oxygenase inhibition by non-steroid anti-inflammatory agents (Whittle, 1983). It is relevant to the endogenous role of these prostanoids that the haemorrhagic damage induced by aspirin or indomethacin is preceded by focal structural changes of the basement membrance of capillary and post-capillary endothelial cells, leading to destruction of the microvessels (Robins, 1980; Rainsford 1983). Mucosal application of the topical irritant ethanol also induces primary microvascular injury, and prevention of endothelial damage and vascular stasis may be a major mechanism by which prostaglandins can protect against the subsequent necrotic damage (Guth et al. 1984; Szabo et al. 1985).

Nitric Oxide

Endothelial cells also release another highly labile humoral vasodilator substance, originally known as endothelium-derived relaxing factor (EDRF), which mediates the vascular relaxation induced by agents such as acetylcholine (Furchgott and Zawadski 1980; Furchgott, 1984). It is now known that nitric oxide (NO), formed by endothelial cells from the amino acid L-arginine, accounts for the biological properties of EDRF (Palmer et al. 1987, 1988; Khan and Furchgott, 1987; Ignarro et al. 1987; Kelm et al. 1988).

The enzyme NO synthase generates NO from the terminal guanidino-nitrogen atoms of L-arginine, through a process in which molecular oxygen is also incorporated (Palmer et al. 1988; Palmer and Moncada, 1989, Leone et al. 1991). The constitutively expressed NO synthase enzyme is calcium, calmodulin and NADPH dependent, although a calcium-independent inducible isoform has been identified that can be expressed following incubation with endotoxin and cytokines in phagocytic cells (Hibbs et al. 1987, 1988; Marletta et al. 1988; Stuehr et al. 1989), in vascular tissue (Busse and Mulsch, 1990; Radomski et al, 1990) and in lung, liver and gut tissue (Knowles et al. 1990; Salter et al, 1991).

The formation of NO from L-arginine by a calcium-dependent constitutive NO synthase in rat gastric mucosal tissue has been demonstrated using a spectrophotometric technique (Whittle et al. 1991). In a further study on the cellular distribution of NO synthase in the rat gastric mucosa, epithelial cells separated by elutriation demonstrated high levels of constitutive enzyme activity as determined by the conversion of radiolabelled L-arginine to the NO co-product citrulline (Brown et al. 1992). This may reflect a non-vascular role for NO in the modulation of mucus or bicarbonate secretion from these cells, which, as in vascular tissue (Gruetter et al. 1979; Moncada et al. 1991), may involve activation of guanylate cyclase and elevation of cyclic guanosine monophosphate (GMP).

The formation of NO is selectively inhibited by L-arginine analogues such as N^G-monomethyl-L-arginine (L-NMMA) shown originally in in vitro studies on vascular tissue (Palmer et al. 1988b; Rees et al. 1989). Studies in the rabbit, rat and guinea-pig in vivo demonstrated that L-NMMA increased systemic arterial blood pressure, an effect reversed by L-arginine but not by the enantiomer, D-arginine, suggesting that endogenous NO biosynthesis from L-arginine can modulate resting vascular tone in vivo (Rees et al. 1989b; Whittle et al. 1989; Aisaka et al. 1989; Gardiner et al. 1990). Local infusion of L-NMMA also increased peripheral vascular tone in man (Vallance et al. 1990), while studies with other L-arginine analogues that inhibit NO biosynthesis, such as the more potent N^G-nitro-L-arginine methyl ester (L-NAME), have confirmed the importance of NO in the regulation of systemic arterial blood pressure (Rees et al. 1990).

Studies using hydrogen gas clearance have demonstrated that intravenous administration of L-NMMA dose-dependently reduced resting gastric mucosal blood flow (Pique et al. 1989). These effects were not shared by D-NMMA, while L-arginine but not D-arginine reversed these actions. Subsequently, using laser Doppler flowmetry, both L-NMMA and L-NAME have been shown to reduce resting mucosal blood flow (Tepperman and Whittle, 1992).

Studies on the mucosal hyperaemia induced by intravenous infusion of pentagastrin demonstrated that this response could be attenuated by concurrent infusion of L-NMMA or L-NAME (Warner et al. 1990). However, since mucosal blood flow may be altered by changes in the rate of acid secretion, it is important to determine concurrent changes in acid output. In such a study, pretreatment with a low dose of L-NMMA reduced the elevation of mucosal blood flow by 65% but had no significant effect on the plateau rates of acid secretion induced by pentagastrin, thus indicating an effect on the microcirculation independent of secretory modulation (Pique et al. 1992). A higher dose of L-NMMA, which both reduced resting mucosal blood flow and abolished the hyperemic response, induced a small but significant inhibition of pentagastrin-stimulated acid output. In contrast, however, administration of this dose of L-NMMA during stable rates of pentagastrin-stimulated acid output had no such effect on acid secretion, yet substantially reduced mucosal blood flow (Pique et al. 1992).

These findings therefore suggest that, whereas NO is a prime mediator of the blood flow changes associated with secretion, inhibition of NO biosynthesis has no direct effect on the stimulation of acid secretion; studies with other secretagogues as well as using isolated parietal cells will provide further evidence. Recent studies have, however, demonstrated the involvement of NO in the process by which acute administration of endotoxin can inhibit acid secretion, but the mechanism is as yet unknown (Martinez-Cuesta et al. 1992).

Interactions of Prostanoids and NO with Sensory Neuropeptides

Vasodilator sensory neuropeptides, predominantly calcitonin-gene-related peptide, that are stored and released from primary afferent neurones in the gastric mucosa (Green and Dockray, 1988) are also considered to play an important role in the preservation of mucosal integrity. Thus, depletion of sensory neuropeptides by chronic administration of capsaicin, which does not itself injure the gastric mucosa, greatly augments the damage induced by a number of ulcerogenic agents (Szolesanyi and Bartho, 1981; Holzer and Sametz, 1986; Holzer 1991; Esplugues et al. 1989; Esplugues and Whittle, 1990).

Recent studies have demonstrated that morphine adminstration, which prevents neuropeptide release from sensory neurones, or capsaicin pretreatment can attenuate the protective properties of PGE_2 and its 16,16-dimethyl analogue against acute gastric challenge (Esplugues and Whittle, 1991; Esplugues et al. 1992). Such findings indicate an interaction between these protective mediators in the modulation of mucosal integrity. Furthermore, the mucosal injury induced by indomethacin is augmented in capsaicin-pretreated rats, which again demonstrates such interactions between endogenous protective sensory neuropeptides and prostanoids (Holzer and Sametz, 1986; Whittle et al. 1990).

In studies on the interactions of these mediators with endogenous NO, administration of L-NMMA induced acute gastric mucosal injury over a 45-min period in rats pretreated with indomethacin, in doses of either agent that themselves did not provoke acute mucosal injury. Likewise, L-NMMA induced extensive haemorrhagic mucosal injury in rats chronically pretreated with capsaicin. Furthermore, L-NMMA induced deep haemorrhagic necrosis involving virtually all of the mucosal area in rats pretreated concurrently with both indomethacin and capsaicin (Whittle et al. 1990). Such findings indicate a crucial interaction between endogenous NO, sensory neuropeptide and prostanoids, all of which appear to subserve a modulator function in the regulation of gastric mucosal integrity. These mediators may not only exert local vasodilator actions on the microcirculation that are essential for adequate microvascular blood flow under physiological conditions, but may act to enhance or preserve endothelial cell function and continuity, especially under conditions of challenge.

The mucosal protective actions of a PGE_2 analogue against ethanol-induced injury do not, however, appear to depend on endogenous NO, since they were not inhibited by N^G-nitro-L-arginine (Konturek et al. 1992), although the protection induced by the anti-ulcer compounds carbenoxolone and sucralfate was attenuated by this inhibitor of NO synthesis (Peskar et al. 1991; Konturek et al. 1992). Moreover, other recent studies have shown that the protective actions against ethanol-induced injury of acute intraluminal instillation of capsaicin, which releases neuropeptides following initial stimulation of the sensory neurones (Holzer and Lippe, 1988; Holzer et al. 1990), are attenuated by N^G-nitro-L-arginine (Peskar et al. 1991). This finding again implies interactions between neuropeptides and NO in the mechanisms subserving mucosal protection.

It is possible that neuropeptides originating from the afferent sensory neurones in the vicinity of the microvessels are involved in the regulation of release of the endothelium-derived mediators. Recent studies have shown that depletion of sensory neuropeptides greatly augments the fall in mucosal blood flow induced by L-NMMA and L-NAME (Tepperman and Whittle, 1992). Furthermore, the acute increase in mucosal blood flow following instillation of capsaicin into the gastric lumen is abolished by concurrent administration of L-NAME (Whittle et al. 1992). This may reflect physiological interactions in the modulation of microvascular tone between NO and sensory neuropeptides, either directly on vascular smooth muscle or by the involvement of NO in the local vascular neuromodulator processes.

Endothelins

Vascular endothelial cells synthesize a 21-residue peptide known as endothelin-1 (ET-1) which exhibits vasoconstrictor actions both in vitro and in vivo (Yanagisawa et al. 1988; Inoue et al. 1989). Local intra-arterial infusion of picomole quantities of ET-1 has been demonstrated to induce substantial gastric mucosal vasocongestion and haemorrhagic injury in the rat (Whittle and Esplugues, 1988). Furthermore, intravenous infusion of ET-1 has been shown to augment mucosal damage induced by intragastric instillation of enthanol or acid (Wallace et. al. 1989a).

Endothelin-1-like immunoreactivity has been demonstrated in the rat gastric mucosa in both antral and corpus regions (Matsumoto et al. 1989; Takahashi et al. 1990). Much lower levels of immunoreactivity to endothelin-3 (ET-3), which differs from ET-1 by changes in six amino acids (Inoue et al. 1989), have also been found in the rat stomach (Matsumota et al. 1989). ET-1 and ET-3 were found to be equipotent in inducing rat gastric haemorrhage following intravenous infusion, although in vitro ET-1 was at least five fold more potent as a vasoconstrictor in the rat isolated stomach (Wallace et al. 1989b). ET-3 has also been shown to induce small increases in canine gastric vascular resistance following close-arterial infusion (Wood et al. 1992). Local intra-arterial infusion of high doses of ET-3 induced vascular lesions in the rat gastric mucosa that involved the venules and capillaries and potentiated the vascular injury induced by acid and ethanol (Morales et al. 1992). Furthermore, an anti-ET-3 serum was found to reduce the extent of mucosal damage induced by intragastric ethanol, suggesting that acute release of endogenous endothelins are involved in such mucosal injury (Morales et al. 1992).

It is likely that there is an interplay between endothelium-derived mediators with opposing vasoactive properties within the gastric mucosal microcirculation following their release. Indeed, the cyclo-oxygenase inhibitor indomethacin, in doses sufficient to reduce prostacyclin and PGE_2 biosynthesis in the mucosa, substantially increased the haemorrhagic injury induced by local and systemic administration of ET-1 (Wallace et al. 1989a; Whittle and Lopez-Belmonte, 1991). Furthermore, interaction of ET-1 with other local mediators such as sensory neuropeptides is also apparent. Thus, chronic administration of capsaicin to deplete sensory neuropeptides or administration of morphine to prevent neuropeptides release greatly augments damage induced by ET-1 (Whittle and Lopez-Belmonte, 1991). The haemorrhagic mucosal damage induced by local infusion of platelet activating factor (PAF), which involves microvascular injury, is likewise augmented by capsaicin pretreatment or morphine administration (Esplugues et al. 1989), as are the deleterious actions on mucosal blood flow (Pique et al. 1990), suggesting a local interaction of these vasoactive mediators with sensory neuropeptides within the microcirculation.

Protection and Injury by NO Donors

The release of NO from nitrovasodilator agents either following metabolic transformation, as with glyceryl trinitrate (GTN) and isoamyl nitrite, or spontaneously, as with nitroprusside, is responsible for their ability to activate guanylate cyclase, elevate cyclic GMP and relax vascular smooth muscle (Grueter et al. 1979; Ignarro et al. 1981; Feelisch and Noack, 1987; Feelisch, 1991). Following intragastric application, these nitrovasodilators can protect against acute haemorrhagic mucosal injury induced by topical irritants and by intravenous infusion of ET-1 (Kitagawa et al. 1990; MacNaughton et al. 1989). The nitrosothiol, *S*-nitroso-*N*-acetyl-penicillamine (SNAP), which spontaneously liberates NO (Ignarro et al. 1981), has also been demonstrated to protect against acute microvascular injury in the stomach and small intestine induced by PAF or endotoxin following intravenous administration (Boughton-Smith et al. 1990; 1992).

The protective action of locally infused SNAP on the mucosal damage by close-arterial infusion of ET-1 has therefore now been investigated.

Inhibition of ET-1 Damage by a Nitrosothiol

In these studies, male rats were anaesthetised with pentobarbitone, the stomach exposed and the left gastric artery cannulated for the local intra-arterial infusion of ET-1 (human-porcine; peninsula Labs, St. Helens, UK) or SNAP (synthesized in the Department of Medicinal Chemistry, Wellcome Research Laboratories). Acid saline (100 m*M* HCl, 2 ml) was instilled into the gastric lumen. Twenty minutes following termination of the local infusion of ET-1, the stomachs were removed and the area of mucosal damage assessed macroscopically in a randomized manner using computerized planimetry. A butterfly needle was inserted into a tail vein to allow systemic administration of the drugs, and intravenous arterial blood pressure was recorded from a catheter inserted into a carotid artery (Whittle and Lopez-Belmonte, 1991).

Local intra-arterial infusion of ET-1 (2–100 pmol kg^{-1} min^{-1}) for 10 min induced dose-dependent mucosal damage when assessed macroscopically 20 min later (Fig. 1). This damage consisted of areas of mucosal vasocongestion and haemorrhage as described before (Whittle and Esplugues, 1988; Whittle and Lopez-Belmonte 1991). ET-1 (10 pmol kg^{-1} min^{-1} i.a.) induced damage involving $54 \pm 6\%$ of the mucosal area ($n = 8$; $p < 0.01$), whereas the vehicle itself (0.1% bovine serum albumin in saline) did not induce any damage. The use of this vehicle for ET-1, rather than isotonic saline was found to enhance the potency of ET-1 for inducing mucosal damage.

The damage induced by ET-1 (10 pmol kg^{-1} min^{-1}) was significantly reduced ($46 \pm 10\%$, $p < 0.05$) by concurrent local intra-arterial infusion of SNAP (10 μg kg^{-1} min^{-1}) throughout the 30-min experimental period, as shown in Fig 2. Likewise, the mucosal damage induced by a lower dose of ET-1 (5 pmol kg^{-1} min^{-1} i.a. for 10 min) was significantly reduced by the concurrent

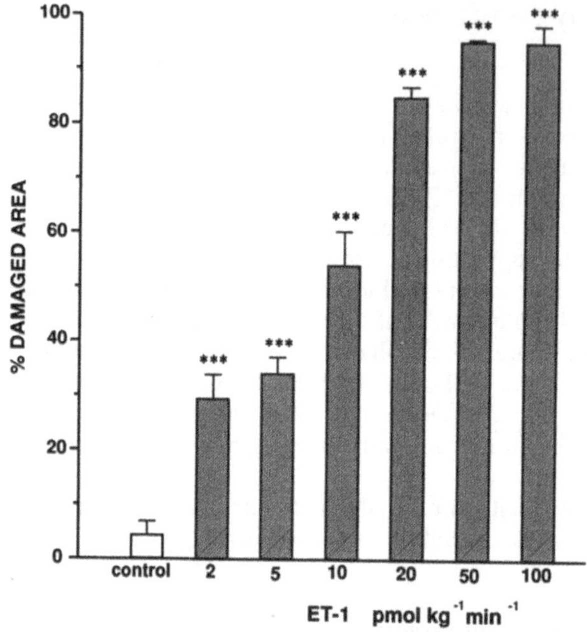

Fig. 1. Gastric mucosal injury induced by close-arterial infusion of endothelin-1 (ET-1; 2–100 pmol kg^{-1} min^{-1} in 0.1% bovine serum albumin). Results, shown as the area of macroscopically assessed damage expressed as a percentage of the total mucosal area 20 min following termination of a 10-min infusion, are given as mean ± SEM of 4–8 experiments per group. ***Significant difference from control vehicle group, $p < 0.001$

local administration of SNAP (5 $\mu g\, kg^{-1}\, min^{-1}$ i.a.) from 34 ± 4% to 16 ± 4% of the total mucosal area ($n = 5$ for each, $p < 0.01$).

Induction of Damage by a Nitrosothiol

By contrast, local infusion of a higher dose of SNAP (20 $\mu g\, kg^{-1}\, min^{-1}$) did not significantly reduce the mucosal damage induced by ET-1(10 pmol $kg^{-1}\, min^{-1}$ i.a.) as shown in Fig. 2. Furthermore, local infusion of SNAP (20 and 40 pmol $kg^{-1}\, min^{-1}$) alone for 30 min itself induced haemorrhagic injury to the mucosa, involving 20 ± 6% and 33 ± 8% of the mucosal area ($n = 6$ and 8, $p < 0.05$ respectively), as shown in Fig. 3.

At the higher local dose of SNAP (40 $\mu g\, kg^{-1}\, min^{-1}$), a fall in systemic arterial blood pressure was observed (Fig. 4), indicating its escape into the systemic circulation. This fall in arterial blood pressure, like the injurious action on the gastric mucosa, was dependent on NO release, since incubation of this thermodynamically and photosensitive NO donor for 48 h at 37 °C in ambient light to deplete its NO content abolished both of these actions (Fig. 4).

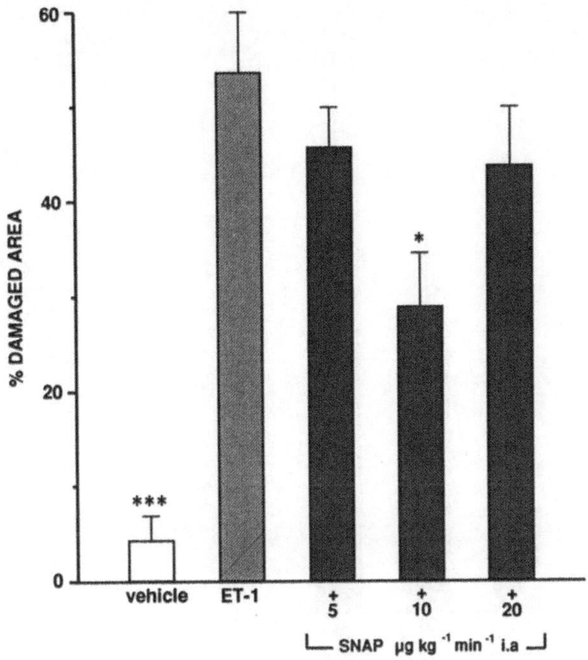

Fig. 2. Effects of concurrent close-arterial infusion of the NO donor *S*-nitroso-*N*-acetyl-penicillamine (SNAP; 5–20 $\mu g\, mg^{-1}\, min^{-1}$) on the gastric mucosal damage induced by ET-1 (10 pmol $kg^{-1} min^{-1}$ for 30 min). Results, shown as the area of macroscopically assessed damage expressed as a percentage of the total mucosal area, are given as mean ± SEM of 4–8 experiments per group. *Significant difference from ET-1 group alone, $p < 0.05$

Conclusions

These findings indicate that local administration of the nitrosothiol SNAP in low doses can protect the gastric mucosa from damage induced by intra-arterial infusion of ET-1. Such actions of the NO donor are likely to reflect vascular interactions between the vasoconstrictor peptide and the locally generated NO in the mucosal microcirculation.

The mucosal injury associated with the spontaneous release of NO from higher doses of this agent may indicate cytotoxic actions of high levels of NO on the microvascular endothelium. Indeed, the excessive production of NO by an inducible NO synthase in endothelial cells is considered to underlie the reduction in viability of these cells in culture following exposure over a 48 h period to endotoxin and the cytokine interferon-α (Palmer et al, 1992), while induction of NO synthesis is also considered to be involved in damage to adenocarcinoma cells (O'Connor and Moncada 1991). In addition, the substantial synthesis of NO by the immunologically induced NO synthase in macrophages accounts for

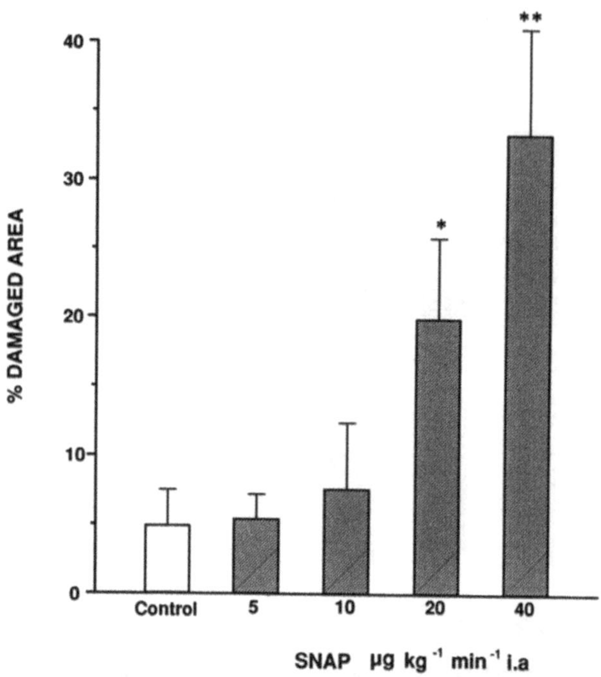

Fig. 3. Induction of gastric mucosal damage by close-arterial infusion of *S*-nitroso-*N*-acetyl-penicillamine (5–40 $\mu g\ kg^{-1}\ min^{-1}$ for 30 min). Results, shown as the area of macroscopically assessed injury expressed as a percentage of the total mucosal area, are given as mean $\pm$ SEM of at least 5 experiments in each group. Significant differences from control (saline infusion): $*p < 0.05$, $**p < 0.01$

the cytotoxic actions against tumour cells (Hibbs et al. 1987, 1988; Drapier et al. 1988).

The induction of NO synthase has also been implicated in the cardiovascular crisis and collapse seen over several hours in both animals and man in endotoxaemia (Nava et al. 1991, Petros et al. 1991; Wright et al. 1992). Furthermore, the microvascular permeability changes, an index of endothelial injury, seen in the rat small and large intestine 4–6 h after endotoxin administration correlate with the induction of a calcium-independent NO synthase over this period (Boughton-Smith et al. 1992). It is possible that local high concentrations of NO, generated from SNAP, may also form tissue-destructive species such as the peroxynitrite and hydroxyl moieties (Beckman et al. 1990) and hence bring about endothelial injury in the microvasculature, leading to mucosal necrosis and ulceration.

It is apparent, therefore, that NO may be involved in both physiological and pathological events in the gastrointestinal mucosa. Thus, endogenous NO plays an important role in the modulation of mucosal blood flow. Furthermore, NO

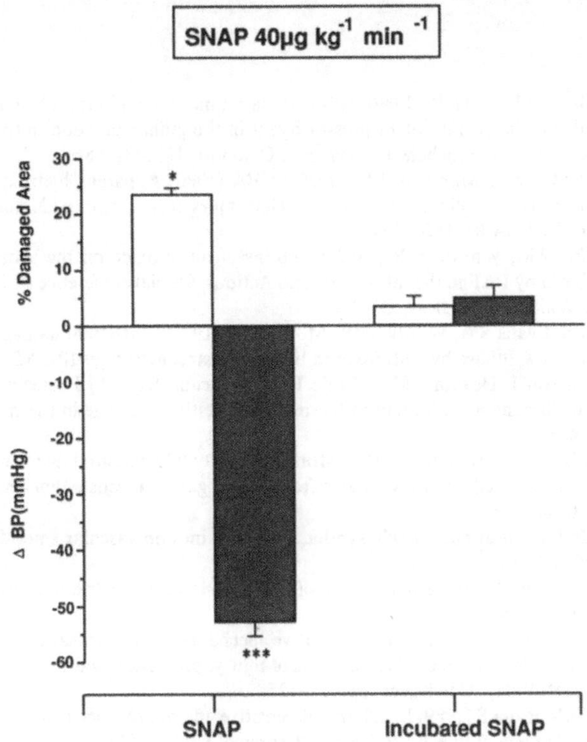

Fig. 4. Effect of incubation of *S*-nitroso-*N*-acetyl-penicillamine (SNAP) for 48 h at 37 °C in ambient light on the induction of gastric mucosal injury and fall in systemic arterial blood pressure following close-arterial infusion (40 μg kg^{-1} min^{-1} for 15 min). Results, shown as area of macroscopically assessed mucosal injury as a percentage of the total mucosal area and change in blood pressure (ΔmmHg), are given as mean $\pm$ SEM of at least 5 experiments in each group. Significant differences from control: *$p < 0.05$, ***$p < 0.0001$

has a key interactive role with other local protective mediators such as the prostanoids and sensory neuropeptides in the physiological regulation of mucosal integrity, and inhibition of its formation can provoke gastric tissue damage, especially under conditions where the synthesis or release of these other mediators is compromised (Whittle et al. 1990). Such interactions between these protective mediators, as well as interactions with proulcerogenic mediators such as ET-1, will need to be considered in the evaluation of mechanisms underlying peptic ulceration. However, as shown in the current study, an excessive, unregulated liberation of NO also has ulcerogenic potential. The factors that regulate the synthesis and release of endogenous NO by both the constitutive enzyme, likely to be involved in physiological processes, and by the inducible enzyme that may underlie certain pathological events, may thus be of significant importance to the understanding of the pathogenesis of ulcer disease.

References

1. Aisaka K, Gross SS, Griffith OW, Levi R (1989) N^G-methylarginine, an inhibitor of endothelium-derived nitric oxide synthesis is a potent pressor agent in the guinea-pig: does nitric oxide regulate blood pressure in vivo? Biochem Biophys Res Commun 160:881–886
2. Beckman JS, Beckman TW, Chen J, Marshall PA, Freeman BA (1990) Apparent hydroxyl radical production by peroxynitrite: implications for endothelial injury from nitric oxide and superoxide. Proc Natl Acad Sci USA 87:1620–1624
3. Boughton-Smith NK, Deakin AM, Whittle BJR (1992a) Actions of nitric oxide on the acute gastrointestinal damage induced by PAF in the rat. Agents and Actions, Special conference issue edited by G.P. Velo, B.J.R. Whittle, M.A. Bray, C3–C9
4. Boughton-smith NK, Berry S, Evans SM, Whittle BJR, Moncada S (1992b) Intestinal damage and the induction of nitric oxide synthase by endotoxin in the rat. Gastroenterology 102:A598
5. Boughton-Smith NK, Hutcheson I, Deakin AM, Whittle BJR, Moncada S (1990) Protective effect of S-nitro-S-acetyl-pencillamine in endotoxin-induced acute intestinal damage in the rat. Eur J Pharmacol 191:485–488
6. Brown JF, Tepperman BL, Handson PJ, Whittle BJR, Moncada S (1992) Differential distribution of nitric oxide synthase between cell fractions isolated from the rat gastric mucosa. Biochem Biophys Res Comm 184:680–685
7. Busse R, Mulsch A (1990) Induction of nitric oxide synthase by cytokines on vascular smooth muscle cells. FEBS Lett 275:87–90
8. Esplugues JV, Whittle BJR (1990) Morphine potentiates of enthanol-induced gastric mucosal damage in the rat. Gastroenterology 98:82–89
9. Esplugues JV, Whittle BJR (1991) Peripheral opioid-sensitive mechanisms of mucosal injury and protection. In: Garner A, O'Brien PE (eds) Mechanisms of injury, protection and repair of the upper gastrointestinal tract. Wiley, Chichester, pp 115–125
10. Esplugues JV, Whittle BJR, Moncada S (1989) Local opioid-sensitive afferent sensory neurones in the modulation of gastric damage induce by Paf. Br J Pharmacol 97:579–585
11. Esplugues JV, Whittle BJR, Moncada S (1992) Modulation by opioids and by afferent sensory neurones of prostanoid protection of the rat gastric mucosa. Br J Pharmacol 106:846–852
12. Drapier J-C, Hibbs JB Jr (1988) Differentiation of murine macrophages to express non-specific cytotoxicity for tumour cells results in L-arginine-dependent inhibition of mitochondrial iron-sulfur enzymes in the macrophage effector cells. J Immunol 140:2829–2838
13. Feelisch M, Noack EA (1987) Correlation between nitric oxide formation during degradation of organic nitrates and activation of guanylate cyclase. Eur J Pharmacology 139:19–30
14. Feelisch M (1991) The biochemical pathways of nitric oxide formation from nitrovasodilators: appropriate choice of exogenous NO donors and aspects of preparation and handling of aqueous NO solutions. J Cardiovas Pharmacol 17 (Suppl. 3): S25–33
15. Furchgott RF (1984) The role of endothelium in the responses of vascular smooth muscle to drugs. Annu Rev Pharmacol Toxic 24:175–197
16. Furchgott RF, Zawadzki JV (1980) The obligatory role of endothelial cells in the relaxation of arterial smooth muscle by acetylcholine. Nature (Lond) 288:373–376
17. Gardiner SM, Compton AM, Bennett T, Palmer RMJ, Moncada S (1990) Control of regional blood flow by endothelium-derived nitric oxide. Hypertension 15:486–492
18. Gerkens JF, Gerber JC, Shand DG, Branch RA (1978) Effect of PGI_2, and PGE_2 and 6-keto-$PGF_{1\alpha}$ on canine gastric blood flow and acid secretion. Prostaglandins 16:815–823
19. Green T, Dockray GJ (1988) Characterisation of the peptidergic afferent innervation of the stomach in the rat, mouse and guinea-pig. Neuroscience 25:181–193
20. Gruetter CA, Barry BK, McNamara DB, Gruetter DY, Kadowitz PJ, Ignarro LJ (1979) Relaxation of bovine coronary artery and activation of coronary guanylate cyclase by nitric oxide, nitroprusside and a carcinogenic nitrosoamine. J Cyclic Nucl Res 5:211–224
21. Guth PH, Paulsen G, Nagata H (1984) Histologic and microcirculatory changes in alcohol-induced gastric lesions in the rat: effect of prostaglandin cytoprotection. Gastroenterology 87:1083–1090
22. Hibbs JB Jr, Vaurin Z, Taintor RR (1987) L-arginine is required for expression of the activated

macrophage effector mechanism causing selective metabolic inhibition in target cells. J Immunol 138: 550–565
23. Hibbs JB Jr, Taintor RR, Vavrin Z, Rachlin EM (1988) Nitric oxide: a cytotoxic activated macrophage effector molecule. Biochem Biophys Res Commun 157:87–94
24. Holzer P (1991) Capsaicin: Cellular targets, mechanism of action, and selectivity for thin sensory neurones. Pharmacol Rev 43:143–201
25. Holzer P, Sametz W (1986) Gastric mucosal protection against ulcerogenic factors in the rat mediated by capsaicin-sensitive afferent neurones. Gastroenterology 91:975–981
26. Holzer P, Lippe IT (1988) Stimulation of afferent nerve endings by intragastric capsaicin protects against ethanol-induced damage of gastric mucosa. Neuroscience 27:981–987
27. Holzer P, Pabst MA, Lippe ITh, Peskar BM, Peskar BA, Livingston EH, Guth PH (1990) Afferent nerve-mediated protection against deep mucosal damage in the rat stomach. Gastroenterology 98:838–848
28. Hutcheson IR, Whittle BJR, Boughton-Smith NK (1990) Role of nitric oxide in maintaining vascular integrity in endotoxin-induced acute intestinal damage in the rat. Br J Pharmacol 101:815–820
29. Ignarro LJ, Buga GM, Wood KS, Byrns RE, Chaudhuri G (1987) Endothelium-derived relaxing factor produced and released from artery and vein is nitric oxide. Proc Natl Acad Sci USA 84:9265–9269
30. Ignarro LJ, Lippton H, Edwards JC, Baricos WH, Hyman AL, Kadowitz PJ, Gruetter CA (1981) Mechanism of vascular smooth muscle relaxation by organic nitrates, nitrites, nitroprusside and nitric oxide: evidence for the involvement of S-nitrosothiols as active intermediates. J Pharmacol Exp Ther 218:739–749
31. Inoue A, Yanagisawa M, Kimura A, Kasuya Y, Miyauchi T, Goto K, Masaki T (1989) The human endothelium family: three structurally and pharmacologically distinct isopeptides predicted by three separate genes. Proc Natl Acad Sci USA 86:2863–2867
32. Kauffman GL, Whittle BJR (1982) Gastric vascular actions of prostanoids and the dual effect of arachidonic acid. Am J Physiol 242:G582–G587
33. Kauffman GL, Whittle BJR, Aures D, Grossman MI (1979) Effects of prostacyclin and a stable analogue 6β-PGI_1 on gastric acid secretion, mucosal blood flow and blood pressure in conscious dogs. Gastroenterology 77:1301–1306
34. Kelm M, Feelisch M, Spahr R, Piper H-M, Noack E, Schrader J (1988) Quantitative and kinetic characterization of nitric oxide and EDRF released from cultured endothelial cells. Biochem Biophys Res Commun 154:236–244
35. Khan MT, Furchgott RF (1987) Additional evidence that endothelium-derived relaxing factor is nitric oxide. In: Rand MJ, Raper C (eds) Pharmacology. Elsevier, New York, pp 341–344
36. Kitagawa H, Tokeda F, Kohei H (1990) Effect of endothelium-derived relaxing factor on the gastric lesion induced by HCI in rats. J Pharmacol Exp Ther 253:1133–1137
37. Knowles RG, Salter M, Brooks SL, Moncada S (1990) Anti-inflammatory glucocorticoids inhibit the induction by endotoxin of nitric oxide synthase in the lung, liver and aorta of the rat. Biochem Biophys Res Commun 172:1042–1048
38. Konturek SJ, Brzozowski T, Radecki T, Piastucki I (1984) Comparison of gastric and intestinal antisecretory and protective effects of prostacyclin and its stable thia-imino-analogue (HOE 892) in conscious rats. Prostaglandins 28:443–453
39. Konturek SJ, Brzozowski T, Majka J, Czarnobilski K (1992) Role of nitric oxide and prostaglandins in sucralfate-induced gastroprotection. Eur J Pharmacol 211:277–279
40. Konturek SJ, Robert A, Hancher AJ, Nezamis JE (1980). Comparison of prostacyclin and prostaglandin E_2 on gastric acid secretion, gastrin release and mucosal blood flow in dogs. Dig Dis Sci 25:673–679
41. Konturek SJ, Radecki T, Brzozowski T, Piastucki I, Dembinska-Kiec A, Zmuda A (1981) Aspirin-induced gastric ulcers in cats. Prevention by prostacyclin. Dig Dis Sci 26:1003–1012
42. Leone AM, Palmer RMJ, Knowles RG, Francis PL, Ashton DS, Moncada S (1991 Constitutive and inducible nitric oxide synthases are L-arginine N^G-C^G-dioxygenases. J Biol Chem 266:23790–23795
43. MacNaughton K, Cirino G, Wallace JL (1989) Endothelium-derived relaxing factor (nitric oxide) has protective actions in the stomach. Life Sci 45:1869–1876

44. Marletta MA, Yoon PS, Iyengar R, Leaf CD, Wishnok JS (1988) Macrophage oxidation of L-arginine to nitrite and nitrate: Nitric oxide is an intermediate. Biochemistry 27:8706–8711
45. Martinez-Cuesta MA, Barrachina D, Pique JM, Whittle BJR, Esplugues JV (1992) The role of nitric oxide and platelet-activating factor in the inhibition by endotoxin of pentagastrin-stimulated gastric acid secretion. Eur J Pharmacol 218:351–354
46. Matsumoto H, Suzuki N, Onda H, Fujino M (1989) Abundance of endothelin-3 in rat intestine, pituitary gland and brain. Biochem Biophys Res Comm 164:74–80
47. Moncada S, Palmer RMJ, Higgs EA (1991) Nitric Oxide: Physiology, pathophysiology and pharmacology. Pharmacol Rev 43:109–142
48. Moncada S, Vane JR (1979) Pharmacology and endogenous roles of prostaglandin endoperoxides, thromboxane A_2, and prostacyclin. Pharmacol Rev 30:293–331
49. Morales RW, Johnson BR, Szabo S (1992) Endothelin induces vascular and mucosal lesions, enhances the injury by HCl/ethanol, and the antibody exerts gastroprotection. FASEB J 6:235–2360
50. Nava E, Palmer RMJ, Moncada S (1991) Inhibition of nitric oxide synthesis in septic shock: how much is beneficial? Lancet 338:1555–15557
51. O'Connor KJ, Moncada S (1991) Glucocorticoids inhibit the induction of nitric oxide synthase and the related cell damage in adenocarcinoma cells. Biochim Biophys Acta 1097:227–231
52. Palmer RMJ, Moncada S (1989) A novel citrulline-forming enzyme implicated in the formation of nitric oxide by vascular endothelial cells. Biochem. Biophys Res Commun 158:348–352
53. Palmer RMJ, Ferrige AG, Moncada S (1987) Nitric oxide release accounts for the biological activity of endothelium-derived relaxing factor. Nature 327:524–526
54. Palmer RMJ, Ashton DS, Moncada S (1988a) Vascular endothelial cells synthesise nitric oxide from L-arginine. Nature 333:664–666
55. Palmer RMJ, Rees DD, Ashton DS, Moncada S (1988b) L-arginine is the physiological precursor for the formation of nitric oxide in endothelium-dependent relaxation. Biochem Biophys Res Commun 153:1251–1256
56. Palmer RMJ, Bridge L, Foxwell NA, Moncada S (1992) The role of nitric oxide in endothelial cell damage and its inhibition by glucorcorticoids Br J Pharmacol 105:11–12
57. Peskar BM, Respondek M, Muller KM, Peskar BA (1991) A role of nitric oxide in capsaicin-induced gastroprotection. Eur J Pharmacol 198:113–114
58. Petros A, Bennett D, Vallance P (1991) Effect of nitric oxide on hypotension in patients with septic shock. Lancet 338:15557–15558
59. Pique JM, Whittle BJR, Esplugues JV (1989) The vasodilator role of endogenous nitric oxide in the rat gastric microcirculation. Eur J Pharmacol 174:293–296
60. Pique JM, Esplugues JV, Whittle BJR (1990) Influence of morphine or capsaicin pretreatment on rat gastric microcirculatory response to PAF. Am J Physiol 258:G352–G357
61. Pique JM, Esplugues JV, Whittle BJR (1992) Endogenous nitric oxide as a mediator of gastric mucosal vasodilatation during acid secretion. Gastroenterology 102:168–174
62. Radomski MW, Palmer RMJ, Moncada S (1990) Glucocorticoids inhibit the expression of an inducible, but not the constitutive, nitric oxide synthase in vascular endothelial cells. Proc Natl Acad Sci USA 87:10043–10047
63. Rainsford KD (1983) Microvascular injury during gastric mucosal damage by anti-inflammatory drugs in pigs and rats. Agents and Actions 13:457–460
64. Rees DD, Palmer RMJ, Moncada S (1989a) Role of endothelium-derived nitric oxide in the regulation of blood pressure. Proc Natl Acad Sci USA 86:3375–3378
65. Rees DD, Palmer RMJ, Hodson HF, Moncada S (1989b). A specific inhibitor of nitric oxide formation from L-arginine attenuates endothelium-dependent relaxation. Br J Pharmacol 96:418–424
66. Rees DD, Palmer RMJ, Schulz R, Hodson HF, Moncada S (1990b) Characterisation of three inhibitors of endothelial nitric oxide synthases in vitro and in vivo. Br J Pharmacol 101:746–752
67. Robert A, Nezamis JE, Lancaster C, Hanchar AJ (1979) Cytoprotection by prostaglandins in rats - Prevention of gastric necrosis produced by alcohol, HCl, NaOH, hypertonic NaCl and thermal injury. Gastroenterology 77:433–443
68. Robins PG (1980) Ultra-structural observations on the pathogenesis of aspirin-induced gastric erosions. Br J Exp Pathol 61:497–504

69. Salter M, Knowles RG, Moncada S (1991) Widespread tissue distribution, species distribution and changes in activity of Ca^{2+}-dependent and Ca^{2+}-independent nitric oxide synthases. FEBS Lett 291:145–149
70. Shea-Donohue T, Nompleggi D, Myers L, Dubois A (1982) A comparison of the effects of prostacyclin and the 15(S) 15-methyl analogs of PGE_2 and $PGF_{2\alpha}$ on gastric parietal and non-parietal secretion. Dig Dis Sci 27:17–22
71. Stuehr D, Gross S, Sakuma I, Levi R, Nathan C (1989) Activated murine macrophages secrete a metabolite of arginine with the bioactivity of endothelium-derived relaxing factor and the chemical reactivity of nitric oxide. J Exp Med 169:1011–1020
72. Szabo S, Trier JS, Brown A, Scnoor J (1985) Early vascular injury and increased vascular permeability in gastric mucosal injury caused by ethanol in the rat. Gastroenterology 88:228–236
73. Szolcsanyi J, Bartho L (1981) Impaired defences mechanism to peptic ulcer in the capsaicin-densensitized rat. In: Mozsik G, Hannien O, Javor T. (eds) Gastrointestinal defence mechanisms. Adv Physiol Sci 29:39–51
74. Takahashi K, Jones PM, Kanse SM, Lam H-C, Spokes RA, Ghatei MA, Bloom SR (1990) Endothelin in the gastrointestinal tract: Presence of endothelin like immunoreactivity, endothelin-1 messenger RNA, endothelin receptors and pharmacological effect. Gastroenterology 99:1660–1667
75. Tepperman BL, Whittle BJR (1992) Endogenous nitric oxide and sensory neuropeptides interact in the modulation of the rat gastric microcirculation. Br J Pharmacol 105:171–175
76. Vallance P, Collier J, Moncada S (1989) Effects of endothelium-derived nitric oxide on peripheral arteriole tone in man. Lancet ii:997–1000
77. Walder CE, Thimermann C, Vane JR (1990) Endothelium-derived relaxing factor participates in the increased blood flow in the response to pentagastrin in the rat stomach mucosa. Proc R Soc Lond [B] 241:195–200
78. Wallace JL, Cirino G, De Nucci G, McKnight W, MacNaughton WK (1989a) Endothelin has potent ulcerogenic and vasoconstrictor actions in the stomach. Am J Physiol 256:G661–666
79. Wallace JL, Keenan CM, MacNaughton WK, McKnight GW (1989b) Comparison of the effects of endothelin-1 and endothelin-3 on the rat stomach. Eur J Pharmacol 167:41–47
80. Walus KM, Pawlik W, Konturek SJ (1980) Prostacyclin-induced gastric mucosal vasodilatation and inhibition of acid secretion in the dog. Proc Soc Exp Biol Med 163:228–232
81. Whittle BJR (1981) Antisecretory actions of prostacyclin and its analogues on the gastric mucosa. In: Lewis PJ, O'Grady J (eds) Clinical pharmacology of prostacyclin. Raven, New York, pp 219–232
82. Whittle BJR (1983) The potentiation of taurocholate-induced rat gastric erosions following parenteral administration of cyclo-oxygenase inhibitors. Br J Pharmacol 80:545–551
83. Whittle BJR, Boughton-Smith NK (1979) 16-Phenoxy prostacyclin analogues-potent, selective anti-ulcer compounds. In: Vane JR, Bergstrom S (eds) Prostacyclin. Raven, New York, pp 159–171
84. Whittle BJR, Lopez-Belmonte J (1991) Interactions between the vascular peptide endothelin-1 and sensory neuropeptides in gastric mucosal injury. Br J Pharmacol 102:950–954
85. Whittle BJR, Vane JR (1987) Prostanoids as regulators of gastrointestinal function. In: Johnston LR (eds) Physiology of the gastrointestinal tract, 2nd edn. Raven New York, vol 1, pp 143–180
86. Whittle BJR, Lopez-Belmonte J, Moncada S (1990) Regulation of gastric mucosal integrity by endogenous nitric oxide: interactions with prostanoids and sensory neuropeptides in the rat. Br J Pharmacol 99:607–611
87. Whittle BJR, Lopez-Belmonte J, Rees DD (1989) Modulation of the vasodepressor actions of acetylcholine, bradykinin, substance P and endothelin in the rat by a specific inhibitor of nitric oxide formation. Br J Pharmacol 98:646–652
88. Whittle BJR, Lopez-Belmonte J, Moncada S (1992) Nitric oxide mediates rat mucosal vasodilatation induced by intragastric capsaicin Eur J Pharmacol 218:339–341
89. Whittle BJR, Boughton-Smith NK, Moncada S, Vane JR (1978) Actions of prostacyclin (PGI_2) and its product 6-oxo-$PGF_{1\alpha}$ on the rat gastric mucosa in vivo and in vitro Prostaglandins 15:955–968
90. Whittle BJR, Higgs GA, Eakins KE, Moncada S, Vane JR (1980) Selective inhibition of prostaglandin production inflammatory exudates and gastric mucosa. Nature 284:271–273

91. Wood JG, Yan ZY, Cheung LY (1992) Relative potency of endothelin analogues on changes in gastric vascular resistance. Am J Physiol 262:G977–G982
92. Wright CE, Rees DD, Moncada S (1992) Protective and pathological roles of nitric oxide in endotoxin shock. Cardiovas Res 26:48–57
93. Yanagisawa M, Kurihara H, Kimura S, Tomobe Y, Kobayashi M, Yazaki Y, Goto K, Masaki T (1988). A novel potent vasoconstrictor peptide produced by vascular endothelial cells. Nature 323:411–415

Gastroduodenal Alkaline Secretion and Its Pathophysiological Significance

A. GARNER

Introduction and Background

Gastric juice is emptied into the duodenum, where neutrality is restored by secretion of alkali from the pancreas. In addition to bulk clearance and neutralisation of gastric acid, it seems likely that gastroduodenal mucosa possesses an intrinsic ability to resist autolytic digestion. The various mechanisms involved in protection and repair in the upper gastrointestinal tract have recently been reviewed in detail [1, 2]. Rapid restitution of the mucosal cell barrier following superficial injury appears to be a ubiquitous response amongst epithelia and is not confined to the stomach or even the gastrointestinal tract. Similarly, repair of deeper lesions such as peptic ulcers occurs by processes analagous to wound healing at other sites. The stomach and duodenum are, however, unique in being the only sites in the body exposed to such extremes of acidity; the parietal cell generates the highest ion gradient encountered in mammalian systems with $[H^+]$ in the lumen, exceeding that in the blood one million times. It is, therefore, not unexpected that gastroduodenal mucosa has well-developed mechanisms which enable it to resist low luminal pH.

Mechanisms responsible for pre-epithelial acid disposal in the surface mucus layer and for maintenance of acid-base balance within the interstitial and intracellular compartments of gastric and duodenal mucosa have all been described. This chapter focuses on the role of mucosal alkaline secretion; the processes of cytoplasmic and interstitial pH regulation have been reviewed elsewhere [3–6]. As a result of the alkaline tide originating from actively secreting parietal cells, the surface cells receive a HCO_3 - enriched blood supply. Secretion of HCO_3 by these cells leads to alkalinisation of the adherent mucus gel layer, which in turn can reduce $[H^+]$ at the mucosal surface. Indeed, at luminal pH 2 and above (10 m*M* HCl and less), a microenvironment near to neutral pH can be maintained adjacent to the apical plasma membrane [7, 8]. Cellular transport of HCO_3 is augmented by passive diffusion of HCO_3 from the interstitium into the lumen via the paracellular route. In fact, free diffusion becomes the predominant mechanism of alkaline "secretion" when there is an increase in mucosal permeability such as that accompanying superficial damage [9, 10].

Basal Rates of Alkaline Secretion

Secretion of alkali can be detected throughout the gastrointestinal tract, as evidenced by titration of unbuffered solutions bathing segments of gut mounted in Ussing-type chambers or perfused in situ (Table 1). The rates of basal alkalinisation tend to reflect passive permeability in any particular region, being highest in "leaky" epithelia such as the ileum and lowest in gastric mucosa, which is considered as a "tight" epithelium characterised by a low passive conductance for ions and a high spontaneous potential difference (PD). Secretory rates seem unrelated to inherent acid resistance in as much as the small intestine, which displays the highest rates of alkalinisation both in vitro and in vivo, is regarded as the least able to withstand detrimental effects of gastric juice. Mucosal protection of the upper gastrointestinal tract against luminal acid is therefore likely to involve factors in addition to an ability to transport HCO_3 into the lumen.

The low rate of HCO_3 transport in the stomach is generally masked by an excess of acid secreted from parietal cells. Specific inhibition of HCl production with H_2 antagonists or H/K-ATPase inhibitors allows detection of a titratable alkalinisation [11]. Gastric alkaline secretion amounts to 5–10% of basal acid output and hence it represents only a minute fraction of the maximal acid output. Rates of alkaline secretion in the antral and fundic regions of the stomach are similar and equate to about 20–30% of output measured from the proximal portion of the duodenum. There is good evidence that secretion of HCO_3 by the stomach is a property of the surface epithelial cells. Whether the secretion of alkali originates from crypt or villus cells in the duodenum has not been finally resolved; while it is generally accepted that intestinal secretion occurs from the crypts, arguments have been presented which suggest that villus cells may be involved in HCO_3 secretion in the duodenum [12].

Mechanisms of Bicarbonate Transport

Uncoupling oxidative phosphorylation or depriving tissues of oxygen inhibits gastroduodenal alkali secretion, indicating its dependence on active cellular metabolism [13, 14]. In contrast to the stomach, where anti-metabolites abolish both secretion and transmucosal PD, agents such as 2,4-dinitrophenol only reduce alkalinisation in the duodenum by 60–70%, implying that the remaining one-third of basal secretion originates from simple diffusion of HCO_3 across the mucosa (Fig.1). Complete removal of HCO_3 from the serosal (blood) side after bathing tissues with a HEPES-containing buffer generally leads to cessation of alkali secretion, suggesting that HCO_3 appearing in the lumen originates in the interstitium [14, 15]. Hence,transport systems must exist to allow HCO_3 to move across both basolateral and apical cell membranes.

The most complete picture of cellular transport has emerged from studies of amphibian proximal duodenum, devoid of Brunner's glands and stripped of

Table 1. Rates of Gastrointestinal luminal alkalinization

Anatomical region	Frog in vitro[a]	Rat in vivo
Stomach (μmol/cm^2 h)	0.23 ± 0.03 (221)	1.2 ± 0.2 (6)
Duodenum (μmol/cm h)	0.67 ± 0.24 (5)	4.7 ± 0.67 (24)
Ileum (μmol/cm h)	2.51 ± 0.37 (5)	10.4 ± 1.71 (12)
Colon (μmol/cm h)	1.13 ± 0.16 (5)	3.8 ± 1.12 (12)

Values are mean ± SEM, with the number of observations in parentheses
[a] Frog data are for *Rana catesbeiana* with the exception of stomach data, which are for *Rana temporaria*

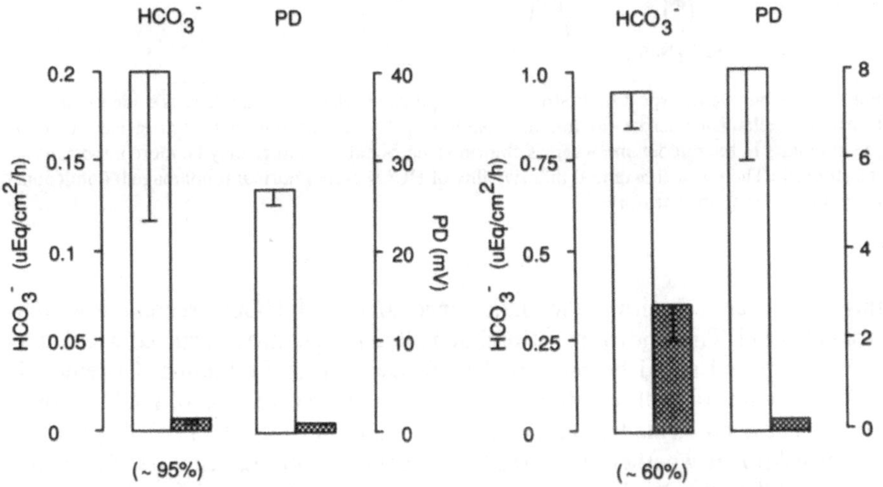

Fig. 1. Inhibition of luminal alkalinisation in the amphibian stomach and duodenum by 2,4-dinitrophenol (2,4 DNP). Addition of 100 μM 2,4-DNP to the serosal bathing solution abolishes gastric alkalinisation and transmucosal potential difference falls to zero. In the proximal duodenum (*righthand panel*) there is a residual alkalinisation equivalent to about 30% of basal rate after treatment with 2,4-DNP reflecting diffusion of HCO_3 from serosal to luminal bathing solutions

external muscle and then mounted in a flux chamber. These studies have led to the model depicted in Fig. 2. Duodenal alkaline secretion is inhibited by ouabain or by removal of either Na or HCO_3 from the serosal bathing solution, suggesting Na-coupled HCO_3 uptake across the basolateral membrane linked to recycling of Na via the Na/K-ATPase [16]. By analogy with electrogenic Cl secretion in the ileum, it was further suggested that accumulated HCO_3 left the cell via conductive channels in the apical membrane. A direct relation between rates of alkaline secretion and the short-circuit current or (lumen-negative) PD is consistent with the presence of an anion conductance.

Whilst electrogenic HCO_3 secretion predominates, Cl/HCO_3 exchange across the apical membrane has also been demonstrated in the duodenum, and

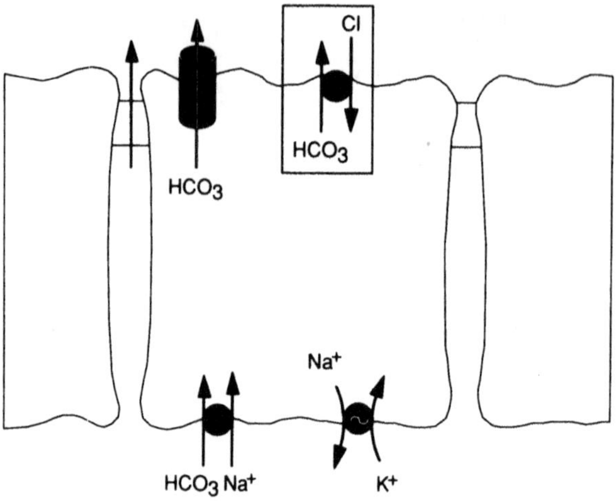

Fig. 2. Bicarbonate transport by gastroduodenal epithelial cells. Although there is evidence for two transport mechanisms across the luminal membrane, it would appear that electrogenic secretion predominates in the duodenum, whereas chloride-bicarbonate exchange may be more important in the stomach. There is a substantial diffusive flux of HCO_3 across normal (undamaged) duodenum via paracellular shunt pathways

this may even constitute the major mechanism of HCO_3 secretion in the stomach [17]. Thus, hormone-stimulated alkaline secretion occurred without a PD change and could be prevented by furosemide or by luminal Cl removal [18]. Existence of both conductive and exchange mechanisms of HCO_3 transport has been confirmed in duodenal apical membrane vesicles [19]. At present, it is not known whether these HCO_3 transporting mechanisms reside in the same or different cells. The precise mechanism or mechanisms of gastric HCO_3 transport remain controversial. Indeed, the two proposed models of a Na-dependent transcellular transport and a Cl-dependent secretion of HCO_3 produced within surface cells may not be mutually exclusive if they reflect subtle species/methodological differences. Finally it is important to realise that Cl remains the predominant anion in gastrointestinal secretions, as would be anticipated solely on the basis of its size; Cl occupies a Van der Vaals volume of 23 A^3 compared with 37 A^3 for HCO_3.

Stimulants and Inhibitors of Alkaline Secretion

There is a large body of experimental evidence which demonstrates that the adenylate cyclase-cAMP pathway is a major intracellular signalling pathway for HCO_3 secretion, at least in the duodenum. Thus,lipophilic analogues of cAMP itself, inhibitors of phosphodiesterase, and agents such as forskolin which activate the cyclase directly have all been reported to stimulate alkaline secretion in the duodenum [18, 20, 21]. Furthermore, a wide variety of different pharmacophores known to elevate intracellular cAMP concentrations, including prostaglandins and β-adrenoceptor agonists, have been found to stimulate duodenal alkalinisation (Table 2). All the above agonists increase transmucosal PD as well as HCO_3 transport, presumably reflecting regulation of apical anion channels by a cAMP-dependent protein kinase. Endogenous prostaglandins appear to regulate basal secretory tone in the duodenum and to mediate the action of many agonists, as evidenced by the inhibitory effect of indomethacin and other cyclo-oxygenase inhibitors. In addition to activation of electrogenic HCO_3 (and presumably Cl) transport, certain hormones such as gastric inhibitory peptide (GIP) and glucagon have been reported to stimulate alkalinisation by an action on electroneutral Cl/HCO_3 exchange [18]. This response is comparable to the effect of carbachol and 16,16-dmPGE2 in gastric fundus.

Experiments in both the stomach and duodenum demonstrate that secretion of alkali is under neural control. Vagal stimulation or sham feeding increases gastroduodenal alkalinisation in laboratory animals and in humans [22, 23]. The rise in gastric alkaline secretion is mediated via a muscarinic action, whereas the duodenal response shows minimal sensitivity to muscarinic agonists and antagonists. However, the peptidergic transmitter vasoactive intestinal polypeptide, which is a potent stimulant of intestinal electrolyte secretion including duodenal luminal alkalinization, may act as a vagal neurotransmitter in the duodenum [12]. Activation of the sympathetic system seems to lead to opposite effects in vitro and in vivo, which probably reflects the predominant influence of blood flow and thus nutrient supply of HCO_3 in the whole animal. Thus, adrenergic agonists stimulate duodenal alkalinisation in vitro by activating β-2 receptors and hence raising cAMP whereas anaesthetised animals there is inhibition of alkaline secretion which appears to be mediated via an α-2 action [24, 25].

The potential protective role of mucosal alkaline secretion is supported by the fact that a range of ulcerogenic agents are capable of inhibiting HCO_3

Table 2. Stimulants of duodenal alkalinization in vitro

Agent	Classification	$IC_{50}(\mu g/ml)$	Efficacy (%)
Prostaglandin E_2	Eicosanoid	0.3	100
Theophylline	PDE inhibitor	50	76
ICI 63197	PDE inhibitor	5	60
Forskolin	Cyclase activator	4	72
Adrenaline	Adrenergic agonist	5	75
Isoprenaline	β-Agonist	5	68
6-Hydroxydopamine	Adrenegic neurotoxin	50	87
2-Chloroadenosine	Purinergic agonist	50	135
Chlordiazepoxide	Anxiolytic	50	86
Dihydropyridazinone	Positive ionotrope	50	41
Dipyridamole	Coronary vasodilator	50	65

Agents were added to the serosal side solution. Efficacy is expressed as the maximum response to a particular agonist as a percentage of the PGE_2-induced maximum in the same tissue. PDE, phosphodiesterase

transport. For example, non-steroidal anti-inflammatory agents, acetazolamide and ethanol have all been reported to inhibit alkalinisation in vitro [17]. In vivo, oral administration of such compounds often leads to a massive rise in luminal alkalinisation due to the increase in mucosal permeability which accompanies damage [9, 26]. A number of drugs with protective or anti-ulcer activity have the ability to enhance rates of luminal alkalinisation without increasing mucosal permeability. The most potent stimulants are E-type prostaglandins such as 15-OH PGEl and 16,16-dmPGE_2,which have been reported to increase alkaline secretion in the stomach and duodenum of a variety of species both in vitro and in vivo [11, 12].

Physiological Significance

There is an enormous imbalance in the comparative rates of acid and alkaline secretions by gastric mucosa. Thus, under conditions of maximum acid output (e.g. preceding a meal), basal alkaline secretion amounts to only about 1% of acid secretion. This imbalance remains very evident in the duodenal bulb even though $[H^+]$ is lower than in the gastric lumen and mucosal alkaline secretion is higher. In order to provide any form of protection aginst luminal acid it is essential that secreted HCO_3 is retained at the mucosal surface. This is achieved by imposition of a mixing barrier, in the form of the thin (ca. 100 μm) layer of mucus glycoprotein gel, between the surface cells and the lumen. Studies using pH-sensitive microelectrodes have demonstrated the effectiveness of this unstirred layer. Hence when luminal $[H^+]$ is of the order of 10 m*M* (i.e. pH 2), the pH at the actual mucosal surface is maintained close to neutrality [7, 8].

Alkaline secretion itself is stimulated by sham feeding as well as by luminal HCl per se [12, 17]. Even allowing for these influences, however, the surface pH gradient collapses when luminal pH falls much below pH 1.8–2.0. In view of the fact that intragastric pH can achieve values below pH1, it is difficult to conceive that the "mucus-bicarbonate barrier" provides anything more than a first line of defence against luminal acid. Indeed, given the inherent impermeability of cell membranes to H^+ ions combined with the existence of effective mechanisms for disposing of any H^+ ions which actually enter the mucosal cells or interstitium, the entire functional significance of this proposed form of defence against luminal acid becomes questionable. It is probably more realistic therefore to consider secretion of HCO_3 as a mechanism of reducing acid concentration locally rather than a system aimed at achieving outright neutrality at the mucosal surface.

Pathological Role in Protection and Repair

The increase in permeability which accompanies mucosal damage is one of the enduring principles in gastric pathophysiology and is central to the concept of a gastric mucosal barrier as proposed by Davenport [27]. Extensive studies have revealed that a wide range of ulcerogens, including aspirin and bile salts, increase gastric mucosal permeability and allow an ultrafiltrate of alkaline-rich interstitial fluid to enter the lumen of the stomach. In the duodenum, even quite modest concentrations of HCl are able to increase the passive permeability of the epithelial cell barrier leading to efflux of interstitial HCO_3 [10, 28]. The much larger secretory efflux accompanying superficial damage provides an extremely efficient means of disposing of quite substantial amounts of acid at the mucosal surface.

Under conditions of mucosal damage, thickness of the unstirred zone at the mucosal surface is also increased considerably by virtue of the shedding of plasma proteins and cellular debris into the adherent mucus layer. This layer (the so-called "mucoid cap") provides a protective shield under which repair of the mucosa can proceed [1, 29]. Repair may be nothing more than the restitution of tight junctional integrity. However, even more severe damage leading to substantial loss of superficial epithelial cells, is also very rapidly repaired by migration of viable cells from within the gastric pits and glands or duodenal crypts [30, 31]. The increase in mucosal permeability which enables flow of plasma HCO_3 into the gastroduodenal lumen also provides a potential pathway for the entry of luminal factors such as EGF into the systemic circulation (Fig. 3). Such a mechanism could underlie the massive increase in

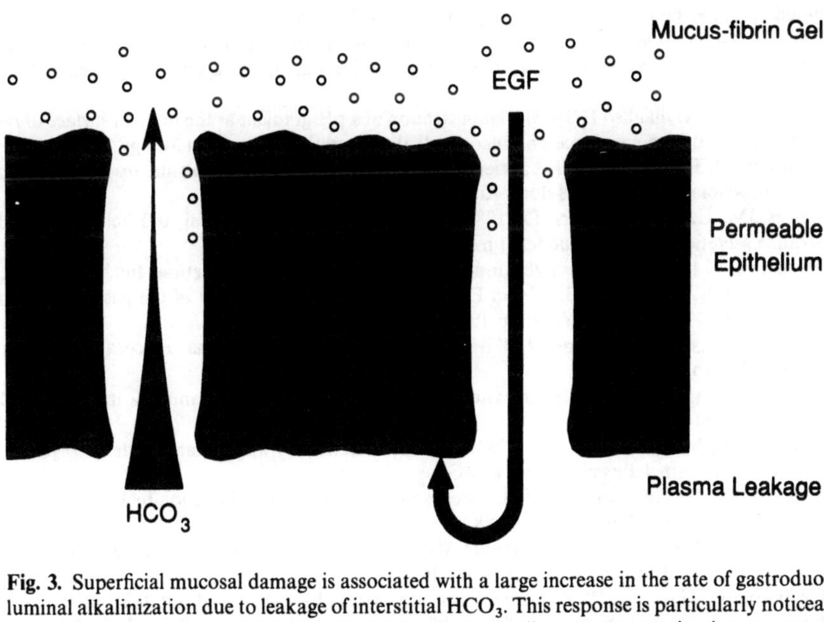

Fig. 3. Superficial mucosal damage is associated with a large increase in the rate of gastroduodenal luminal alkalinization due to leakage of interstitial HCO_3. This response is particularly noticeable in the stomach, because the "tight" epithelial barrier normally prevents passive ion movement. In addition to allowing HCO_3 diffusion into the gastrointestinal lumen, increased mucosal permeability results in bioavailability of luminal EGF,which can gain access to its basolateral receptors and thereby inhibit acid secretion and promote cellular proliferation and differentiation

bioavaliability of EGF which occurs during superficial damage of the gastrointestinal tract [32]. Under these circumstances EGF would gain access to the basolateral-located membrane receptors with which the peptide must interact in order to inhibit acid secretion and stimulate epithelial proliferation and differentiation. Indeed, such a process could explain the conundrum of why EGF is secreted into the lumen of the gut yet is inactive orally. In this regard EGF could be viewed as the "housekeeper" of mucosal protection and repair.

References

1. Garner A, Allen A, Gutknecht J, Yanaka A, Goddard PJ, Silen W, Lacy ER, Bauerfeind P, Starlinger M, Wallace JL (1990) Mechanisms of gastric mucosal defence. Eur J Gastroenterol Hepatol 2:165–188
2. Garner A, O'Brien PE (eds) (1991) Mechanisms of injury, protection and repair of the upper gastrointestinal tract. Wiley, Chichester
3. Machen TE, Paradiso AM (1987) Regulation of intracellular pH in the stomach. Annu Rev Physiol 49:19–33
4. Carter KJ, Saario I, Seidler U, Silen W (1989) Effect of pCO_2 on intracellular pH in in vitro frog gastric mucosa. Am J Physiol 256:G206–G213
5. L Kivilaakso E, FromM D, Silen W (1978) Effect of the acid secretory state on intramural pH of rabbit gastric mucosa. Gastroenterology 75:641–648
6. Starlinger M, Schiessel R (1988) Bicarbonate delivery to the gastro-duodenal mucosa by the blood: its importance for mucosal integrity. Gut 29:647–654
7. Ross IN, Bahari HMM, Turnberg LA (1981) The pH gradient across mucus adherent to rat fundic mucosa in vitro and the effect of potential damaging agents. Gastroenterology 81:713–718
8. Flemstrom G, Kivilaakso E (1983) Demonstration of a pH gradient at the luminal surface of rat duodenum and its dependence on mucosal alkaline secretion. Gastroenterology 84:787–794
9. Konturek SJ, Bilski J, Tasler J, Laskiewicz J (1984) Gastroduodenal alkaline response to acid and taurocholate in conscious dogs. Am J Physiol 247:G149–G154
10. Wilkes JM, Garner A, Peters TJ (1988) Mechanisms of acid disposal and acid-stimulated alkaline secretion by gastroduodenal mucosa. Dig Dis Sci 33:361–367
11. Flemstrom G (1987) Gastric and duodenal mucosal bicarbonate secretion. In: Johnson LR, Christensen J, Jackson MJ, Jacobson ED, Walsh JH (eds) Physiology of the gastrointestinal tract, 2nd edn. Raven, New York, pp 1011–1029
12. Allen A, Flemstrom G, Garner A, Kivilaakso E (1993) Gastroduodenal mucosal protection. Physiol Rev, in press
13. Flemstrom G (1977) Active alkalinization by amphibian gastric fundic mucosa in vitro. Am J Physiol 233:El–E12
14. Simson JNL, Merhav A, Silen W (1981) Alkaline secretion by amphibian duodenum: general characteristics. Am J Physiol 240:G401–G408
15. Takeuchi K, Merhav A, Silen W (1982) Mechanism of luminal alkalinization by bullfrog fundic mucosa. Am J Physiol 243:G377–G388
16. Simson JNL, Merhav A, Silen W (1981) Alkaline secretion by amphibian duodenum: short-circuit current and Na and Cl fluxes. Am J Physiol 240:G472–G479
17. Flemstrom G, Garner A (1989) Secretion of bicarbonate by gastric and duodenal mucosa. In: Forte JG (ed) Salivary gastric and hepatobiliary secretions. American Physiological Society, Bethesda, pp 309–326 (Handbook of physiology, sect 6, vol III)
18. Flemstrom G, Heylings JR, Garner A (1982) Gastric and duodenal HCO_3 transport in vitro: effects of hormones and local transmitters. Am J Physiol 242:G100–G110

19. Brown CDA, Dunk CR, Turnberg LA (1989) Cl-HCO_3 exchange and anion conductance in rat duodenal apical membrane vesicles. Am J Physiol 257:G661–G667
20. Simson JNL, Merhav A, Silen W (1981) Alkaline secretion by amphibian duodenum: effects of DBcAMP, theophylline and prostaglandins. Am J Physiol 241: G528–G536
21. Garner A, Heylings JR, Hampson SE, Stanier AM (1990) Pharmacological profile of duodenal alkaline secretion. Aliment Pharmacol Therap 4:465–476
22. Fandriks L (1986) Vagal and splanchnic neural influences on gastric and duodenal bicabonate secretions. Acta Physiol Scand 128 (suppl 555):1–39
23. Konturek SJ, Kwiecien N, Obtulowicz W, Thor P, Konturek JW, Popiela T, Olesky J (1987) Vagal cholinergic control of gastric alkaline secretion in normal subjects and duodenal ulcer patients. Gut 28:739–744
24. Garner A, Heylings JR, Peters TJ, Wilkes JM (1984) Adrenergic agonists stimulate HCO_3 secretion by amphibian duodenum in vitro via an action on beta-2 receptors. J Physiol 354:34P
25. Nylander O, Flemstrom G (1987) Effect of alpha-adrenoceptor agonists and antagonists on duodenal surface epithelial HCO_3 secretion in the rat in vivo. Acta Physiol Scand 126:433–441
26. Garner A (1978) Mechanisms of action of aspirin on the gastric mucosa of the guinea pig. Acta Physiol Scand 102 (suppl Gastic ion transport):101–110
27. Davenport HW (1972) The gastric mucosal barrier. Digestion 5: 162–165
28. Vattay P, Feil W, Klimesch S, Wenzl E, Starlinger M, Schiessel R (1988) Acid-stimulated alkaline secretion in the rabbit duodenum is passive and correlates with mucosal damage. Gut 29:284–290
29. Wallace JL, Whittle BJR (1986) Role of mucus in the repair of gastric epithelial damage in the rat: inhibition of epithelial recovery by mucolytic agents. Gastroenterology 91:603–611
30. Lacy ER, Ito S (1984) Rapid epithelial restitution of the surface epithelium of in vitro frog gastric mucosa after ethanol injury. Lab Invest 51:573–585
31. Feil W, Wenzl E, Vattay P, Starlinger M, Sogukoglu T, Schiessel R (1987) Repair of rabbit duodenal mucosa after acid injury in vivo and in vitro. Gastroenterology 97:1973–1986
32. Garner A (1993) Therapeutic potential of growth factors and their antagonists. Yale J Biol Med, in press

Role of Lipids and Membrane Biogenesis in the Process of Mucus Secretion*

A. Slomiany and B.L. Slomiany

Introduction

The movement of proteins destined for the cell surface or the organelles distal to endoplasmic reticulum (ER) is carried out by a vesicular transport [1–3]. The biosynthetic, secretory, and endocytic pathways involve the packaging of proteins into transport vesicles that bud off from one membrane and fuse with another. The molecular mechanisms engaged in these complex processes in the formation of intracellular transporters have been studied in many systems, such as semi-intact cells, cell-free systems, and yeast mutants, but only limited progress has been achieved in understanding vesicle biogenesis and vesicle-mediated transport.

In the biosynthetic pathway [3–9], secretory proteins are cotranslationally inserted into the ER. Within the lumen of the ER, proteins are proteolytically processed, glycosylated [10–14], packaged into vesicles and then transported to the Golgi apparatus. A number of cell-free assays, reconstituting steps of intracellular vesicular transport, have been used to determine the requirements for transport, and to purify the proteins that function in vesicle formation, targeting, and fusion. The analyses revealed an immensely complex process that proceeds in number of steps requiring many still unknown factors residing in cytosol or undergoing transient association with intracellular membranes. The first, highly multifactorial step in the intracellular transport from ER is followed by equally complex, or perhaps even more intricate, maturation of the proteins and vesicular membranes in Golgi [15–17]. The structural complexity of the Golgi apparatus, and the specific orientation of the factors and the enzymes involved in Golgi performance, reflect on the multiple functions in the transiting proteins and acquired membrane maturation, recognition, and sorting which must occur in this organelle.

In this review, we discuss recent advances that have been made in understanding the mechanism of protein transport to the lumen of ER, formation of ER-transport vesicles, fusion of the vesicles with Golgi membrane, and transport through the Golgi apparatus. Special emphasis is given to the role of the processes associated with the modification of the protein core of mucus glycoprotein (apomucin) requiring lipid involvement, the function of lipid synthesizing enzymes in the assembly of the apomucin intracellular carriers (vesicles),

* This work was supported by USPHS grant #AA05858-10 from the National Institute on Alcohol Abuse and Alocholism, National Institutes of Health.

and the control of their subsequent fusion with organelles of the secretory pathway by intracellular phospholipases.

Transport of Apomucin to the Lumen of Endoplasmic Reticulum: Cotranslational Translocation

Transport of proteins across the ER membrane is a decisive step in the secretion of gastric mucus glycoprotein (mucin) and of many classes of proteins. The process is initiated by a signal sequence of the apoprotein and mediated by the signal recognition particle (SRP), the SRP receptor, and the signal sequence receptor (SSR) [18–25], but the mechanism by which the peptides subsequently cross the membrane is unknown. One of the hypotheses on the translocation of secretory proteins across ER membrane is that more of ER proteins are involved in the translocation complex [25]. Also, our studies on the transport of apomucin and its cotranslational modifications have led to the identification of an ER integral protein, namely protein fatty acyltransferase (PFAT), responsible for addition of palmitate residue onto, the N-terminal end of apomucin [26–33]. If the enzyme activity of this protein is specifically blocked with monoclonal antibody, the translocation of apomucin across ER membrane is also arrested (Fig. 1). Based on this and previously gathered information, we speculate that

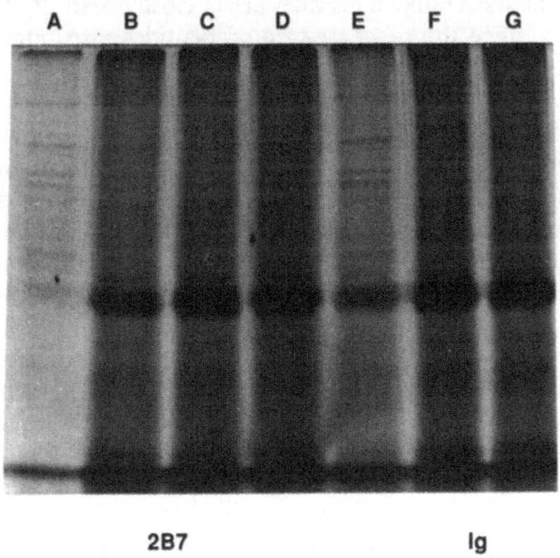

Fig. 1. Effect of anti-PFAT (protein fatty acyltransferase) monoclonal antibody (2B7 MAb) on in vitro translation-translocation of mucus glycoprotein apopeptide. The in vitro translation as described in [21] was performed in the presence of endoplasmic reticular (ER) microsomes (2 A_{280} units per translation mixture) and the translocated apomucin peptides recovered as in [55]. *A*, Translation-translocation mixture without mucin mRNA; *B*, complete translocation mixture; *C–E* complete mixture containing 0.01, 0.1, and 1 μg 2B7 MAb, respectively; *F*, *G*, complete mixture with 0.1 and 1 μg preimmune immunoglobulins (*Ig*). Autoradiography of the translated-translocated apomucin products was performed for 18 h

the protein fatty acyltransferase of ER is directly responsible for the transfer of growing peptide across the membrane.

Palmitoylation before translocation may also be associated with the recognition of apomucin in ER as a candidate for O-glycosylation. Our data indicate that apomucin precursor, after initial N-terminal palmitoylation and transfer to the luminal site of ER, is subjected to systematic O-glycosylation with N-acetylgalactosamine (GalNAc) [27, 30, 32, 34, 35]. Considering the events of the immediate peptide folding, which closely follow the nascent peptide translocation to the lumen of ER [12], this stage appears to be the only feasible moment for complete glycosylation of the peptide chain. The results of the experiments with glycoprotein synthesizing polysomes, immunoprecipitated with monoclonal antibodies recognizing GalNAc, revealed the presence of O-GalNAc containing peptides ranging in size from 6 to 60 kDa [34, 35]. The evidence obtained suggests that the initiated mucin peptides, upon reaching the luminal surface undergo immediate glycosylation. Whether the sequence of these events and secretion of the ER modified apomucin are orchestrated by the initial palmitoylation is still not proven, although a close connection between the rate of palmitoylation and apomucin transport and secretion is apparent.

By examining the protease sensitivity of the luminal peptides and monitoring for palmitate label, it was demonstrated that the protease cannot digest the N-terminal amino acid sequences beyond the fatty acyl residues of the peptides [27, 32]. This resistance to proteolytic degradation could be interpreted as an indication of an immediate and complete systematic O-glycosylation of the nascent peptide, and that the first GalNAc residues are in close proximity to the palmitoylated amino acids, since the protease-treated peptides also retain the fatty acyl substituent [27, 31, 32].

Additional information on the processing of apomucin peptides in ER was obtained from the study with isolated precursors of mucus glycoprotein. Treatment of the completed mucin precursors with trypsin released 8- to 12-kDa peptide which was acylated but devoid of GalNAc residues [28, 32]. This result is consistent with the cytoplasmic orientation of the fatty acyltransferase enzyme [33] which first acylates the N-terminal end of the peptide, and once the translation is completed and the ribosomal subunit dissociated, the C-terminal unprotected segment may be acylated again [35]. The susceptibility of the C-terminal end of the peptide to proteases suggest that the O-glycosylation is terminated as soon as translation is completed, since the 8- to 12-kDa fragment corresponding to the peptide span across the membrane and ribosomal subunit is not substituted with GalNAc [34, 35]. Taken together, these results suggest that O-glycosidic glycosylation is initiated in the rough endoplasmic reticulum [27, 29–32, 34, 35, 37, 38].

At this time, however, although the evidence on the role of N-terminal and C-terminal acylation is not sufficient, it is tempting to speculate that acyl residue directs the peptide to the lumen of ER and serves as the recognition signal for the initiation of the peptide O-glycosylation, whereas the other palmitoyl residues may help localize the apomucin to the plasma membrane or to conceal protein sites which may alter other protein activity [36]. The hypothesis on the role of fatty acylation of proteins and the control of signalling processes was defended in the study of GAP-43 protein that increases guanine nucleotide exchange by heterotrimeric G protein and the activity of which was found to be reversibly blocked by palmitoylation. The results of the studies suggest that palmitoylation controls a cycle of GAP-43 between membrane-bound and -free and conceal sulfhydryl groups, which are required to interact with the α_o subunit of the G protein and activate the second messenger systems.

It has been suggested that protein acylation in ER would not be appropriate for the secretory components, since this modification would lead to the retention of the peptide in the endoplasmic membrane rather than help in its translocation [39]. If, indeed, this was the event, then one should expect the growing peptide

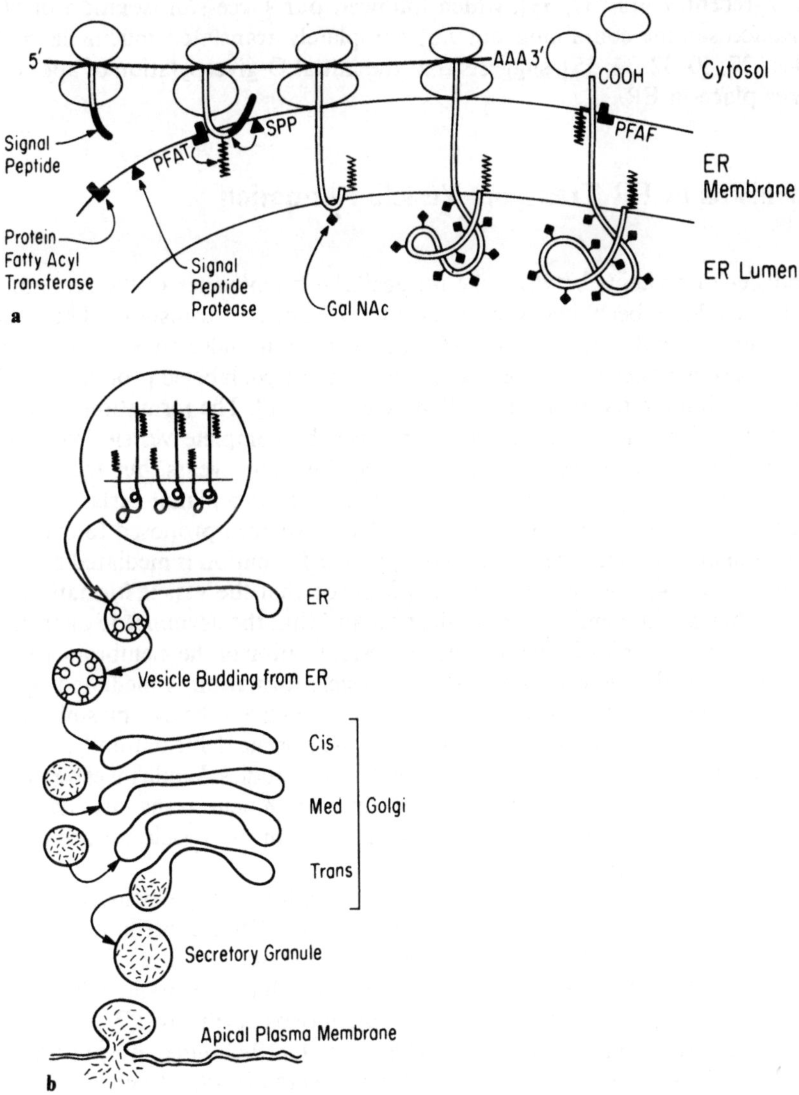

Fig. 2a,b. Proposed pathway of apomucin translation, translocation, and cotranslational modification on the cytoplasmic and luminal site of ER (**a**) and its intracellular vesicular transport (**b**)

by sheer force of the enlargement finding its way to the ER lumen and to appear there in the form of a growing loop until translation is completed (Fig. 2). The model shown in Fig. 2 summarizes the events of the cotranslational translocation and shows several interesting and possibly significant steps in the biosynthetic pathway. It suggests that the peptides entering ER-Golgi secretory pathway are first lipid-linked, a modification occurring on the cytosolic face of the ER membrane. The demonstration that the protein fatty acyltransferase which attaches the fatty acyl has a cytosolic protease sensitive site, tends to support this view [33]. Furthermore, although the site of the initial O-glycosylation is still referred to as Golgi-specific modification, the evidence obtained in recent years [37, 38], which followed our successful isolation of N-acetylgalactosamine-containing but not completely translated mucin nascent peptides [27, 30–32, 34, 35], suggests that the initial O-glycosylation of apomucin takes place in ER.

Mechanisms of ER Transport Vesicle Formation

The transfer of proteins between the intracellular membranes in the secretory pathway has long been believed to occur by vesicular transport. The first evidence for vesicular transport was obtained from pulse-chase studies of pancreatic exocrine cells showing that newly synthesized, labeled protein moved from ER to Golgi apparatus via small vesicles [40, 41]. The formation of such transport vesicles, and a mechanism to release the complete vesicle from the donor membrane, have been studied intensely for many years, but the initial event reflected in the deformation of ER membrane from a planar surface into a curved vesicle remains unknown. Three models have been proposed to explain the mechanism of vesicle formation. In one, vesicle formation is mediated by the cargo molecules [42], in the second it is proposed that the vesicle formation is forced by changes in membrane organization and that the asymmetric distribution of proteins and lipids is responsible for vesiculization of the membrane [43]. In the third model, it is proposed that the vesicle formation is mediated by a protein coat [43] and that the coat proteins recruited from the cytoplasmic face of the membrane provide the driving force for membrane deformation [1–3]. A support for this model has been also obtained in our studies. While investigating the involvement of lipid synthesizing enzymes in mucin transport vesicles biogenesis [44], we observed that they dissociate from the vesicle surface once the membrane is completed.

The enzymes involved in the synthesis of phospholipids, particularly phosphatidylcholine (PC) and phosphatidylethanolamine (PE), contribute a large portion of the proteins that cover the cytoplasmic surface of ER transport vesicles (Fig. 3). Our results with [^{14}C]phosphocholine precursor, which for incorporation into PC requires the intervention of two enzymes (CTP: phosphocholine cytidylyltransferase and 1,2-diacylglycerol: CDP-choline phosphotransferase) showed that over 80% of the label is recovered in PC of newly formed transport vesicles, and 15%–20% remains in the ER membranes which were

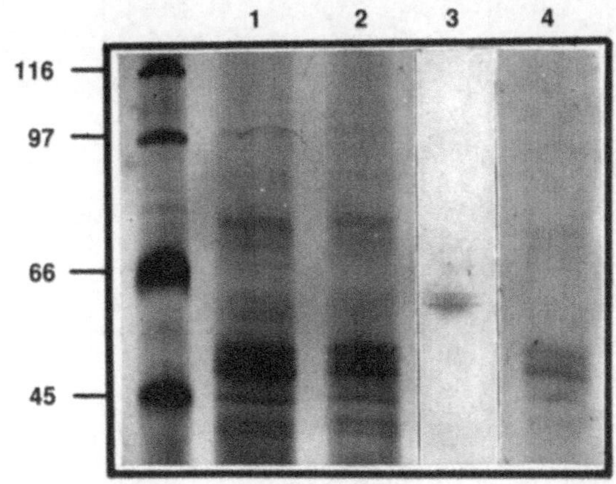

Fig. 3. 7.5% SDS-PAGE and silver staining of the protein components of ER-apomucin transport vesicles. *1, 2* ER transport vesicles before release of lipid synthesizing enzymes: *3* apomucin immunoprecipitated from the vesicles depicted in lane 1; 4 the proteins dissociating from the surface of the vesicle

suggests that the lipid synthesis and vesicle formation are localized to ER areas free of ER integral proteins and which have potential to incorporate the lipid-synthesizing enzyme from the cytosol.

While the completed vesicles are capable of separating from ER, the partially developed transport vesicles remain with maternal membranes, and additional incubation with unlabeled precursors chases about 50% of this label to subsequent batches of vesicles. The partially attached or incomplete vesicles are also observed in electron microscopic studies (Fig. 4). The EM image reveals

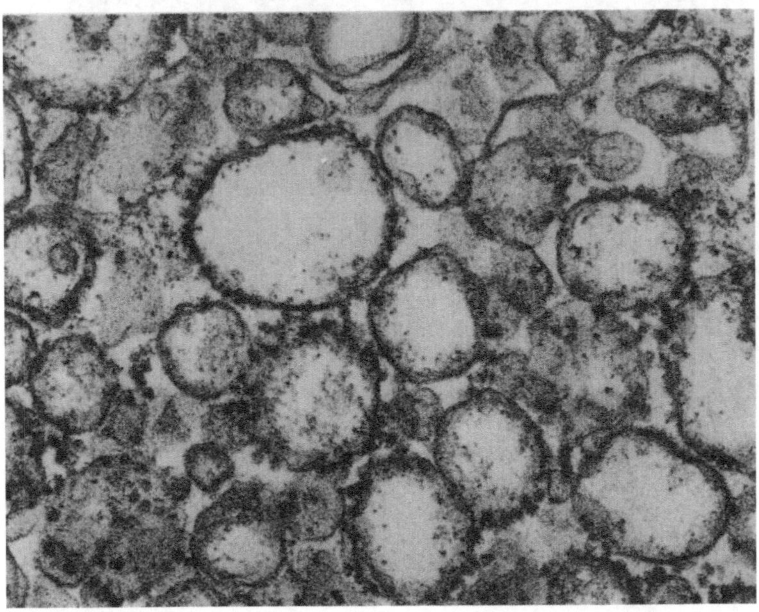

a

Fig. 4a–c. Electron micrographs (× 85000) showing preparation of ER with attached ribosomes (**a**), ER after incubation with ATP, lipid precursors. and cytosol, generating ER transport vesicles (**b**), and preparation of the purified ER transport vesicles (**c**)

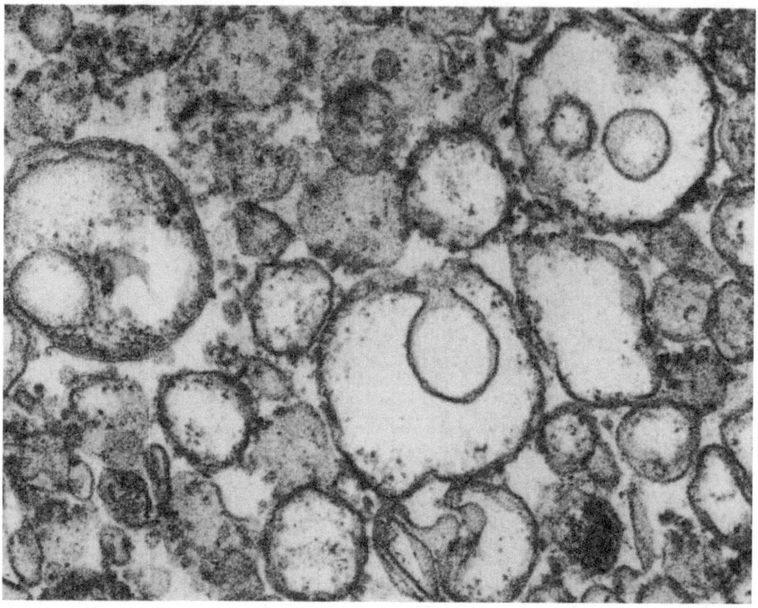

b

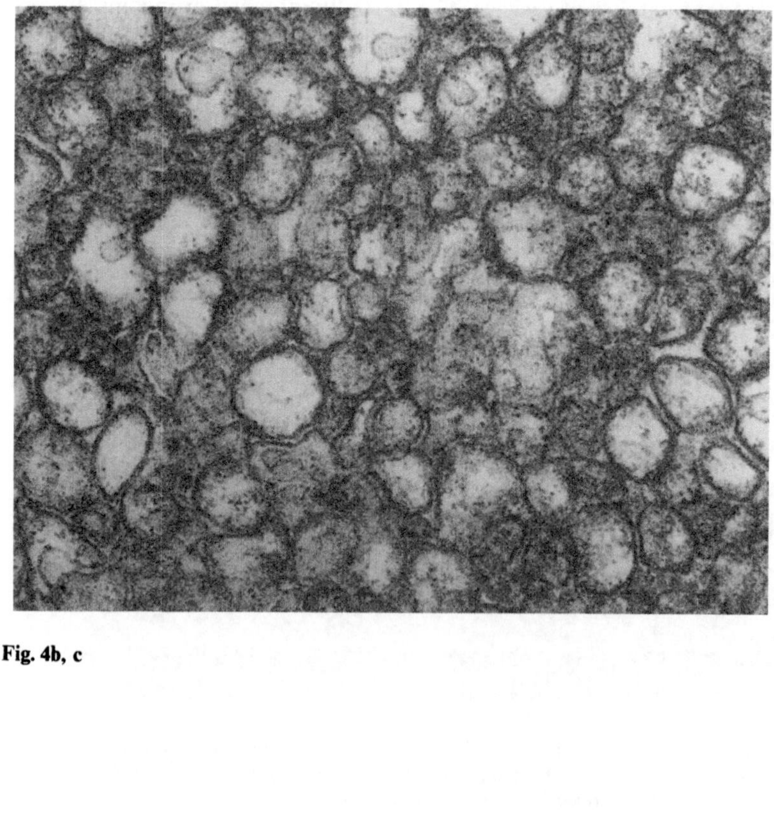

c

Fig. 4b, c

a population of granules 80–100 nm in diameter, and occasional small microsomes with vesicles in the process of synthesis or detachment are also observed.

Protein and Lipid Components of ER Mucin Transport Vesicles

The studies on the protein composition of ER vesicles carrying apomucin cargo have shown enrichment in a number of proteins, of which mucin cargo (60-kDa apomucin) represents only 6%–8% of the total proteins, as estimated by densitometric scanning of the components of ER transport vesicles separated by SDS-PAGE (Fig. 5). The majority of the depicted proteins are found surface-associated and their incubation with lipid precursors (glycerol-3 phosphate, choline, serine, fatty acids, CoA and CTP) results in the synthesis of phosphoglycerides (Fig. 6). As suggested above, these enzymes represent the majority of proteins coating ER vesicles.

The lipid analysis of ER transport vesicles carrying apomucin revealed the presence of phosphatidylcholine (PC), phosphatidylethanolamine (PE), and phosphatidylinositol (PI) (Fig. 7). These three phosphoglycerides account for 95% of lipids in ER transport vesicles. The ceramides contribute 4–5%, sphingomyelin (SM) and phosphatidylserine (PS) are not detectable, while traces of sphingosine are noticed only with ninhydrin staining. In our interpretation

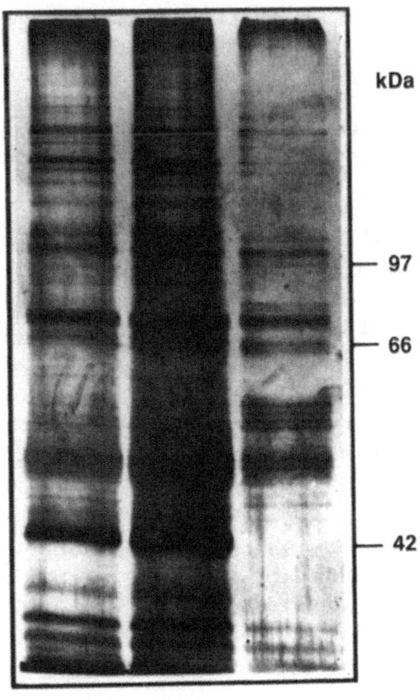

Fig. 5. 7.0% SDS-PAGE and silver staining of ER transport vesicles subjected to the stripping of the surface associated proteins. The middle lane represents ER vesicles before incubation, the left and right lanes depict vesicles incubated at 4°C with 1 M urea and 10 μg/ml brefeldin A for 15 min, respectively. Each incubate contained 10 μg protein

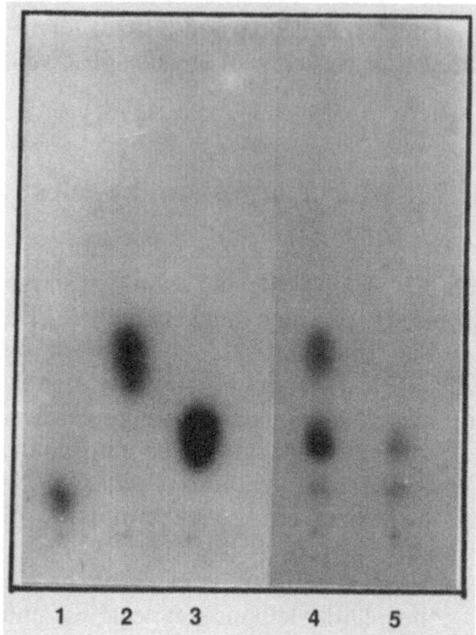

Fig. 6. Enzymatic activity of the proteins associated on the surface of ER transport vesicles. Detection of CTP: phosphocholine cytidylyltransferase activity. *1*, [^{14}C] choline; *2*, CDP- [^{14}C] choline; *3*, [^{14}C] phosphocholine standards; *4*, products derived from incubation of ER transport vesicle proteins with [^{14}C] phosphocholine and CTP; *5*, control, consisting of boiled ER transport vesicle proteins, [^{14}C] phosphocholine, and CTP

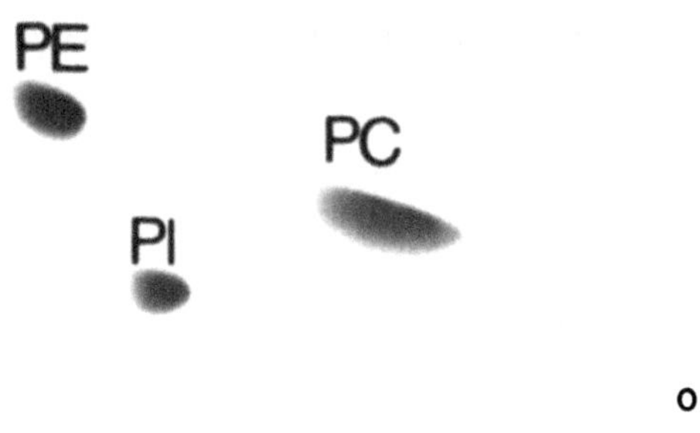

Fig. 7. Lipid composition of ER transport vesicles. Two dimensional thin layer chromatography [63] of ER transport vesicle lipid extract revealed presence of phosphatidylcholine (*PC*), phosphatidylinositol (*PI*), and phosphatidylethanolamine (*PE*)

this suggests that the synthesis of the new promembrane, consisting of three major phosphoglycerides and ceramides, takes place in the areas of ER which undergo vesiculization, packaging with synthesized apomucin and then separation from the maternal membrane. If the lipid synthesis was uniformly spread throughout the ER membrane network, the radiolabeled lipid distribution between ER and the isolated vesicles would be the same. Another argument for the localized growth of ER membrane is that during vesicular transport or even during the in vitro generation of transport vesicles, the resident and integral ER proteins are not exported out of ER (Fig. 8). This is in good agreement with the fact that most of the phosphoglyceride-synthesizing enzymes are only transiently associated with the ER membrane and are released after a desirable concentration of the phospholipid in the membrane is generated. Thus, our hypothesis that the ER transport vesicles are assembled with the aid of lipid-synthesizing enzymes, which retreat to cytosol once the task is completed, is substantiated further. The concept seems even more sensible when combined

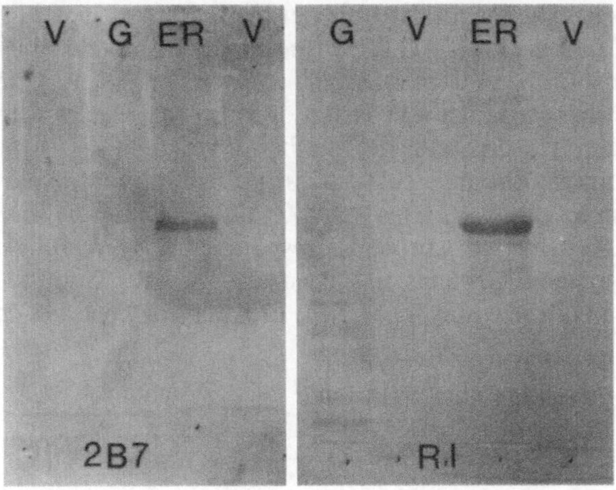

Fig. 8. Fundamental differences between ER and ER transport vesicles. Western blot analysis of the ER, ER transport vesicles (*V*) and Golgi (*G*) proteins with monoclonal antibodies against integral proteins of ER, with 2B7 MAb against PFAT enzyme (*left*) and αR1 MAb against ribophorin I (*right*)

with the findings showing decoating of the vesicles prior to their attachment and fusion with Golgi membrane [1–3].

Other Components of ER Transport Vesicles

Transport and targeting of mature vesicles are critical steps for ensuring the efficiency and specificity of intracellular transport. Studies on polarized cells such as neurons suggest that the transport may be accomplished by translocation along the elements of the cytoskeleton [45, 46], whereas the targeting of the vesicles, direction, and fidelity of the processes are regulated by a large group of mostly unknown proteins [47, 48]. A group of related GTP-binding protein seem to be responsible for the regulation of targeting step [48, 49]. Based on the known activities of the characterized GTP proteins, two potential mechanisms of the small GTP-binding proteins (20–25 kDa) in secretion have been proposed [4–9]. By analogy to the α a subunit of heterotrimeric G-protein of plasma membrane, small GTP-binding proteins may be involved in the amplification or transduction of a signal required for subsequent events in vesicular transport. Interestingly, the Gα-subunit localized to Golgi complex has been implicated in regulating secretion [50].

Several lines of evidence support the role for small GTP-binding proteins in vesicular transport [49, 51, 52]. Firstly, mutation in each of four yeast genes encoding these proteins (ARF1, SAR1, XPT1 and SEC4) results in defects in various steps in secretion. Secondly, in vitro assays that reconstitute steps in intracellular transport requiring GTP are blocked by treatments which inhibit

GTP-binding protein activity. The most compelling evidence implicating GTP proteins in transport was obtained with GTPγS, the nonhydrolyzable GTP analogue which inhibits most of the in vitro transport reactions [1–3, 4, 8]. The addition of GTPγS blocks the uncoating and fusion of transport vesicles with Golgi, resulting in a several-fold increase in the number of vesicles [48].

The protein coat surrounding the accumulated vesicles, in addition to lipid-synthesizing enzymes, contain four proteins of 160, 110, 98, and 61 kDa designated as α, β, γ and δCOP (for "coat protein"), respectively [53]. A soluble protein complex containing these proteins has been also isolated from the cytostol [54], suggesting that they may exist just like the enzymes which

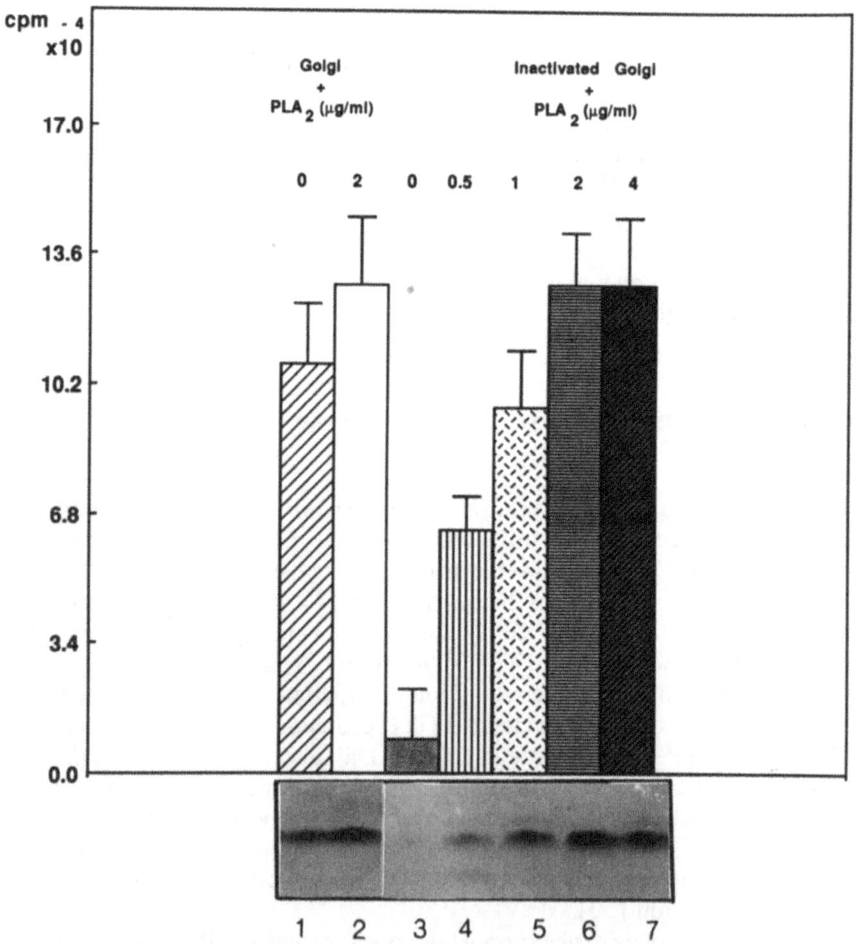

Fig. 9. Effect of fusion promoting phospholipase A_2 fraction on the fusion of ER vesicles with Golgi membranes (*bars*) and transfer of apomucin to Golgi (*bottom panel*). The apomucin, transferred to Golgi of liver, was immunoprecipitated with antimucin 1H7 MAb and subjected to 10% SDS-PAGE and silver staining

assemble membrane, in a dynamic equilibrium between soluble and membrane-bound forms. In addition, our investigations on the cytosolic proteins promoting fusion led to the identification of yet another protein which was found to assist transport, promote fusion of ER-transport vesicles with Golgi, and display phospholipase A_2 (PLA_2) activity [55].

Role of Intracellular Phospholipase A_2 in Vesicular Transport of Apomucin from ER to Golgi

The cytosolic protein fraction was isolated on the basis of its ability to support the transport of apomucin from ER to Golgi, and incorporation of vesicular membrane into Golgi (Fig. 9). The involvement of these proteins in the final event associated with vesicle fusion suggested that the proteins might contribute to the destabilization of the membrane lipid bilayer by transformation of the inert membrane lipids into lysophospholipid fusogens. When fusion-promoting

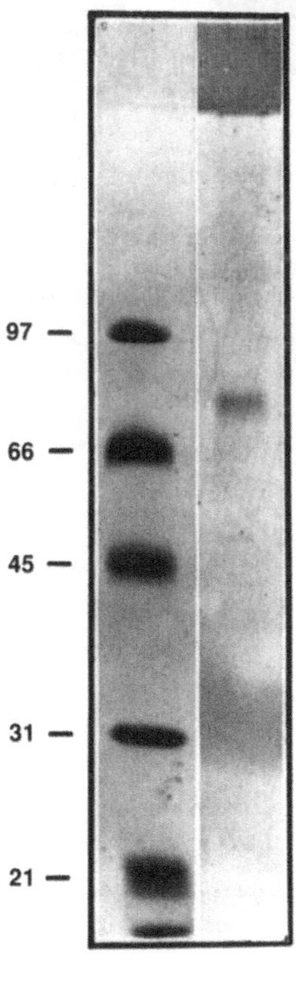

Fig. 10. 7% SDS-PAGE and silver staining of the fusion promoting intracellular 76-kDa phospholipase A_2

fraction, particularly its 76-kDa component (Fig. 10), was incubated with vesicles containing [^{14}C]choline labeled PC, the vesicles were lysed, PC was hydrolysed and the lysophosphatidylcholine was formed (Fig. 11). The evidence obtained with various species of PC labeled at PLA_1-, PLA_2-,PLC-, and PLD-specific positions provided evidence that the isolated protein was a PLA_2 enzyme [55]. Just like vesicle fusion reaction [1–3,48], the PLA_2 activity of the 76-kDa protein was N-ethylmaleimide-(NEM-) and phosphorylation-sensitive (Table 1). The activity and membrane association of the PLA_2 were regulated by

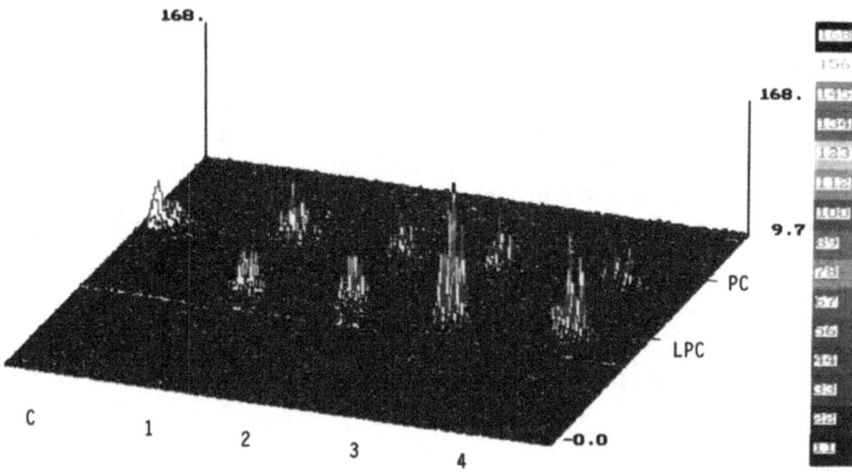

Fig. 11. Generation of lysophosphatidylcholine (*LPC*) from phosphatidylcholine (*PC*) of ER transport vesicles subjected to incubation with 76-kDa phospholipase A_2 for 10 min (*1, 2*) and 20 min (*3, 4*). The ER-transport vesicles containing [^{14}C] choline radiolabeled phosphatidylcholine before incubation are shown at *C*

Table 1. Phospholipase A_2 activity of the 76-kDa protien promoting apomucin transport and ER vesicle fusion with Golgi

Source of the 76-kDa protein or the treatment	PLA_2 activity (μmol/mg min)
Isolated from cytosol and from membranes	3.28 – 22.06 (10)
Isolated from cytosol	0.22 – 1.50 (11)
Stripped from membranes	32.94 – 72.78 (6)
Subjected to phosphorylation	2.39 – 3.39 (3)
Dephosphorylated	77.28 – 82.10 (2)
Treated with 1-m*M* NaF	0
Treated with 1-m*M* NEM	0.10 – 0.12 (2)

NEM, *N*-ethylmaleimide; NaF, natrium fluoride
The numbers in parentheses indicate the number of experiments performed. The activity is expressed in μmol lysophosphatidylcholine (LPC) generated from 1,2-diacyl-sn-glycerol-phospho [^{14}C]choline substrate per milligram PLA_2 protein per minute

phosphorylation and only the membrane-bound form of the protein was active. As has been shown [56], the Golgi membrane receptors and other cytosol-derived components are involved in the process of fusion. The presence of specific 76-kDa PLA_2 receptor on the Golgi membranes would thus guarantee attachment of the cytosolic PLA_2, vesicle fusion, and the vectorial movement of the ER apomucin cargo to Golgi.

Our identification of some of the components constituting the coat protein of ER transport vesicles [44] and the protein supporting and promoting the transport and fusion provide further insight into the complex ER–Golgi transport pathway (Fig. 12). The early events in the transport vesicle formation are NEM-sensitive due to the inhibition of lipid synthesis (Fig. 13). Further effects

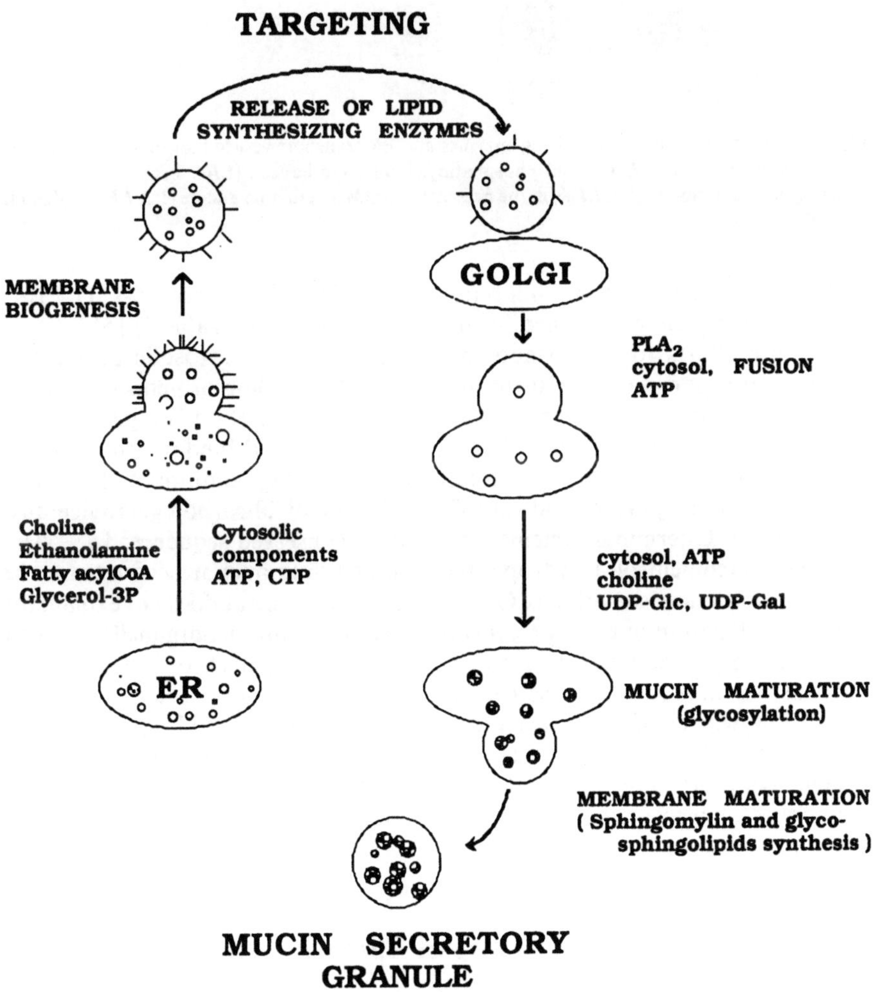

Fig. 12. Proposed model of ER transport vesicle formation and fusion with Golgi, demonstrating the role of lipid synthesizing enzymes and lipid precursors in formation of the vesicles, and the role of intracellular phospholipase A_2 in their fusion with acceptor membrane (Golgi)

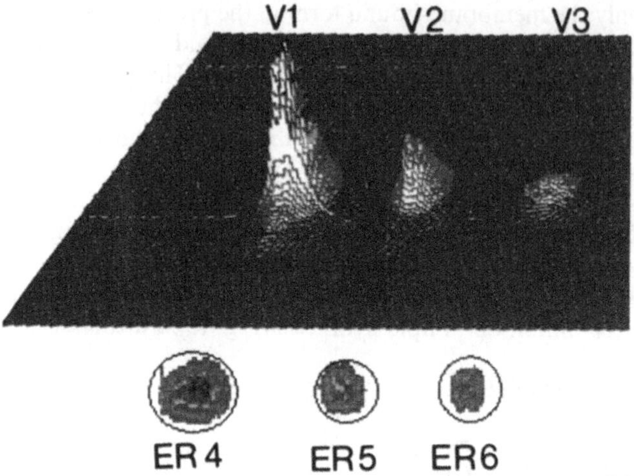

#	net (cts)	net (cpm)
V1	46,190	1,925
V2	8,933	375
V3	4,225	175
ER4	39,847	1,494
ER5	8,344	315
ER6	4,188	158

Fig. 13. Inhibitors of lipid-synthesizing enzymes and ER transport vesicle biogenesis. The amount of vesicles formed (*V1*, *V2*, *V3*) and phosphatidylcholine synthesized (*ER4*, *ER5*, *ER6*) is shown under optimal conditions (*V1*, *ER4*), in the presence of 3m*M* *N*-ethylmaleimide (*V2*, *ER5*) and 3m*M* Zn^{2+} (V3, ER6)

of NEM are related to the inhibition of vesicle fusion, since 76-kDa PLA_2 activity is completely abolished in the presence of NEM (Table 1) [55].

Future efforts to understand the exact role of the cytosolic proteins in vesicular transport are likely to address how GTP-binding proteins specifically associate with different membranes and how this association is regulated. The membrane association of many hydrophilic, small GTP-binding proteins, has been recently shown to depend on fatty acylation [51], addition of 15-carbon farnesyl group to cysteine residue [58], or addition of 20-carbon geranylgeranyl group onto a C-terminal cysteine, specified by conserved sequences [57, 59].

The attachment of a hydrophobic modified lipid anchor accounts for the strong membrane association of GTP-binding proteins, but does not explain the specific localization of these proteins to different membrane organelles or their compartments. Additionally, membrane association must be reversible for proteins which, according to some, recycle through cytosol to secretory vesicles [60]. A knowledge of the events and the proteins which provide specificity and fidelity for each step of the transport will be required to understand how the protein synthesis, transport, and secretion are connected with lipid synthesis, membrane biogenesis, and the formation of polarized membranes in gastric and other epithelia.

Role of Lipids in Mucin Transport Through Golgi

The second key element underlying our current view of transport concerns the role of carrier vesicles in mediating transport through the Golgi complex. The strongest evidence for the existence of a vesicular intermediate in the in vitro transport reaction has been provided by the identification and isolation of the Golgi transport vesicles [61]. In this approach, Golgi fraction prepared from VSV-infected GlcNAc transferase deficient 15B cells ("donor Golgi") were incubated with similar fractions from uninfected wild-type cells ("acceptor Golgi"). Progressive appearance of GlcNAc containing VSV G-protein was interpreted as transfer from mutant "donor" to wildtype acceptor membranes [62]. This transfer has also been divided into two major stages: an early stage, presumed to correlate with the budding of transport vesicles from the donor Golgi, and a late stage reflecting the docking and subsequent fusion of the vesicles with the acceptor Golgi. While transport vesicles seem to represent the most likely mechanism for the transport between compartments, the evidence that vesicles are actually formed is indirect. One cannot exclude the possibility that the G protein moved through tubules connecting the heterologous Golgi stacks. In our studies on Golgi vesicle formation, we have concentrated on the issue of vesicle composition pertaining to whether Golgi carriers contain newly synthesized glycosphingolipids and whether radiolabeled phosphatidylcholine delivered in the form of transport vesicles is utilized for generation of sphingomyelin (SM) [63].

Since the synthesis of sphingomyelin is not observed when ER vesicles are incubated without Golgi or when fusion is blocked, the PC→SM exchange reaction must be specific for the Golgi luminal surface (Fig. 14). Thus, it seems ideal that diglycerides, produced during sphingomyelin formation, which is

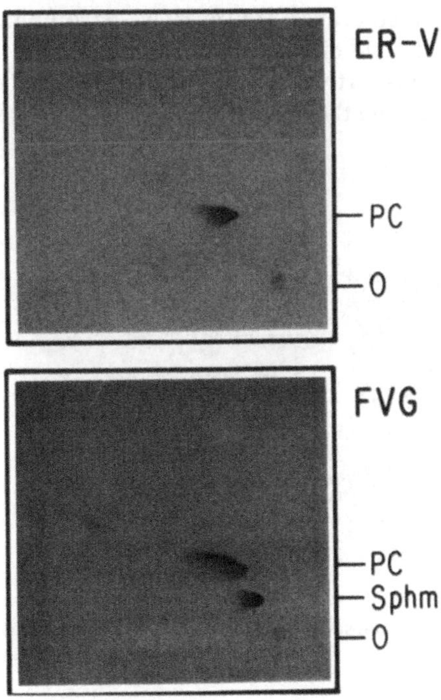

Fig. 14. Utilization of the transport vesicle phosphatidylcholine (*PC*) to synthesize sphingomyelin (*Sphm*) in Golgi. *ER-V*, ER transport vesicles containing [^{14}C] phosphatidylcholine, *FVG*, radiolabeled lipids detected in Golgi after its fusion with *ER-V*

easily and rapidly transferred from one site of the membrane to the other [64–66], can be utilized in the synthesis of phosphatidylcholine or other phosphoglycerides on the cytosolic face of the Golgi membrane. In our study, we tested this possibility by incubating the intact Golgi membranes with CDP-[^{14}C]choline in the cytosol depleted of lipid metabolites. The results revealed that the Golgi membranes without cytosolic source of the substrates to synthesize diglycerides are still able to produce phosphatidylcholine (Fig. 15). In the light of this finding, it appears that the process, otherwise futile (phosphatidylcholine degradation to generate phosphatidylcholine again), allows for the fast lipid transfer and membrane synthesis. Also, our data support the previous studies suggesting that phosphatidylcholine synthesis is not exclusive to ER membranes [67, 68], and it appears that the shuttle of diglycerides from Golgi to ER to synthesize phosphatidylcholine is irrelevant [69].

The findings presented here and the speculations voiced by others [64–69] strongly support the view that the synthesis of phosphatidylcholine (and other phosphoglycerides) on the cytosolic side of Golgi is the only feasible and uncomplicated way to form an asymmetric membrane. The capacity of Golgi membranes to synthesize phosphatidylcholine would guarantee not only a one-to-one ratio of the synthesis on the opposing membrane faces, but would also allow sufficient growth of the outer leaflet to generate vesicles in the shape of spherical structures [70, 71].

Perhaps the fluctuations in the in vitro transport efficiency from ER to Golgi [72] reflect variations in the level of phosphoglyceride substrates, which could differ greatly from that available in vitro. In our assays, the optimal conditions produced up to 33% of the transfer as quantitated in terms of radiolabeled lipids transferred to Golgi membranes. However, we have found that the vesicles which are recovered at the end of the fusion reaction no longer reflect the lipid composition of the ER transport vesicles, but are rather specific for Golgi membranes. This implies that during the incubation of Golgi with ER

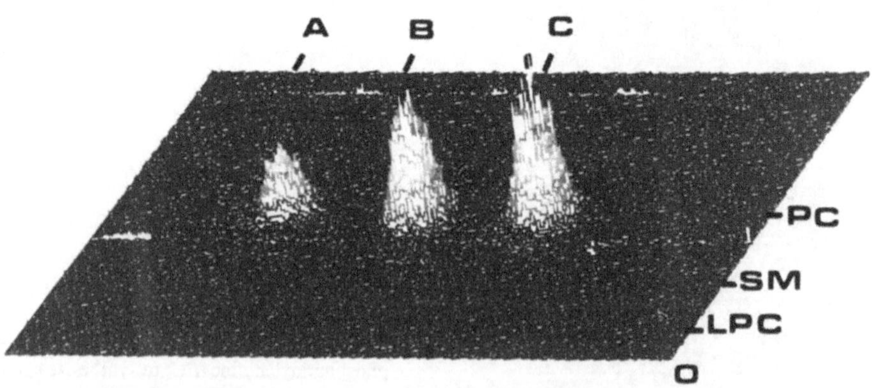

Fig. 15. Potential of Golgi membrane to synthesize phosphatidylcholine (*PC*) without external source of diacylglycerol. Incubation of the intact Golgi membranes with CDP- [^{14}C] choline was performed for 10 min (*A*), 20 min (*B*), and 30 min (*C*)

vesicles, the Golgi transport vesicles are formed and contribute to the pool of the unfused vesicle fraction of the ER origin. Formation of the consecutive batch of vesicles (now derived from Golgi) would account for some discrepancies in calculation of transport efficiency in terms of radiolabeled lipids recovered from the Golgi membranes after fusion. However, it is unlikely that even with this one could have achieved 100% efficiency. At this point, it is more than apparent that many other factors must be brought into play to achieve optimal performance and to account for the fast retrograde transport.

It is possible that the type of vesicle described here is used to deliver some of the protein products to the site of their modification, and to remodel and renew the membranes, whereas the other intracellular transfers are achieved by means of membrane tubules or vesicles which could shuttle between organelles and replace the lost membranes during anterograde transport [69, 73]. Also, one may interpret the results that the vesicles are required in the final stage of packaging of the mature mucins in carriers which become secretory granules, whereas the intra-Golgi intermediates are transferred by tubular network. In our experimental design, it was not possible to assess the other processes or the magnitude of the retrograde transport [69], since the unlabeled Golgi membranes had to be used for the detection of anterograde transport and membrane fusion. Thus, the retrograde transfer, if any, contained mostly unlabeled lipids and hence could not be measured. Also, the flow of phospholipids by means of phospholipid transfer proteins requires further attention [74]. In our opinion, however, the latter mode of compensation against the tide of phospholipids moving as protein packed vesicles is more appealing than vesicular shuttle. One strong argument against the vesicular shuttle is that this process would provide ER membranes with glycosphingolipids (occupying luminal surfaces of Golgi membranes), whereas the transport proteins exchange their lipid cargo with cytosolic domain of the membrane, and thus neither glycosphingolipid nor sphingomyelin are removed during this unilateral removal of phospholipids from Golgi and the delivery of the phospholipids back to the ER.

On the basis of the evidence obtained regarding the conditions for ER vesicle formation and the lipid labeling and composition, we propose that the transport vesicle generation is not only dependent on the action of proteins which are essential for shaping and pinching off the vesicles, but also on the proteins which are phosphoglyceride- and sphingolipid-synthesizing enzymes. Moreover, the lipid complexity of intracellular membranes is achieved gradually by intervention of the lipid core-modifying enzymes of the organelles involved in vesicular transport (Fig. 12).

The next step to reveal the secrets of Golgi is to determine how many Golgi compartments are there, and whether their boundaries are defined by specific proteins, and what is the role of tubules. While much remains to be explored, the incorporation of lipid and membrane biogenesis as one of the primary factors in the vectorial transport for exo- and endocytosis and continuous renewal of cell membrane and its protein components is certainly of primary importance. The relevant conclusion from the reviewed studies is that phospholipid synthesis, membrane biogenesis, and the intracellular transport activities are closely connected events.

Role of Lipids and Biosynthetic Secretory Pathway in Gastric Pathology

The contribution of lipids to cotranslational translocation, reflected in palmitoylation of the nascent peptide, is gaining recognition as a potential regulator of peptide translocation across ER, fusion of transport vesicles with Golgi cisternae [75], and expression of the intermittent activity of the proteins involved in the signal transduction [36]. The connection between secretory activity of gastrointestinal mucus-secreting cells and the activity of protein fatty acyltransferase (PFAT) is apparent when the critical role of the enzyme in the initiation of apomucin transport is considered (Fig. 1). The evidence that decreased activity of PFAT is directly related to the amount of translocated apomucin peptide to ER, together with our earlier findings of reduced PFAT activity in biopsies from patients with chronic gastritis, strongly suggest that the impairment in palmitoylation of apomucin may be responsible for diminished secretion of mucus glycoprotein. Similar although temporary derangement in palmitoylation of apomucin is observed in gastric mucosa treated with ethanol. The PFAT activity is drastically diminished in the presence of 100–120 mM ethanol, and consequently apomucin translocation to the lumen of ER is reduced, and although the Golgi-specific reactions are not affected [75], the amount of secreted mucin is reduced [28]. Both cases illustrate clearly the role of lipids in the initiation of mucin transport and secretion.

In contrast, the PFAT enzyme in cells derived from cystic fibrosis patients displays significantly higher specific activity and shows lower substrate specifi-

Table 2. Protein fatty acyltransferase activity (PFAT) in normal lymphoblasts (N) and lymphoblasts from patients with cystic fibrosis (CF)

Cell line	Specific activity (nmol/mg protein x 30 min)
385 (N)	14.0 – 16.8
856A (N)	7.5 – 9.0
382 (CF)	35.2 – 42.1
552 (CF)	39.3 – 41.0
859C (CF)	26.0 – 35.7

Lymphoblasts from normal cell lines 385 and 856A and cystic fibross cell lines 382, 552 and 859C were cultured and used for PFAT purification. The enzyme activity was measured using the deacylated glycoprotein as substrate. The standard assay mixture contained in 0.1 ml: 100 f4kg deacylated mucus glycoprotein, 35 μM [1-^{14}C] palmitoyl-CoA, 0.25 μg protein, 0.5% Triton X-100, 2 mM dithiothreitol, 25mM NaF, and 100 mM imidazole HCl, pH 7.4

city (Table 2). Cross-experiments with preacylated mucin and the enzyme from patients with cystic fibrosis result in further incorporation of palmitate into the glycoprotein substrate. In our interpretation, the abundance of lipid in mucin from cystic fibrosis patients is responsible for the impaired mucin turnover and obstruction of gastrointestinal and pulmonary tracts [26, 27, 78].

Despite early enthusiasm about the discovery of a cystic fibrosis gene (CFTR protein) [79], the production of the thick, sticky deposits in lungs, gastrointestinal tract and pancreatic ducts cannot be explained on the basis of water and chloride transport abnormalities which are caused by a defect in CFTR protein, and data to support this speculation are lacking. On the other hand, the abnormality exhibited by cystic fibrosis cells reflected in altered exo- and endocytosis [80], the processes closely connected with the vesicular transport and the regulatory mechanisms described herein, particularly with the role of PFAT in the modification of secretory and membrane proteins, may hold the answer to this complex problem in cystic fibrosis.

The alcohol-induced alterations in cells are not limited to the early cotranslational events discussed earlier. Profound biological consequences of the presence of ethanol in the system are also reflected in the variety of changes in activities of membrane-bound enzymes, receptors, and ion channels [81–85], whose function is moderated by the immediate lipid environment created in the membrane. Our studies [86] indicate that membrane biogenesis in the presence of ethanol is significantly modified. Decrease in phosphatidylcholine and ceramide levels and the increase in phosphatidylethanolamine reflect the initial change in membrane composition. Subsequently, repeated rounds of modified vesicle formation and their fusion with plasma membrane lead to a modified cell membrane. Thus, the possibility that ethanol acts on membrane proteins by altering lipids surrounding the channels and receptors [84, 85] gains a new and realistic meaning when combined with our results showing actual changes in membrane biogenesis.

As illustrated by the examples presented, efforts towards reconstituting the intracellular transport of mucin in a fully resolved system coupled with lipid and membrane biogenesis should lead to better understanding of the secretory processes taking place in gastric mucosa in health and disease.

References

1. Balch WE (1989) Biochemistry of interorganelle transport. A new frontier in enzymology emerges from versatile in vitro model system. J Biol Chem 264:16969–16968
2. Goda Y, Pfeffer SR (1989) Cell-free system to study vesicular transport along the secretory and endocytic pathways. FASEB J 3:2488–2495
3. Rothman JE, Orci L (1990) Movement of proteins through the Golgi stock: a molecular dissection of vesicular transport. FASEB J 4:1460–1468
4. Beckers CJM, Balch WE (1989) Calcium and GTP: essential components in vesicular trafficking between the endoplasmic reticulum and Golgi apparatus. J Cell Biol 108:1245–1256

5. Beckers CJM, Plutner H, Davidson HW, Block WE (1990) Sequential intermediates in the transport of protein between endoplasmic reticulum and the Golgi. J Biol Chem 265: 18298–18310
6. Baker D, Hicke L, Rexach N, Schleyer N, Schekman R (1988) Reconstitution of SEC gene product dependent intercompartmental protein transport. Cell 54:335–344
7. Pfeffer SR, Rothman JE (1987) Biosynthetic protein transport and sorting by endoplasmic reticulum and Golgi. Annu Rev Biochem 56:829–852
8. Groesch ME, Ruohola H, Bacon R, Rossi G, Ferro-Novick S (1990) Isolation of functional vesicular intermediate that mediates ER to Golgi transport in yeast. J Cell Biol 111:45–53
9. Graham TR, Emr SD (1991) Compartmental organization of Golgi specific protein modification and vacuolar protein sorting events defined in yeast sec 18 NSF mutant. J Cell Biol 114:207–218
10. Burgess TL, Kelly RB (1987) Constitutive and regulated secretion of proteins. Annu Rev Cell Biol 3:243–293
11. Cutler DF (1988) The role of transport signals and retention signals in constitutive export from animal cell. J Cell Sci 91:1–4
12. Rose JK, Doms RW (1988) Regulation of protein export from endoplasmic reticulum. Annu Rev Cell Biol 4:257–288
13. Warren G (1987) Signals and salvage sequences. Nature 327:17–18
14. Hurtley SM, Helenius A (1989) Protein oligomerization in the endoplasmic reticulum. Ann Rev Cell Biol 5:277–307
15. Mellman I, Simons K (1992) The Golgi complex: in vitro veritas? Cell 68:829–840
16. Slomiany A, Kasinathan C, Slomiany BL (1992) Glycosylation patterns in mucus glycoprotein. Adv Macromol Carbohydr Res (in press)
17. Paulson JC, Colley KJ (1989) Glycosyltransferases, structure, localization and control of cell type specific glycosylation. J Biol Chem 264:17615–17618
18. von Heijne G (1981) On the hydrophobic nature of signal sequences. Eur J Biochem 116:419–422
19. Walter P, Ibrahimi I, Blobel G (1981) Translocation of proteins across endoplasmic reticulum. I. Signal recognition protein binds to in vitro assembled polysomes synthesizing secretory proteins. J Cell Biol 91:545–550
20. Walter P, Blobel G (1981) Translocation of proteins across the endoplasmic reticulum. III. Signal recognition protein (SRP) causes signal sequence dependent and site specific arrest of chain elongation that is released by microsomal membranes. J Cell Biol 91:557–561
21. Walter P, Blobel G (1983) Signal recognition particle: A ribonucleoprotein required for cotranslational translocation of protein, isolation and properties Methods, Enzymol 96:682–691
22. Sanz P, Meyer DI (1989) Secretion in yeast: Preprotein binding to a membrane receptor and ATP-dependent translocation are sequential and separable events in vitro. J Cell Biol 108:2101–2106
23. Rapoport TA (1985) Extensions of the signal hypothesis-sequential insertion model versus amphipathic tunnel hypothesis. FEBS Lett 187:1–10
24. Gilmore R, Blobel G, Walter P (1982) Protein translocation across the endoplasmic reticulum I. Detection in the microsomal membrane of a receptor for the signal recognition particle. J Cell Biol 95:463–469
25. Rothblatt JA, Deshaies RJ, Sanders SL, Daum G, Schekman R (1989) Multiple genes are required for proper insertion of secretory proteins into the endoplasmic reticulum in yeast. J Cell Biol 109:2641–2652
26. Slomiany A, Witas H, Aono M, Slomiany BL (1983) Covalently linked fatty acids in gastric mucus glycoprotein of cystic fibrosis patients. J Biol Chem 258:8535–8538
27. Slomiany A, Zielenski J, Tsukada H, Slomiany BL (1988) Synthesis and cotranslational processing of mucus glycoprotein. In: Mastella G, Quinton PM (eds) Cellular and molecular basis of cystis fibrosis, San Francisco Press, San Francisco, pp 247–261
28. Tsukada H, Zielenski J, Mizuta K,Slomiany BL, Slomiany A (1987) Prostaglandin protection against ethanol induced gastric injury: regulatory effect on mucus glycoprotein metabolism. Digestion 36:201–212
29. Slomiany BL, Tsukada H, Slomiany A (1986) Cotranslational attachment of fatty acids to nascent peptides in gastric mucus glycoprotein. Biochem Biophys Res Commun 141:387–393

30. Slomiany A, Mizuta K, Zalesna G, Tsukada H, Slomiany BL (1988) Cotranslational processing and intracellular transport of rat salivary mucus glycoprotein. Archs Oral Biol 33:807–818
31. Slomiany A, Tsukada H, Zalesna G, Slomiany BL (1988) Cotranslational fatty acylation of mucus glycoprotein. Addition of palmitic acid to peptidyl–tRNA occurs prior to peptide chain completion and release. Int J Biochem 20:1381–1390
32. Zalesna G, Tsukada H, Okazaki K, Slomiany BL, Slomiany A (1989) Synthesis and initial processing of gastric mucin. Biochem Int 18:775–784
33. Kasinathan C, Grzelinska E, Slomiany BL, Slomiany A (1990) Purification of protein fatty acyltransferase and determination of its distribution and topology. J Biol Chem 265:5139–5144
34. Slomiany A, Okazaki K, Slomiany BL (1992) Synthesis and macromolecular organization of gastrointestinal mucin: Evidence for the origin of mucin "link protein". J Clin Gastroenterol 14(1) :S71–S81
35. Slomiany A, Slomiany BL (1992) Synthesis and macromolecular organization of gastrointestinal mucin. J Physiol Pharmacol 43:113–136
36. Sudo Y, Valenzuela D, Beck-Sickinger AG, Fishman M, Strittmatter SM (1992) Palmitoylation alters protein activity: blockade of Go stimulation by GAP-43. EMBO J 11:2095–2102
37. Perez–Vilar J, Hidalgo T, Velasco A (1991) Presence of terminal N–acetylgalactosamine residues in subregions of endoplasmic reticulum is influenced by cell differentiation in culture. J Biol Chem 266:23967–23976
38. Spielman J, Rockley NL, Carraway KL (1987) Temporal aspects of O–glycosylation and cell surface expression of ascites sialoglycoprotein-1, the major cell surface sialomucin of 13762 mammary ascites tumor cells. J Biol Chem 262:269–275
39. Towler DA, Gordon JI, Adams SP, Glaser L (1988) The biology and enzymology of eukaryotic protein acylation. Annu Rev Biochem 57:69–99
40. Palade G (1975) Intracellular aspects of the process of protein synthesis. Science 189:347–358
41. Palade G (1956) Intracisternal granules in the exocrine pancreas. J Biophys Biochem Cytol 2:417–422
42. Roman LM, Garoff H (1985) Revelation through exploitation: the viral model for intracellular traffic. Trends Biochem Sci 10:428–432
43. Sheetz MP, Singer SJ (1974) Biological membranes as bilayer couples. A molecular mechanism of drug-erythrocyte interactions. Proc Natl Acad sci USA 71:4457–4461
44. Slomiany A, Grzelinska E, Kasinathan C, Yamaki K, Palecz D, Slomiany BA, Slomiany BL (1992) Biogenesis of endoplasmic reticulum transport vesicles transferring gastric apomucin from ER to Golgi. Exp Cell Res 201:321–329
45. Burgess TL, Kelly RB (1987) Constitutive and regulated secretion of proteins. Annu Rev Cell Biol 3:243–293
46. Kelly RB (1990) Microtubules, membrane traffic and cell organization. Cell 61:5–7
47. Vale RD (1987) Intracellular transport using microtubul-based motors. Annu Rev Cell Biol 3:347–378
48. Clary DO, Griff IC, Rothman JE (1990) SNAPs, a family of NSF attachment proteins involved in intracellular membrane fusion in animals and yeast. Cell 61:709–721
49. Bourne HR, Sanders DA, McCormick F (1990) The GTPase superfamily: a conserved switch for diverse cell functions. Nature 348:125–132
50. Staw JL, Bruno de Almeida J, Narula N, Holtzman EJ, Ercolani L (1991) A heterotrimeric G protein, Gα1–3, on Golgi membranes regulates the secretion of a heparan sulfate proteoglycan in LLC-PK_1 epithelial cells. J Cell Ciol 114:1113–1124
51. Balch WE (1990 Small GTP-binding proteins in vesicular transport. Trends Biochem Sci 15:473–477.pa
52. Hall A (1990) The cellular functions of small GTP-binding proteins. Science 249:635–640
53. Serafini T, Stenbeck G, Brecht A, Lottspeich F, Orci L (1991) A coat subunit of Golgi-derived non-clathrin-coated vesicules with homology to the clathrin-coated vesicle coat protein β-adaptin. Nature 349:215–220
54. Waters MG, Serafini T, Rothman JE (1991) "Coatomer": a cytosolic protein complex containing subunits of non-clathrin-coated Golgi transport vesicles. Nature 349:248–251
55. Slomiany A, Grzelinska E, Kasinathan C, Yamaki K, Palecz D, Slomiany BL (1992) Function of intracellular phospholipase A_2 in vectorial transport of apoproteins from ER to Golgi. Int J Biochem 24:1397–1406

56. Weidman PJ, Melancon P, Block MR, Rothman JE (1989) Binding of N-ethylmaleimide sensitive fusion protein to Golgi membranes requires both a soluble protein(s) and an integral membrane receptor. J Cell Biol 108:1589–1596
57. Molenaar CMT, Prange R, Galwitz D (1988) A carboxyl-terminal cysteine residue is required for palmitic acid binding and biological activity of the non-related yeast YPT1 protein. EMBO J 7:971–976
58. Lowy DR, Willumsen BM (1989) New clue to Ras lipid glue. Nature 341:389–385
59. Walworth NC, Goud B, Kabcenell AK, Novick PJ (1989) Mutational analysis of SEC4 suggests a cyclical mechanism for the regulation of vesicular traffic. EMBO J 8:1685–1693
60. Goud B, Salminen A, Walworth NC, Novick PJ (1988) A GTP-binding protein required for secretion rapidly associates with secretory vesicles and the plasma membrane in yeast. Cell 53:753–768
61. Orci L, Glick BS, Rothman JE (1986) A new type of coated vesicular carrier that appears not to contain clathrin: its possible role in protein transport within the Golgi stack. Cell 46:171–184
62. Rothman JE, Miller RL, Urbani LJ (1984) Intercompartmental transport in the Golgi complex is a dissociative process: facile transfer of membrane protein between two Golgi populations. J Cell Biol 99:260–271
63. Slomiany A, Grzelinska E, Grabska M, Yamaki K, Tamura S, Kasinathan C, Slomiany BL (1992) Intracellular processes associated with glycoprotein transport and processing. Arch Biochem Biophys 298:167–175
64. Ganong BR, Bell RM (1984) Transmembrane movement of phosphatidylglycerol and diacylglycerol sulfhydryl analogues. Biochemistry 23:4977–4983
65. Pagano RE, Longmuir KJ (1985) Phosphorylation, transbilayer movement and facilitated intracellular transport of diacylglycerol are involved in the uptake of a fluorescent analog of phosphatidic acid by cultured fibroblast. J Biol Chem 260:1909–1916
66. Lipsky NG, Pagano RE (1983) Sphingolipid metabolism in cultured fibroblasts: Microscopic and biochemical studies employing a fluorescent ceramide analogue. Proc Natl Acad Sci USA 80:2608–2612
67. Jelsema CL, Morre DJ (1978) Distribution of phospholipid biosynthetic enzymes among cell components of rat liver. J Biol Chem 253:7960–7971
68. Higgins JA, Fieldsend JK (1987) Phosphatidylcholine synthesis for incorporation into membrane or for secretion as plasma lipoproteins by Golgi membranes of rat liver. J Lipid Res 28:268–278
69. Pagano RE (1988) What is the fate of diacylglycerol produced at the Golgi apparatus? Trends Biochem Sci 12:202–205
70. Malhotra V, Serafini T, Orci L, Glick BS, Block MR, Rothman JE (1989) Purification of a novel class of coated vesicles mediating biosynthetic protein transport through the Golgi stack. Cell 58:329–336
71. de Curtis I, Simons K (1989) Isolation of exocytic carrier vesicles from BHK cells. Cell 58:719–727
72. Beckers CJM, Block B, Glick J, Rothman JE, Balch WE (1989) Vesicular transport between the endoplasmic reticulum and the Golgi stack requires NEM-sensitive fusion protein. Nature 339:397–398
73. Klausner RD, Donaldson TG, Lippincott-Schwartz J, (1992) Brefeldin A: Insights into the control of membrane traffic and organelle structure. J Cell Biol 116 :1071–1080
74. Cleves AE, Mc Gee TP, Whitters EA, Chempion KM, Aitken JR, Dowhan W, Goeld M, Bankaitis VA (1991) Mutations in CDP-choline pathway for phospholipid biosynthesis bypass the requirement for an essential phospholipid transfer protein. Cell 64:789–800
75. Pfanner N, Orci L, Glick BS, Amherdt M, Arden SR, Malhotra V, Rothman JE (1989) Fatty acyl coenzyme A is required for budding of transport vesicles from golgi cisternae. Cell 59:95–102
76. Slomiany A, Jozwiak Z, Liau YH, Slomiany BL (1984) Effect of ethanol on enzymatic sulfation of glycosphingolipids in gastric mucosa. J Biol Chem 259:5792–5796
77. Carter SR, Slomiany A, Gwozdzinski K, Liau YH, Slomiany BL (1988) Effect of ethanol on mucus glycoprotein sulfotransferase from gastric mucosa. J Biol Chem 263:11977–11984
78. Slomiany A, Slomiany BL, Witas H, Zdebska E, Galicki NI, Newman LJ (1983) Lipids of gastric secretion of patients with cystic fibrosis. Biochim Biophys Acta 750:253–260

79. Collins FS (1992) Cystic fibrosis: Molecular biology and therapeutic implications. Science 256:774–779
80. Bradbury NA, Jilling T, Berta G, Sorscher EJ, Bridges RJ, Kirk KL (1992) Regulation of plasma membrane recycling by CFTR. Science 256:530–531
81. Tabakoff B, Hoffman PL (1987) Biochemical pharmacology of alcohol. In: Meltzer HY (ed) Psychopharmacology: the third generation of progress, Raven, New York, pp 1521–1526
82. Hoek JB, Taraschi TF (1988) Cellular adaptation to ethanol. Trends Biochem Sci 13:269–174
83. Pfanner N, Glick BS, Arden SR, Rothman JE (1990) Fatty acylation promotes fusion of transport vesicles with Golgi cisternae. J Cell Biol 110:955–961
84. Stubbs CD, Williams BW, Pryor CL, Rubin E (1988) Ethanol induced modification to membrane lipid structure. Effect on phospholipase A_2 membrane interactions. Arch Biochem Biophys 262:560–573
85. Gies TB, Bertrand C, Landry Y (1988) Membrane phospholipids polar heads influence the coupling of M2 muscarinic receptors to G protein. Neurochem Res 13:737–742
86. Harris RA, Allen AM (1989) Alcohol intoxication: ion channels and genetics. FASEB J 3: 1689–1695
87. Slomiany A, Grabska M, Grzelinska E, Yamaki K, Kasinathan C, Slomiany BA, Slomiany BL (1992) Membrane biogenesis in the presence of ethanol. Alc Clin Exp Res 16:1152–1161

Mucus and Gastric Mucosal Protection*

B.L. SLOMIANY and A. SLOMIANY

Introduction

The ability of gastric mucosa to withstand the corrosive action of acid and pepsin of luminal contents is the most intriguing and yet essential property of the mucosal surface. Although the exact nature of this mechanism remains elusive, the consensus is that the phenomenon is multicomponential in origin. Among the components to which this function is most often ascribed are the viscous and slimy layer of mucus that tenaciously adheres to the epithelial surfaces, the cell membranes of gastric epithelium, and the mucosal blood flow [1–4]. The surface mucus layer exists in a dynamic equilibrium with the preformed intracellular mucus contained within the secretory granules of the surface epithelial and crypt cells, and together these materials form the so-called mucous barrier of the stomach [5, 6]. While the mucus coat provides the first line of mucosal protection, the cell membranes of gastric epithelium along with tight junctions constitute a second line of defense.

Historically, the ability of apical membrane of surface epithelial cells and their tight junctions to physically limit H^+ back-diffusion into the underlying mucosal tissue have been referred to as the "mucosal barrier" [3, 7]. In recent years, however, evidence has been provided that the mucosal integrity is maintained by a combination of such factors as surface mucus and bicarbonate zone, the apical cell membrane, and the mucosal blood flow [5, 8–12]. The multitude of processes occurring in the mucosal elements offer a wide variety of mechanisms of gastric epithelial protection (Fig. 1). These mechanisms under normal physiological conditions, working in concert, assure inherent resistance of the mucosa to injury and this phenomenon is now termed the "gastric mucosal barrier" [13].

While gastric mucosal blood flow is essential in the disposal of intracellular H^+, sustaining Cl^- transport, and transfer of nutrients and oxygen to surface epithelial cells, the initial brunt of luminal insult falls on the mucus layer which constitutes the only physical barrier between gastric lumen and the surface epithelial cells of the mucosa and this is where the battle lines for the preservation of gastric mucosal integrity are drawn [13, 14]. Yet, due to the lack of

*This work was supported by USPHS grant #DK21684-15 from the National Institute of Diabetes and Digestive and Kidney Diseases and grant #AA05858-11 from the National Institute on Alcohol Abuse and Alcoholism, National Institutes of Health

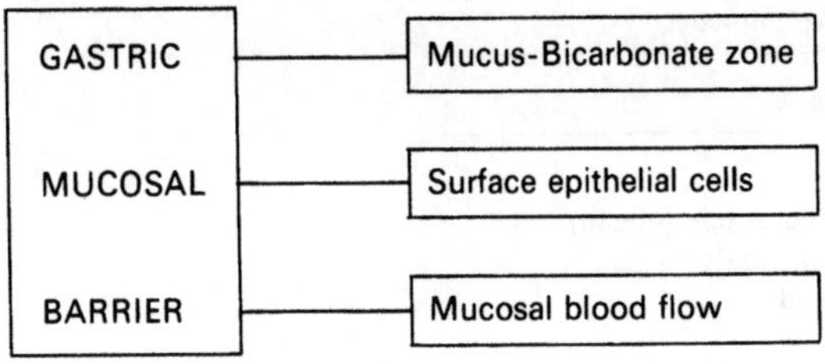

Fig. 1. Elements of gastric mucosal barrier

convincing experimental evidence, acceptance of the importance of mucus in the protection of gastric epithelium varied over the years [15]. Data obtained more recently, however, have begun to show the multitude of protective physicochemical and biological functions of mucus. Included among these are lubrication, waterproofing, hydrogen ion impedance, hydrophobicity, permselectivity, regulation of peptic activity, control of bacterial proliferation, and provision of a milieu for the neutralization of the diffusing luminal acid by the bicarbonate secreted from the epithelial surfaces. As a result, it is becoming increasingly apparent that gastric mucus is an essential part of the mucosal protective network, which is of significance to a variety of processes occurring in the gastrointestinal tract that determine the ability of the individual to successfully resist gastric disease.

Although until recently the disintegration of the mucus coat was attributed exclusively to enhanced activity of the intragastric pepsin and duodenal reflux [1, 16, 17], ample evidence now exists that a bacterial factor, namely infection by *H. pylori* [13, 18, 19], may actually be responsible for the weakening of gastric mucus gel integrity. This chapter offers an insight into the organization and function of gastric mucus coat in health and disease.

Mucus Coat Composition

The coat of mucus which tenaciously adheres to the epithelial surfaces of the gastrointestinal tract is not a single entity, but a heterogeneous mixture of proteins, glycoproteins, and lipids in the form of a gel imbibed with water and electrolytes. The organic constituents amount to 5%–10% of the mucus gel weight and arrive at the mucosal surface through glandular secretion, serum element transudation, and cell exfoliation [20]. Glandular secretions of gastric mucosa contribute mucus glycoproteins, phospholipids, glucoglycerolipids, secretory IgA, and various proteins, including vitamin B_{12}-binding proteins and pepsin. Transudation accounts for the presence in mucus gel of serum glycoproteins, albumin, lipids, and lipoproteins, while the membranes of exfoliating epithelial cells are the source of glycosphingolipids, phospholipids, neutral lipids, and various glycoproteins (Table 1). Compositional data on the organic constituents of human gastric mucus coat indicate that it contains about 65% proteins, 15% carbohydrates, and 20% lipids (Table 2).

Table 1. Origin of constituents of gastric mucus

Origin	Constituent
Glands (secretion)	
	Mucus glycoprotein (mucin)
	Glucoglycerolipids
	Phospholipids
	Secretory IgA
	Vitamin B_{12}-binding proteins
	Pepsin
Serum (transudation)	Albumin
	Serum glycoproteins
	Serum lipoproteins
	Lipids
Cell (exfoliation)	Membrane glycoproteins
	Glycosphingolipids
	Phospholipids
	Proteoglycans

Table 2. Chemical composition of human gastric mucus from healthy individuals and patients with gastric ulcer

Component	mg/100 mg mucus	
	Healthy	Gastric ulcer
Protein	63.7 ± 6.9	68.1 ± 7.2
Carbohydrate	14.8 ± 6.9	12.4 ± 1.0*
Lipids	18.1 ± 1.9	18.8 ± 2.1
Neutral lipids	12.5 ± 1.1	11.7 ± 1.5
Glycolipids	3.4 ± 0.5	4.1 ± 0.6
Phospholipids	2.2 ± 0.3	3.0 ± 0.4*
Covalently bound fatty acids	0.2 ± 0.1	0.2 ± 0.1

Each value represents the mean ± SD of duplicate analyses performed on five individual samples in each group of subjects

Mucus Glycoprotein

The major glycoconjugate of the surface mucus coat is a large, highly glycosylated glycoprotein (Fig. 2), called mucus glycoprotein or mucin [2, 13, 15]. This glycoprotein constitutes 30–40% of the dry weight of the gastric mucus, contains about 85% carbohydrate, 15% protein and 0.3%–0.4% covalently bound fatty acids, and exists in two different molecular weight forms [13]: one a polymer of molecular weight 2000 kDa, and the other of molecular weight 500 kDa and corresponding in size to a pepsin-degraded mucus glycoprotein polymer. The protein core of each mucin form is rich in serine, threonine,

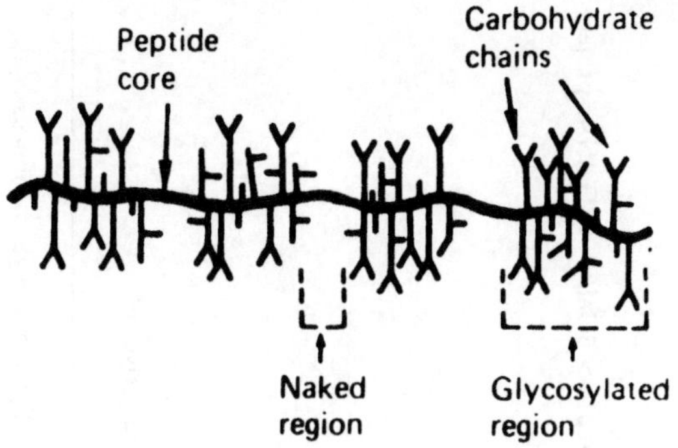

Fig. 2. Linear model of the structure of the gastric mucus glycoprotein

proline, and glycine and exhibits a low content of aromatic and sulfur-containing amino acids [2]. The carbohydrate chains of the glycoprotein are composed of fucose, galactose, *N*-acetylgalactosamine, *N*-acetylglucosamine and sialic acid, and are linked to the protein core through *O*-glycosidic bonds between N-acetylgalactosamine and serine or threonine [22–26]. About 30% of these chains bear a strong negative charge due to the carboxyl group of sialic acid and the presence of the sulfate ester group on the internal residues of *N*-acetylglucosamine and galactose [22, 25, 27]. The chains range in size from 1 to over 20 sugar units arranged in linear or branched fashion,which may contain up to three antennae [22–26]. The terminal carbohydrate sequences of the antennae bear various antigenic determinants, including those which endow the mucin with blood group ABH, Lewis, and Forssman determinants [23–26]. The structural features of carbohydrate chains of gastric mucin are shown in Fig. 3. The covalently bound fatty acids are ester-linked to the protein core of mucin and consist mainly of hexadecanoate and octadecanoate [28–31]. It is estimated that gastric mucus glycoprotein polymer contains about six residues of covalently bound fatty acids and up to 600 carbohydrate chains [6].

Mucus Lipids

Lipids account for up to 25% of the dry weight of gastric mucus and are comprised of neutral lipids, glycolipids, and phospholipids [5, 11, 32, 33]. In human gastric mucus, the lipids contain about 69% neutral lipids, 19% glycolipids, and 12% phospholipids (Table 2). The neutral lipids consist of free fatty acids, cholesterol, cholesteryl esters, and mono-, di-, and triglycerides, while the phospholipids are characterized by a high content of phosphatidylcholine, phosphatidylethanolamine, and sphingomyelin. The glycolipids of human gastric mucus consist mainly of glucoglycerolipids, and also contain up to 15% of glycosphingolipids, mainly glucosyl- and lactosylceramide, derived primarily from the exfoliating cells of gastric epithelium [6, 34].

The glycolipids which appear to be native constituents of gastric mucus, as well as mucous secretions of other parts of the alimentary tract, are glucoglycerolipids. These compounds differ from glycosphingolipids with respect to sugar

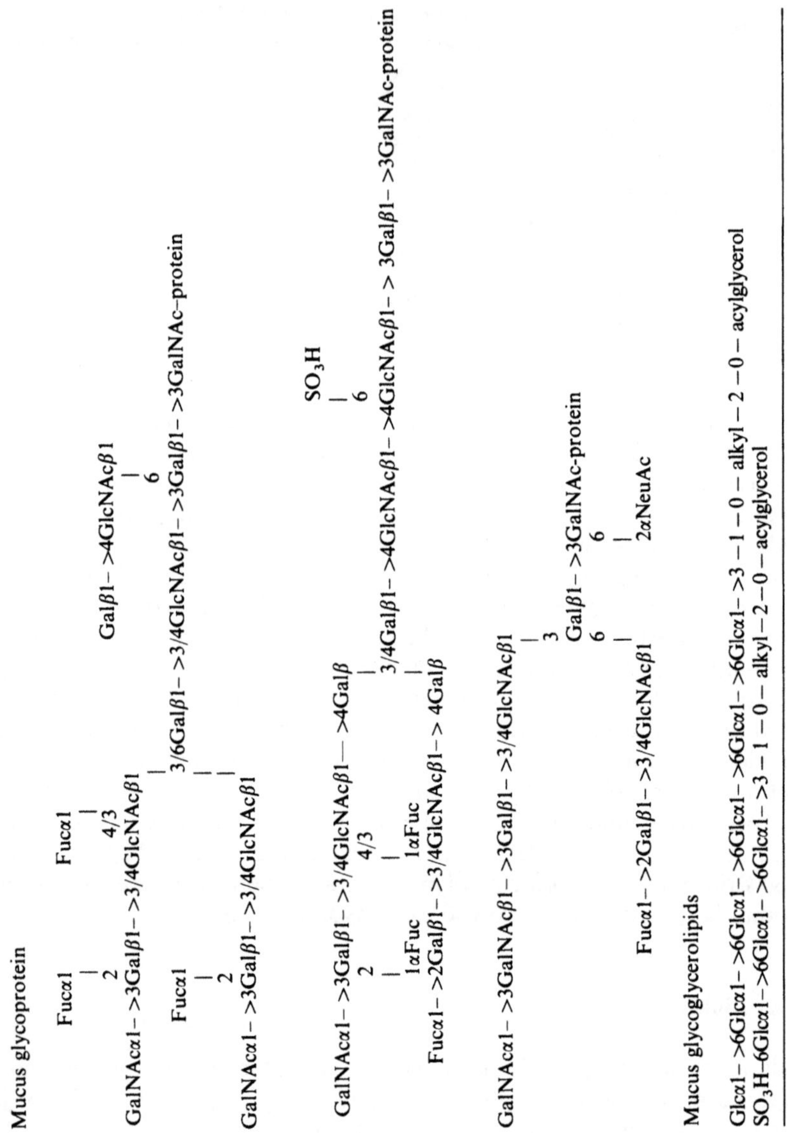

Fig. 3. Typical structures of the carbohydrate chains of mucus glycoproteins and glycolipids of the gastric mucus coat

composition and the nature of their lipid core. While the glycosphingolipids of gastric mucosa are composed of ceramide and one or more sugar residues [35, 36], the glucoglycerolipids found in mucous secretions constitute a group of neutral and sulfated compounds which are composed of a variable number (up to 8) of α(1,6)-linked glucose residues attached to C-3 of the monoalkylmonoacylglycerol lipid core. In sulfated glucoglycerolipids, the sulfate ester group is present at C-6 of the terminal glucose residue [37–39]. The sulfated glucoglycerolipids account for 40–45% of gastric mucus glyceroglucolipids and are represented mainly by tri- and tetraglucosyl compounds, while the neutral glucoglycerolipids of gastric mucus are characterized by the presence of large quantities of hexa- and octaglucosyl compounds (Fig. 3).

Mucus Coat Organization

Understanding the role of the mucus coat in gastric mucosal defense, and how its integrity becomes compromised by the aggressive forces, requires a thorough knowledge of mucus gel organization. The coat covers the gastric epithelium in the form of a continuous transparent layer, varies in thickness from 50 to 400 μm, and shows distinct mesomorphic properties. Unlike rigid gels, gastric mucus flows and anneals if sectioned, undergoes gel-sol transformation in response to changes in the luminal environment, and its strength varies depending upon the nature of interacting molecules. The matrix of the gel arises through noncovalent interaction between mucus glycoprotein polymer molecules [2], each of which consist of alternating glycosylated and nonglycosylated regions (Fig. 2), and the gel-forming properties of gastric mucin depend strongly on its polymeric structure, as proteolytically degraded or thiol reagent-reduced glycoprotein retains little, if any, gelling ability [14]. In addition to polymeric integrity, gel formation involves intra- and intermolecular interactions between the carbohydrate chains.

In the gastric lumen environment, mucus glycoprotein polymer exists in an expanded, highly hydrated form, capable of entering into heterotypic interaction with other constituents of the gel, particularly lipids [5, 6, 40, 41]. Two types of interactions between lipids and mucus glycoprotein can be distinguished within the gastric mucus: one in which lipids remain associated with the glycoprotein through hydrophobic forces and the other in which lipids exist in a covalent linkage with the glycoprotein (Fig. 4). In human gastric mucin, the covalently bound lipids account for 0.3% –0.4% of the glycoprotein dry weight and consist of fatty acids only, while the level of associated lipids reaches values of 21% or higher and their composition is considerably more complex (Table 3). Among the lipid classes found in association with human gastric mucin, the neutral lipids account for 56% of the total lipids, glycolipids 11%, and phospholipids 33% (Table 3).

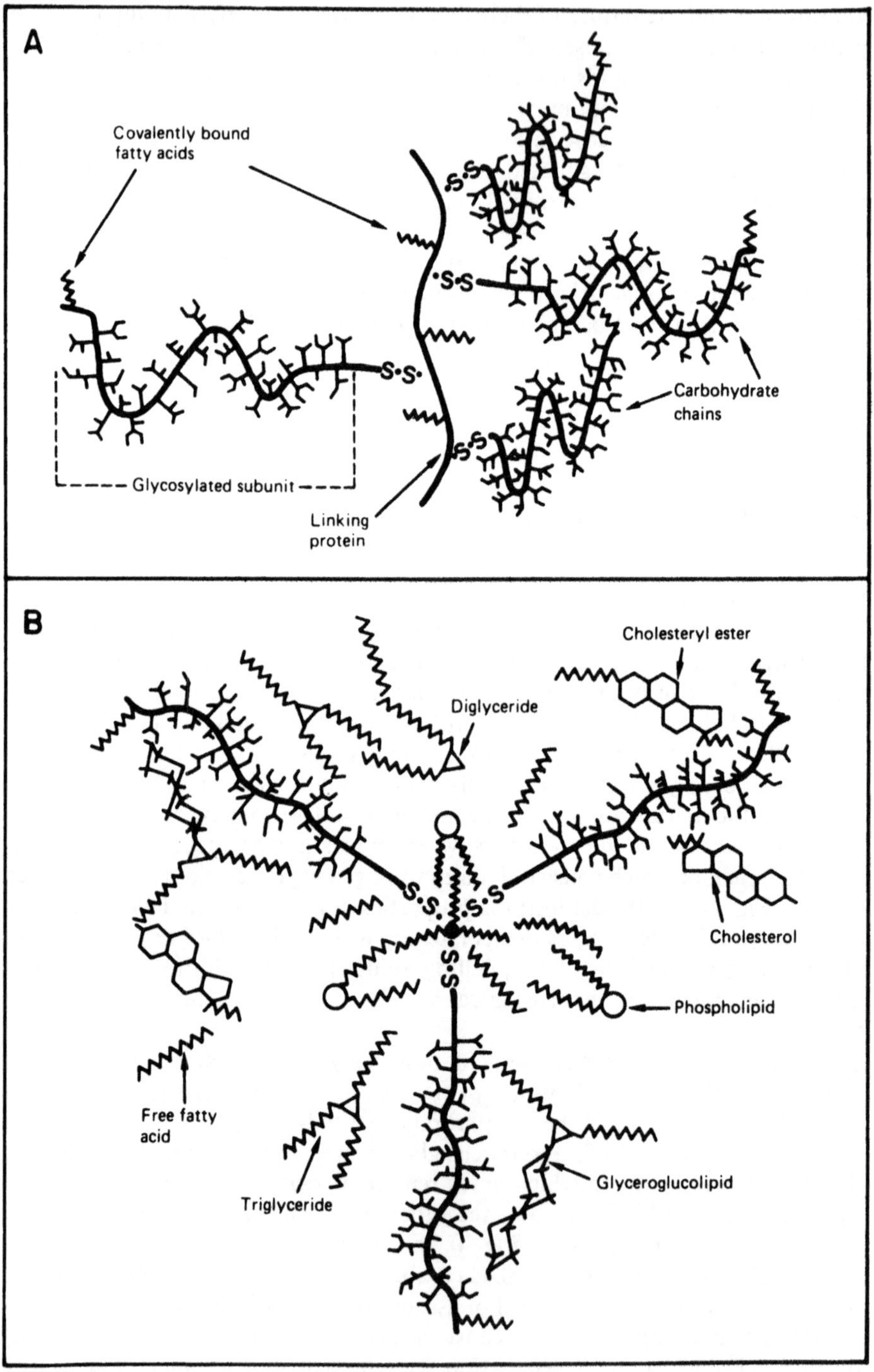

Fig. 4. A, B. Model of gastric mucus glycoprotein-lipid interaction. **A,** side view; **B,** top view.

Table 3. Chemical composition of human gastric mucus glycoprotein from healthy individuals and patients with gastric ulcer

Component	mg/100 mg mucus glycoprotein	
	Healthy	Gastric ulcer
Protein	12.4 ± 2.0	15.6 ± 2.2
Carbohydrate	62.5 ± 5.7	58.3 ± 5.5
Associated Lipids	20.9 ± 2.5	20.4 ± 2.3
Neutral lipids	11.6 ± 1.9	13.4 ± 1.8
Glycolipids	2.4 ± 0.4	2.1 ± 0.4
Phospholipids	6.9 ± 0.8	4.9 ± 0.6*
Covalently bound fatty acids	0.3 ± 0.1	0.1 ± 0.1*

Each value represents the mean ± SD of duplicate analyses performed on five individual samples from each group of subjects

Topography of Lipid–Mucin Interaction

The data on topography of lipids within the mucus glycoprotein polymer indicate that phospholipids interact with the glycoprotein through the non-glycosylated regions, while the interaction with glycolipids and neutral lipids appears to involve the peripheral regions of the glycoprotein molecule that are resistant to proteolytic cleavage [29, 34]. The extent of mucus glycoprotein interaction with the associated lipids is apparently determined by the content and distribution of covalently bound fatty acids [6]. At least four covalently bound fatty acids are present in the nonglycosylated regions of the glycoprotein polymer and one in proximity to the amino terminal of each subunit (Fig. 4). These fatty acids endow the molecule with hydrophobic centers which help to stabilize the extended macromolecular structure of mucus glycoprotein within the mucus coat. Furthermore, studies of gastric mucin topography with fluorescent probes indicate that a substantial number of binding sites in the glycoprotein polymer are buried within the central region of the molecule and become accessible only after reduction of the disulfide bridges.

From this, a concept is emerging according to which mucus glycoprotein polymer through its various hydrophobic and hydrophilic regions forms a dynamic continuum with other components of mucus. This multitude of interactions occurring within the gastric mucus coat ensures the resilience of this protective layer and at the same time makes it very sensitive to any changes in gastric lumen environment, including those taking place in gastropathy.

Multicomponential Nature of Mucus Coat

Although the involvement of gastric mucus proteins and lipids along with mucins in mucosal defense has been recognized since the early 1970s [1, 42], there are differences of opinion as to the way by which these proteins and lipids contribute to the protective function, and some even view the proteins and lipids of mucus coat as impurities [2] which affect detrimentally the physicochemical properties of mucus glycoprotein of the coat (Fig. 5). Others assign the protective function to the socalled "surface active phospholipids" (Fig. 6), supposedly forming an entity separate from other components of the mucus gel [43–45]. There are, however, data which clearly demonstrate that lipids and proteins are an integral part of the mucus gel [6, 13, 34–46, 47], which together with mucin form a dynamic continuum, and that this complex is responsible for the maintenance of gastric mucus coat integrity (Fig. 7). The concept of dynamic organization of the gastric mucus implies that the integrity and strength of the mucus coat could be disrupted not only through mucin degradation, but also through changes in mucus gel proteins and lipids.

Thus, the maintenance of the gastric mucosal defense system depends upon a delicate balance, controlled by factors affecting the elaboration and breakdown of all mucus constituents and not just that of "surface active phospholipids" or, for that matter, mucin only, as has been implied earlier [2, 45].

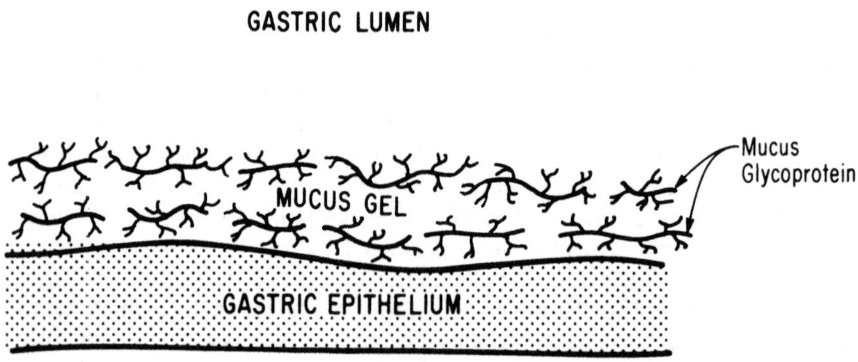

Fig. 5. "Mucin only" model of the gastric mucus barrier

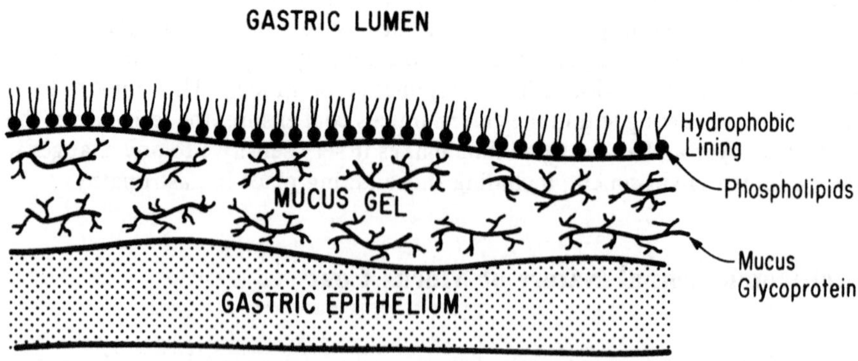

Fig. 6. "Surface active phospholipid" model of the gastric mucus barrier

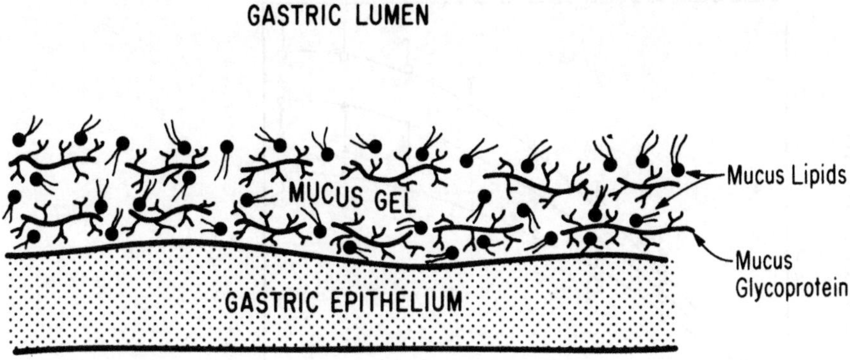

Fig. 7. "Dynamic Continuum" model of the gastric mucus barrier

Function of Mucus Coat Constituents

Extracellular localization and the relative ease with which the underlying epithelium controls the quality of the mucus makes this coat an ideal renewable protective component of the mucosal barrier. Yet, over the years, the protective functions of the mucous coat have been attributed solely to its mucin component (Fig. 5), and the protein and lipid constituents were considered to contribute little, if at all, to the physicochemical properties of this covering [14]. The results of more recent studies, however, demonstrate clearly that such major components of gastric mucus as lipids, albumin, secretory IgA, and fibronectin are capable of affecting many functional properties of mucus coat, such as viscosity and hydrophobicity maintenance, regulation of H^+ impedance, control of proteolytic aggression of pepsin, and management of bacterial proliferation.

Containment of Peptic Activity

The data obtained with lipids indicate that following extraction of associated lipids, the susceptibility of mucus glycoprotein to such bacterial protease as pronase increases by 27%, whereas the treatment of the delipidated and deacylated glycoprotein with pronase leads to its rapid and nearly complete degradation [48]. The effect of lipid removal on the proteolytic activity of pepsin towards gastric mucus glycoprotein is illustrated in Fig. 8. The apparent K_m value for intact mucus glycoprotein prior to removal of lipids was 0.9×10^{-6} *M*, and the glycoprotein following removal of associated lipids gave an apparent K_m value of 1.3×10^{-6}*M*. When the peptic activity assays were performed on the glycoprotein following removal of associated and covalently bound lipids,a K_m value of 2.3×10^{-6} *M* was obtained [29, 34].

Among the constituents of gastric mucus participating directly in the regulation of proteolytic activity of pepsin are sulfated mucus glycoproteins and

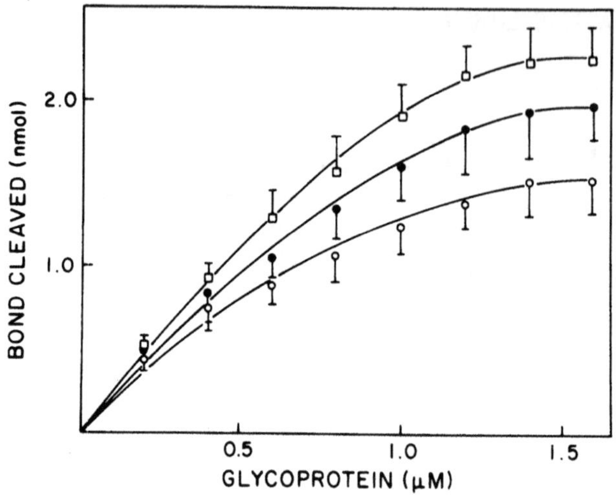

Fig. 8. Proteolytic activity of pepsin toward gastric mucus glycoprotein polymer. ○; Intact mucus glycoprotein. ●; glycoprotein following removal of associated lipids; □ glycoprotein following removal of associated and covalently bound lipids

glucoglycerolipids [49–51]. Moreover, sulfated glyceroglucolipids not only inhibit the proteolytic activity of pepsin, but also are capable of promoting the activation of pepsinogen at higher than normal pH and thus may control pepsin availability [51]. These properties of sulfated glucoglycerolipids and mucus glycoproteins are apparently due to the sulfate ester groups of carbohydrates, since desulfation renders both types of compounds ineffective as inhibitors of peptic activity.

Control of Bacterial Proliferation

The lipids existing in heterotypic and covalent interaction with mucus glycoproteins appear to play a crucial role in determining the properties of mucins, which are directly related to the ability of these glycoproteins to control bacterial adherence and aggregation. For example, salivary mucins of caries-resistant subjects, which are low in associated and covalently bound lipids, exhibit considerably higher bacterial aggregating activity than the lipid-rich mucin of saliva from caries-susceptible subjects [6, 48, 52].Consequently, mucus coat that is low in lipids would be expected to affect adversely mucosal colonization by bacteria, while the lipid-rich mucus could provide a more favorable milieu for bacterial infection.

Quite recently, evidence was obtained that sulfated glycoproteins and glyceroglucolipids of gastric mucus interfere with attachment of *H. pylori* to the mucosa, and that the resistance to the bacteria depends upon the gastric mucosal content of sulfated glycoproteins and glycolipids [13, 53].

Acid Impedance and Permselectivity

Another function of mucus coat constituents that appears to be directly affected by the content of lipids is mucosal permeability to various types of molecules. Studies indicate that the ability of gastric mucus to resist hydrogen ion penetration depends not only on the integrity of its mucin component, but even more on the content and composition of lipids [5, 6, 54–56]. The measurements indicate that extraction of associated lipids reduces the H^+ retardation capacity of gastric mucus glycoprotein by 60%–70%, and that a further 8%–12% loss in H^+ retardation capacity occurs following removal of covalently bound fatty acids (Fig. 9). Among the lipids associated with mucin, the greatest effect on the retardation capacity of mucin is exhibited by phospholipids, followed by glycolipids and neutral lipids [36]. Apparently, lipids associated with the nonglycosylated regions of the mucus glycoprotein molecule are capable of creating a strong hydrophobic environment which impedes the penetration of such hydrophilic substances as HCl. Perhaps that is why animals whose gastric mucosa has a higher content of lipids more easily resist acid challenge [6, 57]. There are also indications that lipids adversely affect the permeability of mucus to larger molecules, such as lactate and glucose [58]. Furthermore, preincubation of mucin with serum albumin or IgA leads to an increase in the ability of the glycoprotein to retard the diffusion of H^+ [56].

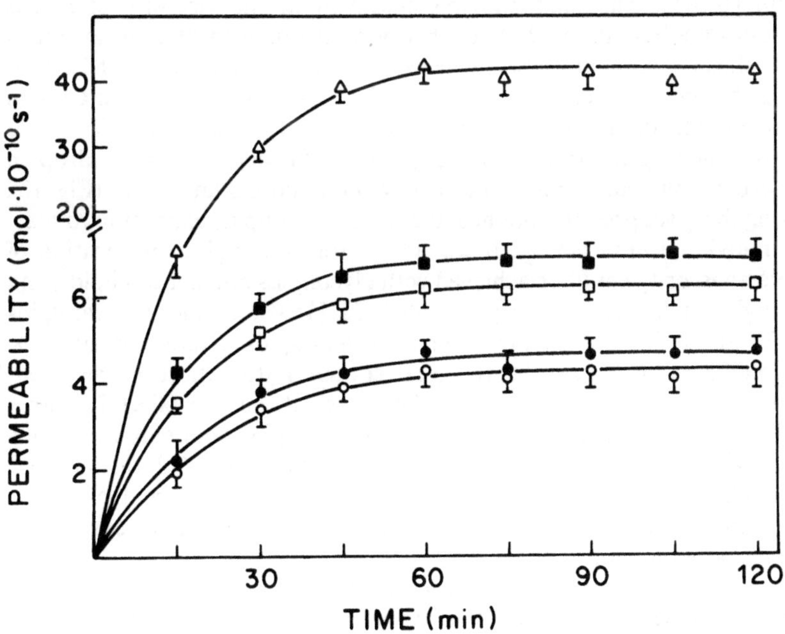

Fig. 9. Effect of lipids on the permeability of gastric mucus glycoprotein to hydrogen ion. ○; Intact mucin; □ mucin following extraction of associated lipids ■; mucin following removal of associated and covalently bound lipids ● lipid-reassociated mucin; △ saline control.

Studies on the diffusion of H^+ in gastric mucin show that the ability of mucus to resist penetration by hydrophilic substances increases with deglycosylation. The changes in acid impedance were most pronounced following the removal of sulfate and sialic acid [34, 39]. These data thus seem to indicate that mucous gel permeability could be influenced by the size and composition of carbohydrate chains of mucin.

Contrary to earlier claims that gastric mucus coat is not permeable to molecules larger than vitamin B_{12}(e.g., myoglobin, molecular weight 17 kDa), studies conducted in a specially constructed permeability chamber [87] revealed that,the mucus layer is permeable to molecules as large as pepsin (38 kDa) and horseradish peroxidase (44 kDa), but the diffusion rate of these molecules through mucus is about 15 times slower than that through the unstirred layer of saline [6, 60]. In contrast to H^+ diffusion, however , the retardation capacity of mucus to these large molecules is not affected by extraction of lipids [60].

Viscoelastic Properties

Although mucus glycoprotein is the only component of mucus coat capable of gel formation, there are strong indications that the viscoelastic properties of mucus are greatly influenced by the content and composition of associated and covalently bound lipids, and such proteins as albumin, secretory IgA and fibronectin [6, 61]. The maximum enhancement in the viscosity of mucus glycoprotein by albumin and IgA, furthermore, is obtained at concentrations similar to those found for these proteins in gastric secretion [62, 63], thus suggesting the physiological significance of the effect. The data obtained with gastric mucin indicate that extraction of associated lipids causes an 80%–85% decrease in mucus glycoprotein viscosity; and a further 35%–40% drop in viscosity occurs following removal of the covalently bound fatty acids (Fig. 10). By allowing the glycoprotein obtained after associated-lipids extraction to react with the individual lipid classes, it was found that the highest restoration of glycoprotein viscosity could be achieved with glycolipids and neutral lipids, and the next highest followed by phospholipids [63]. However, since neutral lipids account for about 50% of the mucus glycoprotein lipids, glycolipids for 35%, and phospholipids for 12%–15%, the greatest quantitative effect on the glycoprotein viscosity is exerted by phospholipids, which has an effect 2.5 times greater than that of neutral lipids and glycolipids. As phospholipids are known to interact with the nonglycosylated regions of mucin [6, 40, 41], the fact that phospholipids have the strongest effect on mucin viscosity may be due to their ability to stabilize the extended macromolecular structure of the glycoprotein in the aqueous environment.

While proteins and lipids exert a significant effect on the physicochemical characteristics of the gastric mucus, it is important to bear in mind that mucin is the only constituent of mucus that is capable of gel formation [2]. This property of mucus glycoprotein arises from its ability to exist in the aqueous environment of the gastrointestinal tract in a hydrated, highly expanded form requiring a

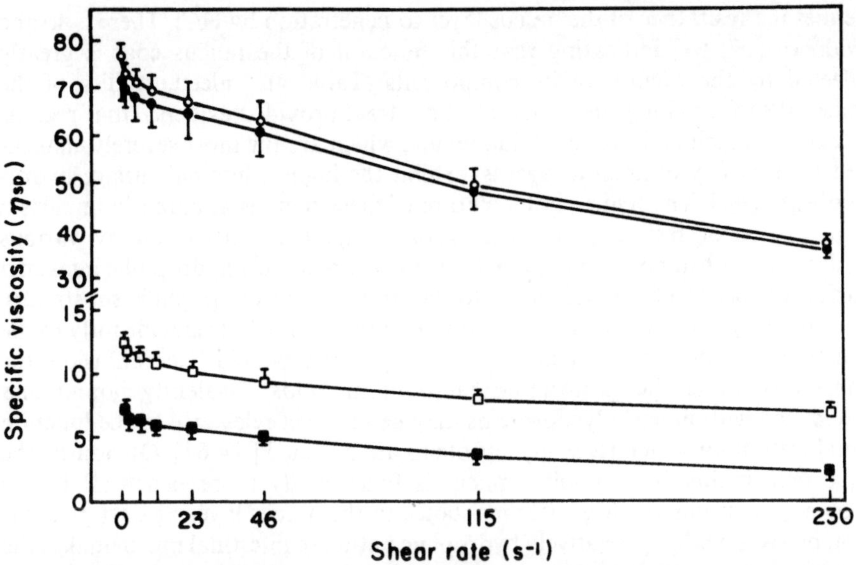

Fig. 10. Effect of associated and covalently bound lipids on the viscosity gastric mucus glycoprotein; ○ Intact mucus glycoprotein; □ glycoprotein following extraction of associated lipids; ■ delipidated glycoprotein following removal of covalently bound fatty acids; ● delipidated glycoprotein following reassociation with associated lipids

large volume. Gel formation apparently occurs as a result of increasing intermolecular interactions driven by a concentration gradient. The gel-forming properties of gastric mucin depend strongly on its polymeric structure, as proteolytically degraded or thiol reagent-reduced glycoprotein retains little, if any gelling ability [2, 63]. In addition to polymeric integrity, gel formation involves intra- and intermolecular interactions between the carbohydrate chains, which create a strongly anionic environment due to the presence of carboxyl and sulfate ester groups [6].

The data on the role of carbohydrates in the maintenance of mucus coat rheology show that viscosity of mucus glycoprotein decreases most drastically following removal of sulfate and sialic acid [34, 59]. A 25% drop in the viscosity of gastric mucin takes place after the cleavage of sulfate ester groups, and an 18% loss in viscosity occurs following removal of sialic acid with neuraminidase. However, the cleavage of peripheral sugars, such as fucose, galactose, or *N*-acetylgalactosamine has a barely discernible effect [34, 59]. On the other hand, extensive deglycosylation (removal of 86% carbohydrate) reduces the glycoprotein viscosity by as much as 40%.

Mucosal Hydrophobicity

Among the physical properties of the gastric mucus coat directly affected by its lipid and protein makeup is the mucosal hydrophobicity, a parameter which defines the resistance of the mucus layer to penetration by HCl. There is strong evidence [57, 64] indicating that this function of the mucus coat is greatly affected by the quality of its components (Table 4). Indeed, studies of the mucosal surface along the gastrointestinal tract provided evidence that regions like the stomach and proximal duodenum, which are the most severely challenged by a variety of noxious agents, exhibit the highest luminal surface hydrophobicity [43]. The hydrophobic nature of these regions apparently imparts a high degree of resistance to their surfaces against penetration by various hydrophilic substances including HCl, while the relatively hydrophilic intestinal surfaces appear to be better suited to the containment of lipophilic substances.

In the light of existing information that lipids contribute significantly to the functional properties of mucins such as impedance of acid back diffusion, the variations along the gastrointestinal tract in lipids covalently bound and associated with mucus glycoproteins may be of direct relevance to the function and location for which these glycoproteins are destined [57, 64]. Obviously, the lipid-rich, highly hydrophobic mucin is functionally more beneficial in the stomach, as it imparts a greater resistance to the mucus layer against penetration by HCl, while the relatively hydrophlic nature of intestinal mucin makes the intestinal region of the gastrointestinal tract better suited than the stomach to the containment of lipophilic bile constituents, but less resistant to acid.

Although the hydrophobicity of the mucosal surface can be directly assessed using the goniometric technique [43–45], evaluation of the hydrophobic characteristics of mucus coat glycoproteins and lipids requires a different approach, namely the use of fluorescent hydrophobic probes. The results obtained using the Bis-ANS probe [47, 65] revealed that the number of binding sites available on the gastric mucin molecule varies depending upon the pH of the environment, being highest at pH 2.0 and lowest at pH 9.0, and that associated lipids and covalently bound fatty acids affect the hydrophobic binding capacity of the glycoprotein (Fig. 11). Analyses of fluorescence titration data showed that the extraction of associated lipids, which are known to interact with mucus glycoprotein polymer mainly through the nonglycosylated regions [6], causes a 30% increase in binding capacity of the glycoprotein for the probe. The

Table 4. Content and composition of mucus glycoprotein and lipid in mucus along the gastrointestinal tract

Location	Mucin (mg/100 mg mucus)	Component (mg/100 mg mucin)			
		Protein	Carbohydrate	Associated lipids	Covalently bound fatty acids
Fundus	13.4	19.1	54.6	23.8	0.4
Antrum	13.2	19.5	54.4	22.5	0.4
Proximal duodenum	8.0	22.7	56.9	15.1	0.3
Distal duodenum	6.8	23.4	56.7	13.4	0.2
Midjejunum	6.9	24.9	58.5	12.3	0.2

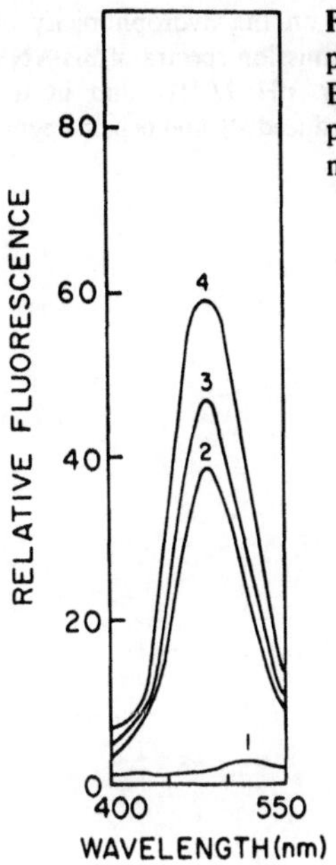

Fig. 11. Effect of associated and covalently bound lipids on the hydrophobicity of gastric mucus glycoprotein. Fluorescence emission spectra of Bis-ANS in 0.10 *M* NaCl/0.05 *M* phosphate buffer, pH 7.0 (1), and in the presence of intact (2), delipidated (4), and delipidated and deacylated (3) mucus glycoprotein

measurements performed on the glycoprotein devoid of covalently bound fatty acid revealed a 26% decrease in the number of hydrophobic sites available for Bis-ANS binding (Fig. 11) demonstrating that covalently bound fatty acids make a considerable contribution to the hydrophobicity of gastric mucus glycoprotein. It should be noted, however, that while the removal of covalently bound fatty acids reduced the hydrophobicity of gastric mucus glycoprotein, the delipidated and deacylated glycoprotein still showed the capacity for Bis-ANS binding.

To ascertain whether these binding sites reside on glycosylated or nonglycosylated regions of the gastric mucin molecule, the glycoprotein was subjected to disulfide bridge reduction and peptic degradation [47, 65]. The data obtained with pepsin-degraded glycoprotein revealed that destruction of the naked protein regions of the mucin molecule essentially abolished the probe binding, whereas the reduction of disulfide bridges resulted in glycoprotein subunits whose number of hydrophobic binding sites were 27% lower than those of the mucin polymer (Fig. 12). These results provide strong evidence that the majority of hydrophobic binding sites exist in the nonglycosylated protease-susceptible regions of the gastric mucus glycoprotein.

The finding that variation in the hydrophobicity of the mucosal surfaces of the gastrointestinal tract results from the interaction of mucus lipids with the glycoprotein is supported by the results obtained with the gastrointestinal tract surface using goniometric procedures [43–45]. The authors of these papers, however, ascribe the hydrophobic properties of the mucosal surface to a separate entity, namely phospholipids supposedly overlying the mucus gel (Fig. 6). As mucus constituents of gastric mucosal barrier form a dynamic continuum

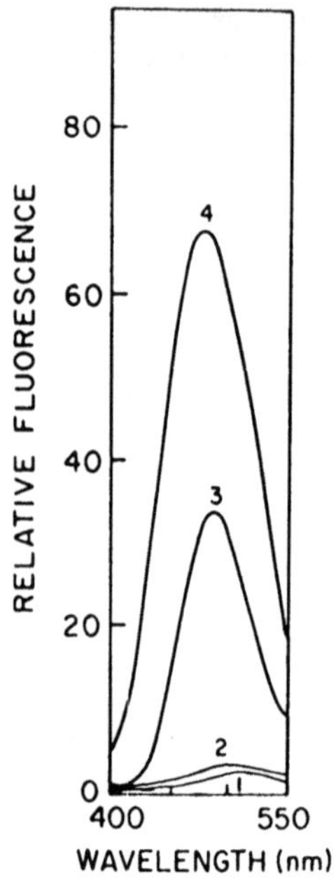

Fig. 12. Effect of proteolytic degradation on the hydrophobicity of gastric mucus glycoprotein. Fluorescence emission spectra of Bis-ANS in 0.10 *M* NaCl/0.05 *M* phosphate buffer, pH 7.0 (1), and in the presence of intact (3), β-mercaptoethanol-reduced (4), and pepsin degraded (2) mucus glyco-protein

(Fig. 7) rather than existing as independent entities, assignment of the protective function either to lipids or mucus glycoprotein alone certainly narrows and distorts the concept of the multicomponential nature of gastric mucosal protection.

Mucus Coat Integrity and Gastric Disease

Although the loss of gastric mucus coat integrity has long been associated with the onset of gastric disease [1–3], this process until recently was attributed primarily to the enhanced activity of intragastric pepsin and the lipolytic enzymes brought by duodenal reflux. This situation has changed drastically in recent years, as evidence was provided that *H. pylori*, a gastric pathogen, through the action of its protease and lipase enzymes may also detrimentally affect the integrity of the gastric mucus.

Changes in Mucus in Gastric Ulcer

Analyses of human gastric mucus [66–69] indicate that in healthy individuals, the mucus coat contains about 64% protein, 15% carbohydrate, 12.5% neutral lipids, 3.4% glycolipids, and 2.2% phospholipids. In patients with gastric ulcer, the coat shows a somewhat higher content of proteins, glycolipids, and phospholipids, but contains less glycoprotein (Table 2). Furthermore, the mucus glycoprotein constituent of the coat from these patients exhibits a higher proportion of the low-molecular-weight mucus glycoprotein form (Fig. 13), which is known to display diminished protective physicochemical properties. Indeed, the measurements of mucus H^+ retardation capacity indicate that patients with gastric ulcer show a 1.5-fold reduction in the ability of the mucus coat to resist acid diffusion (Fig. 14), and display about 60% lower viscosity than the mucus coat in the healthy individuals (Fig. 15).

Considerable differences are also observed in the chemical composition and physical properties of the high-molecular-weight mucus glycoprotein form between the mucus of healthy individuals and patients with gastric ulcer [68, 69]. This glycoprotein from patients with gastric ulcer, while showing a similar

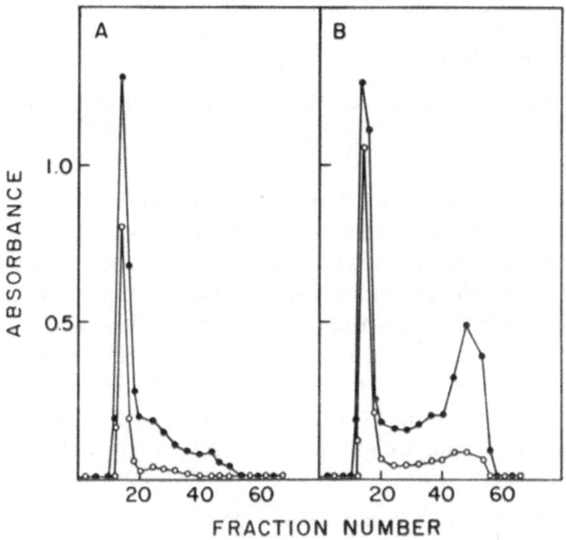

Fig. 13. Mucus glycoprotein molecular forms in human gastric mucus from healthy individuals (**A**) and patients with gastric ulcer (**B**). ○ Protein; ● carbohydrate

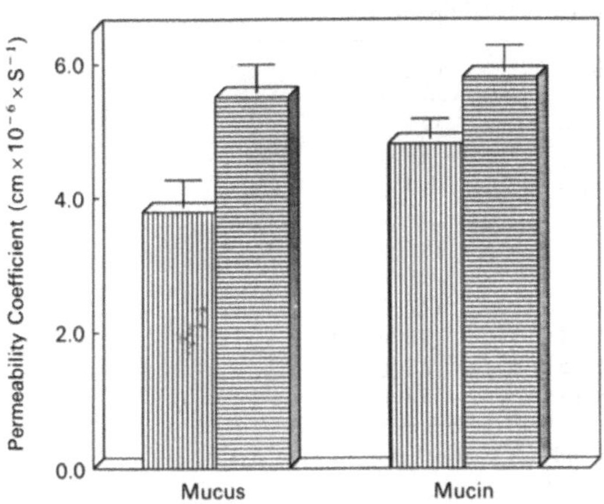

Fig. 14. Hydrogen ion retardation capacity of human gastric mucus and mucus glycoprotein from healthy individuals (||||) and patients with gastric ulcer (≡)

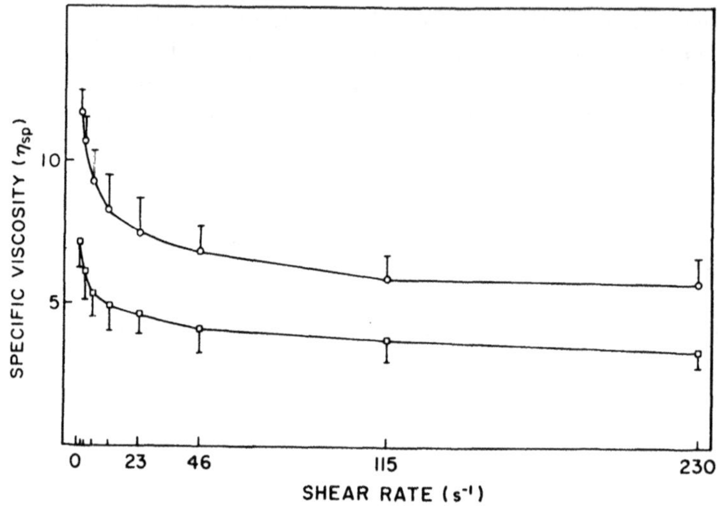

Fig. 15. Viscosity of human gastric mucus from healthy individuals (○) and patients with gastric ulcer (□)

content of protein and carbohydrate, displays a marked decrease in the content of covalently bound fatty acids and the dissociated phospholipids (Table 3). Moreover, the phospholipid composition in the glycoprotein from patients with gastric ulcer differs from that in healthy individuals with respect to the content of phosphatidylcholine, phosphatidylethanolamine, lysophosphatidylcholine, and lysophosphatidylethanolamine (Table 5). The glycoprotein from healthy individuals shows a higher level of phosphatidylcholine and phosphatidylethanolamine, while the content of lysophospholipids is greater among the phospholipids associated with the high-molecular-weight mucus glycoprotein derived

Table 5. Composition of phospholipids associated with gastric mucus glycoprotein in mucus coat of healthy individuals and patients with gastric ulcer

Phospholipid	Percentage of total lipid phosphorus	
	Healthy	Gastric ulcer
Phosphatidylcholine	25.7 ± 2.9	18.4 ± 2.1*
Phosphatidylethanolamine	13.4 ± 1.5	8.5 ± 0.9*
Phosphatidylserine	8.6 ± 0.9	6.1 ± 0.8
Phosphatidylinositol	3.1 ± 0.4	3.5 ± 0.5
Sphingomyelin	18.5 ± 2.0	18.2 ± 2.1
Phosphatidic acid	5.1 ± 0.4	5.0 ± 0.7
Lysophosphatidylcholine	8.3 ± 0.9	17.6 ± 1.9*
Lysophosphatidylethanol amine	6.6 ± 0.8	13.9 ± 1.6*
Diphosphatidylglycerol	3.8 ± 0.5	3.5 ± 0.5
Unidentified	6.9 ± 0.8	5.3 ± 0.7

Each value represents the mean ± SD of duplicate analyses performed on five individual samples from each group of subjects

from gastric mucus of patients with gastric ulcer. As a consequence of these compositional differences, the mucus glycoprotein from patients with gastric ulcer exhibits a 20% reduction in H^+ retardation capacity (Fig. 14), an 80% decrease in viscosity (Fig. 16), and about 40% loss in hydrophobicity (Fig. 17).

While the extent of changes in the physicochemical properties of the gastric mucus coat may vary with the disease, the culminative result is undoubtedly the loss of gastric mucus coat integrity and hence the severe weakening of mucosal defense capacity.

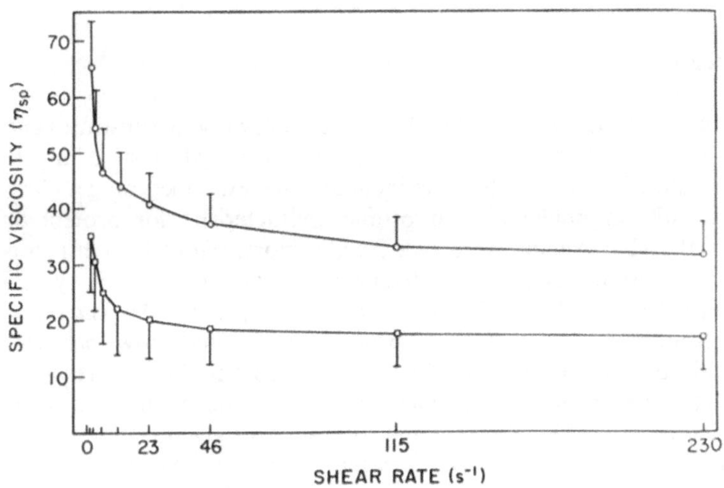

Fig. 16. Viscosity of human gastric mucus glycoprotein isolate from gastric mucus coat of healthy individuals (○) and patients with gastric ulcer (□)

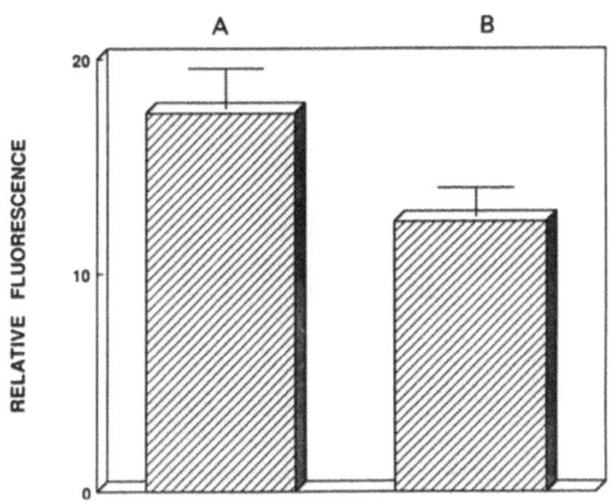

Fig. 17. Hydrophobicity of human gastric mucus glycoprotein purified from gastric mucus coat of healthy individuals (A) and patients with gastric ulcer (B). Fluorescence measurements were conducted with the fluorescent hydrophobic probe Bis-ANS

H. pylori and Gastric Mucus

Although, aside from peptic degradation, the weakening of gastric mucus coat integrity could result from such factors as the reflux of duodenal contents, which are rich in a variety of degradative enzymes, and through the intake of noxious substances such as alcohol, there is an increasing evidence that a bacterium, *H. pylori*, also plays a prominent role in this disruptive process. studies focused on this gastric pathogen demonstrated that it elaborates extracellular enzymes capable of gastric mucus coat glycoprotein and lipid degradation [13, 18, 19, 70–75].

H. pylori Protease

Assays of enzyme activities conducted with a battery of synthetic substrates and gastric mucin established that *H. pylori* does not cause hydrolysis of mucin carbohydrate chains. However, when the incubate was examined on gel chromatography, a shift in mucin elution profile characteristic for proteolytic degradation of the glycoprotein occurred. Furthermore, parallel experiments indicated that the enzyme also caused extensive degradation of such typical protein as albumin [70, 71]. The *H. pylori* protease appears to be associated with a low-molecular-weight ($<$ 50 KDa) protein fraction and shows behavior typical of metalloproteinase [18, 19]. Thus, it is apparent that the result of *H. pylori* protease action on gastric mucin may be the disintegration of the polymeric structure of the glycoprotein and formation of glycopeptides which no longer possess the viscous and gel-forming properties, and exhibit only limited ability for acid impedance. The erosion of mucus glycoprotein polymer, which constitutes the gel matrix, may, indeed, be of dire consequence to the mucosal integrity. Moreover, the challenge on the luminal side by acid and pepsin, and on the mucosal side by *H. pylori* protease, could render the stomach epithelium vulnerable to damage by luminal contents (Fig. 18).

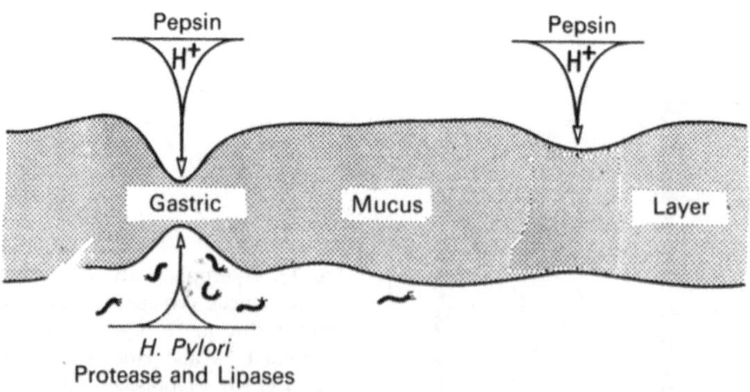

Fig. 18. Concerted action of pepsin and *H. pylori* enzymes on the integrity of gastric mucus coat

H. pylori Lipase

Two lipolytic enzymes, triglyceride lipase and phospholipase A_2, were identified in the extracellular material elaborated by *H. pylori* [72, 73]. The lipase attains its maximum activity at 37°C and a pH of 7.2, while the phospholipase A_2 causes maximum conversion of phosphatidylcholine substrate to free fatty acid and lysophosphatidylcholine at the pH range of 7.0–7.4 and 37°C [18, 19]. The incubation of gastric mucus neutral lipids with *H. pylori* enzymes leads to a 15% increase in free fatty acids, 2.8-fold increase in mono- and diglycerides, and 4.8-fold decrease in triglycerides. The phospholipids of the gastric mucus following incubation with *H. pylori* show the conversion of phosphatidylcholine to lysophosphatidylcholine and of phosphatidylethanolamine to lysophosphatidylehanolamine (Table 6).

As mucus lipids and phospholipids in particular contribute to the integrity and resilience of gastric mucosal defense [6, 13], and are responsible for the

Table 6. Effect of *H. pylori* lipases on lipids of human gastric , mucus coat

Lipid	Control	*H. pylori*
Neutral lipids (% of total neutral lipids)		
Free fatty acids	46.1	61.8
Mono- and diglycerides	4.2	10.9
Triglycerides	25.3	3.8
Phospholipids (% of total lipid phosphorus)		
Phosphatidylcholine	31.7	5.4
Phosphatidylethanolamine	15.6	4.1
Sphingomyelin	11.8	12.1
Lysophosphatidylcholine	13.1	27.4
Lysophosphatidylethanolamine	0.7	13.6

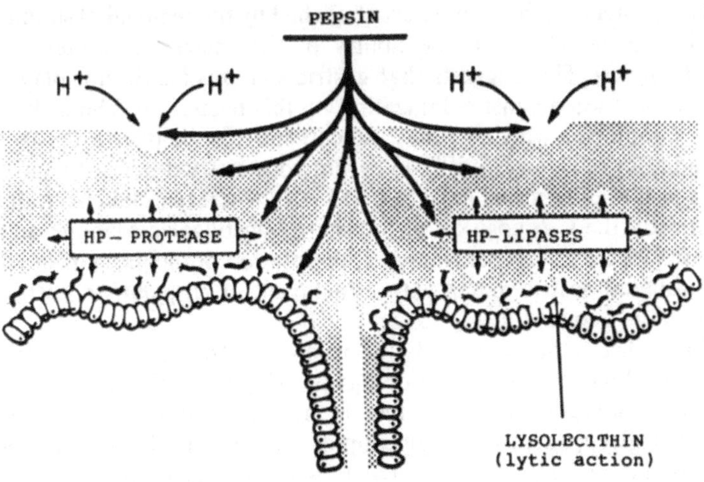

Fig. 19. Aggressive forces affecting the integrity of the gastric mucosal defense

maintenance of the mucus hydrophobicity [43, 47, 55, 65], the alterations in lipids caused by *H. pylori* lipases may be of serious consequence to the mucosal defense. Furthermore, an increase in lysolecithin level due to *H. pylori* phospholipase A_2 offsets the ratio of this lipid to other phospholipids, leading to a drastic change in the lytic activity of the lysophospholipid towards gastric epithelium and the mucus coat [13]. The lipolytic activity of *H. pylori* could, thus, be detrimental at the same time to the mucus layer and the cell membranes of gastric epithelium (Fig. 19).

Role of Gastric Mucin in the Resistance to *H. pylori*

The protective role of mucins as an essential element of mucosal defense against bacterial colonization is well recognized. As a constituent of the mucus layer, these glycoproteins not only pose a passive physical obstacle, but also actively interfere with attachment to the epithelial cell surfaces by many bacteria [6]. Studies indicate that, because of similarities in the structure of their carbohydrate chains to those present on the receptor sites of the cell surface, salivary and gastrointestinal mucins are potent inhibitors of bacterial adherence and show a strong aggregating activity towards a variety of bacteria [15, 76].

The data obtained recently demonstrate that among the constituent of human gastric mucus capable of interfering with *H. pylori* attachment are mucus glycoprotein and glucoglycerolipids [13, 53, 77]. This property of mucin and glycolipids is apparently associated with the acidic component, as the mucin fraction enriched in sialic acid and sulfate showed a 16-fold greater inhibitory titer than the intact mucin. However, while the inhibitory titer of glucoglycerolipid and the glycoprotein can be completely abolished by the removal of sulfate, the desialylation has no effect on the ability of the mucin to inhibit the aggregation of *H. pylori*. This suggests that gastric sialomucins do not play a role in mucosal protection against colonization by this bacterium. The lack of interference by sialomucins with *H. pylori* attachment may be due to the fact that *H. pylori* adhesin recognizes only the carbohydrate structures with sialic acid substituted at C-3 of terminal galactose [13, 78], whereas in mucins sialic acid occupies mostly the C-6 position of internal *N*-acetylgalactosamine and internal galactose [15, 22–27]. A schematic representation of the mechanism of interference by sulfated gastric mucin with attachment of *H. pylori* to gastric mucosal epithelium is depicted in Fig. 20.

These findings clearly point towards the role of gastric sulfomucins and sulfated glucoglycerolipids in the protection against *H. pylori* colonization and suggest that the mucosal resistance to this bacteria may depend upon the mucus content of sulfated glycoproteins and glycolipids. Indeed, the importance of sulfated glycoproteins and glycolipids in the preservation of gastric mucosal integrity is evident from the studies showing that a decrease in the synthesis of sulfated glycolipids accompanies the development of gastritis, and a decline in

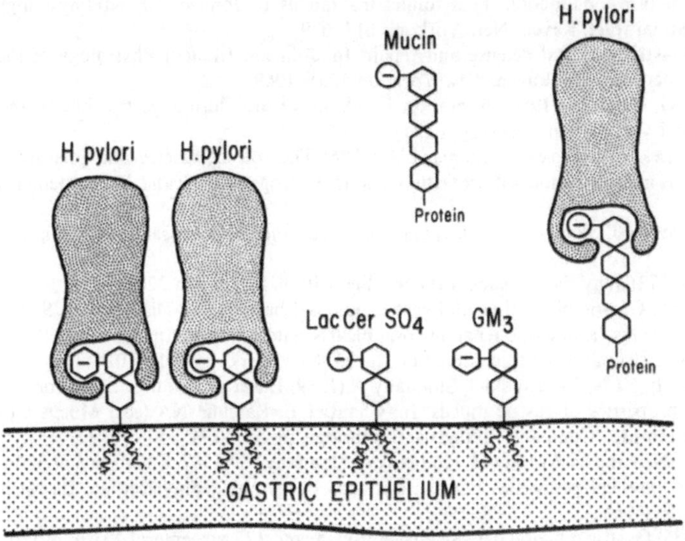

Fig. 20. Mechanism of interference by sulfated gastric mucus glycoprotein in the attachment of *H. pylori* to gastric mucosa.

sulfated mucus glycoprotein content is a prominent feature in the etiology of peptic ulcer [1, 13, 79–81].

Most recent studies indicate that *H.pylori* may be capable of overcoming the mucosal defenses offered by sulfated glycoproteins and glucoglycerolipids of mucus, as the bacterium displays a strong glycosulfatase activity [74, 75]. The data on the enzyme specificity revealed that the sulfatase is capable of removing the sulfate ester groups from *N*-acetylglucosamine-6-sulfate, as well as galactose-6-sulfate [74]. Both these sulfated sugars are known to be present in the carbohydrate chains of gastric mucus glycoproteins [22–27, 35, 81]. The *H. pylori* glycosulfatase is also effective in the desulfation of glucose-6-sulfate, a constituent of gastric mucus gluceroglucolipids [35], but ineffective towards galactosylceramide and lactosylceramide sulfates, which contain the sulfate ester group on C-3 of galactose [35]. These two glycolipids constitute the major sulfated glycosphingolipid species of the cell membranes of gastric epithelium [35, 82], and are known to mediate the *H. pylori* attachment to gastric mucosa [13, 78]. There is also evidence that *H. pylori* interferes with the synthesis and secretion of gastric sulfomucin [83, 84]. This reinforces further the long-held consensus as to the importance of sulfated glycoproteins and glycolipids in the maintenance of gastric mucosal integrity in health and disease.

References

1. Glass GBJ, Slomiany BL (1977) Derangement of biosynthesis, production and secretion of mucus in gastrointestinal injury and disease. In: Elstein M, Parke DV (eds) Mucus in health and disease. Plenum, New York, pp 322–347

2. Allen A (1981) Structure and function of gastrointestinal mucus. In: Johnson LR (ed) Physiology of the gastrointestinal tract. Raven, New York, pp 617–639
3. Silen W (1987) Gastric mucosal defense and repair. In: Johnson LR (ed) Physiology of the gastrointestinal tract, 2nd edn. Raven, New York, pp 1055–1069
4. Szabo S, Pihan G, Triers S (1986) Alteration in blood vessels during gastric injury and protection. Scand J Gastroenterol 21 (suppl 125): 92–96
5. Slomiany BL, Piasek A, Sarosiek J, Slomiany A (1986) The role of surface and preformed intracellular mucus in gastric mucosal protection against hydrogen ion. Scand J Gastroenterol 20:1191–1196
6. Slomiany BL, Sarosiek J, Slomiany A (1987) Gastric mucus and the mucosal barrier. Dig Dis 5:125--145
7. Davenport HW (1972) Why the stomach does not digest itself. Scient Am 226:87–93
8. Jacobson ED (1985) Gastric blood flow and gastric mucosal barrier. Dig Dis Sci 30:77S–80S
9. Flemstrom G (1987) Gastric and duodenal mucosal bicarbonate secretion. In: Johnson LR (ed) Physiology of the gastrointestinal tract, 2nd edn. Raven, New York, pp 1011–1029
10. Slomiany BL, Murty VLN, Piotrowski J, Slomiany A (1989) Effect of antiulcer agents on the physicochemical properties of gastric mucus. In: Chantler E, Ratcliffe NA (eds) Mucus and related topics. Cambridge Company Biologists, Cambridge, pp 179–191
11. Bilski J, Murty VLN, Aono M, Moriga M, Slomiany A, Slomiany BL (1987) Enhancement of the lipid content and physical properties of gastric mucus by geranylgeranylacetone. Biochem Pharmacol 36:4059–4065
12. Turnberg LA (1985) Gastric mucosal defense mechanism. Scand J Gastroenterol 20 (suppl 110): 37–40
13. Slomiany BL, Slomiany A (1991) Role of mucus in gastric mucosal protection. J Physiol Pharmacol 42:147–161 .
14. Allen A (1983) Mucus: a protective secretion of complexity. Trends Biochem Sci 8:163–173
15. Neutra MR, Forstner JF (1987) Gastrointestinal mucus synthesis, secretion and function. In: Johnson LR (ed) Physiology of the gastrointestinal tract, Vol 2, 2nd edn. Raven, New York, vol 2; pp 975–1009
16. Venables CW (1986) Mucus, pepsin and peptic ulcer. Gut 27:233–238
17. Slomiany BL, Glass GBJ, Kojima K, Banas-Gruszka Z, Slomiany A (1982) Effect of lysolecithin on the constituents of gastric mucus. In: Chandler EN, Elder JB, Elstin M (eds) Mucus in health and disease II. Plenum, New York, pp 163–174
18. Slomiany BL, Slomiany A (1992) Mechanism of Helicobacter pylori pathogenesis: focus on mucus. J Clin Gastroenterol 14 suppl 110: 37–40
19. Slomiany BL, Murty VLN, Piotrowski J, Wang SL, Slomiany A (1991) Helicobacter pylori and gastric mucus integrity. In: Menge H et al. (eds) Helicobacter pylori 1990. Springer, Berlin, Heidelberg New York, pp 37–51
20. Slomiany BL, Slomiany A (1984) Lipids of mucous secretions of the alimentary tract. In: Boedeker EG (ed) Attachment of organisms to the gut mucosa. CRC, Boca Raton, vol 2 pp 23–31
21. Slomiany BL, Sarosiek J, Slomiany A (1984) Lipids of salivary and gastrointestinal mucus. NY Med Q 4:124–130
22. Slomiany BL, Meyer K (1972) Isolation and structural studies of sulfated glycoproteins of hog gastric mucosa. J Biol Chem 247:5062–5070
23. Slomiany BL, Zebska E, Slomiany A (1984) Structural characterization of neutral oligosaccharides of human $H^{+}Le^{b+}$ gastric mucin. J Biol Chem 259:2863–2869
24. Slomiany A, Zdebska E, Slomiany BL (1984) Structures of the neutral oligosaccharides isolated from A-active human gastric mucin. J Biol Chem 259:14743–14749
25. Slomiany BL, Meyer K (1973) Oligosaccharides produced by acetolysis of blood group active (A + H) sulfated glycoprotein from hog gastric mucosa. J Biol Chem 248:2290–2295
26. Slomiany BL, Banas-Gruszka Z, Zdebska E, Slomiany A (1982) Characterization of the Forssman-active oligosaccharides from dog gastric mucus glycoprotein isolated with the use of monoclonal antibody. J Biol Chem 257:9561–9565
27. Carter SR, Slomiany A, Gwozdzinski K, Liau YH, Slomiany BL (1988) Enzymatic sulfation of mucus glycoprotein in gastric mucosa. J Biol Chem 263:11977–11984

28. Slomiany BL, Liau YH, Piasek A, Slomiany A (1985) Effect of ethanol on mucus glycoprotein fatty acyltransferase from gastric mucosa. Biochemistry 24:3514–3521
29. Slomiany A, Jozwiak Z, Takagi A, Slomiany BL (1989) The role of covalently bound fatty acids in the degradation of human gastric mucus glycoprotein. Archs Biochem Biophys 229:560–567
30. Slomiany BL, Takagi A, Liau YH, Jozwiak Z, Slomiany A (1984) In vitro acylation of rat gastric mucus glycoprotein with [H] palmitic acid. J Biol Chem 259:11997–12000
31. Slomiany A, Witas H, Aono M, Slomiany BL (1983) Covalently linked fatty acids in gastric mucus glycoprotein of cystic fibrosis patients. J Biol Chem 258:8535–8538
32. Piotrowski J, Bilski J, Nishikawa H, Slomiany A, Slomiany BL (1990) Enhancement in gastric mucus gel qualities with colloidal bismuth subcitrate administration. Eur J Pharmac 184:55–63
33. Slomiany BL, Piotrowski J, Okazaki K, Grzelinska E, Slomiany A (1989) Nature of the enhancement of the protective qualities of gastric mucus by sucralfate. Digestion 44:222–231
34. Slomiany BL, Nadziejko C, Mizuta K, Slomiany A (1988) Role of associated and covalently bound lipids in the physicochemical properties of mucus. In: Mastella G, Quinton P (eds) Cellular and molecular basis of cystic fibrosis. San Francisco Press, San Fransisco, pp 263–279
35. Slomiany BL, Slomiany A (1980) Glycosphingolipids and glyceroglucolipids of glandular epithelial tissue. In: Sweeley CC (ed) Biochemistry of cell surface glycolipids. ACS Symp Ser No 128, pp 150–176
36. Slomiany A, Galicki NI, Kojima K, Banas-Gruszka A, Slomiany BL (1981) Glyceroglucolipids of the mucous barrier of dog stomach. Biochim Biophys Acta 665:88–91
37. Slomiany BL, Slomiany A, Glass GBJ (1977) Glycolipids of the human gastric content: structure of the sulfated glyceroglucolipid. Eur J Biochem 78:33–39
38. Slomiany BL, Slomiany A, Glass GBJ (1977) Characterization of two major neutral glyceroglucolipids of the human gastric content. Biochemistry 18:3954–3958
39. Slomiany BL, Galicki NI, Kojima K, Slomiany A (1980) The neutral and acidic glycerogluco lipids from gastric mucous barrier of rat stomach antrum, body and forestomach. Eur J Biochem 111:259–263
40. Witas H, Sarosiek J, Aono M, Murty VLN, Slomiany A, Slomiany BL (1983) Lipids associated with rat small-intestinal mucus glycoprotein. Carbohyd Res 120:67–76
41. Witas H, Slomiany BL, Zdebska E, Kojima K, Liau YH, Slomiany A (1983) Lipids associated with dog gastric mucus glycoprotein. J Appl Biochem 5:16–24
42. Slomiany A, Yano S, Slomiany BL, Glass GBJ (1978) Lipid composition of the gastric mucous barrier in the rat. J Biol Chem 253:3785–3791
43. Lichtenberger LM, Graziani LA, Dial EJ, Butler BD, Hills BA (1983) Role of surface-active phospholipids in gastric cytoprotection. Science 219:1327–1329
44. Hills BA (1985) Gastric mucosal barrier: stabilization of hydrophobic lining of the stomach by mucus. Am J Physiol 249:G343–G348
45. Kay YC, Lichtenberger LM (1987) Localization of phospholipid-rich zones in rat gastric mucosa: possible origin of a protective hydrophobic luminal lining. J Histochem Cytochem 35:1285–1298
46. Goggin PM, Ahmed H, Northfield TC (1990) Molecular basis for gastric mucosal hydrophobicity. Gastroenterology 98:A48
47. Gwozdzinski K, Slomiany A, Nishikawa H, Okazaki K, Slomiany BL (1988) Gastric mucin hydrophobicity: effects of associated and covalently bound lipids, proteolysis and reduction. Biochem Int 17:907–917
48. Slomiany BL, Murty VLN, Slomiany A, Zielenski J, Mandel ID (1986) Mucus glycoprotein of human saliva: differences in the associated and covalently bound lipids with caries. Biochim Biophys Acta 882:18–28
49. Takagi YM, Hotta K (1979) Characterization of peptic inhibitory activity associated with sulfated glycoprotein isolated from gastric mucosa. Biochim Biophys Acta 584:288–297
50. Slomiany BL, Kojima J, Slomiany A (1982) Peptic inhibitory activity of the glyceroglucolipids from gastric secretion. J Appl Biochem 3:531–534
51. Slomiany BL, Kojima K, Witas H, Slomiany A (1982) Promotion of activation of pepsinogen by glyceroglucolipids. J Appl Biochem 3:531–534
52. Slomiany BL, Murty VLN, Slomiany A (1985) Salivary lipids in health and disease. Progr Lipid Res 24:311–345

53. Piotrowski J, Slomiany A, Murty VLN, Fekete Z, Slomiany BL (1991) Inhibition of H. pylori colonization by sulfated gastric mucin. Biochem Int 24:749–756
54. Sarosiek J, Slomiany A, Takagi A, Slomiany BL (1984) Hydrogen ion diffusion in gastric mucus glycoprotein. Effect of associated and covalently bound fatty acids. Biochem Biophys Res Commun 118:523–531
55. Slomiany BL, Sarosiek J, Takagi A, Slomiany A (1986) Role of mucus in gastric mucosal protection against hydrogen ion. Ann NY Acad Sci 463:351–353
56. Sarosiek J, Slomiany A, Slomiany BL (1983) Retardation of hydrogen ion diffusion by gastric mucus constituents: effect of proteolysis. Biochem Biophys Res Commun 113:1053–1060
57. Kosmala M, Carter SR, Konturek SJ, Slomiany A, Slomiany BL (1986) Mucus glycoprotein secretion by duodenal mucosa in response to luminal arachidonic acid. Biochim Biophys Acta 884:419–428
58. Slomiany BL, Murty VLN, Mandel ID, Zalesna G, Slomiany A (1989) Physicochemical characteristics of mucus glycoproteins and lipids of the human oral mucosal mucus coat. Arch Oral Biol 34:229–237
59. Slomiany BL, Sarosiek J, Slomiany A (1987) Role of carbohydrates in the viscosity and permeability of gastric mucin to hydrogen ion. Biochem Biophys Res Commun 142:783–790.
60. Piasek A, Slomiany A, Slomiany BL (1985) Permselective properties of gastric mucus: effect of lipids. Gastroenterology 88:A1539
61. Slomiany A, Okazaki K, Tamura S, Slomiany BL (1991) Identity of mucin's 118 kDa "link protein" with fibronectin. Arch Biochem Biophys 268:383–388
62. Sarosiek J, Slomiany A, Murty VLN, Slomiany BL (1984) Contribution of proteins and lipids to the rheological properties of gastric mucin. Gastroenterology 86:A1232
63. Murty VLN, Sarosiek J, Slomiany A, Slomiany BL (1984) Effect of lipids and proteins on the viscosity of gastric mucus glycoprotein. Biochem Biophys Res Commun 121:521–529
64. Slomiany BL, Kosmala M, Carter SR, Konturek SJ, Bilski J, Slomiany A (1987) Intestinal mucin release in response to HCl and taurocholate. Comp Biochem Physiol 87A:657–663
65. Slomiany BL, Murty VLN, Piotrowski J, Slomiany A (1988) Role of associated and covalently bound lipids in mucin hydrophobicity: effect of proteolysis and disulfide bridge reduction. Biochem Biophys Res Commun 151:1046–1053
66. Sarosiek J, Piotrowski J, Gabryelewicz A, Slomiany A, Slomiany BL (1988) Changes in macromolecular organization of gastric mucin with peptic ulcer: differences in phospholipids and covalently bound fatty acids. Gastroenterology 94:A398
67. Sarosiek J, Piotrowski J, Gabryelewicz A, Slomiany A, Slomiany BL (1989) Alterations in mucin hydrophobicity and molecular form distribution with peptic ulcer. Gastroenterology 96:A441
68. Ehrlich J, Piotrowski J, Slomiany A, Slomiany BL (1989) Evidence for changes of aggregative properties of mucin in gastric ulcer. Gastroenterology 96:A136
69. Ehrlich J, Piotrowski J, Slomiany A, Slominy BL (1990) Dynamic laser light scattering studies of gastric mucin in health and disease. Gastroenterology 98: A68
70. Slomiany BL, Bilski J, Sarosiek J, Murty VLN, Dworkin B, VanHorn, K, Zielenski J, Slomiany A (1987) Campylobacter pyloridis degrades mucin and undermines gastric mucosal integrity. Biochem Biophys Res Commun 144:307–314
71. Sarosiek J, Slomiany A, Slomiany BL (1988) Evidence for weakening of gastric mucus integrity by Campylobacter pylori. Scand J Gastroent 23:585–590
72. Slomiany BL, Nishikawa H, Piotrowski J, Okazaki K, Slomiany A (1989) Lipolytic activity of Campylobacter pylori: effect of sofalcone. Digestion 43:33–40
73. Slomiany BL, Kasinathan C, Slomiany A (1989) Lipolytic activity of Campylobacter pylori: effect of colloidal bismuth subcitrate (De–Nol). Am J Gastroent 84:506–510
74. Slomiany BL, Murty VLN, Piotrowski J, Liau YH, Sundaram P, Slomiany A (1992) Glycosulfatase activity of H. pylori toward gastric mucin. Biochem Biophys Res Commun 183:506–513
75. Murty VLN, Piotrowski J, Morita M, Slomiany A, Slomiany BL (1992) Inhibition of H. pylori glycosulfatase activity towards gastric sulfomucin by nitecapone. Biochem Int 26:1091–1099
76. Beachy EH (1981) Bacterial adherence: adhesin-receptor interactions mediating the attachment of bacteria to mucosal surface. J Infect Dis 143:325–345
77. Piotrowski J, Slomiany BL, VanHorn K, Sengupta S, Slomiany A (1990) Sulfated mucins and sucralfate inhibit hemagglutination of erythrocytes by C. pylori. Gastroenterology 98:A107

78. Slomiany BL, Piotrowski J, Samanta A, VanHonr K, Murty VLN, Slomiany A, Slomiany BL (1989) Campylobacter pylori colonization factor shows specificity for lactosylceramide sulfate and GM_3-ganglioside. Biochem Int 19:929–936
79. Azuumi Y, Ohara S, Ishihara K, Okabe H, Hotta K (1980) Correlation of quantitative changes of gastric mucosal glycoprotein with aspirin induced damage in rats. Gut 21:533–536
80. Murakami S, Mori Y (1984) Changes in the incorporating activity of ^{35}S-sulfate into gastric sulfated glycoproteins in the rat with erosion by restraint and water immersion. Jpn J Pharmac 35:279–286
81. Slomiany BL, Liau YH, Tsukada H, Mizuta K, Rosenthal WS, Slomiany A (1987) Sulfation of glycolipids by human gastric mucosa in disease. Digestion 36:246–252
82. Slomiany A, Jozwiak Z, Liau YH, Slomiany BL (1984) Effect of ethanol on the enzymatic sulfation of glycosphingolipids in gastric mucosa. J Biol Chem 259:5792–5796
83. Liau YH, Lopez RA, Slomiany A, Slomiany BL (1992) Helicobacter pylori lipopolysaccharide effect on the synthesis and secretion of sulfated gastric mucin. Biochem Biophys Res Commun 184:1411–1417
84. Slomiany BL, Liau YH, Lopez RA, Czajkowski A, Piotrowski J, Slomiany A (1992) Effect of H. pylori lipopolysaccharide on the synthesis and secretion of gastric mucin. Biochem Int 27:687–697

Gastric Mucosal Blood Flow and Its Role in the Pathogenesis of Acute and Chronic Ulceration*

C. PIASECKI

Introduction

In the oft-quoted equation describing the balance between aggressive and defensive factors, adequate mucosal blood flow is an absolutely vital requirement for maintaining all biochemical defensive mechanisms. Clinically local failure of blood supply is suspected whenever necrotic lesions occur singly and in the same area, as is the case in coronary thrombosis or cerebral infarction. On this basis a failure of blood supply has been suspected in the case of chronic gastric and duodenal ulcers ever since Virchow suggested in 1853 that emboli might occlude gastric arteries [1]. The most striking feature of chronic ulcers is their singularity and localisation to the lesser curvature and first part of the duodenum. Within the lesser curvature there is an increasing incidence from the oesophageal towards the pyloric end, with maximal incidence in the incisural area [2]. Duodenal ulcers occur on the anterior or posterior walls of the first 4 cm, uncommonly on the superior "cap", and rarely on the inferior wall. Since infarction at the same site is usually due to occlusion of end-arteries, studies in the early part of this century sought evidence for such a mechanism. Thus, in 1908 Mayo first described the well-known phenomenon now called "Mayo's anaemic spot" [3], where traction produced by pulling the stomach downwards and to the left at operation results in pallor on the anterior wall of the 1st inch (2.5 cm) of the duodenum, which disappears when the tension is relaxed. In 1911 Wilkie [4] suggested the pallor was due to traction on the supraduodenal artery, which according to his studies was an end-artery. However, Kirk [5], whilst confirming the existence of "Mayo's anaemic spot", reported that the force of traction was taken up by connective tissues which became taut, leaving the vessels patent.

Wilkie's statement that the supraduodenal artery was an end-artery is erroneous, because his drawings show that he had examined only the subserous branches of the artery, and not the branches of the submucosal plexus. In the middle of the century a number of post-mortem injection studies of the gastric

*The various studies described here have been carried out with grants from the Peter Samuel Royal Free Fund and the Wellcome Trust. Thanks are due to the following publications for permission to reproduce illustrations: *Journal of Anatomy*, Kluwer Publications, *Gastroenterology*, *Current Science*, *Journal of Physiology and Pharmacology*.

vessels in man [6–11] demonstrated a rich anastomotic plexus at the submucosal level between all the vessels entering through the external muscle. Vessels approaching in the mesenteries pierce the external muscle and divide, forming a rich submucosal plexus in all regions. Mucosal arteries arise from the submucosal plexus and after piercing the muscularis mucosae they ramify in the mucosa. It was found that in the lesser curvature and in the first 2.5 cm of the duodenum, the submucosal plexus is poorer than elsewhere in terms of having fewer and smaller vessels. However, the efficiency of the submucosal collaterals, even of those in the lesser curvature, was demonstrated by Somerville [12] and Wood [13], who ligated 90% of the blood supply to the stomach without any incidence of necrosis. These studies dealt a blow to the hypothesis of infarction by occlusion of end-arteries.

We reinvestigated the arterial supply to the human stomach during the 1970s in greater detail than had been done so far, and found end-artery systems of two types [14–16]. One of these has an extraordinary correlation with chronic peptic ulceration; the other is diffusely distributed throughout the stomach. Recently we found that contraction of muscle layers through which these vessels pass can occlude them, causing necrosis and ulceration [17]. Finally, we worked out the number and duration of muscle spasms that were necessary to induce ulceration in this way [18]. These latter physiological studies were performed in animals but the results are applicable to the human stomach because of the anatomical similarity in patterns of blood supply. These studies comprise evidence for an infaractive pathogenesis which accounts for both mechanical initiation and localisation of ulcers. It is compatible with current views of aggressive and defensive factors, which we feel are more likely to be involved in determining exacerbation or healing after the lesion has formed.

Blood Supply to the Stomach

Basic Pattern

The basic pattern of the blood supply is illustrated in Figs. 1 (upper only) and 2, which show how vasa recta piercing the external muscle divide and join up to form an extensive plexus between muscle and mucosa, i.e. in the loose submucosal tissue. Small mucosal arteries arise from this plexus, pierce the muscularis mucosae layer of muscle, and each supplies a discrete patch of mucosa. Note that the central parts of Figs. 1 and 2 show an exception to this pattern, described below. The poverty of vascularity in the lesser curvature found by previous authors is localised still further. In the lesser curvature there is a quantitative decrease in the number and calibre of anastomosing vessels from the cardiac to the pyloric part, with a similar decrease in the duodenum from the second part to the pylorus, i.e. the plexus is least in the pyloric third of the lesser curvature and in the first 2.5 cm of the duodenum. However, our studies brought to light two new and important features [14, 15], outlined below.

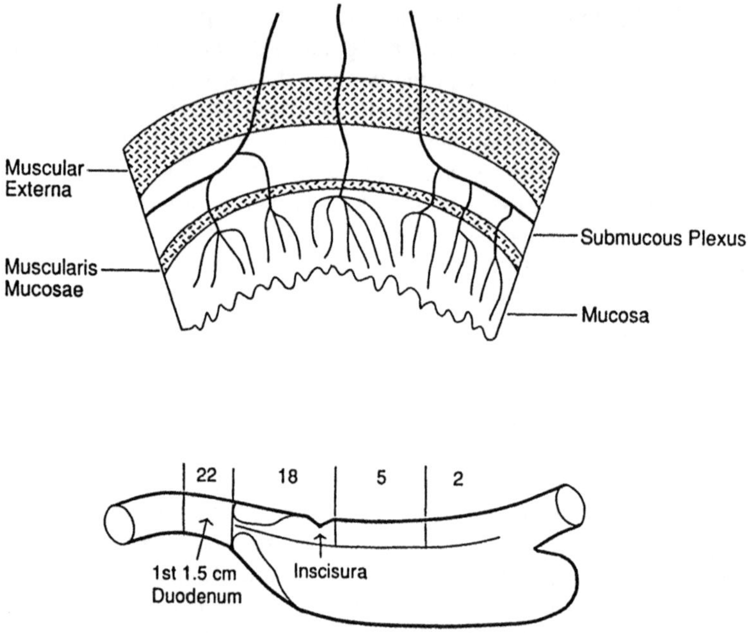

Fig. 1. *Upper*: Transverse section showing the blood supply in the lesser curvature and adjoining walls in man. On each side, normal inputs form a submucous plexus, and mucosal arteries pass through one muscle layer, the lamina muscularis mucosae. The central part shows an exception to the usual pattern which is found only in some individuals, a single mucosal end-artery of extramural origin in the centre which passes through both layers of muscle. *Lower*: Distribution of 47 end-arteries of extramural origin found in 10 out of 21 human specimens. Note the resemblance to the distribution of chronic peptic ulcers

Existence of Special End-Artery Systems in the Ulcer-Bearing Areas in Man

The most significant finding in our studies was that in the areas of poorest plexus, some individuals have no plexus at all. The mucosa underlying these patches is supplied by mucosal arteries which arise outside the stomach wall, pierce the external muscle as well as the muscularis mucosae, and each supplies 2–12 mm^2 surface area of mucosa. They do not connect with the submucosal plexus nor with other mucosal arteries in the mucosa, and so appear to be end-arteries (central areas of Figs. 1 and 2). They are found only in the lesser curvature and first part of the duodenum and we call them "mucosal end-arteries of extramural origin". The lower part of Fig. 1 shows the distribution of 47 such vessels found in 10 out of 21 human specimens. There is a remarkable correspondence between the distribution of such end-arteries and the distribution of chronic gastric and duodenal ulcers. This gives an anatomical basis for the localisation of chronic ulcers and suggests that the existence of such end-arteries may be an indispensable feature for initiating chronic ulceration. However, since these stomachs did not have ulcers and their owners had no

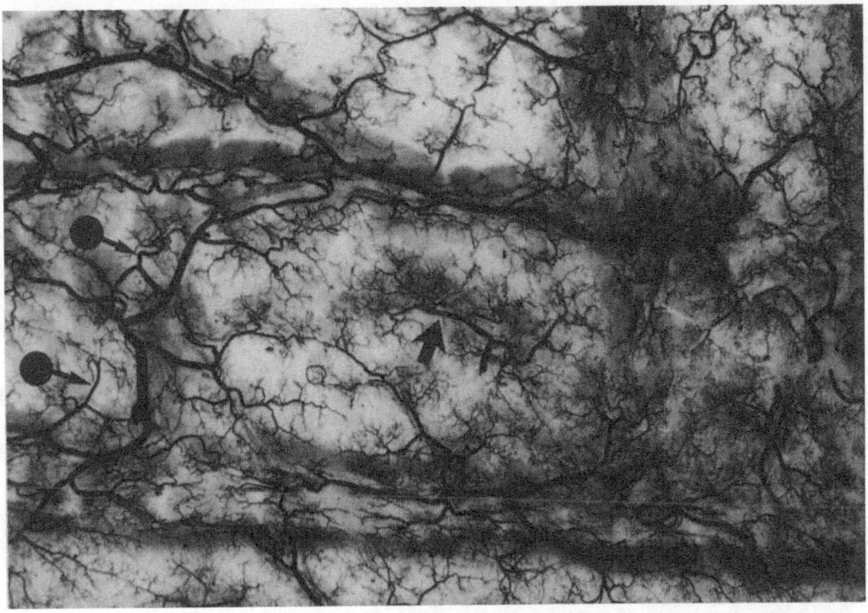

Fig. 2. Plan view of submucous plexus of arteries from the lesser curvature of a human non-ulcerated stomach. External muscle has been removed so that perforating input vessels have been cut. Mucosal arteries (*black round discs with arrows*) arise from this plexus and divide to supply the mucosa. Note the mucosal artery of extramural origin in the centre (*arrow*), supplying a large area of mucosa, and having no connection with the submucous plexus. ×6

history of ulceration, a second factor causing occlusion is necessary but was clearly not operative in these individuals.

The fact that some individuals do not have such end-arteries explains why some people are not prone to peptic ulcers, and this could account for familial occurrence, geographical distribution and changes in incidence over time. The initial size of ulcers could be determined by the fact that two or more such end-arteries are found side by side, but their extension after formation could be dependent on secondary aggressive factors acting at the ulcer margin, such as acid or *H. pylori* infection thrombosing exposed capillaries.

A search for an in vivo model of such end-arteries in a host of laboratory animals [19] revealed that such vessels were occasionally present in guinea-pigs and rabbits on the lesser or greater curvatures. This different distribution does not discount such vessels from being involved in human ulceration, because ulceration is dependent on both the existence of end-arteries and their obstruction by a second dynamic mechanism. We were unable to perform physiological studies in these models as it was impossible to find these occasionally occuring vessels in vivo.

Most Ordinary Mucosal Arteries are End-Arteries

There has always been discussion in the literature as to whether there is any anastomosis between capillary beds of adjacent mucosal arteries within the mucosa. We examined this problem using careful stereomicroscopy with micromanipulation of human stomachs, and found an almost total absence of anastomoses [14, 19]. What early workers thought were anastomoses were in fact "overlapping" capillaries. In a certain plane of view the clear, unfilled intervals between mucosal capillary beds are easily visible (Fig. 3). An identical pattern with lack of anastomoses between mucosal arteries exists in most laboratory animals, particularly in the guinea-pig, which we therefore chose for in vivo studies of this question.

We ligated 33 individual gastric mucosal arteries in guinea-pigs. This resulted in necrosis of the whole thickness of the mucosa in the area supplied by each vessel in 25 out of the 33 cases [16] (Fig. 4). Thus, three-quarters of mucosal

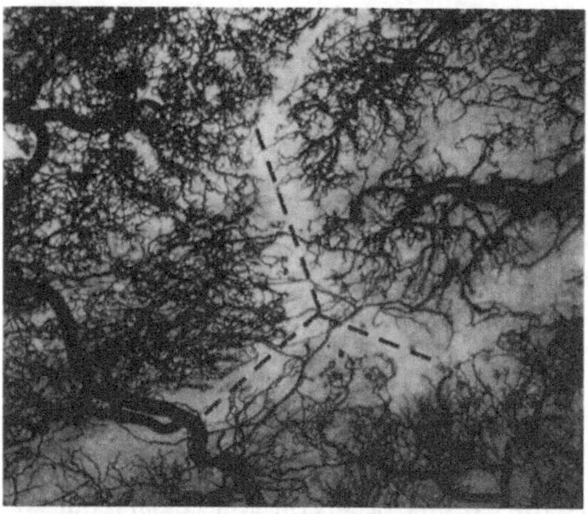

Fig. 3. At higher power, capillaries from one mucosal artery are seen not to connect up with capillaries from adjacent mucosal arteries, along an unfilled (*dotted*) line (the vessels crossing this line belong to the submucosal connective tissue plexus which is at a different level) × 10

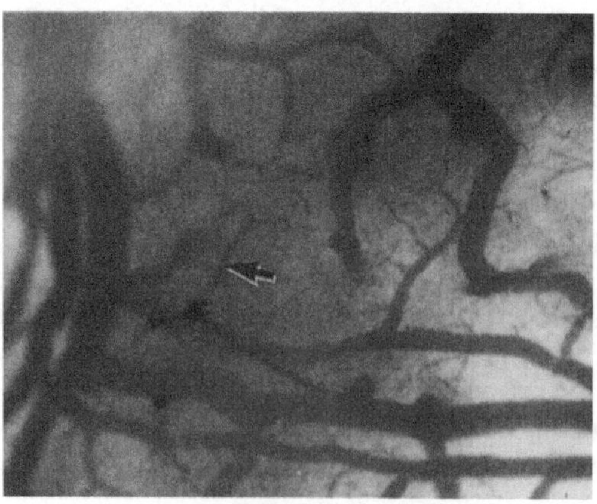

Fig. 4. Transilluminated stomach wall of guinea-pig, showing submucosal plexus and mucosal arteries and veins. Note one mucosal artery has been ligated (*arrow*)

arteries are end-arteries in this species. When two or three adjacent mucosal arteries were ligated, necrosis resulted in 95%, indicating that in the single ligations the remaining quarter of arteries survived because of an effective functional anastomosis from neighbouring vessels. Existing suspicions that ordinary mucosal arteries might be functional end-arteries were thus confirmed. In contrast to those special end-arteries in the lesser curvature, we have here a second type of end-artery existing throughout the stomach, each one supplying a small patch of mucosa. Hence, the required structural basis for infarction is present throughout the stomach, and the infarction mechanism can thus be invoked to explain the initiation of multiple acute ulcers.

Vulnerability of Mucosal End-Arteries to Temporary Obstruction

We ascertained the end-artery status of a particular muscosal artery by obstructing it and noting the degree of reduction of blood flow in the mucosa, using a special modified oxygen electrode applied to the mucosa [20, 21]. Preliminary experiments in which each artery was ligated permanently showed that immediately after ligation a fall of more than 92% indicated end-artery status (since necrosis resulted), whilst falls of 50–74% indicated the existence of a functional anastomosis (since the mucosa survived) [18].

Using the guinea-pig model, we temporarily obstructed mucosal arteries for given periods using a snare, and allowed 3 h recovery for histological necrosis to occur. In single obstruction experiments, necrosis began to occur following a 30-min obstruction. However, the results of shorter multiple obstructions were much more interesting. Necrosis began to occur in some cases after only four occlusions of 5 min duration, repeated at 1-min intervals. It always occurred after four 10-min occlusions. The necrosis was caused by thrombosis occurring in the vessel at the site of obstruction. After the third 5-min occlusion, we were able to detach the thrombus by moving the vessel. However, after the fourth occlusion the thrombus could not be moved on and the blockage became permanent. Whilst pulling a snare might appear unphysiological and unlikely to occur in life, we will show below that contraction of external muscle or of muscularis mucosae also causes complete obstruction of arteries and veins, so the snare technique does mimic real events.

Conclusion From the Above Studies on Vessels

To summarise the above studies, we have demonstrated the existence of two types of end-arteries in the stomach. The first are those found only in the lesser curvature and first part of the duodenum. They arise outside the wall and so have to pierce two layers of muscle on their way to supply the mucosa – the external muscle and the muscularis mucosae. Some individuals do not have such vessels. The second type are the usual mucosal arteries found throughout the organ, and since these arise from the sub-mucosal plexus within the wall, they pierce only the muscularis mucosae. We have shown that the second type of end-artery is vulnerable to short periods of obstruction, and it is very likely that this also applies to the first type, since the latter have no anastomoses with neighbouring vessels either.

Two mechanisms might cause obstruction of both types of arteries. One is vasoconstriction, which is a feature in stress (Alexis St Martin's mucosa became pale when he was mentally stressed); the other is that the arteries may be externally occluded by spasm of the muscle layers through which they pass. Inspection of Fig. 1 (upper) shows that the muscularis mucosae is in a position to obstruct both types of end-artery, whilst the external muscle could only obstruct the first type found in the lesser curvature and antrum (shown in the centre of the figure). Whilst not denying the role of vasoconstriction, we feel the evidence is strong for the occlusive factor being focal spasm of muscle layers, and we now outline the evidence supporting this mechanism.

Role of the External Muscle in Occluding End-Arteries in the Lesser Curvature

In 1969, Oi et al. [22] found that in man two-thirds of gastric ulcers lie beneath thickened bundles of external muscle bordering the lesser curvature. Another thickening exists in the circular layer in a position suggestive of the incisura angularis. The close relationship between the site of 63 gastric ulcers and the thickened muscle bundles is shown in Fig. 5, and strongly suggests that the external muscle plays a role in determining the site of ulceration.

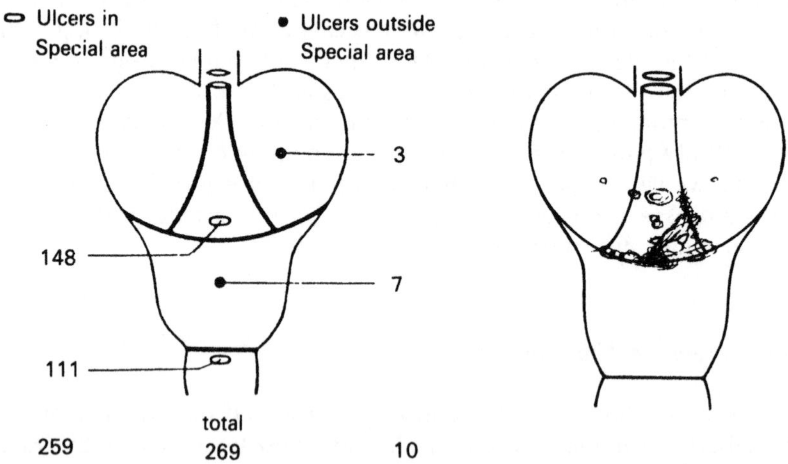

Fig. 5. *Left*: Location of chronic gastric and duodenal ulcers in relation to thickened muscle bundles. Two *vertical curving lines* within the stomach indicate muscles bordering the margins of the lesser curvature, whilst the *horizontal curving line* indicates thickened muscle at the incisura. The *lowest horizontal line* indicates the pylorus. *Right*: Distribution of 64 chronic gastric ulcers found in 60 specimens selected at random. Circles show shape as well as location of ulcers found on the musculature. (From [22])

We studied the effect of contracting external muscle on vessels piercing it at the borders of the lesser curvature in ferrets and guinea-pigs (unpublished study). Peristaltic waves induced by stimulating the cut distal vagus completely obstructed both arteries and veins passing through the muscle (Fig. 6). This effect has also been reported by Livingstone et al. [23]. We were unable to produce tonic contractions at one site, but the slowest wave caused arterial occlusion lasting 7 s. Simultaneous measurements with the oxygen electrode showed zero blood flow in the underlying mucosa. This was surprising, for it indicated that if compensation occurs via the submucosal plexus it does not occur instantaneously.

Radiological studies performed by Orator [24] showed that in man the peristaltic wave tends to "stand still" at the incisura whilst the rest of it sweeps round the greater curvature (because of the greater length of this part), thus providing an association between the sites of most prolonged contraction and the most frequent sites of gastric ulceration. Unfortunately, Orator did not state the maximum duration of contraction at the incisura, but since our 5-min obstructions of end-arteries repeated several times in animals caused ulceration, it could be assumed that similar durations of spasm in the human would also cause ulceration in individuals having end-arteries at that site. Such prolonged contractions or focal spasms are consistent with recent studies demonstrating abnormal motility in active ulceration [25, 26].

Barbara et al. [26] reviewed the evidence for abnormal motility and concluded that the predominant state is one of hypomotility. It is possible that in hypomotility there is a slowing down of contraction, so that foci of spasm might remain for prolonged periods. Read [27] implied that this may occur in the duodenum, saying, "the major abnormality in duodenal ulceration is that the normal coordinated antral duodenal contractions are replaced by more complex non-propagated duodenal wave forms", i.e. suggesting static focal spasm of external musculature.

a

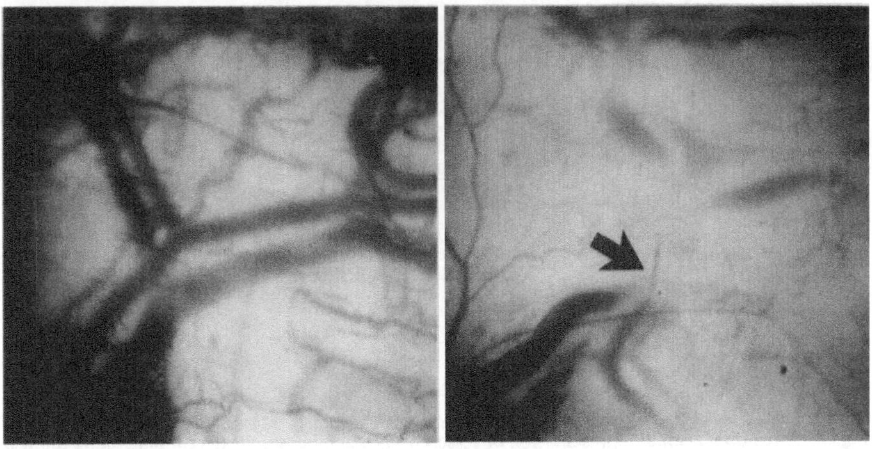

b

Fig. 6a, b. Transilluminated gastric wall in ferret before (**a**) and during (**b**) vegally stimulated contraction of muscle. Note compression of both arteries and veins to occlusion by the contracting muscle at the point where they penetrate the muscle (*arrow*)

On the other hand, recent studies in animals favour hypermotility as being important in ulcerogenesis. Thus, in dogs chronic gastric ulcers have been induced by stimulating the muscle with implanted electrodes [28]. In stress produced by cold and restraint [29], or by hypothalamic stimulation, ulceration was associated with contractions that were increased fourfold in duration and amplitude [30, 31]. This problem may be explained by the probability that in hypermotile states, foci of spasm may exist which would be undetected by the currently available methods of measuring muscle tone.

Role of Muscularis Mucosae in Obstructing Mucosal Arteries

In contrast to the external muscle, which can obstruct the end-arteries of extramural origin confined the ulcer-bearing area, the muscularis mucosae, because of its position, can obstruct all mucosal arteries throughout the stomach (see Fig. 1). In 1953 Walder first suggested this might occur. We have recently been able to study spontaneous focal contractions of the muscularis mucosae in anaesthetised guinea-pigs. On occasions such contraction was sufficiently prolonged to result in ulceration of the underlying mucosa whilst the rest of the mucosa remained healthy [17].

The use of the guinea-pig in experimental studies, however, requires explanation of one anatomical difference between this species and man. Inspection of Figs. 1 and 7 shows that in man the submucosal plexus is in the submucosa, so that mucosal arteries arising from it pierce the whole thickness of the muscularis mucosae prior to entering the mucosa. Mucosal arteries are therefore liable to be

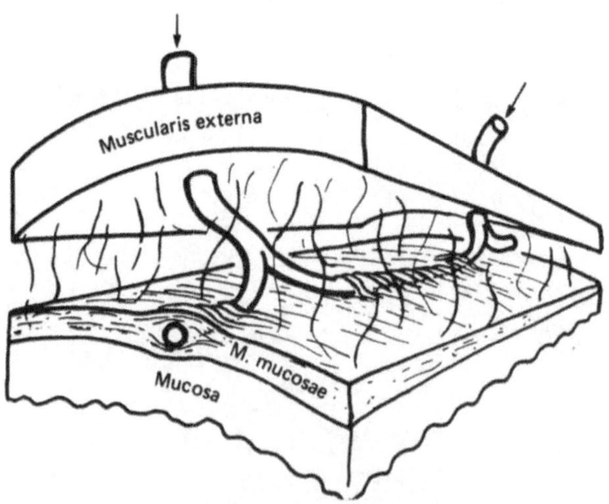

Fig. 7. Three-dimensional representation of vessels of the submucosal plexus running along tunnels within the muscularis mucosae in guinea-pig. Contraction of lamina muscularis mucosae in this pattern explains the appearance shown in Figs. 9 and 10

compressed by contraction of the muscle, but the submucosal plexus vessels will not be affected. In the guinea-pig (as also in the rabbit and the rat), both the submucosal plexus and the origins of mucosal arteries are embedded within the muscularis mucosae. Thus, contraction of the muscle will compress both submucosal vessels and mucosal arteries. This effect is seen in Figs. 8 and 9.

We observed the effect by removing a small piece of external muscle and observing the vasculature by transillumination [17]. Foci were visible in which veins and arteries were irregularly compressed. It must, however, be stressed that such foci were visible through the muscle before its removal, though the muscle had to be removed to obtain a clear view for photography. Cutting the muscle increased the effect. It is also important that such foci were surrounded by areas with normal circulation, even within the area denuded of muscle and transilluminated. It can thus be concluded that, whilst the effect was due to the stress of surgery, the exact localisation of foci was not determined by local procedure, but rather by an intrinsic spasm confined to areas of a particular size. In the most severe degree, all small arteries and veins were completely absent (Fig. 8). In less severe cases, veins were completely devoid of blood, with a sudden cut-off at the point where they entered the muscularis mucosae, whilst arteries were clearly flattened by transverse bands, a picture quite different from intrinsic vasoconstriction and highly suggestive of external compression (Fig. 9c). The phenomenon was not due to extrinsic pressure, since it was present before the light guide touched the tissue. As is expected in an area of contracting

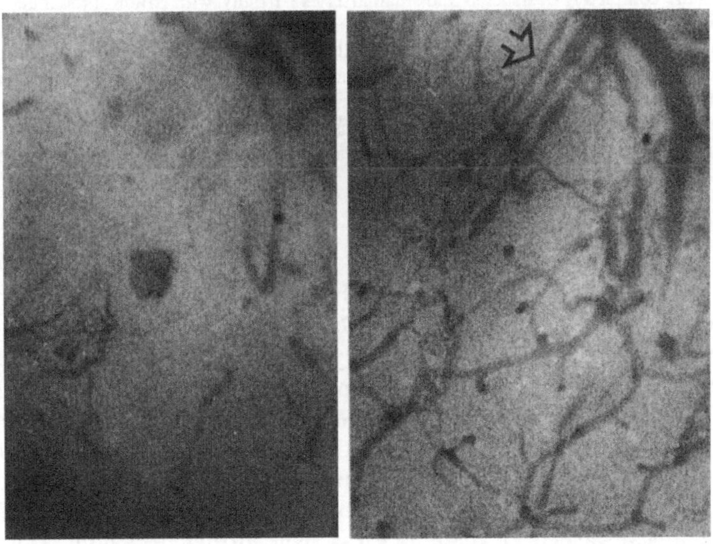

a b

Fig. 8a, b. Transilluminated gastric submucosa/mucosa after removal of external muscle, to show a focus of ischaemia with almost total absence of vessels (**a**) and reappearance of a nearly normal circulation (**b**) 5s after mechanical stimulation of luminal surface. The dark rounded patch in the centre of **a** is an artefact. The two pictures show exactly the same area, as can be verified by the position of the vessels. Note that the three parallel vessels indicated by an *arrow* in **b** are completely absent during a spasm (**a**). Granularity is due to exposure of 1600 ASA film at 3200 ASA. X40

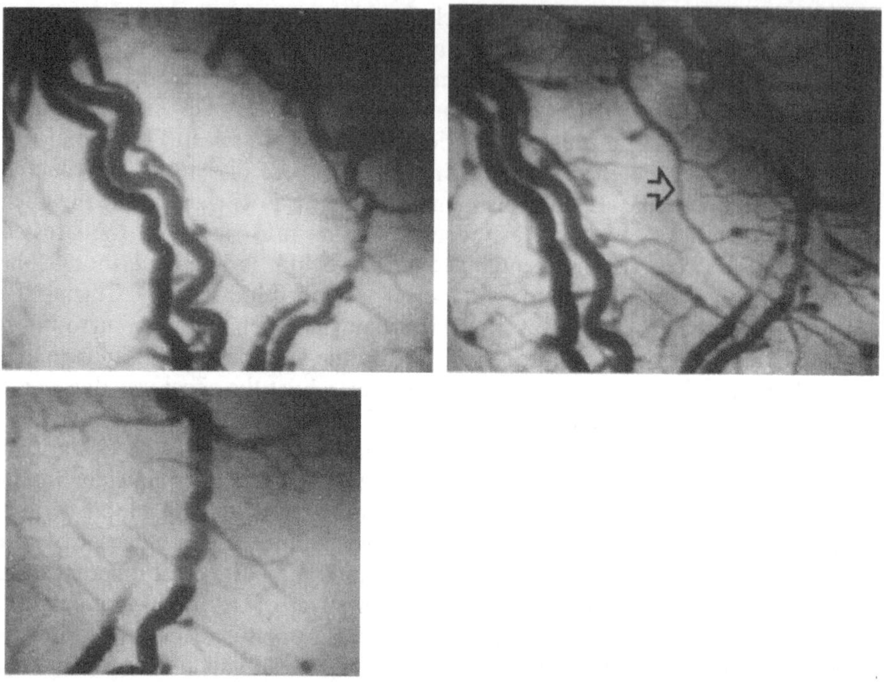

a b c

Fig. 9a. Submucosa. Gastric submucosal vessels immediately after exposure, showing a focus in which small veins are completely obstructed and small arteries partially, with pallor of the mucosa. X40 **b** Five seconds after mechanical stimulation of mucosa. Note appearance of a venous network invisible in **a**, more prominent small arteries and less pallor of mucosa. Note also the diminished tortuosity of the two largest parallel vessels in the picture. The vein indicated by an *arrow* was completely obstructed in **a**. Vessels now appear normal under conditions of the experiment. X40. **c** This is an enlarged view of the lower right corner of **a**. Transverse bands appear partially to constrict the large artery running from top to bottom. The accompanying vein is completely obstructed and its stem is visible at the top of the picture. X80

muscle, the size of the area exhibiting this "spasm" was shrunk by 27% compared to its size when later relaxed, and this was manifested at the time of spasm by tortuosity of unaffected vessels (Fig. 9a, b). This phenomenon is new to the literature and we conclude it could only be caused by the muscularis mucosae, the only remaining muscle in the prepared area. The concomitant pallor of the mucosa is consistent with compression of the mucosa induced by prolongations of muscularis mucosae into the mucosa [32]. Simultaneous recording of oxygen delivery to the pale mucosa showed severe ischaemia, oxygen content being only 2%–5% of that when the spasm effect had passed off.

A most significant aspect of these foci was their further behaviour. If left undisturbed they usually disappeared spontaneously within 3–5 min (whereupon a normal circulation reappeared), but they could also be abolished in 3–5 s by gentle mechanical stimulation of the mucosal surface. Indeed, manipulation performed to produce the best possible illumination abolished the effect, and this explains why many workers have missed seeing this phenomenon. On the other hand, in 5 out of 25 cases the foci could not be abolished by mechanical stimulation. They remained and were observed for 3 h, whereupon the underlying mucosa had full-thickness necrosis, in contrast to surrounding areas which had normal mucosa underlying uncompressed vessels. Continuous observation showed that in these cases thrombosis had occurred in the obstructed arteries and veins in the first 20 min.

Clinical Implications of the Function of the Muscularis Mucosae in Acute and Chronic Ulceration

The function of the muscularis mucosae is unknown, but its prolongations into the mucosa indicate that it may compress the mucosa in order to pump out secretions from the glands into the gastric lumen. The above study shows that in the absence of motility this may happen at the expense of occluding the circulation. In the presence of continued stress, it may be prolonged in susceptible subjects to the point at which thrombosis of perforating vessels occurs and results in necrosis. This has great clinical implications. During normal peristaltic activity, movements of opposing surfaces of an empty stomach or of food rubbing against the mucosa will tend to reverse any tendency to spasm of the muscularis mucosae. Conversely, reduced movements will favour spasm and ischaemia. Since hypotonia and slow emptying have been shown to occur in stress and in chronic ulceration [25, 26], they can be regarded as ulcerogenic factors in so far as their influence on the muscularis mucosae is concerned. Thus, the cycle of events leading to acute ulceration could be physical or mental stress inducing hypotonia and patchy contraction of the muscularis mucosae. This obstructs the circulation, and if contractions of 5 or more minutes' duration are repeated, an acute ulcer will result. This mechanism is likely to occur in acute ulceration due to stress, such as in hypothalamic lesions or burns. It can also be invoked for the induction of chronic ulcers, for two reasons. Firstly, on anatomical grounds the special end-arteries of extramural origin in the ulcer-bearing area pass through the lamina muscularis mucosae as well as the external muscle. Secondly, it has always been considered by some that chronic ulcers may begin as acute ones, the chronicity being due to continued aggressive factors. Continued periodical stress, preferentially affecting the lesser curvature and antrum, and perhaps exacerbated by infection with *H. pylori*, will make an acute gastric ulcer chronic until rest and medication stop the process. According to the only study performed on human gastric muscularis mucosae, this muscle is thickest in the lesser curvature and its contractions in this region are stronger and more prolonged than in other regions [33].

Suggested Pathogenesis of Acute and Chronic Ulceration

We have presented evidence that some individuals have large end-arteries whose distribution closely mimics that of chronic ulcers, and also that many ordinary mucosal arteries are functional end-arteries. Repeated compressions of such vessels, each lasting 5 min, are sufficient to produce ulceration. Such compression can occur from contraction of external muscle or of the muscularis mucosae. Whilst such spasm of external muscle remains conjectural, we have seen acute stress causing focal spasm of muscularis mucosae, resulting in ischaemia and ulceration in an animal model. If the results from animal studies are extrapolated to man, there exists evidence for every step of the following sequence:

Stress → Prolonged repeated muscle spasm → Obstructed circulation → Ischaemia → Breakdown of mucosal barriers → Ulceration

If the spasm involves the external musculature and the patient is unfortunate enough to have end-arteries of extramural origin, necrosis will occur in the underlying area. Its further history will depend on the existence or otherwise of continued initiation and the anti-healing effects of gastric contents and infection by *H. pylori*. If the spasm is of the muscularis mucosae and the stress is a single episode, acute ulceration will occur wherever the foci of spasm exist. It is interesting to observe that contraction of external muscle has been implicated in the acute experimental ulceration in rats induced by cold restraint stress, indomethacin and cysteamine.

This postulated pathogenesis accounts for the localisation and initiation of lesions. It is totally compatible with the well-established mechanisms of breakdown of mucosal barriers, with acidity and *H. pylori* preventing healing and with therapeutic regimens designed to promote healing. There is, however, one missing step in this sequence, which may prove to be a fruitful line of future investigation: namely, whether ulcer patients develop abnormally prolonged focal spasm of external muscle or muscularis mucosae immediately preceding ulceration. In view of the fact that stress produces various forms of muscle spasm, e.g. that causing headache or spastic colon, it is possible or even likely it also causes spasm of gastric musculature.

Possible New Approaches to Treatment and Prevention

A new approach to treatment could be development of drugs that will relax stress-induced spasm, which, as we suggest, might be the most important cause of initiation and recurrence. It could be based on pharmacological intervention in the mechanisms of contraction of the muscularis mucosae. This may involve stimulating the reflex whereby mucosal nerve endings relax the muscularis mucosae as shown in our experiments. This reflex is probably mediated by the recently described capsaicin-sensitive nerves [34], and may involve leukotrienes [35] and opioid receptors [36]. A very similar segmental constriction of submucosal veins has been shown to occur with leukotriene C4 and ethanol [36–38], so that the effect of these substances on the gastric circulation may be mediated in part by the muscularis mucosae, and the concomitant mucosal stasis and increased permeability may be secondary effects.

References

1. Virchow R (1853) Historisches, Kritisches und Positives zur Lehre der Unterleibsaffektionen. Virchow Arch Pathol Anat Physiol 5:623
2. Ivy AC, Grossman MI, Bachrach WH (1950) Peptic ulcer. Churchill, London
3. Mayo WJ (1908) Anaemic spot on the duodenum. Surg Gyn Obst 6:600
4. Wilkie DPD (1911) Blood supply to the duodenum with special reference to the supraduodenal artery. Surg Gyn Obst 13:399–405
5. Kirk RM (1968) Site and localisation of duodenal ulcers: a study at operation. Gut 9:414–419
6. Reeves TB (1920) Study of arteries to the stomach and duodenum, and their relation to ulcer. Surg Gyn Obst 30:374–385
7. Barlow TE, Bentley FH, Walder DN (1951) Arteries, veins and arteriovenous anastomoses in the human stomach. Surg Gyn Obst 93:657–671
8. Disse H (1903) Uber die Blutgefasse menschlichen Magenschleimhaut, besonders über die Arterien derselben. Arch Mikros Anat 63:512–531
9. Jatrou S (1920) Über die arterielle Versorgung des Magens und ihre Beziehung zum Ulcus ventriculi. D Z Chir 159:196–223
10. Hoffman L, Nather K (1921) Zur Anatomie der Magenarterien. Arch Klin Chir 115:650–671
11. Berlet K (1923) Über die Arterien des menschlichen Magens und ihre Beziehungen zur Aetiologie und Pathogenese des Magengeschwürs. Z Pathol 30:472–489
12. Somervell TH (1945) Physiological gastrectomy: the operation of ligature of the arteries of the stomach to relieve hyperacidity, to prevent hyperacidity and to prevent recurrent ulceration after gastroenterostomy. Br J Surg 33:146–152
13. Wood WQ (1949) Treatment of peptic ulceration by vascular ligation. Arch Surg 48:455–462
14. Piasecki C (1974) Blood supply to the human gastroduodenal mucosa with special reference to ulcer bearing areas. J Anat 118:295–335
15. Piasecki C (1971) A possible vascular factor in the aetiology of duodenal ulceration. Br J Surg 58(9):660–662
16. Piasecki C, Thrasivoulou C, Rahim A (1989) Ulcers produced by ligation of individual gastric mucosal arteries. Gastroenterology 97:1121–1129
17. Piasecki C, Thrasivoulou C (1991) Focal spasm of gastric muscularis mucosae can induce focal ischaemia and ulceration. Gut 32(10):1246
18. Piasecki C, Thrasivoulou C (1992) Durations of complete focal mucosal ischaemia required to produce gastric ulceration. Eur J Gastroenterology Hepatology. 4:487–493
19. Piasecki C, Wyatt C (1986) Patterns of blood supply to the gastric mucosa. A comparative study revealing an end-artery model. J Anat 149:21–39
20. Piasecki C (1981) A new method for the assessment of gut viability. Br J Surg 68:319–322
21. Piasecki C (1985) First experimental results with the oxygen electrode as a local blood flow sensor in canine colon. Br J Surg 72:452–453
22. Oi M, Ito Y, Jumagi F, Yoshida K et al. (1969) A possible dual control system in the origin of peptic ulcer. A study on ulcer location as affected by mucosa and musculature. Gastroenterology 57:280–293
23. Livingstone EH, Howard T, Passaro EP, Guth PH (1990) Effect of gastric contractions upon gastric mucosal blood flow. Gastroenterology 98:A187
24. Orator V (1925) Cited by Ivy AC, Grossman, MI, Bachrach WH (1950) In: Peptic ulcer. Churchill, London, p 519
25. Yabana T, Yachi A (1988) Seminars on gastric mucosal injury VI: stress induced vascular damage and ulcer. Dig Dis Sci 33:751–761
26. Barbara L, Strangehellini V, De Giogio R, Paternico A, Corinaldesi R (1988) Gastrointestinal motility in pathological conditions. Chel R, Bovero E, Pandolfo N (eds), Gastric motility. Raven, New York, pp 83–94
27. Read NW (1991) The role of gastroduodenal motor activity in peptic ulceration. Halter F, Garner A, Tytgat G (eds), Mechanisms of peptic ulcer healing: Falk symposium 59. Kluwer, Lancaster

28. Quist G, Dormandy J, Brown C, Sloane D, Scott G (1974) The experimental production of gastric ulcers by induced muscle spasm. Br J Surg 61:259–63
29. Garrick T, Leung FW, Buack S, Hirabayashi K, Guth PH (1986) Gastric motility is stimulated but overall blood flow is unaffected during cold restraint in the rat. Gastroenterology 91:141–8
30. Garrick T, Grijalva C, Trauner M (1990) High amplitude contractions are necessary for lateral hypothalamic lesion and tail shock mucosal injury. Gastroenterology 99:A1213
31. Ueki A, Takeuchi K, Okabe S (1988) Gastric motility is an important factor in the pathogenesis of indomethacin-induced gastric mucosal lesions in rats. Dig Dis Sci 33:209–16
32. Leeson CR, Leeson TS, Paparo AA (1985) Textbook of histology. Saunders, Philadelphia, p 337
33. Walder DN (1953) The muscularis mucosae of the human stomach. J Physiol 120:373–82
34. Holzer P, Pabst M, Lippe I et al. (1990) Afferent nerve-mediated protection against deep mucosal damage in the rat stomach. Gastroenterology 98:838–848
35. Whittle BJR, Oren-Wolman N, Guth PH (1985) Gastric vasoconstrictor actions of leukotriene C_4, $PGF2^{\alpha}$, and thromboxane mimetic U-46619 on rat submucosal microcirculation in vivo. Am J Physiol 248:G580–586
36. Esplugues JV, Whittle BJR (1990) Morphine potentiation of ethanol-induced gastric mucosal damage in the rat. Gastroenterology 98:82–89
37. Bou-Abboud CF, Wayland H, Paulsen G, Guth PH (1988) Microcirculatory stasis precedes tissue necrosis in ethanol-induced gastric mucosal injury in the rat. Dig Dis Sci 33(7) :872–877
38. Oates PJ, Hakkinen JP (1988) Studies on the mechanisms of ethanol induced gastric damage in rats. Gastroenterology 94:110–121

Growth Factors in Gastric Mucosal Integrity, Protection and Healing of Acute and Chronic Ulcerations

S.J. Konturek, T. Brzozowski, J.W. Konturek, and B.L. Slomiany

Introduction

The maintenance of gastric mucosal integrity in the adverse environment of luminal contents depends upon the delicate balance of numerous factors which control the mucosal defense lines, such as mucus and alkaline secretion, mucosal hydrophobicity, richness of mucosal blood flow, maintenance of mucosal sulfhydryls, rapid restitution of epithelial cells, proliferation of mucosal cells, and tissue repair. Primary among these are epidermal growth factor (EGF), transforming growth factor-α (TGF-α), platelet-derived growth factor (PDGF), and basic fibroblast growth factor (bFGF). These factors have been identified in the gastric mucosa and found to exhibit the protective, mitogenic, and angiogenic activities that appear to be essential for the proliferation of cells in the normal mucosa as well as for the reepithelialization, repair, and healing processes occurring in the damaged or ulcerated mucosa.

Although growth factors differ in structure, origin, and sensitivity to luminal degradation, the common mechanism of their action on target cells is the interaction with specific high-affinity membrane receptors [1–4]. The binding of growth factors to their receptors generates a signal that is amplified and transduced to activate cytoplasmic regulatory proteins, which then alter gene expression and induce the biological responses. In the case of EGF, TGF-α and PDGF, the ligands bind to the same receptors on the target gastric mucosal cells. This binding results in the activation of intrinsic receptor tyrosine kinase and autophosphorylation of receptor, followed by an increase in the activity of ornithine decarboxylase and the tissue content of polyamines, which appear to be central events in mediating the biological effects of EGF, TGF-α and PDGF (Fig. 1).

The pharmacological agents such as sucralfate, colloidal bismuth compounds, and aluminium-containing antacids (Al-antacids), which are capable of protecting the growth factors from acid-pepsin degradation in the gastric lumen, may influence the binding of these factors to their receptors [4] in the mucosa or affect the expression of the receptors, and this may alter the biological action of growth factors on the gastric mucosa.

In this review we describe the biochemical and physiological mechanisms underlying the protective and ulcer-healing effects of growth factors and their interaction with drugs that are protective for the mucosa.

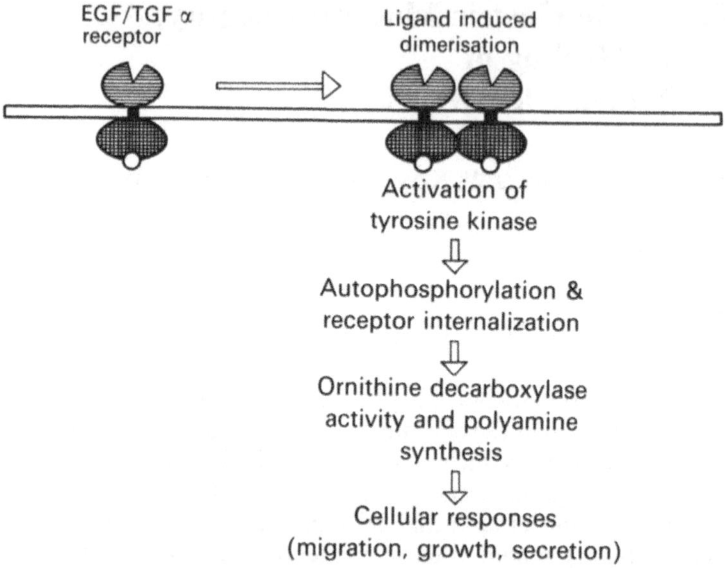

Fig. 1. The action of growth factors such as epidermal growth factor (EGF) or transforming growth factor-α (TGF-α) includes binding to a common receptor, activation of tyrosine kinase, and autophosphorylation of receptor, with subsequent intracellular signal transduction involving increased activity of ornithine decarboxylase and synthesis of polyamines, leading to final cellular responses

Growth Factors in the Gastric Mucosa: Origin and Spectrum of Biological Action

Gastric Mucosal Growth and Its Control

Gastric mucosa is one of the most rapidly proliferating tissues in the body [5]. Migration, proliferation, and growth of mucosal cells are balanced by continuous cell loss through exfoliation, so that under normal conditions the population of mucosal cells is maintained in a dynamic steady state. Because of the rapid turnover of mucosal cells, any imbalance between cell growth and cell loss, e.g., after exposure to topical irritants, may lead to mucosal injury, erosion, or ulceration.

The growth of the mucosa is controlled by a variety of factors including nutrients, nerves, and some nongastrointestinal hormones such as growth hormone and certain gut hormones, especially gastrin and somatostatin. Polypeptide growth factors, particularly EGF, TGF-α, PDGF, and bFGF, may also be involved and be brought into play, mainly following mucosal damage, to facilitate mucosal cell restitution, repair, and healing through endocrine or local paracrine or luminal pathways [5] (Fig. 2).

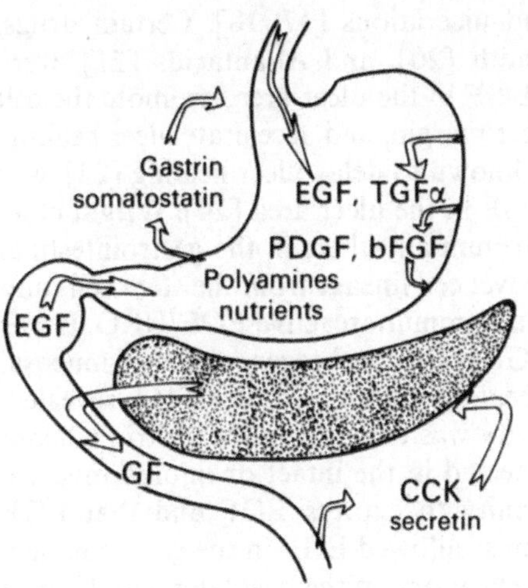

Fig. 2. Mucosal growth promoting factors acting on the gastric mucosa from a luminal site (e.g., EGF, polyamines, nutrients) and by paracrine (e.g., TGF-α) and endocrine routes (e.g., gastrin, somatostatin)

Certain antiulcer drugs may also affect mucosal growth, either by stimulating the release of growth-promoting gut hormones such as gastrin (e.g., histamine H_2-receptor antagonists or proton pump inhibitors) or by enhancing the receptor expression of EGF and other polypeptide growth factors (e.g., sucralfate) [4].

Epidermal Growth Factor, Transforming Growth Factor-α, Platelet-Derived Growth Factor, and Basic Fibroblast Growth Factor in the Gastric Mucosa

EGF is a 53-amino acid polypeptide that was originally discovered by Cohen [6] in mouse salivary glands and then found to resemble the structure and biological actions of urogastrone [7], which was detected a long time ago [8] in urine of pregnant women and shows a beneficial effect on healing of experimental ulcers; the common name EGF/URO has been proposed.

In the digestive system, EGF has been detected in large quantities in the salivary glands, Brunner's glands, and the pancreas [9–13]. It is stored in the tubular or ductal cells and released in the saliva or duodeno-pancreatic secretion, so the EGF present in the gastric lumen originates mainly from the salivary secretion [12–14].

EGF-like immunoreactivity has also been detected in the gastric mucosa, but it is not clear whether it is normally produced locally in the mucosa or simply absorbed from the gastric lumen [11, 12, 15]. Swallowed EGF secreted by salivary glands could bind to the mucosal receptors, become internalized, and then be detected as immunoreactivity in mucosal extracts. Since EGF mRNA was not detected in gastric mucosal samples [16], the EGF immunoreactivity in the mucosa must originate from salivary EGF present in the gastric contents. Chronic gastrointestinal ulcerations were, however, reported to be accompanied by an increased expression of EGF and EGF receptors, especially within the area of mucosal lesions and ulcerations [17, 18]. Certain drugs, such as sucralfate [19], colloidal bismuth [20], and Al-antacids [21], were found to enhance the accumulation of EGF in the ulcer area, promote the cell proliferation and angiogenesis at the ulcer margin, and accelerate ulcer healing. Treatment with indomethacin, which is known to delay ulcer healing [22], was shown to reduce the accumulation of EGF in the ulcer area [20]. Wright et al. [23] showed that the ulceration of epithelium anywhere in the gastrointestinal mucosal induces the development of a novel cell lineage from the stem cells and this lineage contains and secretes abundant immunoreactive EGF/URO. It was proposed that a major in vivo role of EGF is the local regeneration of mucosal cells at the ulcer margin and ulcer healing. Recent studies [16] revealed, however, that little EGF immunoreactivity was detected in the gastric mucosa and no EGF mRNA expression was detected in the intact or injured mucosa, indicating that this mucosa has no ability to express EGF and that EGF observed in the ulcer area originates from swallowed EGF in the gastric lumen.

The demonstration of specific EGF receptors on the basolateral and apical membranes of the gastric proliferative zone cells [16] indicates that these cells may be the targets of the restitution and proliferation stimulating actions of EGF present in the gastric lumen.

The major form of growth factor in the gastric mucosa was found to be TGF-α, which is a 50-amino acid polypeptide sharing about a 35% sequence homology, a common receptor, and a nearly identical spectrum of biological activity with EGF [16, 24–26]. Mucosal damage markedly increases TGF-α mRNA expression and results in local production and release of TGF-α into the gastric lumen, suggesting that TGF-α, not EGF, is the major growth factor produced in the intact and injured gastric mucosa [16]. The demonstration of the expression of TGF-α and its receptors throughout the gastric mucosa invites the speculation that local production of TGF-α could play a part in the stomach's defense against various forms of mucosal injury, by inhibiting acid secretion and by stimulating cell migration and later cell proliferation to accelerate tissue repair and healing.

Another growth factor that could be implicated in the maintenance of mucosal integrity is platelet-derived growth factor (PDGF), a glycoprotein composed of two peptide chains (A and B) linked by disulfide bonds [27]. The two chains can be assembled to give three isoforms; PDGF-AA, PDGF-AB and PDGF-BB. Each of these isoforms binds to different receptors whose distribution varies from cell type to cell type. PDGF constitutes the major mitogenic activity in platelets and shows a similar spectrum of biological action to EGF, including direct stimulation of growth of connective tissue cells, proliferation of endothelial and epithelial cells, mucosal repair, and wound or ulcer healing.

PDGF may be the first growth factor released locally in the area of gastric lesions by platelets and macrophages [27]. It has been reported that PDGF mRNA is expressed in the gastric mucosa [28], and the specific receptors for PDGF have been identified in the gastric mucosal cell membranes [4]. Recent studies indicate that PDGF given orally reduces the severity and number of acute gastric mucosal lesions produced by indomethacin [29] and accelerates the healing of acute duodenal lesions induced by cysteamine [30].

bFGF, a 146-amino acid polypeptide, was also demonstrated in the intact and damaged mucosa and proposed to participate in mucosal repair, particularly when this labile peptide is protected from acid degradation in the gastric lumen by antiulcer agents such as sucralfate or antacids [31]. This peptide is produced by a variety of cells, including fibroblasts, endothelial cells, and smooth muscle cells, and stored in extracellular matrix to be released upon tissue damage or remodeling and to stimulate locally the proliferation of these cells [32–35]. The role of bFGF in mucosal repair has yet to be proven, but recent studies of Folkman et al. [31] suggest that bFGF plays a crucial role in angiogenesis in the granulation tissue at the ulcer bed. Our studies indicate that omentum, which exhibits a marked expression of bFGF and which has a prodigious ability to stimulate angiogenesis, accelerates ulcer healing when attached to the serosa covering the ulcer area, and this acceleration is similar to that obtained with administration of exogenous bFGF [36]. The relative contribution of each of the growth factors encountered in the stomach in the maintenance of mucosal integrity, growth, repair, and healing requires further studies.

Involvement of Growth Factors in the Function and Integrity of Gastric Mucosa

EGF and TGF-α administered parenterally in vivo are very potent inhibitors of gastric acid secretion [26], but these peptides have been detected only in minute concentrations in the blood, present partly as a free plasma peptide and partly bound to platelets. Studies in vitro on the isolated gastric glands or parietal cells confirmed that EGF and TGF-α are direct inhibitors of acid production induced by histamine and other secretagogues [26, 38]. The inhibition of acid production is very rapid and does not require continuous exposure to EGF or TGF-α as in the case of stimulation of cell proliferation by these factors, suggesting that the transduction of signal from the receptors to the acid transport system in the parietal cells is very rapid [37]. The receptors involved in this inhibition are located on the basolateral membrane of parietal cells [1, 18, 37], so they may not be readily accessible to EGF present in the gastric lumen even in high concentrations [12–15]. In contrast, TGF-α is produced locally in the intact and damaged gastric mucosa in amounts several times higher than EGF [15, 16], so it might affect gastric acid secretion by acting in a paracrine manner on the parietal cells. This action could explain a marked but transient suppression of acid secretion in mucosa exposed to various irritants and damaging agents.

Since it is unlikely that growth factors other than TGF-α are released in amounts physiologically important enough to affect gastric acid secretion, there is considerable interest in the luminal effects of endogenous EGF delivered to the stomach in saliva or local effects of PDGF and bFGF released in the gastric mucosa. EGF, TGF-α, and PDGF are acid-stable and relatively resistant to pepsin degradation [7], so they are attractive candidates for participation in the mucosal integrity, even without affecting gastric acid secretion (Fig. 3). The spectrum of their biological effects include the stimulation of mucus-alkaline

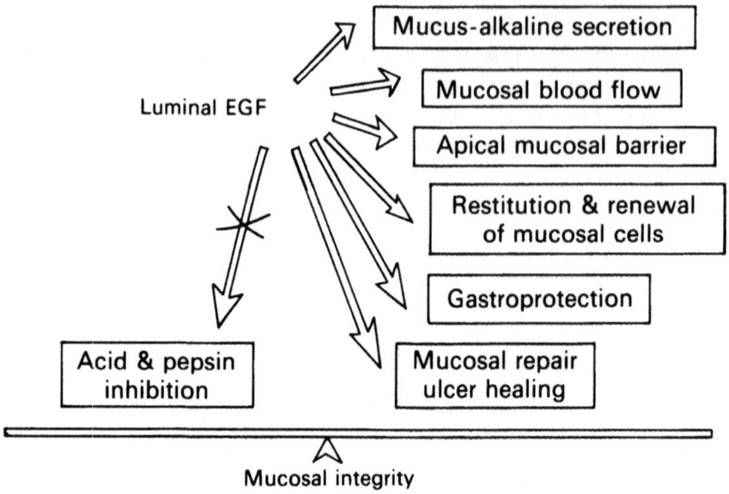

Fig. 3. Luminal EGF in the stomach does not affect gastric acid secretion but exhibits growth promoting, protective, and ulcer-healing effects

secretion, strengthening of the apical mucosal barrier to acid and pepsin back-diffusion, increase in mucosal blood flow, stimulation of rapid restitution of and renewal of mucosal cells, protection of the stomach against various topical irritants and ulcerogens, and acceleration of the healing of acute and chronic of gastric ulcerations [39].

All biological effects of EGF and related peptides are mediated by specific receptors on the target cells [1–4]. It is of interest that the activation of EGF receptors in the mucosal cells leads to stimulation of calcium channel activity through phosphorylation of channel proteins [40, 41]. Calcium is an important regulatory element in many cellular processes [42] including cell integrity and secretion, so certain biological effects of EGF could be related to the activation of the calcium channel by this peptide (Fig. 4). The influx of calcium into the

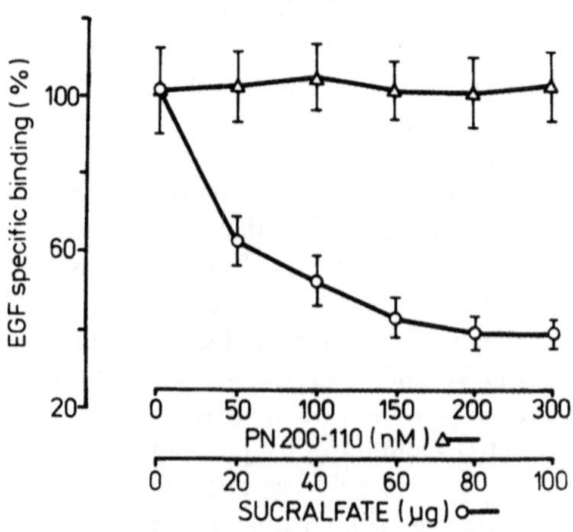

Fig. 4. Effect of sucralfate on EGF binding to gastric mucosal calcium channel protein. The channel protein prior to binding assay was preincubated at room temperature for 30 min either with 0–100 μg sucralfate or 0–300 n*M* PN200-110, a calcium channel antagonist

mucosal cells caused, for instance, by exposure of these cells to ethanol may result in a calcium imbalance and cell damage [43]. The ability of sucralfate to reduce the calcium uptake through inhibition of the EGF-stimulated gastric mucosal calcium channel may explain, at least in part, the protective activity of this drug.

Role of Growth Factors in Gastric Protection

The hypothesis that salivary EGF participates in the maintenance of mucosal integrity, tissue repair, and healing of gastric mucosal injury is supported by studies on salivectomized rats. These rats have atrophic gastric mucosa [44] and show an absence of adaptive cytoprotection to mild irritants [45, 46] and delayed healing of acute and chronic gastric ulcerations that may be reversed by oral or parenteral EGF as well by TGF-α and PDGF [47–49]. Salivectomy increases the susceptibility of gastric mucosa to the formation of acute lesions by various irritants or stress [45, 46] (Fig. 5). Furthermore, the removal of salivary glands reduced the ability of the gastric mucosa to adapt to various ulcerogens such as aspirin, mild irritants, or stress [50]. The reduction in gastric EGF after salivectomy was accompanied by a decrease in DNA synthesis and DNA

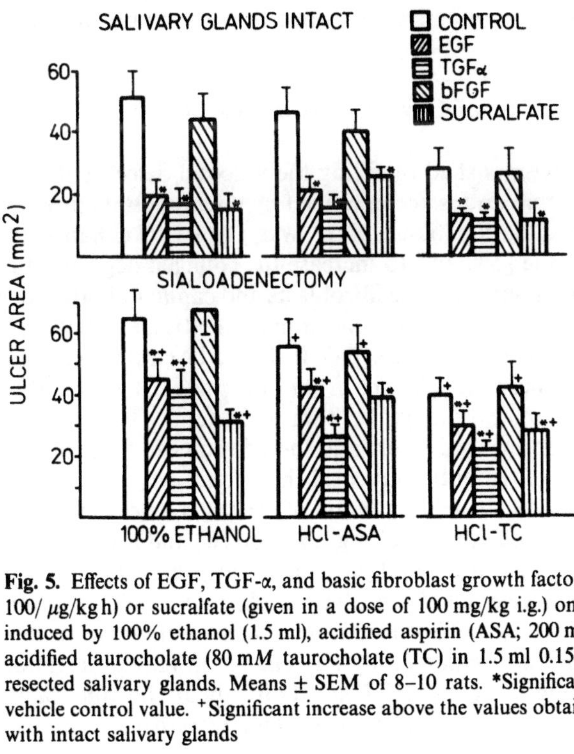

Fig. 5. Effects of EGF, TGF-α, and basic fibroblast growth factor (bFGF) (infused s.c. in a dose of 100/ μg/kg h) or sucralfate (given in a dose of 100 mg/kg i.g.) on the area of acute gastric lesions induced by 100% ethanol (1.5 ml), acidified aspirin (ASA; 200 mg/kg in 1.5 ml 0.15-m*M* HCl) or acidified taurocholate (80 m*M* taurocholate (TC) in 1.5 ml 0.15-m*M* HCl) in rats with intact or resected salivary glands. Means ± SEM of 8–10 rats. *Significant ($P < 0.05$) decrease below the vehicle control value. +Significant increase above the values obtained in similar experiments in rats with intact salivary glands

contents [44, 46, 49],suggesting that the decrease in the mucosal growth-promoting action of EGF is responsible for the increased sensitivity of the mucosa to damaging agents and the loss of gastric adaptation. Administration of exogenous EGF restores in part the resistance of gastric mucosa to the action of various irritants [51, 52].

The importance of endogenous EGF, TGF-α, or PDGF in the protection of gastric mucosa has been emphasized by numerous investigators. EGF given parenterally prevented the formation of acute mucosal lesions induced by various ulcerogens such as absolute ethanol, acidified aspirin, bile acids, or stress [39, 46, 52]. This protection was also observed by some investigators after intragastric administration of these growth factors [29, 51], but it was less pronounced and occurred when gastric lesions were produced by less severe ulcerogens such as acidified aspirin, taurocholate, or stress, but not necrotizing agents such as absolute ethanol [52]. Administration of bFGF failed to protect the mucosa against any topical irritant or ulcerogen [53], indicating that this peptide, unlike other growth factors, does not exhibit any protective activity.

The role of luminal EGF in gastric protection is supported by studies with removal of salivary glands leading to a dramatic fall in EGF content in gastric lumen [39, 44–46]. The salivectomy did not result in the formation of spontaneous gastric lesions, but greatly augmented the production of ulcerations by various ulcerogens (cysteamine) [51] and topical irritants (aspirin, bile acids, 100% ethanol) [52]. Because the intragastric application of saliva-containing EGF or EGF alone prevented the formation of the lesions, it has been postulated that EGF in saliva is an active gastroprotective component [44].

Role of Growth Factor in Healing of Chronic Gastric Ulceration

The healing of an ulcer is accomplished by filling the mucosal defect with cells migrating from the ulcer margin and is accompanied by inflammation, proliferation, and formation of granulation tissue. EGF was shown to enhance the formation of granulation tissue [53] and to increase the collagen deposition in this tissue [54]. In the proliferation step, the fibroblasts and capillary buds move from the ulcer margin (healing zone) and from the granulation tissue, resulting in the repair of the defect with connective tissue [54]. It should be emphasized that healing of chronic gastric ulcers is distinct from the previously described mucosal protection against acute damage by topical irritants. The mucosal protection involves the deeper mucosal layers and there is no need for extensive cell renewal and restoration of the entire mucosal thickness.

As mentioned previously, the beneficial action of urogastrone on healing of chronic peptic ulcerations was recognized a long time ago [8] and it was clearly unassociated with its gastric inhibitory and gastroprotective activity [49, 52]. EGF was also reported to accelerate the healing of chronic duodenal ulcers induced by cysteamine in rats [48]. This acceleration was comparable to that caused by cimetidine but not accompanied by any change in gastric secretion (whereas cimetidine was), suggesting that EGF acted directly on the mucosa via promotion of cell replication in the healing zone and reepithelialization of mucosal defect. EGF and other growth factors enhanced ulcer healing while salivectomy delayed the healing process [49], and this delay could be reversed by the addition of growth factors to salivectomized rats [47–49]. The finding that EGF and other growth factors administered orally enhanced ulcer healing and reversed the delay of healing in salivectomized animals as well as normalizing mucosal growth emphasizes the important role of cell renewal in EGF-induced promotion of the healing process (Fig. 6).

We showed that the induction of ODC activity and increased polyamine synthesis are probably involved because blocking of ornithine decarboxylase (ODC) by difluoromethyl ornithine (DFMO) almost completely reversed the acceleration of ulcer healing by EGF [46, 55, 56].

As EGF accumulates in the ulcer bed, either bound to the fibrin-rich material at the ulcer crater or produced locally due to the appearance of a novel EGF-secreting cell lineage [23], it is likely that it promotes local cell renewal and proliferation at the ulcer margin and the formation of the granulation tissue that supplies connective tissue and microvessels (angiogenesis) to the mucosal scar.

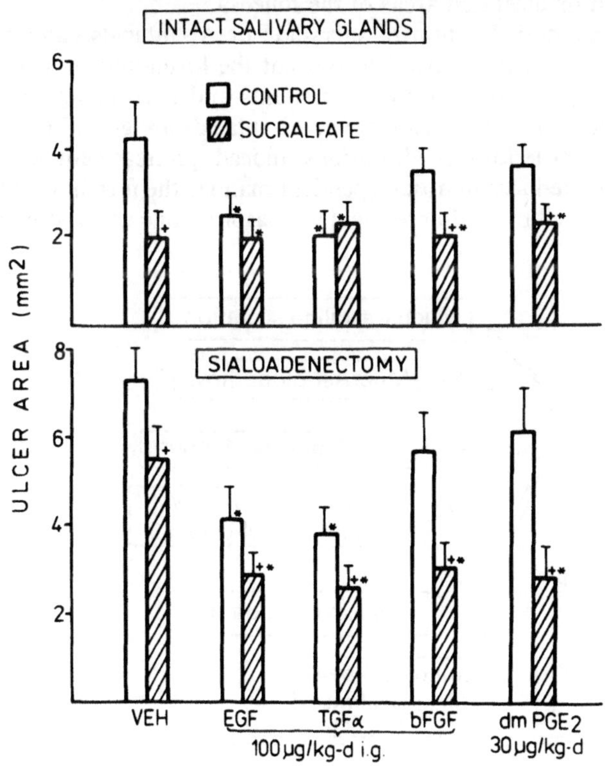

Fig. 6. The area of gastric ulcers in rats with intact and resected salivary glands and treated with EGF, TGF-α, bFGF (100 µg/kg day i.g.) or 16, 16-dimethyl PGE_2 (30 µg/kg i.g.) without or with sucralfate. Means ± SEM of 8–10 rats. *Significant decrease below the value obtained with vehicle. [+]Significant decrease below the value obtained in tests without sucralfate

Interaction of Growth Factors with Gastroprotective Drugs

Gastric Protection and Ulcer Healing Induced by Drugs

Sucralfate, an aluminium salt of sulfated disaccharide-sucrose, colloidal bismuth subcitrate (De-Nol) and Al-antacids (Maalox 70) are widely used antiulcer drugs because they accelerate ulcer healing but do not reduce gastric acid secretion [58]. Their mechanism of action is not clear, except that they cover the surface of the gastric mucosa and bind to the ulcer bed. After acidification such as occurs after intragastric administration, sucralfate and Al-antacids become viscous and adhesive substances tightly bound to eroded or ulcerated mucosa. In eroded areas the surface epithelial cells are lost, and positively charged uncovered tissue proteins attract the negatively charged drug's particles (Fig. 7).

Formation of a protective barrier by sucralfate or Al-antacids over injured, eroded, or ulcerated mucosa together with the inhibition of pepsin activity and adsorption of pepsin and bile salts was initially postulated as the major mechanism of their healing action. The main site of sucralfate action was claimed to be the eroded or ulcerated areas of the mucosa.

The concept of a "band-aid" action of sucralfate or Al-antacids cannot, however, explain the ability of these drugs to prevent the formation of acute mucosal injury induced by a variety of topical irritants and necrotizing substances, because in all these instances sucralfate or Al-antacids are given before the development of mucosal lesions or ulcerations. Indeed, pretreatment with sucralfate and Al-antacids reduces in dose-dependent manner the formation of acute mucosal lesions induced by acid-dependent (e.g., aspirin, bile acids, stress)

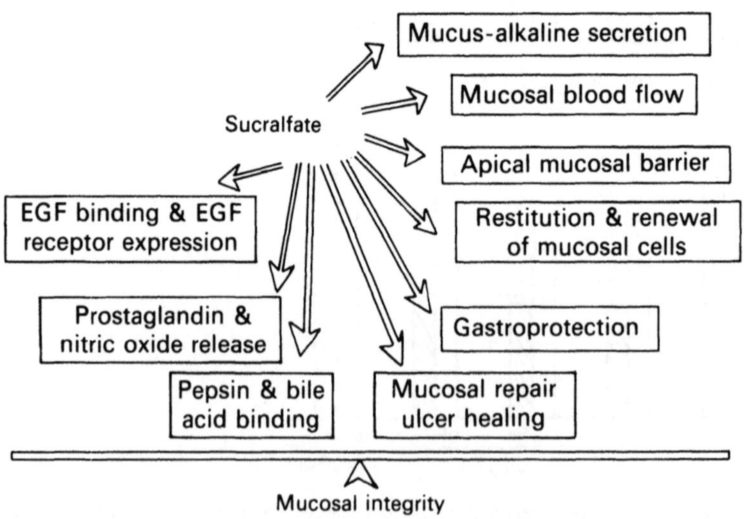

Fig. 7. Spectrum of biological effects of sucralfate (on *right*) and possible mechanisms of action of this drug (on *left*) resulting in the maintenance of mucosal integrity

and acid-independent (e.g., absolute ethanol) ulcerogens. This protective activity depends upon the presence of acidic pH in the gastric lumen and the acidification of sucralfate or Al-antacids greatly augments the protective properties of these drugs.

Implication of Prostaglandins, Nitric Oxide and Growth Factors in Gastroprotective Activity of Gastroprotective Drugs

Sequential analysis of the mucosal changes showed that sucralfate or Maalox 70 did not prevent the excessive exfoliation of surface epithelium caused by topical irritants, but protected deeper mucosal layers, including the proliferative zone cells and mucosal microvessels. The morphological and functional features of protection of the gastric mucosa against ethanol-induced necrosis are similar to these obtained with prostaglandin, suggesting that endogenous prostaglandins mediate, at least in part, the protective action of these drugs.

The mucosal microvasculature plays a vital role in supplying the mucosa with oxygen and nutrients. Gastroprotective drugs were reported to increase gastric mucosal blood flow both in normal and in injured mucosa. Although the protection of gastric microvasculature and increased blood flow to the mucosa could be partly reversed by pretreatment with indomethacin and, therefore, attributed to the endogenous prostaglandins, recent studies suggest that these effects of sucralfate and Al-antacids may also be mediated by endogenous nitric oxide (NO), another locally acting vasodilating and mucosal-protective substance. Blocking of NO synthase by L-nitro-arginine analog reversed the gastroprotective and hyperemic effects of sucralfate and Al-antacids, and concurrent administration of L-arginine but not D-arginine restored their protective activity against ethanol or aspirin damage (Fig. 8).

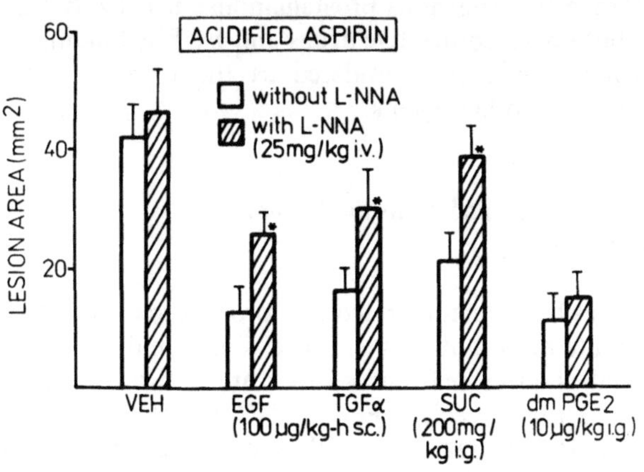

Fig. 8. Enhancement of aspirin-induced gastric mucosal lesions by the administration of *N*-nitro-*L*-arginine (L-NNA) in rats treated with growth factors, sucralfate or dimethyl PGE_2. Means ± SEM of 8–10 rats. *Significant increase above the value obtained in rats without administration of L-NNA

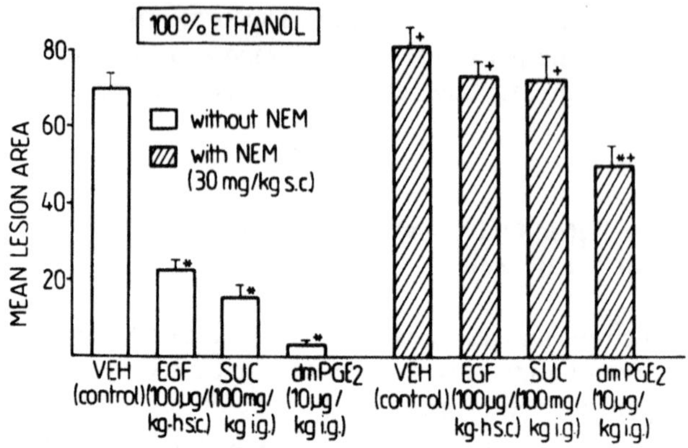

Fig. 9. Effects of subcutaneous administration of *N*-ethylmaleimide (NEM) on ethanol-induced gastric lesions in rats treated with vehicle, EGF (100/µg/kg h s.c.), sucralfate (100 mg/kg i.g.) or dimethyl PGE_2 (10 µg/kg i.g.). Means ± SEM of 8–10 rats. *Significant decrease below the vehicle control value. ⁺Significant increase above the value obtained in rats without pretreatment with NEM

It is of interest that the NO system seems also to participate in the gastroprotection bestowed by growth factors such as EGF or TGF-α, indicating again that the protective mechanism of these factors on the gastric mucosa involves mediators similar to those induced by sucralfate. In contrast to growth factors, the gastroprotection induced by exogenous methylated PGE_2 analog does not appear to be mediated by the NO system (Fig. 8).

The gastroprotective activity of gastroprotective drugs as well as EGF against ethanol damage can also be eliminated by pretreatment with *N*-ethylmaleimide (NEM), the sulfhydryl alkylator (Fig. 9). Since this agent also reversed the protection afforded by exogenous prostaglandins, it is likely that the first biological effect of both gastroprotective drugs and EGF is binding to endogenous sulfhydryls, which could be considered as the common final mediator in mucosal protection by other agents.

Interaction of Gastroprotective Drugs and Growth Factors in Mucosal Repair and Ulcer Healing

Experimental studies in animals have demonstrated that prolonged exposure of the gastric mucosa to sucralfate or Al-antacids produces functional and morphological changes in normal or ulcerated mucosa that are indistinguishable from those evoked by growth factors, especially EGF and TGF-α [58]. Furthermore, the addition of sucralfate to treatment with growth factors greatly enhances the ulcer-healing potency of these factors, both in rats with intact and those with removed salivary glands (see Fig. 6).

New data on mucus secretion indicate that sucralfate, like EGF or TGF-α, is capable of initiating the chain of events linking extracellular signals to intracellular responses. They activate a cascade of regulatory protein phosphorylation, the process closely associated with cellular proliferative activities. Slomiany et al. [2–4], who characterized the EGF receptors in gastric mucosa [3], also demonstrated that the administration of sucralfate results in an increase in gastric expression of EGF and TGF-α receptors (Fig. 10). Gastric mucosal cell membranes isolated from the stomach of rats receiving sucralfate twice daily for 3 consecutive days (100 mg/kg) revealed an over 50% increase in specific EGF and TGF bindings compared to those in vehicle-treated controls. Examination of protein tyrosine phosphorylation patterns using anti-phosphotyrosine antibody revealed that EGF, TGF-α and PDGF caused a marked increase in protein phosphorylation and the phosphoprotein profiles obtained with EGF were quite similar to those obtained with TGF-α or PDGF. This indicates that these growth factors exert their action through a common receptor in gastric mucosal cells.

The demonstration that gastric mucosal cell membranes from the stomach exposed to sucralfate show a significant increase in EGF, TGF-α- and PDGF-specific receptor binding attests to the effect of sucralfate on mucosal cell proliferation. Until now this effect has been attributed solely to the drug's ability to bind growth factors and to prolong their luminal availability. Indeed, sucralfate and Maalox were found to be capable of coprecipitating with EGF, TGF-α, PDGF, and bFGF in a pH-dependent manner, so that with a decrease in pH below 4.5, such as occurs in the gastric lumen [19–21], most luminal growth factors are bound to sucralfate or Maalox (Fig. 11). This binding of luminal EGF (delivered to the stomach in saliva) or TGF-α, PDGF, and bFGF (produced locally by gastric mucosa) seems to be an important factor, since sucralfate and Maalox also chelate selectively with proteinaceous material in the eroded or ulcerated mucosa to form a dense coating in the ulcer bed [58]. This is supported by the observation that radiolabeled EGF or TGF-α introduced into a stomach treated with sucralfate or Maalox accumulates in higher amounts in the ulcer area than in untreated stomach. Nexo and Poulsen [59] first reported in an autoradiographic study that the ulcerated mucosa exhibited much higher concentrations of labeled EGF than the intact mucosa. Our results

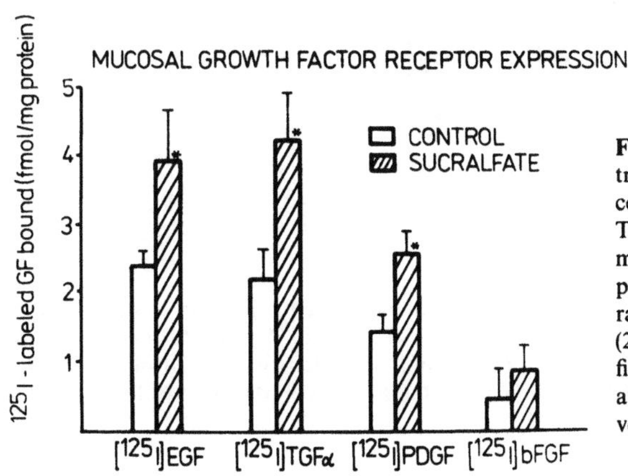

Fig. 10. Effects of prolong administration of sucralfate on gastric mucosal receptor expression for EGF, TGF-α, PDGF, or bFGF. Gastric mucosal cell membranes were prepared from the stomachs of groups of rats receiving sucralfate for 3 days (200 mg/kg day). Means ± SEM of five experiments performed in duplicate. *Significant increase above the vehicle control values

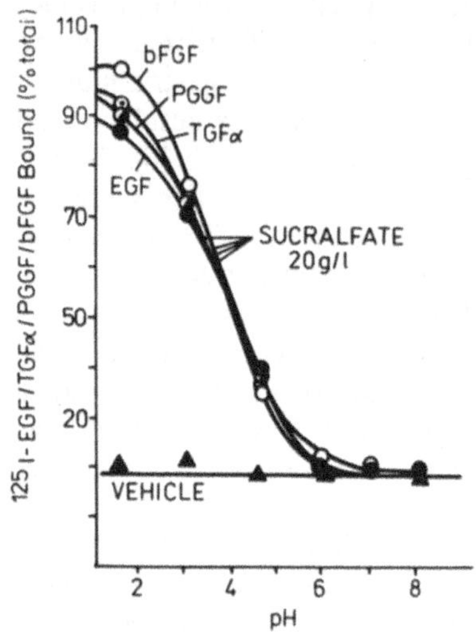

Fig. 11. Binding of labeled EGF, TGF-α, PDGF, or bFGF by sucralfate (20 g/l) or vehicle solution adjusted to pH ranging from 1.5 to 8.0. The results are expressed as a percentage of total labeled growth factor added to the solution

[19–21] confirmed higher concentrations of EGF in the ulcer area than in the intact mucosa in rats treated with sucralfate or Maalox (Fig. 12). This accumulation of EGF in the ulcer bed could originate from the expression of a higher number of specific receptors for these growth factors as well as from the binding of these factors to the proteins in the ulcerated mucosa. An important role of

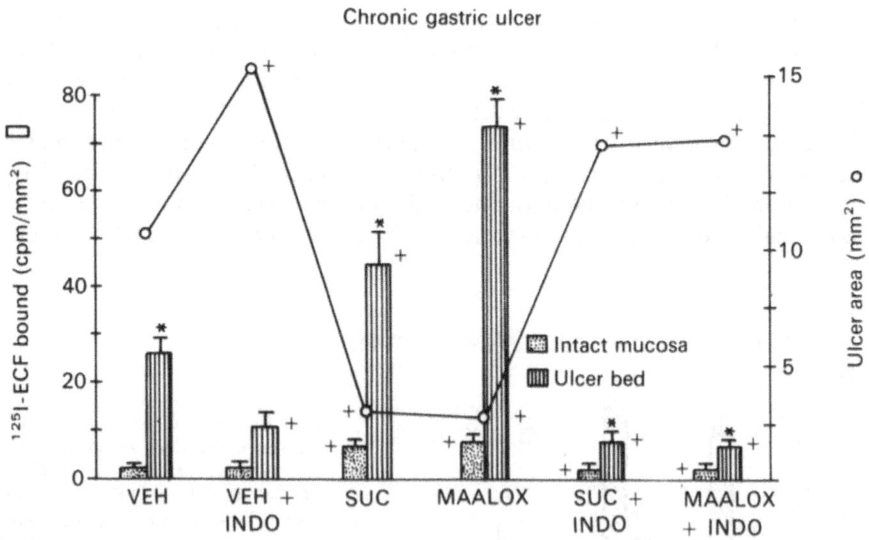

Fig. 12. The accumulation of EGF in the intact mucosa and in the ulcer bed in rats treated with vehicle (saline), indomethacin (2 mg/kg day), sucralfate (400 mg/kg day) or Maalox (2 ml/day) without or with indomethacin (2 mg/kg i.p.). The area of gastric ulcers is also shown. *Significant increase above the value obtained in the ulcer bed. $^{+}$Significant change as compared to the value in vehicle-treated rats.

interaction of sucralfate or Al-antacids and EGF is evidenced by the finding that salivectomy reduced the ulcer-healing effect of these drugs and the addition of EGF restored the healing effect of sucralfate in salivectomized rats [19, 20]. Administration of indomethacin delayed ulcer healing, as reported previously [21, 22]. The major factor in this delay is probably the reduction in the accumulation of EGF material in the ulcer area, because the amount of the labeled EGF bound to the ulcer bed in indomethacin-treated animals without or with addition of sucralfate or Maalox was significantly less than that in rats without administration of indomethacin (Fig. 12).

Role of Growth Factors and Gastroprotective Drugs in Angiogenesis at the Ulcer Bed

Angiogenesis and neovascularization is a central event in wound healing, and gastric erosions and ulcerations are not dissimilar from chronic wounds. Studies of healing of wounds show that the production of granulation tissue, composed of delicate matrix of fibroblasts and capillaries, starts with the release of a variety of growth factors originating first from the platelets in the form of PDGF and then from the macrophages [27, 32]. Fibroblasts and capillaries develop together, being stimulated by locally released growth factors. Among these factors, basic FGF appears to be the most potent stimulant of proliferation of endothelial cells. It may be released from its store in extracellular matrix due to tissue damage and act locally to enhance angiogenesis and fibroplasia.

Basic FGF is a very labile polypeptide and may quickly undergo degradation in the gastric lumen by acid and pepsin. Sucralfate and Maalox have a high affinity to bFGF and protect bFGF from degradation in the acid milieu that would be normally found in the stomach. This protective property of sucralfate in relation to bFGF probably explains the intense angiogenesis observed in the chorioallantoic membrane of the chick embryo or rabbit cornea with implanted sucralfate or sucralfate-bFGF pellets [31].

Folkman and his coworkers [31] provided evidence that bFGF is present in significantly higher amounts in the ulcer bed of sucralfate-treated rats than in vehicle-treated animals. They also showed that other anti-ulcer drugs such as cimetidine result in an increase in the level of bioactive bFGF by virtue of reducing gastric acid content and the degradation of bFGF in the ulcer bed. A unified concept was proposed according to which endogenous bFGF has a central role in ulcer healing and various anti-ulcer drugs accelerate the healing process, presumably by longer survival of endogenous bFGF. It should be emphasized that bFGF should be first released from its storage in the extracellular matrix before interaction with its receptors on target cell plasma membrane and the stimulation of proliferation of fibroblasts and endothelial cells. No direct evidence was provided that such release occurs at the ulcer bed during the healing process, and, therefore, it is not clear when sucralfate could interact with bFGF in the time course of ulcer healing.

References

1. Forgue-Lafitte M-E, Kobari L, Gespach C, Chamblier M-C, Rosselin G (1984) Characterization and partition of epidermal growth factor-urogastrone receptors in gastric glands isolated from young and adult guinea pigs. Biochim Biophys Acta 798:192–198
2. Slomiany BL, Liu J, Yao P, Wu-Wang CY, Keogh JP, Wang SL, Slomiany A (1990) Characterization of the epidermal growth factor receptor in the gastric mucosa. Digestion 47:1981–1990
3. Bielanski WJ, Keogh JP, Wang SL, Lui SL, Konturek SJ, Slomiany A, Slomiany BL (1991) Transforming growth factor α binds to the epidermal growth factor receptor in gastric mucosa. Biochem Int 25:419–427
4. Slomiany BL, Lin J, Keogh JP, Piotrowski J, Slomiany A (1992) Enhancement of gastric mucosal epidermal growth factor and platelet-derived growth factor receptor expression by sucralfate. Gen Pharmac 23:715–718
5. Johnson LR (1988) Gastrointestinal mucosal growth. Physiol Rev 68:455–490
6. Cohen S (1962) Isolation of mouse submaxillary gland protein accelerating incisor eruption and eyelid opening of newborn animals. J Biol Chem 237:1155–1162
7. Gregory H (1975) Isolation and structure of urogastrone and its relationship to epidermal growth factor. Nature (Lond) 257:325–327
8. Sandweiss DJ, Friedman MHF (1942) Is the beneficial effect of urine extract on M-W ulcers due to gastric secretory depressant in urine? Am J Dig Dis 9:166–169
9. Heitz PV, Kasper M, Noorden SV, Polak JM, Gregory H, Pearse AGE (1978) Immunohistochemical localization of urogastrone to human submandibulary glands. Gut 19:408–443
10. Kasselber AG, Orth DN, Gray ME, Stahlman MT (1985) Immunocytochemical localization of human epidermal growth factor/urogastrone in several human tissues. J Histochem Cytochem 33:315–322
11. Poulsen SS, Nexo E, Olsen PS, Hess J, Kirkegaard J (1986) Immunohistochemical localization of epidermal growth factor in rat and man. Histochemistry 85:389–394
12. Olsen PS, Kirkegaard P, Poulsen SS (1984) Adrenergic effects on exocrine secretion of rat submandibular epidermal factor. Gut 25:1234–1240
13. Konturek JW, Bielanski W, Konturek SJ, Bogdal J, Oleksy J, Rovati L (1989) Distribution and release of epidermal growth factor in humans. Gut 30:1189–1200
14. Konturek SJ, Bielanski W, Konturek JW, Oleksy J, Yamazaki J (1989) Release and action of epidermal growth factor on gastric secretion in humans. Scand J Gastroenterol 24:485–492
15. Cartlidge SA, Elder JB (1989) Transforming growth factor alpha and epidermal growth factor levels in normal human gastrointestinal mucosa. Br J Cancer 60:657–660
16. Polk WH, Dempsey PJ, Russall WE, Brown PI, Beaucham RD, Bernard JA, Coffey RJ (1992) Increased production of transforming growth factor α following acute gastric injury. Gastroenterology 102:1467–1474
17. Tarnawski A, Stachura J, Durbin T, Gergely H (1991) Expression of epidermal growth factor receptor in rat gastric oxyntic mucosa. J Clin Gastroenterol 13:(Suppl 1):S109–113
18. Hansson H-A, Hong L, Helander HF (1990) Changes in gastric EGF, EGF receptors and acidity during healing of gastric ulcer in the rat. Acta Physiol Scand 138:241–242
19. Konturek SJ, Brzozowski T, Bielanski W, Warzecha Z, Drozdowicz D (1989) Epidermal growth factor in the gastroprotective and ulcer healing actions of sucralfate in rats. Am J Med 86 (Suppl): 32–37
20. Konturek SJ, Dembinski A, Warzecha Z, Bielanski W, Brzozowski T, Drozdowicz D (1988) Epidermal growth factor (EGF) in the gastroprotective and ulcer healing action of colloidal bismuth subcitrate. Gut 29:894–902
21. Konturek SJ, Brzozowski T, Drozdowicz D, Dembinski A, Nauert Ch (1990) Healing of chronic gastroduodenal ulcers by antacids. Role of prostaglandins and epidermal growth factor. Dig Dis Sci 35:1121–1129
22. Wang JY, Yamasaki S, Takeuchi K, Okabe S (1989) Delayed healing of acetic acid-induced gastric ulcers in rats by indomethacin. Gastroenterology 96:393–402
23. Wright NA, Pike C, Elia G (1990) Induction of a novel epidermal growth factor: secretin cell lineage by mucosal ulceration in human gastrointestinal stem cells. Nature (Lond) 343:82–85
24. Derynck R (1986) Transforming growth factor α, structure and biological activities. J Cell Biol 32:293–304

25. Derynck R (1988) Transforming growth factor α. Cell 54:593–595
26. Konturek SJ, Brzozowski T, Majka J, Dembinski A, Slomiany A, Slomiany BL (1992) Transforming growth factor α and epidermal growth factor in protection and healing of gastric mucosal injury. Scand J Gastroenterol 27:649–655
27. Raines EW, Sporn-Pope DF, Ross R (1990) Platelet-derived growth factor. In: Sporn MB, Roberts AB (eds) Peptide growth factors. Springer, Berlin Heidelberg New York, pp 173–262 (Handbook of experimental pharmacology, vol 95)
28. Bennett C, Peterson IM, Corbishley CM, Luqmani YA (1989) Expression of platelet-derived growth factor and epidermal growth factor receptor encoded transcripts in human gastric tissues. Cancer Res 49:2104–2112
29. Guglietta A, Hervada T, Nardi RV, Lesch CA (1992) Effect of platelet-derived growth factor BB on indomethacin-induced gastric lesions in rats. Scand J Gastroenterol 27:673–676
30. Vattay P, Gyomber E, Morales RE, Szabo S (1991) Effects of orally administered platelet-derived growth factor (PDGF) on healing of chronic duodenal ulcers and gastric secretion in rats. Gastroenterology 100:A180
31. Folkman J, Szabo S, Stovroff M, McNeilp LW, Shing Y (1991) Duodenal ulcer. Discovery of a new mechanism and development of angiogenic therapy that accelerates healing. Ann Surg 214:414–425
32. Burgess AW, Sizerland AM (1990) Growth factors and the gut. J Gastroenterol Hepatol 5 (suppl 1):10–21
33. Baird A, Esch F, Mormede P, Veno N, Ling N, Bohlem P, Ying SY, Wehrenberg WP, Guillemin R (1986) Molecular characterization of fibroblast growth factor: Distribution and biological activities in many tissues. Recent Prog Horm Res 42:143–205
34. Vlodavsky I, Folkman J, Sulliman R (1987) Endothelial cell-derived basic fibroblast growth factor. Synthesis and deposition into subendothelial extracellular matrix. Proc Natl Acad Sci USA 84:2292–2296
35. Gospodarowicz D (1990) Fibroblast growth factor. Clin Orthop 257:231–248
36. Konturek SJ, Brzozowski T, Pawlik W, Stachura J (1992) Omentum and basic fibroblast growth factor (bFGF) in healing of chronic gastric ulcers. Gastroenterology 102:A101
37. Gregory H, Thomas CE, Young JA, Willshire IR, Garner A (1988) The contribution of the C-terminal undecapeptide sequence of urogastrone-epidermal growth factor to its biological action. Regul Pept 22:217–226
38. Konturek SJ, Cieszkowski M, Jaworek J, Konturek JW, Brzozowski T, Gregory H (1984) Effects of epidermal growth factor on gastrointestinal secretions. Am J Physiol 246:G580
39. Konturek JW, Brzozowski T, Konturek SJ (1991) Epidermal growth factor in protection, repair and healing of gastroduodenal mucosa. J Clin Gastroenterol 13:(suppl 1):388–397
40. Peppelenbosch MP, Tertoden LGF, deLaat SW (1991) Epidermal growth factor-activated calcium and potassium channels. J Biol Chem 266:19938–19944
41. Slomiany BL, Lin J, Slomiany A (1992) Platelet-derived growth factor activation of gastric mucosal calcium channels. Biochem Biophys Res Commun (in press)
42. Hosey MM, Lazdunski M (1988) Calcium channels pharmacology, structure and regulation. J Membr Biol 104:81–105
43. Tarnawski A, Brzozowski T, Gergely H, Sekkon S, Krause WJ (1990) The role of calcium in injury of isolated gastric gland cells. Acta Physiol Pol 41:84–85
44. Tepperman BL, Soper BD (1990) Effect of sialoadenectomy on gastric mucosal integrity and growth in the rat. Dig Dis Sci 35:943–949
45. Tepperman BL, Soper BD, Morris GP (1987) Effect of sialoadenectomy on adaptive cytoprotection in the rat. Gastroenterology 97:123–129
46. Konturek PK, Brzozowski T, Konturek SJ, Dembinski A (1990) Role of epidermal growth factor (EGF), prostaglandins and sulfhydryls in stress-induced gastric lesions. Gastroenterology 99:1607–1615
47. Olsen PS, Poulsen SS, Therkelsen K, Nexo E (1986) Effects of sialoadenectomy and synthetic human urogastrone on healing of chronic ulcers in rats. Gut 27:1443–1449
48. Olsen PS, Poulsen SS, Therkelsen K, Nexo E (1986) Oral administration of synthetic human urogastrone promotes healing of chronic duodenal ulcers in rats. Gastroenterology 90:911–917
49. Konturek SJ, Dembinski A, Warzecha Z, Brzozowski T, Gregory H (1988) Role of epidermal growth factor in healing of chronic gastroduodenal ulcers in rats. Gastroenterology 94:1300–1307

50. Konturek SJ, Brzozowski T, Stachura J (1992) Adaptation of the gastric mucosa to stress. Role of prostaglandins and epidermal growth factor. Scand J Gastroenterol (in press)
51. Olsen PS, Poulsen SS, Kirkegaard P, Nexo A (1984) Role of submandibular saliva and epidermal growth factor in gastric cytoprotection. Gastroenterology 87:103–108
52. Konturek SJ, Brzozowski T, Dembinski A, Warzecha Z (1989) Gastric protective and ulcer-healing action of epidermal growth factor. In: Garner A, Whittle BJR (eds) Advances in drug therapy of gastrointestinal ulceration. Wiley, London, pp 261–273
53. Laato M, Niinikoski J, Gerdin B, Lebel L (1986) Stimulation of wound healing by epidermal growth factor, a dose-dependent effect. Ann Sug 203:379–381
54. Buckley A, Davidson JM, Kamerath CD, Woodward SC (1987) Epidermal growth factor increases granulation tissue formation dose-dependently. J Sug Res 43:322–328
55. Bielanski W, Brzozowski T, Majka J, Szlachcic A, Ott W, Konturek SJ (1992) Fibroblast growth factor (bFGF) in gastroprotection and ulcer healing. Interaction with sucralfate. Gastroenterology 102:A42
56. Brzozowski T, Konturek SJ, Majka J, Dembinski A, Drozdowicz D (1992) Epidermal growth factor, polyamines and prostaglandins in healing of stress-induced gastric lesions in rats. Dig Dis Sci 37 (in press)
57. Marcuard SP, Silverman JL, Finley JL, Seidel ER (1992) Ornithine decarboxylase activity during gastric ulcer healing in dogs. Dig Dis Sci 37, 1015–1019
58. Konturek SJ, Konturek JW (1989) Gastroprotection by nonprostaglandin substances. In: Hollander D, Tarnawski AS (eds) Gastric cytoprotection. A Clinician's Guide. Plenum, New York, pp 197–214
59. Nexo E, Poulsen SS (1987) Does epidermal growth factor play a role in the action of sucralfate? Scand J Gastroenterol 22 (Suppl 127):45–49

Cellular Mechanisms of Gastric Ulcer Healing

A. TARNAWSKI

Introduction

An ulcer is a deep necrotic lesion in gastroduodenal mucosa involving the entire mucosal thickness and penetrating through the muscularis mucosae (Fig. 1) [1]. It develops as a result of a marked imbalance between aggressive factors (such as hydrochloric acid, pepsin, lysolecithin, ethanol, nonsteroidal antiinflammatory drugs, (NSAIDs), and *H. pylori* infection) present in the gastric (or duodenal) lumen and the mucosal defensive mechanisms listed in Table 1 [2–4]. Numerous

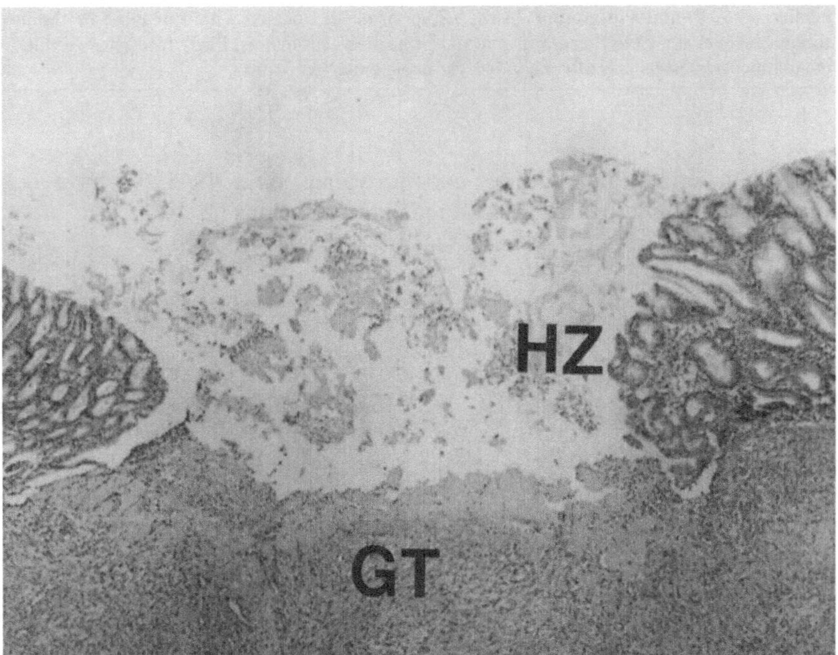

Fig. 1. Photomicrograph of 5-day-old gastric ulcer produced in rat by serosal application of acetic acid. *HZ*, Healing zone at the ulcer margin; *GT*, granulation tissue at the ulcer bottom. (From [7], p. S151)

Table 1. Mucosal Defensive Mechanisms After Tarnawski et al. [49]

1. *Unstirred layer of mucus and bicarbonate.* This first line of defense is very important, because it maintains a "neutral" (pH close to 7.0) microclimate at the luminal surface of the surface epithelial cells, while in the gastric lumen pH is often between pH 1.0 and 3.0.
2. *The surface epithelial cells* (second line of defense) are able to secrete mucus and bicarbonate and generate prostaglandin. Due to the presence of phospholipids on their surfaces, these cells are hydrophobic, "repelling" acid and water-soluble damaging agents. Surface epithelial cells interconnect by tight junctions, forming a "barrier" preventing back diffusion of acid and pepsin.
3. *Continuous mucosal cell renewal* from the progenitor cells in the mucosal proliferative zone enables replacement of damaged or aged surface epithelial ceils. Usually it takes 3–5 days to completely replace the surface epithelium, while it takes months to replace the glandular cells. Superficial injury to the surface epithelium is restituted within a few hours by migration of the cells from neck area.
4. "*Alkaline tide*". Parietal cells secreting hydrochloric acid into the gastric gland lumen concurrently secrete bicarbonate into the lumen of adjacent microvessels. Then bicarbonate is transported upward, contributing to the "neutral" microclimate at the luminal surface.
5. *Mucosal microcirculation through the microvessels* supplies oxygen and nutrients to the entire mucosa and removes toxic substances. Microvascular endothelium generates vasodilators such as prostacyclin and nitric oxide, which protect the gastric mucosa against injury and oppose mucosal damaging action of vasoconstrictors such as leukotriene C_4 and endothelin.
6. *Continuous generation of prostaglandin E_2 (PGE_2) and prostacyclin (PGI_2)* by the mucosa is crucial for the maintenance of mucosal integrity. Almost all the mucosal defensive mechanisms are stimulated or facillitated by endogenous or exogenous prostaglandins. Neutralization of endogenous mucosal prostaglandins with antibodies results in formation of gastric and intestinal ulcerations.
7. *Sensory nerve* stimulation leads to the release of neurotransmitters such as calcitonin gene-related peptide (CGRP) and substance P in the nerve terminals, located within or close to the large submucosal vessels. CGRP exerts a mucosal protective action, most likely through vasodilation of submucosal vessels possibly mediated via nitric oxide generation.

factors – genetic, neural, humoral, and iatrogenic (e.g., NSAIDs) – have been implicated in the etiology of gastroduodenal ulcerations [2–4].

Ulcer Development

Originally, Virchow postulated in 1853 that vascular factors and impaired mucosal circulation (and thus ischemia) play a critical role in the development of gastroduodenal ulcers [5]. Recent experimental studies have fully supported Virchow's contention. Piasecki [6] demonstrated that ligation of gastric submucosal arteries or their prolonged occlusion by contraction of muscularis mucosae and/or muscularis propria is the basis of the ulcer formation. In our experimental study on development of experimental, acetic acid-induced gastric ulcer in rats [7], we found that within 5–15 min after acetic acid application, thrombi developed in submucosal vessels and collecting venules, leading to microvascular stasis and resultant ischemic mucosal necrosis (Table 2).

This study clearly demonstrated that the vascular and microvascular changes are the earliest events in the development of experimental gastric ulcer.

These vascular changes cause mucosal ischemia, free radical formation, cessation of nutrient delivery which all result in mucosal necrosis [7]. During the acute stage of ulceration, the mucosa and submucosa become necrotic and attract polymorphonuclear leukocytes and macrophages [1, 7], and eventually necrotic portions of the mucosa detach and/or are removed by scavenging macrophages within 24 h [7]. By 48 h necrosis involves the muscularis mucosae. By 72 h, the ulcer undergoes transition into the "chronic" stage, characterized histologically by the presence of granulation tissue at the ulcer base and the appearance of a distinct ulcer margin at the adjacent nonnecrotic mucosa (Table 2).

Table 2. Time sequence[a] of mucosal changes during formation and development of acetic acid-induced gastric ulcer in rat. (From [7], p. 156)

1 min:
- Vasodilation of large submucosal veins and arteries and overlying mucosal collecting venules
- Focal edema of submucosa
- Mucosal swelling of stromal tissue, but surface epithelial cells and glands look normal

15 min (additional changes):
- Blood clots in submucosal dilated veins
- Marked edema of submucosa
- Delineated areas of mucosal swelling and deterioration of surface integrity in affected area

1 h (additional changes):
- Blood clots in submucosal arteries
- Clearly disintegrating surface with desquamating surface epithelial cells
- Cellular depletion of the glandular mucosa

3 h (additional changes):
- More pronounced disintegration of the mucosa. Transition zone between necrotic and normal mucosa involves 2–4 glands
- Accumulating of polymorphonuclear leukocytes in submucosal vessels and in the submucosa
- Beginning of detachment of larger necrotic masses from the necrotic mucosa

24 h:
- Generalized tissue necrosis and sloughing from the ulcer crater
- Necrosis involves muscularis propria
- Prominent inflammatory infiltration of serosa

48 h:
- Craters free of necrotic tissue
- Necrotic and purulent muscularis propria
- Purulent serosa

72 h:
- Granulation tissue covers the ulcer bottom
- Some ulcers ruptured through the serosa
- "Chronic" appearance of ulcerations
- Granulation tissue often penetrates into surroundings, especially the pancreas
- Mucosa at the ulcer margin forms transitional healing zone

120 h:
- Large amount of granulation tissue at ulcer craters
- Increased mitotic activity in transitional zone
- Cells in transitional zone poorly differentiated (most likely dedifferentiated)

[a]Time refers to time after application of acetic acid

Majority of studies on ulcer healing have utilized different experimental models, e.g., surgical resection, thermal cauterization, cryoprobes, laser, or submucosal or serosal application of acetic acid. All these models showed striking similarities in the morphologic evolution and stages of ulcer healing [7–14], which indicates that once an ulcer develops, it goes through the same common stages of healing. It also appears that gastric ulcer healing has many similarities to and follows the same general principles as the wound healing process [15].

Ulcer Healing

Ulcer healing, i.e., the reconstruction of the mucosal architecture, is an active process of filling the mucosal defects with proliferating and migrating epithelial cells and connective tissue components. Ulcer healing is a very complex process, requiring the interaction of different tissue and cellular systems. The following factors and/or morphologic structures play an important role in ulcer healing (Fig. 2), [1, 7, 11, 12, 14,16–18].

Luminal Factors

Clinical and experimental experience indicate that inhibition of acid secretion and thus reduction of aggressive factors such as hydrochloric acid and pepsin

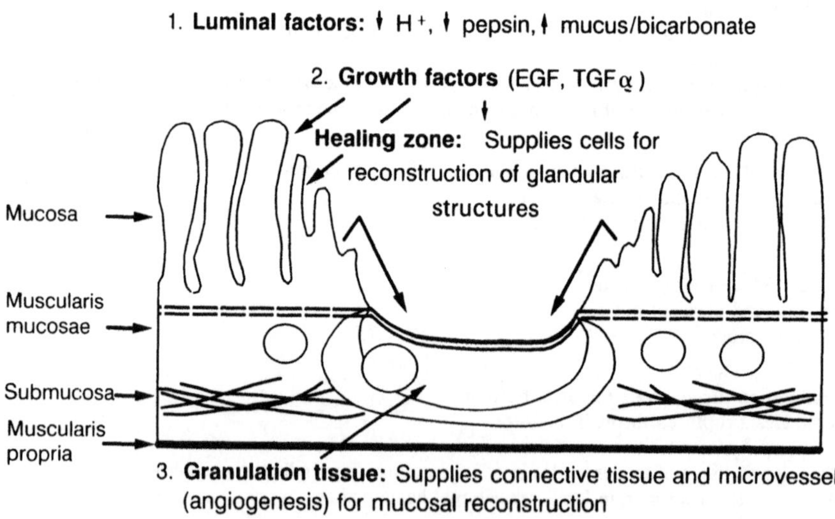

Fig. 2. Ulcer healing process and factors affecting ulcer healing. Healing of the ulcer is accomplished by filling the mucosal defect with, first, cells migrating from the healing zone and replicating [under influence of epidermal growth factor (*EGF*) and transforming growth factor-α (*TGFα*)], and, second, connective tissue cells including microvessels originating from the granulation tissue. (From [35], p. S44). The growth and proliferation of connective tissue cells and endothelial cells (angiogenesis) is under control of fibroblast growth factor family (especially basic FGF) and other cytokines

accelerates ulcer healing. Such mechanisms are the basis and account for the therapeutic action of acid-inhibitory drugs (H_2-receptor antagonists and omeprazole) [16]. Mucus and bicarbonate secretion may also be important in the ulcer healing process, because the mucus/bicarbonate layer may protect newly formed cells against acid and pepsin digestion [17, 18].

Mucosa of the Ulcer Margin

Mucosa at the ulcer margin forms a characteristic "healing" zone which undergoes striking changes in structure and cellular composition. The glands

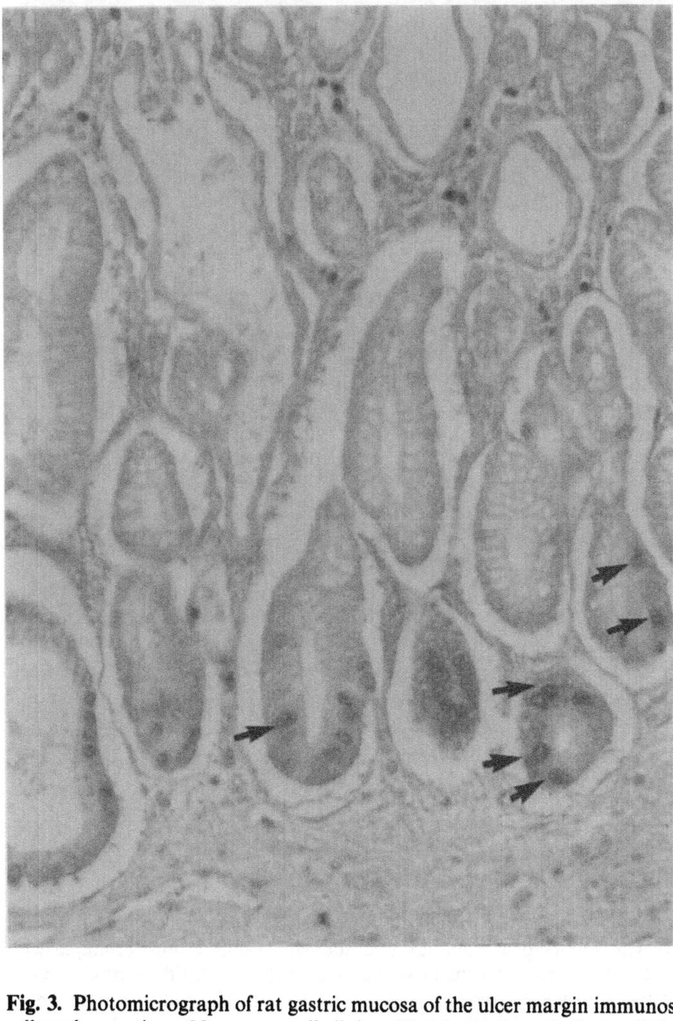

Fig. 3. Photomicrograph of rat gastric mucosa of the ulcer margin immunostained for proliferating cell nuclear antigen. Numerous cells lining dilated glands at the base of ulcer margin with stained nuclei (*arrows*) are in the S phase of the cellular cycle. This reflects increased cell proliferation at the ulcer margin

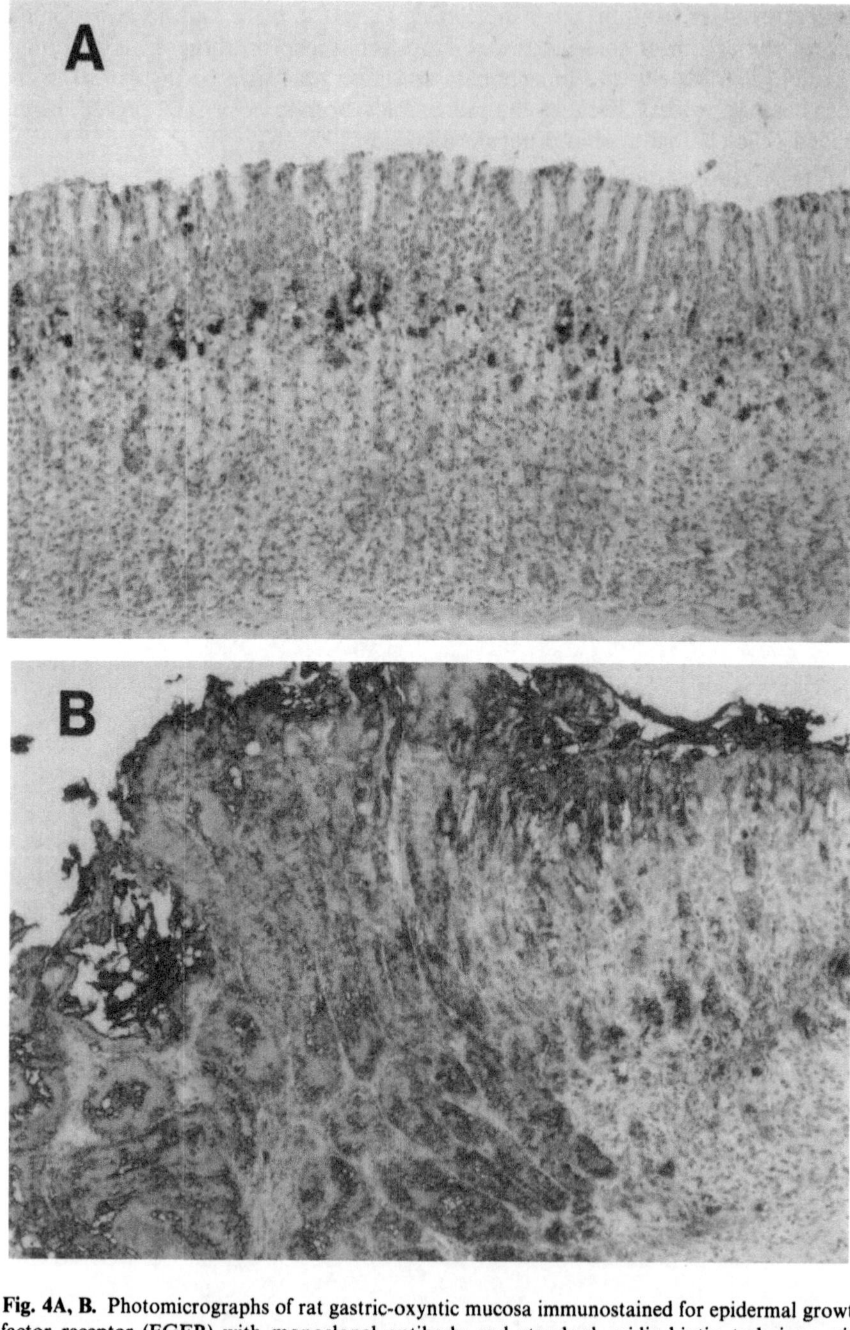

Fig. 4A, B. Photomicrographs of rat gastric-oxyntic mucosa immunostained for epidermal growth factor receptor (EGFR) with monoclonal antibody and standard avidin-biotin technique with aminoethyl carbazole as a chromogen. **A** Normal oxyntic mucosa shows EGFR reaction in some neck cells of the proliferative zone and in some parietal cells. **B** Mucosa of the ulcer margin 7 days after ulcer induction shows increased EGFR expression. The cells showing EGFR expression occupy the entire mucosal thickness. (From [22], p. 697)

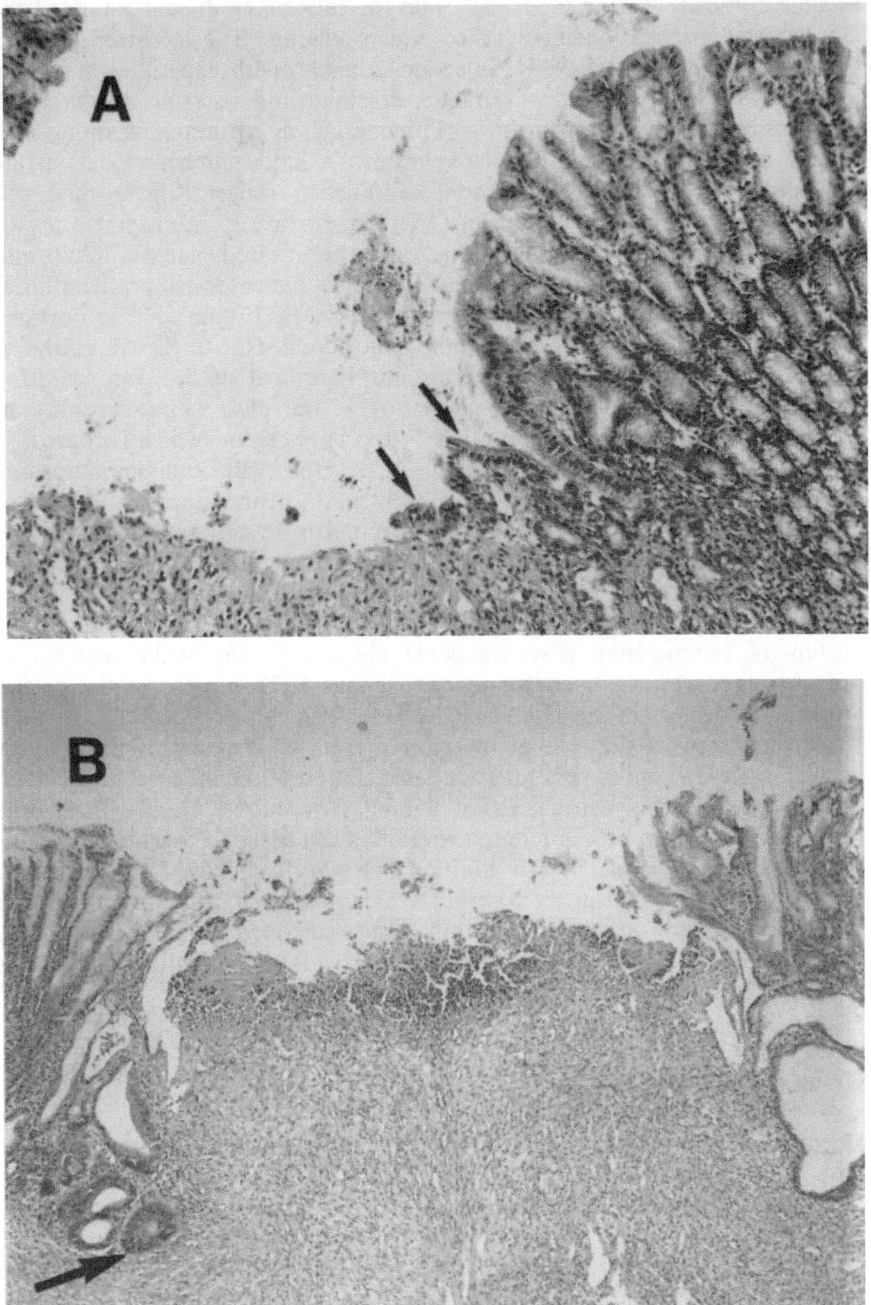

Fig. 5A, B. Photomicrographs of the gastric ulcer margin. **A** Cells from the healing zone migrate (*arrows*) onto granulation tissue to cover the ulcer base. **B** Poorly differentiated cells budding into the granulation tissue (*arrow*) to form new glandular structures. (From [35], p. 545)

become cystically dilated [7, 11, 12], and the cells lining dilated glands of the ulcer margin become dedifferentiated and proliferate. The increased proliferation can be demonstrated by injecting animals (with experimental gastric ulcers) with [^{3}H]thymidine or bromodeoxyuridine and assessing cellular DNA synthesis by autoradiography (for [^{3}H]thymidine) or by immunostaining with specific antibody against bromodeoxyuridine. A large number of cells at the ulcer margin express also proliferating cell nuclear antigen (Fig. 3) which is a 36-kDa auxiliary protein (cyclin) of DNA polymerase δ, an enzyme vital for DNA replication [19]. Synthesis of this protein begins in the later G_1 phase and peaks during the S phase of the cellular cycle. The increased cell proliferation is most likely initiated by epidermal growth factor (EGF) and/or transforming growth factor-α (TGF-α), which are mitogenic peptides for the gastric epithelial cells [20]. This is supported by immunohistochemical studies demonstrating that the cells lining dilated gastric glands at the ulcer margin display an enormous increase in expression of EGF and its receptor (which is shared by TGF-α) 1–7 days after ulcer induction [21, 22] (Fig. 4B). Radioimmunoassay study demonstrated increased EGF concentration in the mucosa of the ulcer margin [21]. The source of EGF is either luminal, from salivary glands [23, 24], or it is locally synthesized by the cells of regenerating glands [25]. Thus, EGF and its receptor play an important role in this phase of ulcer healing. This is further underscored by the fact that exogenous EGF and TGF-α accelerate healing of experimental gastroduodenal ulcers [24, 26], while removal of salivary glands (a major source of endogenous EGF present in the gastric lumen) delays ulcer healing [23, 24].

Proliferation of the cells at the ulcer margin is very important for ulcer healing, since it supplies cells for reepithelialization of the mucosal surface and reconstruction of the gastric mucosal glandular structures [11, 17]. These cells migrate from the ulcer margin onto the granulation tissue to cover (reepithelialize) the ulcer base (Fig. 5A). In addition, the poorly differentiated cells from cystically dilated glands at the base of the ulcer margin (healing zone) bud into the lamina propria and/or into granulation tissue, forming tubules (Fig. 5B). These tubules undergo transformation into glands that eventually will communicate with the gastric lumen.

Granulation Tissue

During the chronic stage of ulceration, granulation tissue develops at the ulcer base [1, 7]. It consists of proliferating connective tissue cells – macrophages, fibroblasts, endothelial cells (Fig. 6A) – which form microvessels through the process of angiogenesis (Fig. 6B) [27]. Granulation tissue is an important component of the ulcer healing process because it supplies microvessels for restoration of the microvasculature within the mucosal scar and connective tissue cells for the restoration of the lamina propria. The granulation tissue undergoes continuous remodeling and changes in cellular composition. Initially, inflammatory cells and macrophages are abundant, while at the later stages fibroblasts predominate [1]. The growth of granulation tissue and generation of

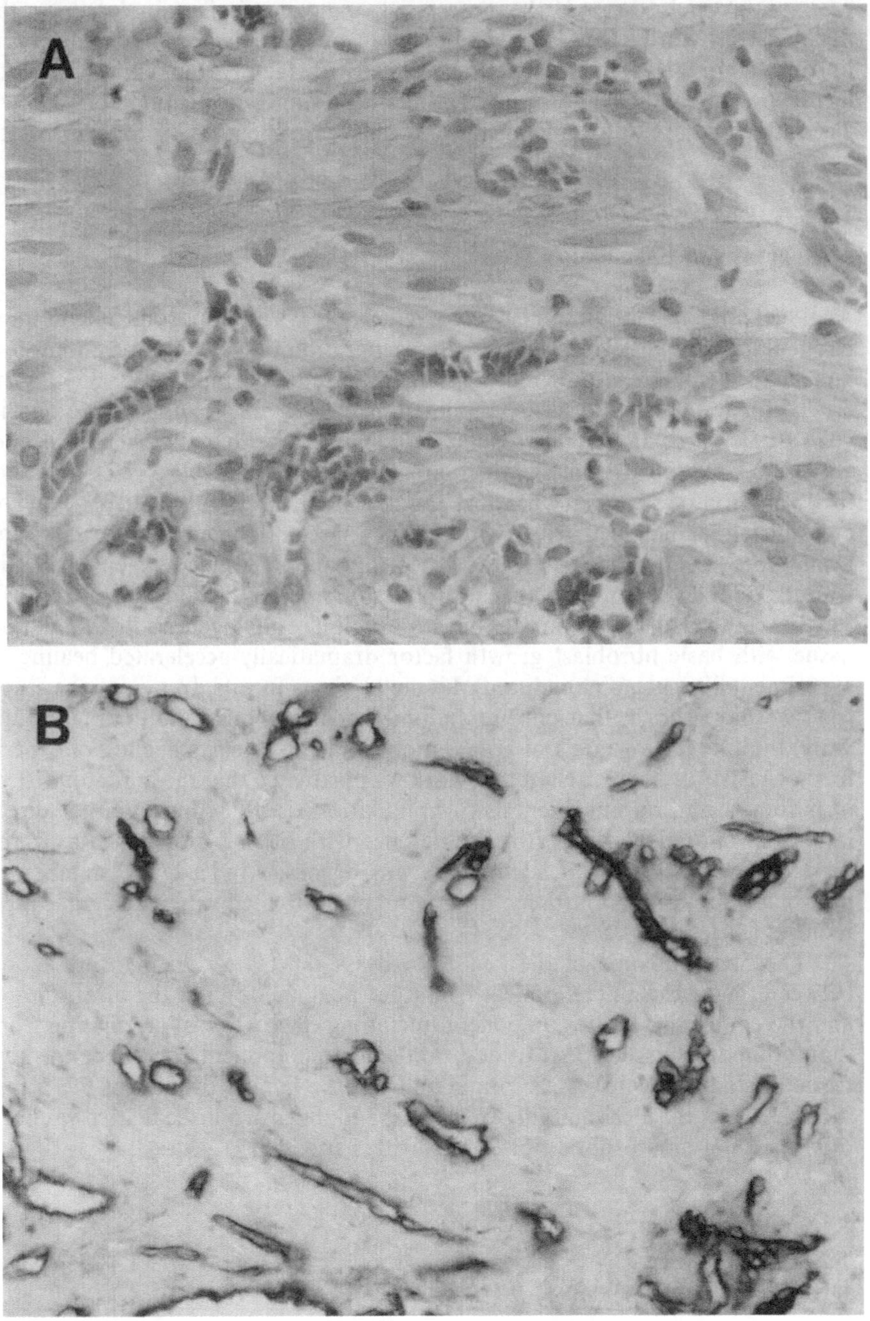

Fig. 6A, B. Photomicrographs of granulation tissue at the ulcer base. **A** Granulation tissue contains numerous fibroblasts and numerous microvessels generated in the process of angiogenesis. H&E staining. **B** Immunostaining for laminin (basement membrane component) outlines numerous vessels and microvessels in granulation tissue

new microvessels through the process of angiogenesis is stimulated by the fibroblast growth factors [28], and possibly by other factors, including basic fibroblast growth factor, platelet-derived growth factor, transforming growth factor, prostaglandins, and/or interleukin-1 and tumor necrosis factor [29–31]. The latter two are mitogenic mediators, which are chemotactic for fibroblasts.

Angiogenesis in Granulation Tissue

Angiogenesis – formation of new microvessels – plays an important role in morphogenesis, wound healing, and tissue regeneration [1, 15, 27]. It is an important component of the repair of acute gastric mucosal injury [32, 33] and is crucial for the healing of gastroduodenal ulcers [29, 28]. From in vivo and in vitro studies, including our own data [32, 33], it is clear that angiogenesis occurs via a series of sequential steps which are summarized in Table 3 [27]. Through the formation of a capillary network, angiogenesis in granulation tissue facilitates nutrient and oxygen delivery to the ulcer base and therefore is crucial to the healing process. It has been demonstrated that an increase in oxygen tension in wounds doubles or triples collagen production and epithelial cell growth [15].

Folkman et al. [28] reported that stimulation of angiogenesis in granulation tissue with basic fibroblast growth factor dramatically accelerated healing of experimental (cysteamine-induced) duodenal ulcers in rats. In a previous study [34] we have shown that chronic indomethacin administration (1 mg/kg i.p., daily) inhibits angiogenesis in granulation tissue and delays healing of experimental gastric ulcers in rats. In that work we postulated that the inhibitory effect of indomethacin on angiogenesis in granulation tissue is due to either direct inhibition of angiogenesis or by interference with other factors (such as fibroblast growth factors) which stimulate angiogenesis. Indeed, the number of fibroblasts in granulation tissue of indomethacin-treated rats was significantly reduced [34].

The final outcome of the healing process reflects a dynamic interaction between the epithelial component from the "healing" zone at the ulcer margin and the connective tissue component (including microvessels) originating from the granulation tissue [35]. In addition, some components of the connective tissue (including microvessels) originate from the lamina propria of the transitional zone at the ulcer margin. An increased number of mitotic figures has been reported in lamina propria fibroblasts at this site [11].

Table 3. Angiogenesis: sequence of events. (From [27])

1. Degradation of microvascular basement membrane
2. Endothelial cell migration into perivascular space (sprouting) and proliferation
3. Formation of microvascular tube
4. Formation of anastomoses, lumina, and basement membrane
5. Formation of capillary network

Scar Contraction

Tissue contraction appears to be an important phase of wound healing. Recent observations have indicated that contraction of granulation tissue may be a permissive factor in gastric ulcer healing [36].

Role of Extracellular Matrix in Ulcer Healing

Extracellular matrix (ECM) components such as fibronectin, laminin, and collagens play an important role in cell attachment, migration, proliferation, and differentiation [37–39]. Recent studies have demonstrated that during repair of tissue injuries, including skin and corneal ulcers, pulmonary and myocardial infarction, and liver regeneration [40–43], ECM plays a critical role in forming structural support for regenerating cells and in contributing to cell proliferation, migration, and differentiation [37, 43, 44]. Fibronectin is the most important component of ECM, because it is a link molecule between cells and the ECM [38, 39]. It has extensive codistribution with collagen type III and affects the formation and maturation of connective tissue, including granulation tissue. Recent reports suggest a therapeutic role for topical application of fibronectin in promoting healing of chronic skin and corneal ulcers [45, 46]. The addition of fibronectin to skin wounds enhances the healing process, possibly by linking fibroblasts to collagen fibrils and mediating wound contraction during the advanced stage of healing [45].

Laminin and collagen type IV are two major basement membrane proteins. They serve as adhesive proteins promoting the attachment of various types of cells to the extracellular matrix [37]. In previous studies [27, 32–34] we found that angiogenesis is important for the gastric mucosal repair process and for ulcer healing. ECM components are involved in formation of the basement membranes of capillary and arterial endothelium and smooth muscles cells and promote angiogenesis [37, 38].

In a recent study [47] we analyzed the distribution of fibronectin, laminin, and collagen types III and IV in the gastric mucosa and granulation tissue sequentially during healing of experimental gastric ulcers. This study demonstrated that fibronectin expression increased progressively from the initial healing stage (4 days) through scar formation (10–21 days). It was localized in the lamina propria of dilated regenerating glands at the ulcer margin and in the developing granulation tissue. The increased expression of fibronectin persisted in the ulcer scar for 21 days. Laminin and collagen type IV were expressed in the basement membrane of regenerating glands. Their expression rose markedly at 10–21 days, mainly in regenerating microvessels. This study demonstrated that expression of ECM components is significantly increased during ulcer healing and persists after the ulcer has healed [47]. Strong expression of the ECM components at the base of the ulcer margin indicates close interaction between granulation tissue and the epithelial cells of the ulcer margin in the process of reepithelization during ulcer healing. Finally, strong expression of ECM components in and around regenerating capillary vessels in granulation tissue suggests their participation in angiogenesis [47].

Factors Affecting Ulcer Healing

As discussed above, a number of factors appear to influence ulcer healing: luminal factors (H^+ secretion, pepsin, mucus, bicarbonate) as well as growth factors, angiogenic factors, oxygen, and nutrient supply. In addition, macrophages, platelets, lymphocytes, and mast cells seem to participate in the repair mechanisms. While the role of these latter cells and platelets in wound healing is well recognized, little information, if any, is available regarding their mechanisms of action in ulcer healing.

Quality of Ulcer Healing

Assessment of gastric ulcer healing is usually based on a visual examination by endoscopy in patients, or on evaluation of the ulcer size in experimental studies, not on histologic and ultrastructural assessment of subepithelial mucosal reconstruction. This approach has led to the assumption that the mucosa of grossly "healed" gastric and/or duodenal ulcers returns to normal, either spontaneously or following treatment [35]. In a previous study [48] we demonstrated that the reepithelialized mucosa of grossly "healed" experimental gastric ulcers has prominent histologic (Fig. 7) and ultrastructural abnormalities: reduced height, marked dilation of gastric glands, poor differentiation and/or degenerative changes in glandular cells, increased connective tissue, and disorganized microvascular network. These morphologic abnormalities are accompanied by functional changes such as reduced mucosal oxygenation (A. Tarnawski and J. Sarfeh, unpublished data) and increased microvascular permeability (F. Halter, personal communication).

While it is known that gastric ulcers tend to recur at the same location [49], the reason for this has not been clear. It seems likely that the prominent abnormalities found in the subepithelial mucosa of grossly "healed" gastric ulcers might interfere with mucosal defense and may predispose these specific mucosal areas to subsequent damage and ulcer recurrence when ulcerogenic factors are present [35, 48]. Therefore, the quality of mucosal structure restoration may be the most important factor in determining future ulcer recurrence. If this is truly the case, then many therapeutic regimens may be in need of re-evaluation. Although a number of pharmacologic agents are known to affect the rate of gastric ulcer healing, it is unknown what effect these same agents might have on the quality of ulcer healing, i.e., on mucosal architecture reconstruction, because observations have been based predominantly on superficial visual inspection.

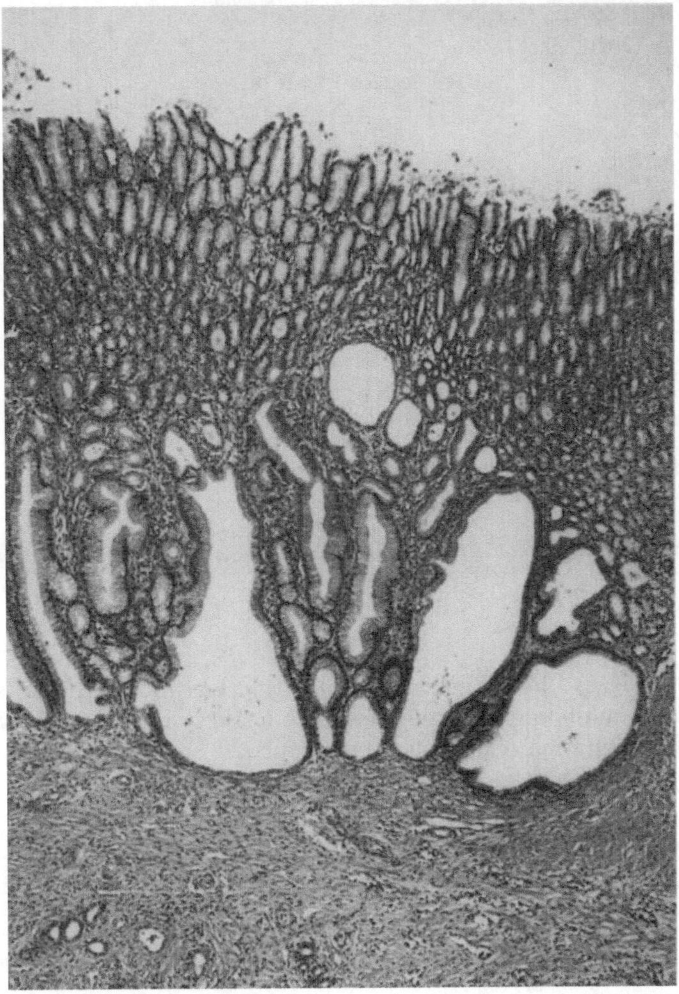

Fig. 7. Photomicrograph of the gastric mucosa from the area of grossly healed ulcer, 4 months after ulcer induction. The subepithelial mucosa exhibits dilation of the gastric glands

Pharmacological Factors Affecting Quality of Ulcer Healing

In a recent study [34], we demonstrated that chronic administration of a relatively low dose of indomethacin (1 mg/kg) not only significantly delayed healing of experimental gastric ulcer in rats, but also impaired the overall quality of ulcer healing, distorting restoration of mucosal architecture and blocking the differentiation and maturation of glandular epithelial cells (Fig. 8). Moreover, indomethacin treatment significantly reduced the number of fibroblasts, collagen fibers, and microvessels (reflecting inhibition of angiogenesis) in

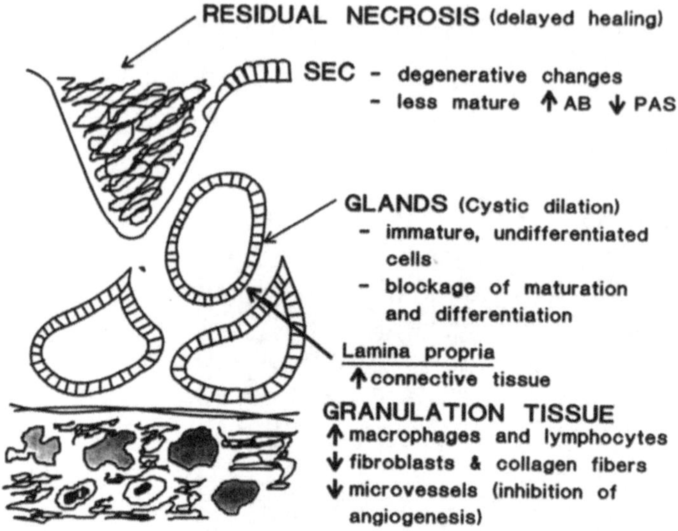

Fig. 8. The effect of indomethacin on healing of acetic acid-induced gastric ulcer in rat. *SEC*, surface epithelial cell. (From [34])

granulation tissue (Fig. 8) [34]. Whether the latter effect of indomethacin is indirect (through an inhibiton of angiogenesis) or a direct one on cellular differentiation and maturation remains to be determined.

References

1. Robbins SL, Cotran RS, Kumar V (eds.) Healing and repair in robbins pathologic basis of disease. Saunders, Philadelphia, pp 71–86
2. Richardson CT (1985) Pathogenetic factors in peptic ulcer disease. Am J Med 79(2C):1–7
3. Isenberg JI (1981) Peptic ulcer. Dis Mon Dec:1–58
4. Lam SK (1984) Pathogenesis and pathophysiology of duodenal ulcer. Clin Gastroenterol 13:447–472
5. Virchow R (1853) Historisches, Kritisches und Positives zur Lehre der Unterleibesaffektionen. Virchow Arch Pathol Anat Physiol 5:281–386, 632
6. Piasecki C (1992) Evidence for an infarctive pathogenesis of acute and chronic gastroduodenal ulceration. J Physiol and Pharmacol 43:99–112
7. Tarnawski A, Hollander D, Stachura J, Krause WJ, Eltorai M, Dabros W, Gergely H (1990) Vascular and microvascular changes – key factors in the development of acetic acid-induced gastric ulcers in rats. J Clin Gastroenterol 12(Suppl 1):S148–157
8. Okabe S, Roth JLA, Pfeiffer CJ (1971) A method for experimental, penetrating gastric and duodenal ulcers in rats. Dig Dis 16:277–284
9. Halter F, Barbezat GO, Van Hoorn-Hickman R, Van Hoorn WA (1980) Healing dynamics of traumatic gastric mucosal defects in the normal and hyperacid stomach. Dig Dis Sci 25:916–920
10. Blom H (1983) Cimetidine and parietal cell regeneration in experimental wounds in rat gastric mucosa. A light and electron microscopic study. Scand J Gastroenterol 18:853–857

11. Helpap B, Hattori T, Gedigk P (1981) Repair of gastric ulcer. A cell kinetic study. Virchows Arch [A] 392:159–170
12. Helander HE (1983) Morphologic studies on the margin of gastric corpus wounds in the rat. J Submicrosc Cytol 15(3):627–643
13. Geboes K, Rutgeerts P, Vantrappen G, Desmet V (1984) The influence of 15(R)-15 methyl PGE_2, methyl ester, on Nd:YAG laser-induced gastric ulcers. Gastrointestinal Endoscopy 30:173–178
14. Inauen W, Wyss PA, Kayser S, Baumgartner A, Schurer-Maly CC, Koelz HR, Halter F (1988) Influence of prostaglandins, omeprazole, and indomethacin on healing of experimental gastric ulcers in the rat. Gastroenterology 95:636–641
15. Hunt TK (1991) The principles of wound healing. In: Halter F, Garner A, Tytgat GNT (eds) Mechanisms of peptic ulcer healing. Falk Symposium No 59. Kluwer, Dordrecht, pp 1–12
16. Freston JW (1990) Overview of medical therapy of peptic ulcer disease. Gastroent Clin North Am 9(1) :121–140
17. Shorrock CJ, Rees WDW (1989) Bicarbonate secretion and alkaline microclimate. In: Hollander D, Tarnawski A, Gastric cytoprotection. Plenum, New York, pp 91–108
18. Allen A, Hunter AC, Mall A (1989) Mucus secretion. In: Hollander D, Tarnawski A, (eds) Gastric Cytoprotection. Plenum, New York, pp 75–90
19. Bravo R, Frank R, Blundell PA, MacDonald-Bravo H (1987) Cyclin/PCNA is the auxiliary protein of DNA polymerase delta. Nature 326:515–517
20. Burgess AW (1989) Epidermal growth factor and transforming growth factor. Br Med Bull 45:401–424
21. Lee H, Hansson H-A, Norstrom E, Hellander HF (1991) Immunoreactivities for epidermal growth factor (EGF) and for EGF receptors in rats with gastric ulcer. Cell Tissue Res 265: 211–218
22. Tarnawski A, Stachura J, Durbin T, Sarferh IJ, Gergely H (1992) Increased expression of epidermal growth factor receptor during gastric ulcer healing in rats. Gastroenterology 102:695–698
23. Skov Olsen P, Poulsen SS, Therkelsen K, Nexo E (1986) Effect of sialoadenectomy and synthetic human urogastrone on healing of chronic gastric ulcers in rats. Gut 27:1443–1449
24. Konturek SJ (1990) Role of growth factors in gastroduodenal protection and healing of peptic ulcers. Gastroenterol Clin N Am 19:41–65
25. Wright NA, Pike C, Elia G (1990) Induction of a novel epidermal growth factor – secreting cell lineage by mucosal ulceration in human gastrointestinal stem cells. Nature 343:82–85
26. Konturek SJ, Brzozowski T, Majka J, Dembinski A, Slomiany A, Slomiany BL (1992) Transforming growth factor alpha and epidermal growth factor in protection and healing of gastric mucosal injury. Scand J Gastroenterol 27:649–655
27. Tarnawski A, Hollander D, Stachura J, Gergely H, Krause WJ, Sarfeh IJ. Role of angiogenesis in healing of experimental "gastric ulcer". In: Halter F, Garner A, Tytgat GNJ, (eds) Mechanisms of Peptic Ulcer Healing. Falk Symposium 59. Kluwer, Dordrecht, pp 165–171
28. Folkman J, Szabo S, Stovroff A, McNeil P, Li W, Shing Y (1991) Duodenal ulcer. Discovery of a new mechanism and development of angiogenic therapy that accelerates healing. Ann Surg 214:414–427
29. Leibovich SJ, Polverini PJ, Shepard HM, Wiseman DM, Shively V, Nuseir N (1987) Macrophage-induced angiogenesis is mediated by tumous necrosis factor-α. Nature 329:630–632
30. Klagsburn M (1988) Angiogenesis factors. In: Ryan US (ed) Endothelial cells, vol II. CRC Press, Boca Raton, pp 37–50
31. D'Amore PA, Braunhut SJ (1988) Stimulatory and inhibitory factors in vascular growth control. In: Ryan US (ed) Endothelial cells, vol II. CRC Press, Boca Raton, pp 13–36
32. Tarnawski A, Hollander D, Stachura J, Sarfeh IJ, Gergely H, Krause WJ (1989) Angiogenic response of gastric mucosa to ethanol injury is abolished by indomethacin. Gastroenterology 96:A505
33. Tarnawski A, Hollander D, Stachura J, Sheffield M, Gergely H, Krause WJ (1990) Angiogenic response of damaged gastric mucosa – a prostaglandin mediated process? Gastroenterology 98:A136
34. Tarnawski A, Stachura J, Douglass TG, Krause WJ Gergely H, Sarfeh IJ (1991) Indomethacin impairs quality of experimental gastric ulcer healing: a quality histologic and ultrastructural

analysis. In Graner A, O'Brien P (eds) Mechanisms of injury, protection and repair of the upper gastrointestinal tract. Wiley, London, pp 521–531
35. Tarnawski A, Stachura J, Krause WJ, Douglass TG, Gergely H (1991) Quality of gastric ulcer healing-a new, emerging concept. J Clin Gastroenterol 13 (Suppl 1): S45–47
36. Ogihara Y, Okabe S (1991) Effects of ornoprostil on the healing of acetic acid-induced gastric ulcer in rats. In: Halter F, Garner A, Tytgat GNJ (eds) Mechanisms of Peptic Ulcer Healing. Falk Symposium 59. Kluwer, Dordrecht, pp 151–163
37. Martin GR, Timpl R (1987) Laminin and other basement membrane components. Annu Rev Cell Biol 3:57–85
38. Ruoslahti E, Pierschbacher MD (1987) New perspectives in cell adhesion: RGF and integrins. Science 238:491–497
39. Clark RAF, Della Pelle P, Manseau E, Lanigan JM, Dvorak HF, Colvin RB (1982) Blood vessel fibronectin increases in conjunction with endothelial cell proliferation and capillary in growth during wound healing. J Invest Dermatol 79:269–276
40. Couchman JR, Austria MR, Woods A (1990) Fibronectin-cell interactions. J Invest Dermatol 94(Suppl 6):S7–S14
41. Brotchie H, Wakefield D (1991) Fibronectin: structure, function and significance in wound healing. Australasian J Dermato 31(1):47–56
42. Luomanen M, Virtanen I (1991) Fibronectins in healing incision, excision and laser wounds. J Oral Pathology Med 29(3):133-138
43. Martinez-Hernandez A, Delgado FM, Amenta PS (1991) The extracellular matrix in hepatic regeneration. Localization of collagen types I, III, IV, laminin, and fibronectin. Lab Investig 64(2):157–166
44. Humphries MJ, Obara M, Olden K, Yamada KM (1989) Role of fibronectin in adhesion, migration, and metastasis. Cancer INvest 7(4):373–393
45. Colvin RB (1989) Fibronectin in wound healing. In: Mosher DF (ed) Fibronectin. Academic, San Diego, pp 213–254
46. Kim KS, Oh JS, Kim IS, Jo JS (1990) Topical fibronectin treatment in persistent corneal epithelial defects and corneal ulcers. Korean J Ophthalmol 4(1):5–11
47. Lu S-Y, Tarnawski A, Stachura J, Thillai I (1992) Sequential expression and distribution of fibronectin, laminin and collagen III and IV during experimental gastric ulcer healing. Gastroenterology A116:192
48. Tarnawski K, Hollander D, Krause WJ, Dabros W, Stachura J, Gergely H (1990) "Healed" experimental gastric ulcers remain histologically and ultrastructurally abnormal. J Clin Gastroenterol 12(Suppl 1):S139–147
49. Tarnawski A, Erickson RA (1991) Sucralfate-24 years later: current concepts on its protective and Therapeutic actions. Europ J Gastroenterol Hepatol 3:795–810

Role of bFGF and Angiogenesis in Ulcer Healing and the Treatment of Gastritis

S. Szabo, S. Kusstatscher, and M. Stovroff

Introduction

The prevention and therapy of gastric and duodenal ulcers, until recently, have been virtually restricted to neutralization of intraluminal acid or reduction of HCl secretion. The introduction of the concept of gastric cytoprotection in the late 1970s and 1980s promised a new approach, but the results were mainly disappointing since gastroprotection only referred to the prevention of *acute* hemorrhagic gastric erosions and had nothing to do with the treatment of *chronic* gastric and duodenal ulcers. Nevertheless, the existing alternatives to the acid-oriented approach were reviewed in the late 1980s [1] and were exemplified by the efficacy of locally acting antiulcer drugs such as sucralfate and colloidal bismuth, which brought about rapid duodenal ulcer healing without suppression of gastric acidity [2–4]. Recent studies have also suggested that the ulcer relapse rate was lower after treatment with sucralfate than following the healing achieved with antisecretory drugs [5].

Growth Factors and Angiogenesis

A conceptually new approach to ulcer prevention and treatment has become a reality with the availability of growth factors which stimilate the cellular and paracellular components of ulcer healing. Contrary to the *indirect* approach to ulcer treatment via acid suppression, when the ulcer is left alone to heal itself, growth factors *directly* stimulate ulcer healing, most of the time without suppression of the basic physiologic function of the stomach, i.e., acid and pepsin secretion. Among the components of ulcer healing, the production of new blood vessels, i.e., angiogenesis, and granulation tissue, i.e., proliferation of fibroblasts, monocytes, and deposition of collagen, are the most important. Namely, epithelial regeneration and restitution will complete the restoration of mucosal architecture if the necrotic ulcer crater with acute and chronic inflammation is replaced with dense granulation tissue which provides a solid framework for epithelial restoration.

Growth factors exert a variable degree of specificity, e.g., epidermal growth factor (EGF) is virtually specific for epithelial cell proliferation, while basic fibroblast growth factor (bFGF), in addition to stimulating fibroblasts, is the most potent mitogen for vascular endothelial cells, but also affects epithelial and smooth muscle proliferation [6]. bFGF also stimulates neuronal regeneration, thus influencing the restoration of virtually all the elements needed to replace the lost tissue in gastric or duodenal ulceration. Since angiogenesis or neovascularization is one of the most important processes in ulcer healing, and bFGF is the most potent angiogenic peptide so far isolated, we hypothesized that bFGF might exert potent ulcer healing properties.

We review here our most recent data on the additive and synergistic interaction between bFGF and cimetidine in the treatment of chronic duodenal ulcer [7] as well as on the synergistic interaction between bFGF and sucralfate in the treatment of chronic chemically induced gastritis in rats [8].

Additive Interaction Between bFGF and Cimetidine in Ulcer Healing

Our previous studies demonstrated that oral treatment of rats with the naturally occurring bFGF or its acid-resistant mutein bFGF-CS23, in which the second and third cysteines are replaced by site-specific mutagenesis by serines [9], accelerated the healing of chronic cysteamine-induced duodenal ulcers [10–12]. On molar basis the antiulcer effect of bFGF (100 ng/100 g) was about 1 million times more potent than that of cimetidine (10 mg/100 g), and was achieved without suppression of gastric acid or pepsin secretion.

The aim of the study was to investigate the effect of joint treatment with bFGF and H_2-antagonists on ulcer healing. In this and most of the previous studies we used the acid-resistant mutein bFGF-CS23 (Takeda Chemical Industries). Sprague-Dawley female rats (195–285 g) were maintained on Purina Laboratory chow and tap water ad libitum throughout the study and received cysteamine-HCl (25 mg/100 g) intragastrically three times on the first day. On the third day laparotomy was performed under ether anesthesia and rats were randomized to six groups (a–f; $n = 8$–12) with homogeneously severe ulcers (perforated or penetrated into the liver or pancreas) and treated twice daily for 3 weeks with the following given intragastrically: (a) vehicle citrate buffer (0.05*M*, pH 7.0) (controls); (b) bFGF 10 ng/100 g; (c) bFGF 50 ng/100 g; (d) cimetidine (Smith Kline Beecham) 10 mg/100 g; (e) cimetidine (10 mg/100 g) + bFGF (10 ng/100 g); (f) cimetidine (10 mg/100 g) + bFGF (50 ng/100 g).

Autopsy was performed on the 21st day and the ulcer size was measured in two of its largest diagonals and its surface calculated by the ellipse formula. The results were confirmed by computerized stereomicroscopic planimetry. Ulcer healing was evaluated by light microscopy and histochemistry. The size of ulcers was analyzed by one-way analysis of variance, unpaired Student's t-test, and Mann-Whitney U-tests. The ulcer sizes were: (a) 10.3 ± 1.8; (b) 3.6 ± 1.0 ($p < 0.05$); (c) 2.3 ± 0.2 ($p < 0.01$); (d) 4.8 ± 1.4 ($p < 0.05$); (e) 1.4 ± 0.5 ($p < 0.01$); and (f) 1.3 ± 0.4 ($p < 0.01$) (Fig. 1). The difference was also significant

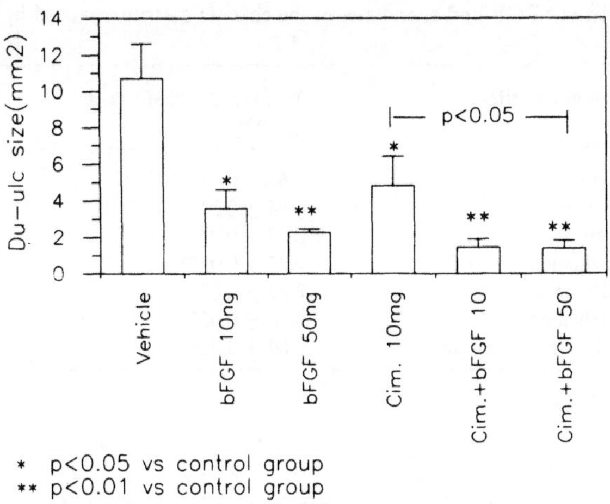

Fig. 1. The effect of bFGF and cimetidine on the healing of chronic cysteamine-induced duedenal ulcers in rats

($p < 0.05$)between cimetidine alone and cimetidine + bFGF (50 ng/100 g), and that between cimetidine and cimetidine + bFGF (10 ng/100 g) was at the border of significance ($p = 0.06$).

The histologic and histochemical evaluation of ulcers also revealed major differences. In the control vehicle-treated rats, most of the ulcers demonstrated necrotic crater with acute and chronic inflammation and surrounding *hypovascular* granulation tissue. Ulcers in cimetidine-treated rats had similar qualitative features, except the ulcers were usually smaller (see above). Duodenal sections from rats treated with bFGF-CS23 alone or in combination with cimetidine revealed dense granulation tissue with enhanced angiogenesis and minimal acute and chronic inflammation if the epithelial and mucosal reconstruction were not complete. In healed ulcers, histologic signs of smooth muscle regeneration were also evident, often with focal serosal signs of chronic, localized peritonitis, indicating previous perforation.

Chronic Gastritis and Synergism Between bFGF and Sucralfate

In contrast to the plethora of models of acute gastric mucosal injury and the few animal models of chronic gastric and duodenal ulcers, virtually no rat model of chronic diffuse erosive gastritis existed until recently. We found, as a follow-up to our investigations [13] on the gastroprotective role of sulfhydryls (SH), that ingestion of low concentrations of SH alkylators (e.g., 0.1 % iodoacetamide) in the drinking water induced severe, diffuse acute and chronic erosive gastritis in rats [14]. The lesions in the mucosa of the glandular stomach contain initially acute inflammatory cells such as leukocytes, mostly replaced by lymphocytes, plasma cells, and macrophages in the chronic stage of gastritis, which resembles

Table 1. Effect of oral administration of bFGF and sucralfate on the chronic gastritis induced by iodoacetamide in rats

Treatment	Chronic gastritis	Wet weight of stomach (g/100 g)
Control	Absent	0.66 ± 0.01
Vehicle	Extensive	0.84 ± 0.01
Sucralfate (5 mg/100 g)	Extensive	0.82 ± 0.03
bFGF-CS23 (25 ng)	Mild/healed	0.77 ± 0.02**
bFGF-wild (25 ng)	Extensive	0.82 ± 0.02
bFGF-wild + Sucralfate	Mild/healed	0.70 ± 0.02*
bFGF-CS23 + Sucralfate	Hardly detectable/healed	0.64 ± 0.02*

*$p < 0.001$ vs. vehicle; **$p < 0.005$ vs. vehicle.

the human alcoholic gastritis. We used this new animal model of gastritis to investigate the additive or synergistic therapeutic interaction of bFGF and sucralfate.

In these experiments after induction of gastritis by the SH alkylator 0.1% iodoacetamide in drinking water for 1 week, 60 rats were randomized to receive either (a) native bFGF-w (25 ng/100 g); (b) a site-specific mutated acid stable bFGF-CS23 (25 ng/100 g); (c) sucralfate in low dose (5 mg/100 g), or (d) combinations of these agents by gavage twice daily. Untreated rats received vehicle only. All the rats except controls remained on drinking water containing iodoacetamide for one more week. At autopsy on the 14th day macroscopic and histologic involvement of gastric glandular mucosa was quantified, and wet and dry stomach weights were obtained.

The results (Table 1) demonstrate that only acid-resistant bFGF was effective ($p < 0.05$). Neither native bFGF nor sucralfate had any effect at that low dose on chronic gastritis. Both native bFGF and the acid-resistant mutein in combination with sucralfate at a low dose were more efficient in the repair of mucosal injury and siginificantly more effective than either of these agents alone ($p < 0.001$). Thus, bFGF and sucralfate may act synergistically in healing of chronic erosive gastritis.

Summary

Recent results with bFGF, the most potent endothelial mitogen, and animal models of chronic duodenal ulcer and chronic gastritis demonstrate that stimulation of angiogenesis and other wound healing processes may represent a *new* and *direct* approach to accelerate the healing of chronic gut lesions: namely, daily oral treatment of rats with bFGF accelerated the healing of chronic duodenal ulcers induced by cysteamine. The potent antiulcer effect of bFGF was accompanied by prominent angiogenesis in the ulcer bed and not associated with inhibition of gastric secretion. Low doses of bFGF and cimetidine seem to exert additive or synergistic action in ulcer healing. bFGF in synergism with sucralfate also accelerated the healing of chemically induced subacute and chronic gastritis. Thus, the naturally occurring healing bFGF may be a new endogenous mediator *and* a pharmacologic tool in ulcer healing and in the natural history of gastritis.

References

1. Szabo S, Bynum TE (1988) Alternatives to the acid-oriented approach to ulcer disease: does 'cytoprotection' exist in man? A new classification of antiulcer agents. Scand J Gastroenterol 23:1–6
2. Yamamoto O, Okabe S (1987) Effects of sucralfate on healing of chronic gastric ulcers in rats. In: Szabo S, Mozsik G (eds) New pharmacology of ulcer disease. Experimental and new therapeutic approaches. Elsevier, New York, pp 413–423
3. Hollander D, Tarnawski A (1987) Protective effect of sucralfate on the gastric mucosa mediated by endogenous prostaglandins. In: Szabo S, Mozsik G (eds) New pharmacology of ulcer disease. Experimental and new therapeutic approaches. Elsevier, New York, pp 404–412
4. Pickard R (1987) Review of the clinical efficacy of De-Nol. In: Szabo S Mozsik G (eds) New pharmacology of ulcer disease. Experimental and new therapeutic approaches. Elsevier, New York, pp 128–136
5. Lam SK, Hui WM, Lau WY, Branicki FJ, Lia CL, Lok ASF, Ng MMT, Fok PJ, Poon GP, Choi TK (1987) Sucralfate overcomes the adverse effect of cigarette smoking on duodenal ulcer healing and prolongs subsequent remission. Gastroenterology 92:1193–1201
6. Folkman J, Klagsburn M (1987) Angiogenic factors. Science 235:442–447
7. Kusstatscher S, Folkman J, Nagy L, Szabo S (1992) Additive effect of fibroblast growth factor (bFGF) and cimetidine on chronic duodenal ulcer healing in rats. Gastroenterology 102:A169
8. Stovroff M, Vattay P, Marino B, Szabo S, Folkman J (1991) Healing of experimental gastritis by oral fibroblast growth factor. Surg. Forum 42:174–175
9. Seno K, Sasada R, Iwane K, Sudo K, Kuroko T, Ito K, Igarashi I (1988) Stabilizing basic fibroblast growth factor using protein engineering. Biochem Biophys Res Commun 151:701–708
10. Szabo S, Vattay P, Morales RE, Johnson B, Kato K, Folkman J (1989) Orally administered bFGF mutein: effect on healing of chronic duodenal ulcers in rats. Dig Dis Sci 34:1323
11. Folkman J, Szabo S, Vattay P, Morales RE, Pinkus G, Kato K (1990) Effect of orally administered bFGF on healing of chronic duodenal ulcers, gastric secretion and acute mucosal lesions in rats. Gastroenterology 98:A45
12. Szabo S, Folkman J, Vattay P, Morales RE, Kato K (1991) Duodenal ulcerogens: effect of FGF on cysteamine-induced duodenal ulcer. In: Halter F, Garner A, Tytgat GNJ (eds) Mechanisms of peptic ulcer healing. Kluwer, London, pp 139–150
13. Dupuy D, Raza A, Szabo S (1989) The role of endogenous nonprotein and protein sulfhydryls in gastric mucosal injury and protection. In: Szabo S, Pfeiffer CJ (eds) Ulcer disease: new aspects of pathogenesis and pharmacology. Boca Raton, CRC, pp 421–434
14. Szabo S, Trier JS, Brown A, Schnoor J (1984) Sulfhydryl blockers induce severe inflammation gastritis in the rat. Gastroenterology 86:1271

Helicobacter pylori: Pathogenic Mechanisms

F.A. Wyle, K.J. Chang, and A. Tarnawski

Introduction

H. pylori is a bacterium which colonizes the gastric mucosa. In 1896, Salomon described spiral organisms in stomachs of man and animals [1]. It was not until 1983, when Warren and Marshall first reported the isolation of a spiral bacterium from gastric biopsies of patients with gastritis [2, 3], that the dramatic expansion of information on *H. pylori* (Hp) began. Its worldwide distribution and high prevalence make it one of the commonest infections in mankind [4, 5]. Hp infection is associated with chronic type B gastritis, duodenal and gastric ulcer, and gastric carcinoma [6, 7] (Tables 1 and 2).

H. pylori and Chronic Type B Gastritis

It is now widely accepted that Hp is the cause of chronic type B gastritis. The worldwide distribution as well as the age-specific prevalence rates of the latter mirror the occurrence of Hp infection. Isolation rates from the gastric mucosal biopsies in patients with chronic type B gastritis between 64 % and 100 % have been reported [6, 7]. The reports of voluntary ingestion of Hp producing chronic gastritis [8], together with the fact that Hp is never present in gastric mucosa without underlying pathologic changes, indicate a causal role for this infection. Most investigators and clinicians are convinced that Koch's postulates have been met. Treatment with antimicrobial agents leads to the clearing of the bacteria from the antral mucosa, which is always accompanied by histologic improvement of the gastric inflammation.

H. pylori and Peptic Ulcer Disease

There is a close correlation between duodenal ulcer and the presence of Hp in the antral mucosa [6, 7]. It has been generally accepted that there is a strong association between duodenal ulcer and antral gastritis, in that all patients with a duodenal ulcer will have concomitant chronic type B gastritis in the distal part

Table 1. Incidence of *H. pylori* infection in gastroduodenal diseases

Chronic type B gastritis	88%–100%
Duodenal ulcer	85%–100%
Gastric ulcer	64%–97%
General population in industrialized countries	~ 1% per year
General population in nonindustrialized countries	~ 1.5% per year

Table 2. Incidence of *H. pylori* infection in gastric carcinoma

Study	Cancer patients (%)	Control subjects (%)	Odds ratio
Parsonnet et al. [12]	84	61	3.6
Nomura et al. [10]	94	76	6.0
Forman et al. [13]	69	47	2.8

of their stomach. There is good evidence of an extremely high prevalence of gastric metaplasia in the duodenum of patients with duodenal ulcer. One must consider that the changes seen in the stomach with Hp infection may predispose the duodenum to the development of gastric metaplasia. It is, therefore, highly probable that, as with gastritis, there is a concomitance between duodenal ulcer and gastric metaplasia. Duodenal ulcer associated gastric metaplastic cells frequently have attached Hp. It follows, then, that the processes that allow Hp to contribute to the development of active chronic gastritis, also apply to chronic duodenitis and, ultimately, duodenal ulcers.

Gastric ulceration in peptic ulcer disease has long been recognized to occur in the setting of active chronic gastritis or chronic atrophic gastritis. It is well established that gastric ulcers develop, in terms of peak occurrence, at least a decade later in life than duodenal ulcers. Hp again has an obvious close association to gastric ulcers relating to the underlying gastritis. If one eliminates gastric ulcers associated with nonsteroidal anti-inflammatory drugs, aspirin, and duodenal-gastric reflux, then peptic gastric ulcers probably have the same Hp correlations as do duodenal ulcers.

H. pylori and Gastric Cancer

To examine any possible relationship of Hp to gastric cancer, one has to look for a common denominator. As indicated above, there is substantial proof of the involvement of Hp in type B gastritis. What then is the relationship of gastritis to gastric cancer? Chronic type B gastritis is known to antedate the development of gastric carcinoma [9], and some investigators consider this type of gastritis is a precancerous lesion. Countries in which gastric cancer prevalence is high also have high rates of gastritis. There have been a number of studies showing a high prevalence of Hp in gastric carcinoma [10–13].

Gastric Physiology

The gastric surface epithelial cells are in the first line of the mucosal defense (Fig. 1). They secrete mucus and bicarbonate which form an unstirred mucus-bicarbonate layer, maintaining a neutral pH microclimate. They produce prostaglandins which are important for maintaining musocal integrity. Surface epithelial cell hydrophobic cell membranes resist acid, pepsin, and other water-soluble toxic substances. Parietal cells secrete HCl into the foveolar lumen and, concurrently, bicarbonate into the contiguous microvessels. It is transported to the surface epithelium to contribute to the neutral microenvironment. The integrity and repair of the gastric mucosa is dependent upon the mucus neck stem cells, which are essential for the continuous renewal of specialized epithelial cells. Not only is the replacement of rapidly aging surface epithelial cells vital for maintaining mucosal integrity, but it is essential to repair damage to the epithelium from external noxious substances. The microvasculature provides nutrients and oxygen to the mucosa while removing metabolic endproducts and

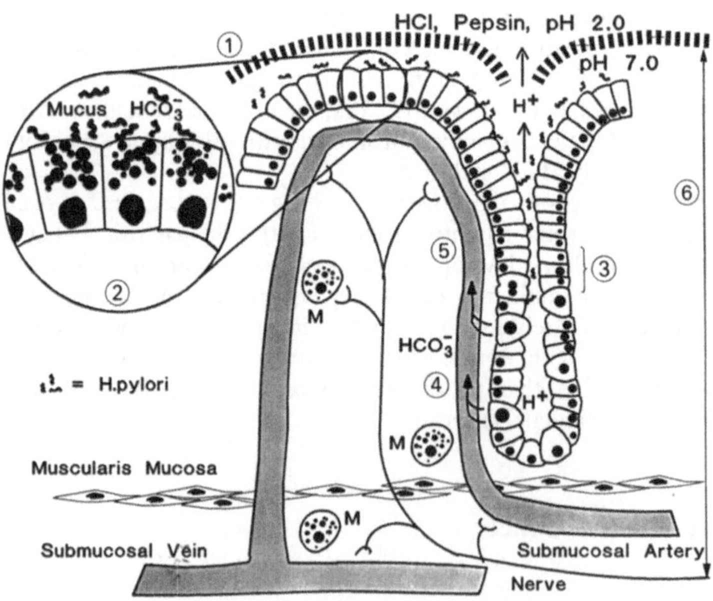

Fig. 1. Mucosal defense mechanisms and *H. pylori. H. pylori* along with HCl and pepsin are defended by *1*, an unstirred layer of mucus and biocarbonate; *2*, surface epithelial cells, *3*, parietal cells; *4*, mucosal cell renewal, *5*, microvasculature; and *6*, prostaglandin generation

toxic substances, as well as being a conduit for inflammatory cells necessary for the removal of necrotic material from the submucosa. G-cells are an essential component of the gastric endocrine system, producing gastrin in response to a complex set of stimuli. Gastrin functions in stimulation of parietal cells and acid secretion.

Mucus Gel and *H. pylori*

The mucus gel is an important mucosal defense mechanism. Its integrity serves to allow acid from parietal cells to reach the lumen while at the same time protecting mucosal cells from low luminal pH. The maintenance of the pH gradient across gastric mucus and the bicarbonate-neutralized microenvironment at the cell surface are important elements in cell protection. The mucus barrier prevents or retards back diffusion of H^+ ions and pepsin.

Since Hp lives in and under the gastric mucus gel, the relationship with and the effects of this organism upon this protective layer have been of interest. Alterations in the mucus gel have been described in gastric diseases [14, 15]. There have been reports that significant changes in the properties of the gastric mucus gel are induced by Hp extracellular enzymes. Hp has been shown to produce protease and lipase which can degrade mucin and change its barrier properties [16–18]. A decrease in mucus structure has been described and thought to be favorable for penetration and movement of motile Hp [19]; mechanisms invoked include the local effect of ammonia generated by Hp urease and changes in epithelial cell turnover rate.

Gastritis, Inflammation, and *H. pylori*

The mechanisms by which Hp produces gastritis are still a matter of some speculation. One can gain valuable insights to this question by examining some of the observations made about Hp-induced gastritis. When carefully looked for, Hp is identified in a high proportion of gastric biopsies showing chronic type B gastritis. It is not seen in so-called specific gastritis, such as Menetrier's disease, lymphoid hyperplasia, Crohn's gastritis, eosinophilic gastritis, and granulomatous gastritis [20]. Several studies note the close histologic relationship of overlying Hp and an underlying picture of active chronic gastritis [20–23]. others report close correlation with the degree of active polymorphonuclear leukocyte (PMN) infiltration and the density of overlying Hp [24–30]

How Hp induces such an inflammatory response is not yet clear. The organisms are most often found in two locations on the gastric mucosa: in the mucus gel itself and attached to the surface epithelial cells. There appears to be a predilection for the organisms to migrate into the gastric pits and, as demonstrated ultrastructurally, to attach to the apical cell membrane near the tight junctions [31]. From these locations on the mucosa, the Hp organisms can actively, or passively (through cell death), release chemotactic products. Such factors would be absorbed into the mucosa and attract the inflammatory cells of acute response. Another possible mechanism of attracting inflammatory cells might be through the toxic effect that Hp would have on the gastric epithelial cell, wherein they would release chemotactic factors to induce inflammation. Since the infection is persistent, it would also promote the immigration of mononuclear cells (chronic inflammatory response). Such inflammation would continue over time, producing the histologic picture of active chronic type B gastritis. Over the years, the inflammation may worsen, leading to ulcer formation, or may abate, leading to chronic gastritis and eventually mucosal atrophy. It has been well demonstrated that the eradication of Hp leads to the resolution of the active PMN inflammatory cellular infiltrate in the lamina propria initially, and eventually to disappearance of the mononuclear cell infiltrate. The mucosa can return to normal. The potential for this acute and chronic inflammation to alter the function of the gastric epithelium is obvious. This becomes apparent when one considers that Hp-induced gastritis almost certainly continues for many years [32, 33] and in most cases remains asymptomatic [34].

The potency of mediators of either acute or chronic inflammation is widely recognized. The ability of granulocytes, lysosomal enzymes, and proteins to promote cell alterations and death is well known [35]. The presence of PMNs as the characteristic cell in active chronic gastritis indicates the severity of the inflammatory process in the mucosa. The question of the role of the ubiquitous mononuclear cells in this process has recently been examined. Mucosal production of tumor necrosis factor α (TNFα) and interleukin-6 was increased in patients with Hp-related chronic gastritis [36, 37]. Those with an active (PMN infiltration) histologic picture had higher levels of TNFα than those with an inactive histology. It has been shown that soluble proteins extracted from Hp can activate monocytes and macrophages to produce interleukin-1 and TNFα [38]. Even the activity of neutrophils can be modified by cytokines [39]. These observations may explain the findings that T-cell density and expression of HLA-DR on epithelial cells are increased in chronic type B gastritis [40, 41]. With regards to the plasma cells present in the mucosa of gastritis patients, local mucosal production of both IgG and IgA has been well described [42, 43].

The fact of the extremely close association of both active and inactive gastritis with Hp infection of the gastric mucosa is well accepted. What remains to be explained is how gastritis maintains a "steady state" without progression in the majority of infected patients. Why some patients progress to duodenal or gastric ulcers and others to gastric carcinoma or nonulcer dyspepsia also needs further explanation.

H. pylori Adherence to Gastric Cells (Specific Receptors)

The high specificity of Hp for gastric epithelial cells is well known and implies a specific adhesin-receptor interaction. The attachment to surface epithelium cells has been associated with an underlying change in the cell membrane structure

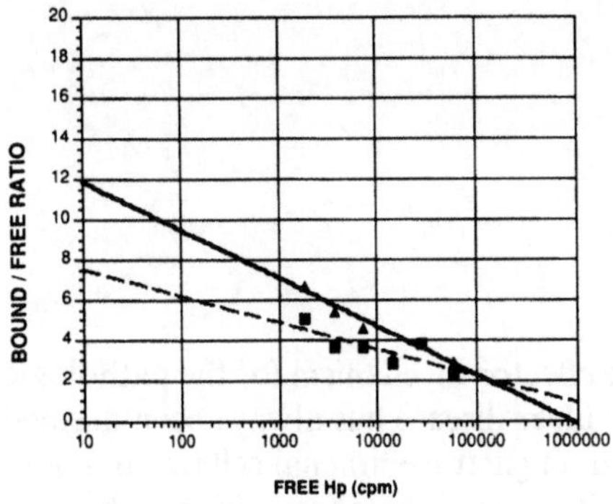

Fig. 2. Scatchard plot of *H. pylori* adherence to Kato III cells in vitro. Two strains (one *dashed* line and one *solid* line) demonstrate different binding avidities

leading to the formation of adherence pedestals [44, 45]. Thickening of glycocalyx of the Hp is often seen. Evans et al. [46] showed the presence of antibody to Hp *N*-acetylneuraminyl-lactose CFA in patients infected with Hp, indicating that this putative fibrillar adhesin is produced in vivo. They also noted that only 75% of infected patients had detectable antibody to this antigen; the explanation of this remains to be determined. Our group has investigated the specificity of adherence by Hp to gastric cells [47] and has found strain variation in coefficients of adherence (Fig. 2). The importance of Hp adherence remains to be determined. Teleologically, adherence to epithelial cells serves two purposes: one, it permits the organism to firmly attach to its niche and establish itself, and secondly, it permits the maintenance of close contact with its "target" cell. Such proximity is essential for the efficient functioning of the Hp toxic virulence factors. In such a posture, Hp enzymes and toxins can easily influence the functions of the adjacent epithelial cell.

H. pylori Exotoxins and Gastroduodenal Diseases

We know from extensive investigations that Hp produces extracellular substances which can exert an action on various cells in vitro (Table 3). The important issue is, what are the in vivo effects of these substances. What can one expect them to do to the epithelial cells and how would those cellular effects work with respect to gastritis and peptic ulcer disease.

There are subtle differences in gastritis with regard to active and chronic disease, to antral localization versus diffuse spread, duodenitis and its relation to gastritis and gastric metaplasia, and the effects of time and chronicity. All these differences may be due to Hp strain variations. Out of all the people infected and with chronic gastritis relatively few get peptic ulcer, because only few infecting strains have all the necessary virulence factors. Moreover, the Hp host, man, may be endowed with variations in receptor numbers or avidity, in inflammatory responses, in cellular sensitivity or insensitivity to virulence factors. These influences along with Hp strain variation may produce the variety of clinical manifestations seen in Hp-associated disease.

Table 3. *H. pylori* exotoxins

Urease
Cytotoxins
Protease
Phospholipase A_2
Platelet-activating factor

While the role of inflammation as the effector mechanism for the pathologic abnormalities seen in gastritis and peptic ulcer disease has always been deemed important, the direct effect of Hp infection on gastric epithelial cell function and physiology has not until recently been given much emphasis. Many observations of epithelial cell abnormalities made over the past several years can be interpreted as resulting from a direct Hp activity. Careful light microscopic examinations reveal surface epithelial cell changes including disintegration, loss of apical mucus, epithelial pits, and microerosion [48]. Well described are the ultrastructural changes in epithelial cells associated with Hp colonization; these include loss of microvilli, depletion of mucus granules, development of intracytoplasmic vacuolization, and disruption of intercellular junctional complexes [49–52]. Hp does not appear to have or has only minimally invasive properties, unlike most other pathogenic bacteria. Although the subject of some debate, the invasion of epithelial cells has been described by ourselves [53] and others [49, 51, 22, 52], this probably represents a rare event and is probably not a pathogenic mechanism of Hp.

The role of extracellular enzymes and toxins produced by Hp remains to be fully clarified. Hp is reported to be one of the most efficient producers of urease of any bacterial species [54–56]. Urease is viewed as a protective mechanism for Hp. In the digestion of urea, ammonia is produced, which can neutralize acid and provide a more conductive microclimate for this acid-sensitive organism. This enzyme, through ammonia production, has been said to cause mucus to be disintegrated [19]. Similarly, such ammonia was found to be toxic for gastric epithelial cells in vitro, decreasing their viability [57]. Thus, urea has been held potentially responsible for some of the changes seen in Hp-associated gastritis.

Hp also produces a cytotoxin, which is suggested as a major virulence factor. The cytotoxin was first described by Johnson and Lior [58]. Leunk greatly extended the observations on the cytotoxin by demonstrating its capacity to induce the intracellular vacuolization of eukaryotic cells in vitro [59, 60]. There is clear evidence that the cytotoxin is distinct from urease by both molecular size and activity [61, 59]. It is important to point out that the Hp cytotoxins described by different groups are not identical in either molecular size or effects on indicator cells [60, 62–64]. Vacuolation of gastric cells in vivo by Hp have been reported in the gnotobiotic pig [65] and in infected humans [66]. There is clear evidence that Hp cytotoxins are secreted by infecting organisms in vivo; cytotoxin-neutralizing antibodies can be detected in the serum of patients infected with toxin-producing strains [67, 68]. Cover and Blaser [62] have purified the 87000 kDa cytotoxin and have identified corresponding neutralizing antibodies in sera of Hp-infected persons. They noted structural terminal amino acid sequences similar to ion-transporting ATPases. This would indicate that the cell membranes of gastric epithelial cells might be the target of Hp cytotoxin. Our laboratory recently found that Hp cytotoxin can inhibit DNA replication at concentrations below that needed for vacuolization and can do so within 2 h of exposure [69]. One very important part of the Hp cytotoxin story is the fact that not all strains produce exotoxin(s). Several investigators have reported that cytotoxin production is found in only 50%–60% of strains isolated, and that cytotoxin-positive strains are isolated more frequently from patients with peptic ulcer than from those with only gastritis [59, 63, 70, 44]. The potential for the cytotoxins of Hp to be intimately involved in the pathophysiology of gastritis and peptic ulcer disease is quite significant; the in vivo mechanisms of action remain to be clarified.

There are other potential or putative virulence factors secreted by Hp. Lipolytic activity [71] and phospholipase A_2 [72, 73] have been found in significant concentrations in Hp. The finding of high levels of phospholipase A_2 and lysolecithin in gastric fluids of Hp-infected patients supports the concept that this may be involved in the development of Hp-related diseases. The secretion of the inflammatory mediator, platelet-activating factor, by Hp has recently been demonstrated [74]. Platelet-activating factor has previously been shown to be ulcerogenic to the gastric mucosa [75, 76], thus adding to the list of potential Hp virulence factors.

Schwartz' paradigm of aggressive and defensive factors in peptic ulcer disease may also apply to potential pathogenic mechanisms employed by Hp-associated chronic active gastritis and peptic ulcer disease (Fig. 3).

The classical aggressive factors of acid and pepsin may be influenced by Hp infection. Chronic Hp infection induces a state of chronic hypergastrinemia, most notable in the postprandial period [77–80]. There seems to be a re-set in the feedback of acid on gastrin inhibition. The hypergastrinemia is not suppressed by normal increases in gastric acid. Ammonia production by Hp-urease in the antrum is hypothesized to prevent G-cell acid suppression, resulting in gastrin overproduction [77, 80]. Alternatively, Hp exotoxins or chronic inflammation in the antrum may cause G-cell membrane receptors to yield less feedback inhibition to acid. Hypergastrinemia was seen to normalize when Hp

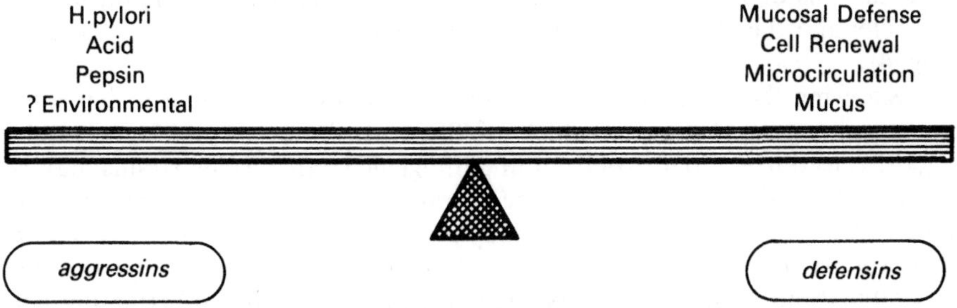

Fig. 3. Pathogenesis of peptic ulcer disease. Current view of the balance between aggressive factors and defensive factors in the human stomach

infection was treated and organisms eradicated [80]. Duodenal ulcers often occur in the presence of antral chronic active gastritis and increased parietal cell mass. The increased acid secretion could produce gastric metaplasia of the duodenum, which permits Hp to colonize the duodenal mucosa, whereas gastric ulcer is not associated with increased acid secondary to widespread chronic gastritis, which leads to a diminution of the parietal cell mass and increased back diffusion of H^+ ion.

Pepsin has recently attracted renewed interest as an important aggressive factor in peptic ulcer disease [81]. Elevations of pepsinogens I and II have been correlated to Hp infection of the gastric mucosa [82, 83, 84]. Elevated levels of pepsinogen has been known to be associated with chronic gastritis [85, 86]. Children successfully treated for Hp infection have shown a return to normal of their elevated pepsinogen levels [84]. Here again we have a perturbation of another aggressive factor which might contribute to the development of Hp-associated peptic ulcer disease.

Conclusion

As has been described, Hp possesses the necessary accoutrements for pathogenicity. One can see the pieces of the puzzle, but how the pieces fit together remains unclear. The question that continues to shadow Hp and its causality role in gastroduodenal disease needs to be addressed: "If Hp is a major factor in the development of gastroduodenal disease, why do relatively few of the many patients infected get peptic ulcer disease?" Another standard query is, "Why can 50%–80% of a population become chronically infected with Hp and yet remain healthy?" There is a hypothesis that can explain these apparent dilemmas. It points out that Hp is not a homogeneous species but is composed of a large number of strains that differ in their virulence characteristics [87]. The variation in cytotoxin production among strains isolated from patients with and without ulcer disease is a prime illustration of this concept.

In addition, the question of physical contact between an Hp organism and an epithelial cell needs to be more fully explored. The avidity of Hp adherence to mucosal cells depends on both the adherence properties of the organism (one variable) and the receptor properties of the epithelial cell (a second variable) (Fig. 4).

Knowing the large array of virulence mechanisms available to Hp, variations among strains as to which of these attributes they possess would, logically, lead to a broad spectrum of pathogenic strains. Some strains may be saprophytic and benignly inhabit the antral mucosa for years producing only mild chronic gastritis. Other strains may possess a "full set" of virulence factors and produce severe recurrent duodenal ulcer disease. They may do this through a combination of engendering hypergastrinemia and/or down-regulating epithelial membrane receptors for epithelial growth factor and/or depressing mucosal prostaglandin synthesis. Another group of strains may be equipped to

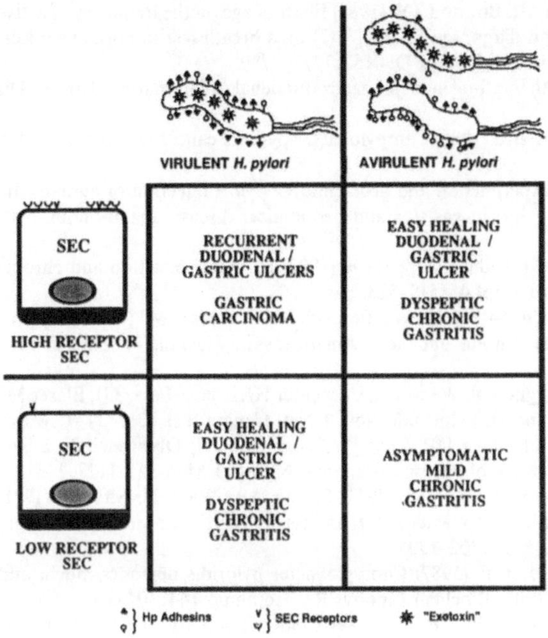

Fig. 4. Proposed pathogenic relationship between *H. pylori* adhesins and gastric surface epithelial cells. *SEC*, surface epithelian cell

produce chronic active gastritis over years without ulcer development; this could lead to eventual atrophic gastritis and gastric carcinoma.

Finally, one should not forget the Hp host, man. We are all aware of the fantastic genetic diversity of man. In the case of gastroduodenal disease, man may be endowed with variations in receptor numbers or avidity, in inflammatory responses, in cellular sensitivity or insensitivity to virulence factors. These influences along with Hp strain variation may produce the variety of clinical manifestations seen in Hp-associated disease. We are faced with an exciting challenge: how to rearrange the pieces of the pathophysiology of gastritis and peptic ulcer disease.

References

1. Salomon H (1896) Ueber das Spirillum des Saugetiermagens und sein Verhalten zu den Belegzellen. Zentralbl Bakt (Naturwiss) 19:433–443
2. Warren JR, Marshall B (1983) Unidentified cured bacilli on gastric epithelium in active chronic gastritis. Lancet i:1273
3. Marshall BJ (1983) Unidentified curved bacilli on gastric epithelium in active chronic gastritis. Lancet ii:1273–1275
4. Goodwin CS, Armstrong JA, Marshall BJ (1986) Campylobacter pyloridis, gastritis and peptic ulceration. J Clin Pathol 39:353–365

5. Graham DY, Klein PD, Opekun AR, Boutton TW (1988) Effect of age on the frequency of active Campylobacter pyloridis infection diagnosed by the [^{13}C] urea breath test in normal subjects and patients with peptic ulcer disease. J Infect Dis 157:7777–7780
6. Blaser MJ (1990) H. pylori and the pathogenesis of gastroduodenal inflammation. J Infect Dis 161:626–633
7. Tytgat GNJ, Rauws EAJ, De Koster E (1988) Campylobacter pylori. Scand J Gastroenterol 155 (suppl): 68–81.
8. Morris A, Nicholson G (1989) Experimental and accidental C. pylori infection of humans. In: Blaser MJ (ed) Campylobacter pylori in gastritis and peptic ulcer disease. Igaku-Shoin, New York, pp 61–72
9. Sipponen P, Kosunen TU, Valle J, Riihela, Seppala K (1992) H. pylori infection and chronic gastritis in gastric cancer. J Clin Pathol 45:319–323
10. Nomura A, Stemmermann GN, Chyou PH, Kato I, Perez-Perez GI, Blaser MJ (1991) H. pylori infection and gastric carcinoma among Japanese Americans in Hawaii. N Engl J Med 325:1132–1136
11. Talley NJ, Zinsmeister AR, DiMagno EP, Weaver A, Carpenter HA, Perez-Perez GI, Blaser MJ (1991) Gastric adenocarcinoma and H. pylori infection. J Natl Cancer Inst 83:1734–1739
12. Parsonnet J, Friedman GD, Vandersteen DP, Chang Y, Vogelman JH, Orentreich N, Sibley (1991) H. pylori infection and the risk of gastric carcinoma. N Engl J Med 325:1127–1131
13. Forman D, Newell DG, Fullerton F, Yarnell JWG, Stacey AR, Wald N, Sitas F (1991) Association between infection with Helicobacter pylori and risk of gastric cancer: evidence from a prospective investigation. BMJ 302:1302–1305
14. Slomiany BL, Bilski J, Sarosiek J et al. (1987) Campylobacter pyloridis degrades mucin and undermines gastric mucosal integrity. Biochem Biophys Res Commun 144:307–314
15. Slomiany BL, Nishikawa H, Piotrowski J et al. (1989) Lipolytic activity of Campylobacter pylori: effect of sofalcone. Digestion 43:33–40
16. Yuonan F, Pearson J, Allen A et al. (1982) Changes in the structure of the mucus gel on the mucosal surface of the stomach in association with peptic ulcer. Gastroenterology 82:817–831
17. Slomiany BL, Slomiany A (1991) Role of mucus in gastric mucosal protection. J Physiol Pharmacol 42:149–163
18. Slomiany BL, Kasinathan C, Slomiany A (1989) Effect of colloidal bismuth subcitrate on the lipolytic activity of Campylobacter pylori. Gastroenterol 84:1273–1277
19. Sidebotham RL, Baron JH (1990) Hypothesis: H. pylori, urease, mucus, and gastric ulcer. Lancet 335:193–195
20. Morris A, Maher K, Thomsen L, Miller M, Nicholson G, Tasman-Jones C (1988) Distribution of Campylobacter pylori in the human stomach obtained at postmortem. Scand J Gastroenterol 23:257–264
21. Hazell SL, Hennessy WB, Borody TJ, Carrick J, Ralston M, Brady L, Lee A (1987) Campylobacter pyloridis gastritis II: distribution of bacteria and associated inflammation in the gastroduodenal environment. Am J Gastroenterol 82:297–301
22. Back GE, Gourley WK, Lee WK et al. (1986) Relation of Campylobacter pyloridis to gastritis and peptic ulcer. J Infect Dis 153:664–669
23. Price AB, Levi J, Dolby JM et al. (1985) Campylobacter pyloridis in peptic ulcer disease: microbiology, pathology, and scanning electron microscopy. Gut 26:1183–1188
24. Satoh K, Kimura K, Yoshida Y, Kasano T, Kihira K, Taniguchi Y (1991) A topographical relationship between H. pylori and gastritis: Quantitative assessment of H. pylori in the gastric mucosa. Amer J Gastroenterol 86:285–291
25. Karttunen T, Niemela S, Lehtola J et. al (1987) Campylobacter-like organisms and gastritis: Histopathology, bile reflux, and gastric fluid composition. Scand J Gastroenterol 22:478–486
26. Queiroz DMM, Barbosa AJA, Nendes EN et al. (1988) Distribution of Campylobacter pylori and gastritis in the stomach of patients with and without duodenal ulcer. Am J Gastroenterol 83:1368–1370
27. Bayerdorffer E, Oertel H, Lehn N et al. (1989) Topographical association between active gastritis and Campylobacter pylori colonization. J Clin Pathol 42:834–839
28. Stolte M, Eidt S. Ohnsmann A (1990) Differences in H. pylori-associated gastritis in the antrum and body of the stomach. Z. Gastroenterol 28:229–233

29. Steininger H, Schneider U, Bartz K, Simmler B (1989) Campylobacter pylori und Gastritis – Besiedelungsdichte und Grad der Entzundung. Semiquantitative und morphometrische Untersuchung. Leber Magen Darm 19:70–78
30. Collins JSA, Sloan JM, Hamilton PW, Watt PCH, Love AHG (1989) Investigation of the relationship between gastric antral inflammation and Campylobacter pylori using graphic tablet planimetry. J Pathol 158:281–285
31. Goodwin CS, Armstrong JA, Marshall BK (1986) Campylobacter pyloridis gastritis and peptic ulcerations. J Clin Pathol 39:353–365
32. Siurala M, Varis K, Wiljasalo M (1966) Studies of patients with atrophic gastritis: a 10–15 year follow up. Scand J Gastroenterol 1:40–48
33. Siurala M, Isokoski M, Varis K, Kekki M (1968) Prevalence of gastritis in a rural population. Bioptic study of subjects selected at random. Scand J Gastroenterol 3:211–223
34. Dooley CP, Cohen H, Fitzgibbons PL, Mauer M, Appleman MD, Perez-Perez GI, Blaser MJ (1989) Prevalence of H. pylori infection and histologic gastritis in asymptomatic ons. N Engl J Med 321:1562–1566
35. Weiss SJ (1989) Tissue destruction by neutrophils. N Engl J Med 320:365–376
36. Crabtree JE, Shallcross TM, Heatley RV, Wyatt JI (1991) Mucosal tumour necrosis factor α and interleukin-6 in patients with H. pylori associated gastritis. Gut 32:1473–1477
37. Engstrand L, Scheynius A, Pahlson C, Grimelius L, Schwan A, Gustavsson S (1989) Association of Campylobacter pylori with induced expression of class II transplantation antigens on gastric epithelial cells. Infect Immun 57:827–832
38. Mai UEH, Perez-Perez GI, Wahl LM, Wahl SM, Blaser MJ, Smith PD (1991) Soluble surface proteins from H. pylori activate monocytes/macrophages by lipopolysaccharide-independent mechanism. J Clin Invest 87:894–900
39. Steinbeck MJ, Roth JA (1989) Neutrophil activation by recombinant cytokines. Rev Infect Dis 11:549–568
40. Papadimitriou CS, Iaachim-Velogianni EE, Tsianos EB, Moutsopoulos HM (1988) Epithelial HLA-DR expression and lymphocyte subsets in gastric mucosa in type B chronic gastritis. Virchows Arch (A) 413:197–204
41. Lambert JR, Borromeo M, Korman MG, Hansky J (1987) Role of Campylobacter pyloridis in non-ulcer dyspepsia. A randomized controlled trial. Gastroenterology 91:1488
42. Rathbone BJ, Wyatt JI, Worsley BW, Shires SE, Trejdosiewicz LK, Heatley RV, Losowsky MS (1986) Systemic and local antibody responses to Campylobacter pyloridis in non-ulcer dyspepsia. Gut 27:M2–647
43. Rathbone BJ, Heatley RV (1989) Immunology of C. pylori infection. In: Blaser MJ (ed.) Campylobacter pylori in gastritis and peptic ulcer disease. Igaku Shoin, New York pp 135–140
44. Hessey SJ, Spencer J, Wyatt JL et al. (1990) Bacterial adhesion and disease activity in Helicobacter associated chronic gastritis. Gut 31:134–138
45. Smoot DT, Mobley HLR, Gillian T et al. (1989) Pedestal formation of H. pylori with gastric epithelial cells in vitro may require actin polymerization. Gastroenterology 5:A127
46. Evans DJ, Evans DG, Smith KE, Graham DY (1989) Serum antibody responses to the *N*-acetylneuraminyllactose-binding hemagglutinin of Cambylobacter pylori. Infect Immun 57:664–667
47. Wyle FA, Tarnawski A, Wadington S (1990) Pathogenesis of H. pylori gastric disease: the role of adherence. Amer J Gastroent 85:1243
48. Hui PK, Chan WY, Cheung PS, Chan JK, Ng CS (1992) Pathologic changes of gastric mucosa colonized by H. pylori. Hum Pathol 23:548–556
49. Kazi JL, Sinniah R, Zaman V, Ng ML, Jafarey NA, Alam SM, Zuberi SJ, Kazi AM (1990) Ultrastructural study of H. pylori-associated gastritis. J Pathol 161:65–70
50. Hazell SL, Lee A, Brady L, Hennessy W (1986) Campylobacter pyloridis and gastritis: association with intercellular spaces and adaptations to an environment of mucus as important factors in colonization of the gastric epithelium. J Infect Dis 153:658–663
51. Chen XG, Correa P, Offerhaus J et al. (1986) Ultrastructure of the gastric mucosa harboring Campylobacter like organisms. Am J Clin Pathol 86:575–582
52. Bode G, Malfertheiner P, Ditschneit H (1988) Pathogenetic implications of ultrastructural finding in C. pylori related gastroduodenal disease. Scand J Gastroenterol 23:25–39

53. Wyle FA, Tarnawski A, Schulman D, Dabros W (1990) Evidence for gastric mucosal cell invasion by C.pylori: an ultrastructural study. J Clin Gastroent 12 (suppl 1) :92–98
54. Dick JD (1990) Helicobacter (Campylobacter) priori priori: a new twist to an old disease. Annu Rev Microbiol 44:249–269
55. Rauws EAJ, Tytgat GNJ (1989) Campylobacter pylori. WC den Ouden, Amsterdam
56. Blaser MJ (1990) Epidemiology and pathophysiology of Campylobacter pylori infections. Rev Infect Dis 12 (suppl 1) :4–4–59
57. Smoot DT, Mobley HLT, Chippendale GR, Lewison JF, Resau JH (1990) Helicobacter pylori urease activity is toxic to human gastric epithelial cells. Infect Immun 58:1992–1994
58. Johnson WM, Lior H (1986) Production of heat-labile cytotoxin by Campylobacter pyloridis. Adv Intern Med 34:B234
59. Leunk RD, Johnson PT, David BC, Kraft WG, Morgan DR (1988) Cytotoxic activity in broth-culture filtrates of Campylobacter pylori. J. Med Microbiol 26:93–99
60. Leunk RD (1991) Production of a cytotoxin by H. pylori. Rev Infect Dis 13 (suppl 8) :S686–689
61. Cover TL, Puryear W, Perez-Perez GI, Blaser MJ (1991) Effect of urease on HeLa cell vacuolation induced by H. pylori cytotoxin. Infect Immun 59:1264–1270
62. Cover TL, Blaser MJ (1992) Purification and characterization of the vacuolating toxin from H. pylori. J Biol Chem 267:10570–10575
63. Cover TL, Dooley CP, Blaser MJ (1990) Characterization of and human serologic response to proteins in Helicobacter pylori broth culture supernatants with vacuolizing cytotoxin activity. Infect Immun 58:603–610
64. Guerrant RI, Barrett LJ, Marshall BJ (1991) Cytotoxin production by Campylobacter pylori. In: Ruiz-Palacios G (ed.) Campylobacter V. Mexico City, Instituto Nacional de la Nutricion
65. Eaton KA, Morgan DR, Krakowka S. (1989) Campylobacter pylori virulence factors in gnotobiotic piglets. Infect Immun 57:1119–1125
66. Tricottet V, Bruneval P, Vire O, Camilleri JP, Bloch R, Bonte N, Roge J (1986) Campylobacter-like organisms and surface epithelium abnormalities in active, chronic gastritis in humans: an ultrastructural study. Ultrastruct Pathol 10:113–122
67. Leunk RD, Ferguson MA, Morgan DR, Low DE, Simor AE (1990) Antibody to cytotoxin in infection by H. pylori. J Clin Microbiol 28:1181–1184
68. Cover TL, Cao P, Blaser MJ (1991) Neutralization of H. pylori cytotoxin-induced HeLa cell vacuolation by human sera. Gastroenterology 100:A570
69. Chang K, Fujiwara Y, Wyle F, Tarnawski A (1992) H. pylori toxin inhibits growth and proliferation of cultured gastric cells — Kato III. J Phys Pharm (in press)
70. Figura N, Guglielmetti P, Rossolini A, Barberi A, Cusi G, Musmanno RA, Russi M, Quaranta S (1989) Cytotoxin production by *Campylobacter pylori* strains isolated from patients with peptic ulcers and from patients with chronic gastritis only. J Clin Microbiol 27:225–226
71. Slomiany BL, Kasinathan C and Slomiany A (1989) Lipolytic activity of Campylobacter pylori: effect of colloidal bismuth subcitrate (De-No1). Amer J Gastroent 84:1273–1277
72. Langton SR, Cesaarco SD (1992) H. pylori associated phospholipase A_2 activity: a factor in peptic ulcer production? J Clin Pathol 45:221–224
73. Raedsch R, Stiehl A, Waldherr R, Pasch B, Kommerell B (1988) Elevated concentrations of not amidated and secondary bile acids and lysolecithin in gastric juice in the presence of Campylobacter pylori. Gastroenterology 94:A257
74. Denizot Y, Sobhani I, Rambaud JC, Lewin M, Thomas Y, Benveniste J (1990) PAF-acether synthesis by H. pylori. Gut 31:1242–1245
75. Rosam AC, Wallace JL, Whitde BJR (1990) Potent ulcerogenic actions of platelet-activating factor on the stomach. Nature 319:54–56
76. Wallace JL, Whittle BJR (1986) Picomole doses of platelet-activating factor predispose the gastric mucosa to damage by topical irritants. Prostaglandins 31:989–998
77. Levi S, Beardshell K, Haddad G, Playford R, Ghosh P, Calam J (1989) Campylobacter pylori and duodenal ulcers: the gastrin link. Lancet 1:1167–1168
78. Smith JTL, Pounder RE, Evans DJ, Graham DY, Evans DG (1989) Inappropriate 24 hour hypergastrinemia in asymptomatic C. pylori infection. Gut 30:A732–A733
79. Karnes WE, Ohning GV, Sytnik B, Kim SWR, Walsh JH (1991) Preservation of pH inhibition of gastrin release in subjects with H. pylori. Rev Infect Dis 13:S665–S670

80. Graham DY, Opekun A, Lew GM, Evans Jr DJ, Klein PD, Evans DG (1990) Ablation of exaggerated meal-stimulated gastrin release in duodenal ulcer patients after clearance of H. (Campylobacter) pylori infection. Am J Gastoenterol 85:394–398
81. Samloff IM (1989) Peptic ulcer: The many proteinases of aggression. Gastroenterology 96 (suppl): 586–595
82. Veenendaal RA, Biemond I, Pena AS, van Duijn W, Kreuning J, Lames CBHW. (1992) Influence of age and H. pylori infection on serum pepsinogens in healthy blood transfusion donors. Gut 33:452–455
83. Asaka M, Kimura T, Kudo M, Takeda H, Mitani S, Miyazaki T, Miki K, Graham DY (1992) Relationship of H. pylori to serum pepsinogens in an asymptomatic Japanese population. Gastroenterology 102:760–766
84. Oderda G, Vaira D, Holton J, Dowsett JF, Ansaldi N (1989) Serum eosinogen I and IgG antibody to Campylobacter pylori in non-specific abdominal pain in childhood. Gut 30:912–916
85. Samoff IM, Varis K, Ihamaki T, Siurala M, Rotter JI (1982) Relationships among serum pepsinogen I, serum pepsinogen II, and gastric mucosal histology. Gastroenterology 83:204–209
86. Westerveld BB, Pals G, Lamers CBHW, Defize J, Pronk JC, Frants RR (1987) Clinical significance of pepsinogen A isozymogens, serum pepsinogen A and C levels, and serum gastrin levels. Cancer 59:952–958
87. Wyle FA, Chang KJ (1993) H. pylori: are they different from one another/? Eur J Gastroent Hep (in press)

Gastric Diseases and Treatment

Epidemiology of Ulcer Disease

A. SONNENBERG and G.S. SONNENBERG

Introduction

The aim of this review is to give an account of the epidemiology of ulcer disease. In accordance with this aim, the natural course of ulcer disease, its risk factors, and their interaction with the normal physiology of the upper gastrointestinal tract will be presented. Lastly we will describe the temporal and geographic variations of ulcer disease. To help readers keep their bearings and make the various areas of ulcer epidemiology more accessible, at the start of each section we have posed a question directed at the central issue in that section.

Why Do We Study Epidemiology?

The science of epidemiology is concerned with the behavior of illnesses in human populations and the factors that influence this behavior [1]. An epidemiologist is interested in the temporal, geographic, social, and demographic variations of a particular disease in order to be able to draw conclusions from these data about the causes of the disease. In addition, the expectation is that the study of epidemiology will produce some clinically useful findings, on which prevention and better treatment can be based.

Natural Course of Ulcer Disease

What Is the Natural Course of Ulcer Disease?

The first distinction to be made is between gastric and duodenal ulcers. These two types of ulcer have different natural courses [2]. Gastric ulcers affect men and women equally; nowadays most gastric ulcer patients are 60 years old or more. In about 20%–30% of gastric ulcer patients the ulcer heals spontaneously within 4–6 weeks, and in about 40% it recurs within a year. Duodenal ulcers, on the other hand, affect men twice as often as women, and duodenal ulcer patients are on average 10–20 years younger than gastric ulcer patients. Duodenal ulcers have a higher rate of spontaneous healing than gastric ulcers, but unfortunately they also have a higher rate of recurrence. In about half the patients they heal spontaneously within 4 weeks, and in about 80% they recur within a year.

Why Are the Two Ulcer Types Given a Common Name?

The reason two diseases with different courses and localizations are referred to under a common name such as "ulcer disease" or "peptic ulcer" is historic. It was not until the beginning of this century that gastric and duodenal ulcers were recognized as separate diseases and classified correspondingly in the international classification of diseases. Secondly, these diseases both have similar clinical symptoms [2–4]. Patients with both types of ulcer complain of epigastric pain, nausea, and discomfort, which can lead to weight loss. Although pain on an empty stomach, especially at night and in the early hours of the morning, is characteristic of duodenal ulcers, it is also occasionally described by patients with gastric ulcers. Gastric and duodenal ulcers can lead to similar complications. The ulcer may penetrate into adjacent organs, e.g., pancreas or bile duct. Both ulcer types are associated with hemorrhage and can lead to perforation of the abdominal cavity. After healing has taken place, scarring in the area of the ulcer wound can lead to pyloric stenosis. Simply because of the narrower diameter of the organ concerned, this complication is seen more frequently in association with duodenal than with gastric ulcers. Lastly, and perhaps the most important reason, is the peptic effect of the gastric juice, which plays a central part in both types of ulcer. "No acid, no ulcer" [5]. This phrase by K. Schwartz applies to both types of ulcer, and in both types the healing rate can be doubled by inhibiting acid secretion. Another fact that emphasizes the importance of acid is that the recurrence rate can be reduced to a third by decreasing nocturnal acid secretion.

Risk Factors for Ulcer Disease

What Are the Exogenous Risk Factors for Ulcer Disease?

On the subject of risk factors, one must distinguish between those for gastric and those for duodenal ulcers. In addition, there is a distinction between risk factors that delay healing of the ulcer in the acute stage and those that promote the formation of an ulcer in the first place or its tendency to recur. However, in practice it is not always possible to classify a risk factor as definitely one or the other on the basis of the available data. We will illustrate this with some examples.

Smoking is a risk factor particularly for duodenal ulcers; it has only a subordinate part to play in gastric ulcers [6]. Smoking affects both ulcer formation and healing. Cigarette smokers develop duodenal ulcers about twice as often as nonsmokers. They also have a much higher recurrence rate; in many studies the recurrence rate among nonsmokers receiving no medication was just as high as among smokers receiving long-term prophylactic treatment with histamine$_2$-antagonists [7]. In patients receiving no medication, smoking doubles the length of time taken for spontaneous healing.

Aspirin, i.e., acetylsalicylic acid, is a risk factor especially for gastric ulcers [8, 9]. Persons who for whatever reason have to take more than 1 g aspirin per day over a long period of time have a ten- to twentyfold higher risk of developing a gastric ulcer. Other nonsteroidal anti-inflammatory drugs such as indomethacin or ibuprofen are associated with a two or three times higher risk. The risk seems to relate chiefly to formation of the ulcer; apparently healing is less affected. Any negative effect is at least cancelled out by antacid treatment and is no longer statistically or epidemiologically significant.

The last important exogenous risk factor is *H. pylori*, which, if it infects the gastric or duodenal mucosa, influences the formation, healing, and tendency to recur of both types of ulcer [10–13]. One hundred percent of patients with duodenal ulcers (except for those in whom there is another cause, e.g., Zollinger-Ellison syndrome or aspirin consumption) have evidence of *H. pylori* infection. Seventy percent of gastric ulcers are associated with *H. pylori*. Both types of ulcer heal when the bacteria are eradicated by treatment with antibiotics. With these high percentages, however, it should not be forgotten that colonization of the upper gastrointestinal tract by *H. pylori* is often found in the normal (i.e., ulcer-free) population, and indeed increases with age. *H. pylori* is found in 50 % of the normal population aged over 50 years.

What Effect Does Stress Have on the Formation of an Ulcer?

For ethical and methodological reasons, it is very difficult to study the effects of stress in the formation of an ulcer. Even today we still lack (apart from a couple of meagre indicators) convincing, patholophysiologically acceptable proof of the influence of stress on the development of an ulcer. We do not believe that ulcer patients have a particular, psychologically abnormal character which could be clearly identified by appropriate psychological testing. On the other hand, there are persuasive case studies showing how a massive stress situation has led to formation of a ulcer. For example, during the German bombing of London in the Second World War, a rise in ulcer disease was seen [14]. It is conceivable that a subgroup of ulcer patients react to exogenous stress situations with an increase in acid secretion [15]. That would mean that they show a particular response to stress, without necessarily having any other psychological peculiarities. There are people who react to stress with abdominal cramps and diarrhea. Others blush in awkward situations. It is not difficult to imagine other people who might have a tendency to a kind of "gastric blushing," made up of increased acid secretion, disturbed motility, or other reactions of the upper gastrointestinal tract. However, this is all speculative at present; we have little evidence as yet to support such hypotheses.

Are There Any Endogenous Risk Factors for Ulcer Disease?

In addition to the exogenous risk factors, which result from the environment, there probably also exist several endogenous, i.e., congenital or physiologically based factors that promote the development of ulcer disease (Fig. 1). In general, patients with ulcers often have a family history of ulcers, a disposition towards gastric ulcers being inherited separately from a disposition towards duodenal ulcers [16]. However, it may be that the accumulation of ulcer disease in a single family is partly also due to orofecal spread of *H. pylori* infection within the same household (see below). Blood group O occurs 1.4 times more often in duodenal ulcer patients than in healthy subjects [17]. The reason for this is still unknown.

In the long term, healthy subjects with an elevated rate of acid secretion are at higher risk of developing a duodenal ulcer later in life [18]. Pepsinogen, a precursor of the protein-digesting enzyme pepsin in the gastric juice, is synthesized in the chief cells of the gastric mucosa. During the synthesis, a small portion of the synthesized pepsinogen leaks into the blood instead of into the gastric lumen, and its presence there can be demonstrated by radioimmunological methods. Half of all patients with a duodenal ulcer have elevated serum concentrations of pepsinogen [19]. This phenomenon may be an expression of increased synthesis of pepsin. It has been suggested that a gene responsible for producing hyperpepsinogenemia is inherited in an autosomal dominant fashion [20]. Besides this, leakage of pepsinogen into the blood stream is also an expression of mucosal inflammation. When the gastric *H. pylori* infection has been successfully treated with antibiotics, the surface gastritis recedes and serum concentrations of pepsinogen drop [21].

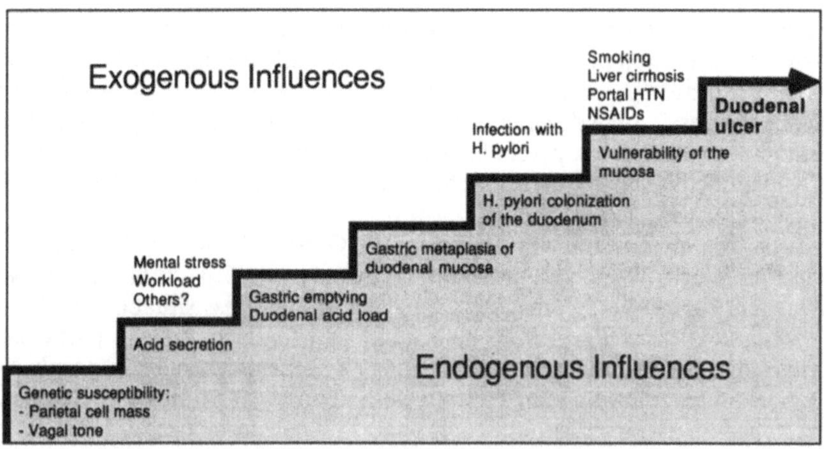

Fig. 1. Interaction between exogenous and endogenous risk factors in the development of duodenal ulcer. Each step symbolizes one development towards duodenal ulcer

In addition to these examples of endogenous predisposing factors for ulcer disease, there are other risk factors in which endogenous and exogenous influences interact. A typical example of these is alcohol consumption. Portal hypertension of any origin is associated with a threefold higher risk of either type of ulcer [22]. Since alcohol abuse is the most frequent cause of liver cirrhosis and consequently also of portal hypertension, it is obvious that excessive alcohol consumption promotes the formation of ulcers. However, it is important to stress that it is only via the development of liver cirrhosis that alcohol promotes the formation of an ulcer. Alcohol alone has no influence on ulcer formation; in moderate amounts it may even have a beneficial effect on the development and healing of ulcers [23, 24].

Temporal, Geographic, and Demographic Variations in Ulcer Disease

What Are the Temporal Variations in Ulcer Disease?

Until the last century ulcer disease was extremely rare. Not until the beginning of the nineteenth century did it enter medical awareness, when young girls and women "in the bloom of life," as chroniclers wrote, suddenly complained of severe abdominal pain, sometimes vomited blood, and then died within 24 or 48 h [25]. At autopsy, a lesion was often found, looking like a hole punched through the gastric wall – i.e., a perforated gastric ulcer. The disease had such a dramatic course and its patient population was so characteristic that it seems most unlikely that this disease entity, had it existed at the time, would have escaped the observation of all the excellent physicians produced by the eighteenth century. Rather, we must assume that a new, hitherto unobserved disease really had appeared. As the nineteenth century wore on, ulcer disease continued to spread and started to appear in men as well. Later a new type of ulcer was seen, the duodenal ulcer, which mainly affected men. Since most of the men concerned were among those of an age to bear arms and liable to be called up for military service during the First World War, state institutions developed an interest in discovering how to overcome this by now relatively frequent condition. During the first half of the twentieth century, ulcer disease at times affected 5%–10% of the population [26, 27]. Men developed gastric ulcers twice as often and duodenal ulcers as much as four times as often as women. Duodenal ulcers had taken over from gastric ulcers as the most frequent ulcer type. Events took a new turn in the 1960s, when the incidence of ulcer disease began to take a downward trend [28–31]. This trend began in the younger age groups, and accordingly the average age of ulcer patients started to go up. The downtrend has continued to this day. It was steepest in relation to duodenal ulcers and among men, so that gastric ulcers and ulcer disease in women have become proportionately more frequent again, although overall both types of ulcer and both sexes have been affected by the downtrend.

Are There Any Other Social or Demographic Characteristics of Ulcer Disease?

Up until halfway through this century, ulcers were more common among the urban than among the rural population [32, 33]. On a worldwide scale, ulcers were a disease of the western industrialized nations. Not until during the past two decades do ulcers seems to have affected urban populations in Asia and Africa as well. In the industrialized nations ulcers were chiefly a disease of the working classes [34–38]. The higher social classes rarely suffered from ulcers. A typical example is given by the foreign workers (*Gastarbeiter*) in Germany and Switzerland, imported for heavy manual labor from the start of the 1960s, among whom the incidence of duodenal ulcers reached near-epidemic proportions at a time when these ulcers were clearly on the wane in the native German and Swiss populations [35, 39].

Could Differences in Smoking and Drinking Habits Have Caused These Epidemiological Effects?

Genetic mechanisms and endogenous risk factors are ruled out from the start as explanations of these temporal variations, because the genetics and physiological reaction patterns of a population cannot change in such a short space of time. Other, exogenous factors must be considered instead. Cigarette smoking began gradually around 1880 [40]. The highest cigarette consumption was reached by the male population born between 1915 and 1920. These are the men who went away to fight in the Second World War and were later exposed to the smoking film heroes of the 1940s and 1950s. Smoking did not come into fashion among women until 1920, and was on the increase until the 1970s. Although the general reduction in smoking habits in the last two decades is one factor that has contributed to the fall in ulcer disease, taken as a whole the long course of ulcer disease from the beginning of the nineteenth century and the shorter and rather different course of cigarette smoking do not coincide.

The first aspirin was on sale in Germany in 1899. Since then, the use of nonsteroidal anti-inflammatory drugs has been continually on the increase. The course of this development does not fit with the temporal and geographic changes in the history of ulcer disease either.

Does the Epidemiology of *H. pylori* Explain the Variations in the History of Ulcer Disease?

Although *H. pylori* can survive in the outside environment, the most frequent route of infection seems to be by orofecal contamination or interpersonal contact [41, 42]. This is suggested by the accumulation of infected persons within one family and the relatively high incidence of ulcers among gastroenterologists, who are occupationally more exposed than others to material from the gastrointestinal tract. Since infection, once it has occurred, is for life, and spontaneous elimination of the bacteria does not occur, the prevalence of ulcers naturally increases with age. The prevalence is in negative correlation to family income and education. In general, lower social class and unhygienic conditions are associated with a higher rate of infection. Men and women are infected with equal frequency. In Asian and African countries, the infection rates can reach between 50 % and 100 % even in children – rates which in Europe are only ever seen in adults.

Gastric infection with *H. pylori* seems to play an important part in duodenal ulcer, gastric ulcer, and cancer of the stomach [41, 42]. The participation of a bacterium in the development of three diseases could be responsible for their undergoing similar temporal and geographic variation (Fig. 2). In unhygienic conditions, infection takes place during childhood. A chronic stomach infection of 40–60 years leads to diffuse atrophic gastritis. Additional exogenous factors such as a diet rich in salt and deficient in fruit and vegetables could promote the development of intestinal metaplasia, mucosal dysplasia, and stomach cancer. Further, as yet unknown immunological and genetic factors may also have a part in this process [43]. Under better hygienic conditions infection with *H. pylori* does not take place until adulthood. Although a similar chain of cause and effect is set in action as in childhood infection, the atrophic transformation of the gastric mucosa is less extreme and the gastritis does not usually continue for long enough to cause the development of stomach cancer. After partial atrophic transformation, the gastric mucosa secretes less acid than in a healthy

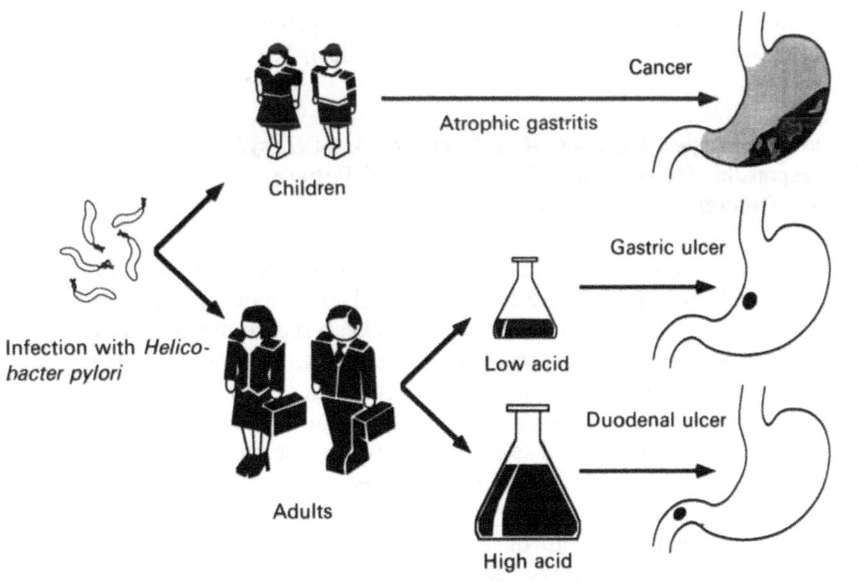

Fig. 2. Interaction between age at infection with *H. pylori* and amount of acid secreted, in relation to clinical outcome

person, but it is still enough to cause ulceration of the mucosa that has been weakened by infection. Finally, in an adult with a high rate of acid secretion, *H. pylori* principally colonizes the antrum. The overacidic milieu in the body of the stomach appears to be deleterious for growth of the bacteria. Possibly as protection, duodenal mucosa that is exposed to large amounts of gastric acid undergoes gastric metaplasia. This transformation of the duodenal mucosa allows the *H. pylori* to leave the stomach and colonize the duodenum. The resulting duodenitis combined with high acid secretion promotes the development of duodenal ulcers. If the bacteria do succeed, in the course of the chronic infection, in colonizing the mucosa of the body of the stomach, the initial diffuse antral gastritis develops into multifocal atrophic gastritis. Atrophy of the acid-producing mucosa reduces acid secretion, leading in the medium term to the appearance of a gastric ulcer to replace the duodenal ulcer, and in the long term to a general reduction in the tendency of either ulcer type to recur – i.e., the ulcer disease has "burned out" [44, 45].

In the nineteenth century, the hygienic conditions in Europe and North America were poor, and most people became infected with *H. pylori* during childhood. Stomach cancer remained a rare disease, since few in the population reached the age of 60 years or more. As life expectancy increased, so did the incidence of stomach cancer. As, with increasing urbanization, social reform, and the foundation of modern bacteriology, hygiene became a matter of general concern, infection became delayed until adulthood. Stomach cancer became rarer, while the incidence of peptic ulcers rose massively. As the twentieth century went on, infection was further delayed to later in life, and then began to fall off altogether. This age-specific trend would explain why the average age of ulcer patients has risen during the course of the twentieth century. The rise and fall of ulcer disease, and its affecting ever older age groups, reflect the probability in successive generations of becoming infected during adulthood with *H. pylori.*

Could One Single Exogenous Risk Factor Such as *H. pylori* Be Responsible for the Entire Epidemiological Pattern of Two Different Types of Ulcer?

Some of the statements made in the previous paragraph are at present to a large extent speculative and require further clinical and epidemiological proof. To date, we still do not know why ulcer disease takes a recurrent course when the *H. pylori* infection and resulting changes are chronic. One possible explanation could be other exogenous influences that temporarily throw the delicate interplay of defensive and aggressive factors out of equilibrium. For example, acute, short-term stimulation of acid secretion due to mental stress of other exogenous factors could promote the development of a recurrence [46]. It is probable that additional factors besides the age at which infection occurs and the amount of secreted acid determine who develops stomach cancer, a gastric ulcer, or a duodenal ulcer, and who stays healthy.

It is possible that physical labor and consumption of salt in the diet are two additional risk factors that have left their mark in the epidemiology of ulcer disease [47]. Physical labor stimulates acid secretion [48–50]. Epidemiological data from Germany and England show a close, i.e., statistically significant, relationship between physical labor and incidence of duodenal ulcer [51, 52]. The historical course of ulcer disease coincides with the history of heavy physical labor (Fig. 3) [53]. During the course of industrial expansion and urbanization around the turn of the century, the proportion of the population engaged in heavy physical labor increased massively. Not until the mechanization and automation of labor that occurred towards the end of this century have the numbers involved in heavy labor dropped again. That ulcer disease was at first found most frequently in urban, i.e., industrial centers, that it affected men most, especially those of the working classes, and the way in which it suddenly rose in European *Gastarbeiter* could be further evidence for this hypothesis.

Consumption of dietary salt is probably another risk factor that plays a role especially in gastric ulcers and cancer of the stomach. Patients with either of these often, in addition to the stomach lesion, suffer from hypertensive diseases [22]. Coronary heart disease and cerebrovascular disease occur more frequently in patients with gastric cancer or ulcer than in subjects without these conditions. This suggests that a high salt consumption plays a role in all these diseases, hence the epidemiological clustering of these diseases in the same patient group. Moreover, there is a statistically significant correlation between the geographic distribution of salt consumption and gastric cancer or gastric ulcer (Fig. 4) [54–58]. In countries where salt consumption is low, gastric cancer, gastric ulcer, and hypertensive disease are relatively rare, while in countries where salt consumption is high, all three diseases are common. Today, these chiefly include

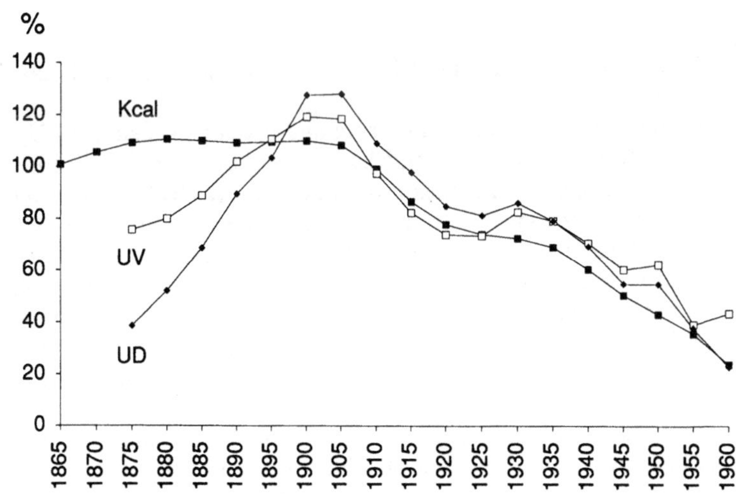

Fig. 3. Evolution over time of ulcer-related mortality and workload in Germany during the past 100 years (data from [53]). *Abscissa*: Date of birth; *ordinate*: standardized ulcer-related mortality and workload. The 100 % value on the ordinate corresponds to the mean of all birth cohorts. Each curve connects the standardized data for individual birth cohorts. *UD*, Duodenal ulcer; *UV*, gastric ulcer; *Kcal*, cumulative lifetime workload, measured in kilocalories

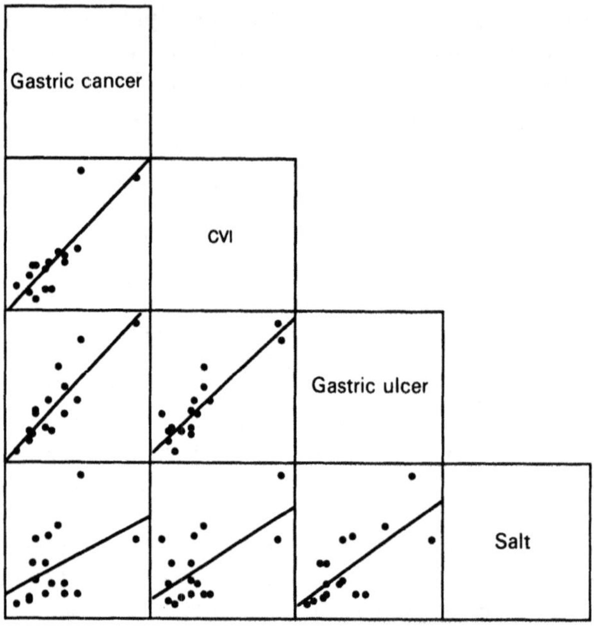

Fig. 4. Linear correlations between mortality in men from gastric cancer, cerebrovascular insult (*CVI*), gastric ulcer, and salt consumption in 16 countries (data from [57]). Each dot represents one country

countries where a lot of salt is still used for preserving fish, such as Japan, Portugal, and Spain.

From ancient times, salt was valued as a rare and precious substance [59]. It could be mined only in a few places and had to be transported over long distances. Apart from mining, the only means to obtain salt was by boiling water containing a high concentration of salt. This entailed burning wood, itself a valuable commodity. Apart from the expenses of production and transport, the cost of salt was still further increased by the state monopoly on it, with high taxes. In France, for example, the salt tax (*la gabelle*) was not abolished until the Revolution. In addition to direct consumption, the chief use of salt was in the preservation of food. Not until the second half of the twentieth century was it replaced in this role by the refrigerator. It is possible that the sudden availability of salt, together with its initially increased and then reduced consumption, had some part in the historical variations of gastric ulcers and gastric cancer.

Physical labor and salt consumption are two examples of how historical developments may have influenced the course of ulcer disease. No doubt there are other exogenous and endogenous risk factors of whose significance we know little. The attraction of epidemiology lies in the attempt to discover such connections. However, they have to be tested in prospective clinical studies and experimental investigations before they can be regarded as proved.

References

1. Mausner JS, Kramer S (1985) Epidemiology: an introductory text, 2nd edn. Saunders, Philadelphia
2. Blum AL, Sonnenberg A, Börsch G (1990) Epidemiologie, natürlicher Verlauf und Risikofaktoren der Ulkuskrankheit. In: Bauerfeind P, Blum AL (eds) Ulkusalmanach 1 + 2, 2nd edn. Springer, Berlin Heidelberg New York, pp 11–47
3. Soll AH (1989) Duodenal ulcer and drug therapy. In: Sleisenger MH, Fordtran JS (eds) Gastrointestinal disease: pathophysiology, diagnosis, management. Saunders, Philadelphia, pp 814–879
4. Richardson CT (1989) Gastric ulcer. In: Sleisenger MH, Fordtran JS (eds) Gastrointestinal disease: pathophysiology, diagnosis, management. Saunders, Philadelphia, pp 879–909
5. Schwartz K (1910) Über penetrierte Magen- und Jejunalgeschwüre. Bruns Beitr Klin Chir 67:96–128
6. US Department of Health and Human Services (1990) The health benefits of smoking cessation: a report of the Surgeon General. Rockville, Maryland, DHHS Publication no. (CDC) 90-8416, pp 429–442
7. Sontag S, Graham DY, Belsito A, Weiss J, Farley A, Grunt R, Cohen N, Kinnear D, Davis W, Archambault A, Achord J, Thayer W, Gillies R, Sidorov J, Sabesin SM, Dyck W, Fleshler B, Cleator I, Wenger J, Opekun A Jr (1984) Cimetidine, cigarette smoking, and recurrence of duodenal ulcer. N Engl J Med 311:689–693
8. Langman MJS, Brooks P, Hawkey CJ, Silverstein F, Yeomans N (1991) Non-steroidal anti-inflammatory drug associated ulcer: epidemiology, causation and treatment. J Gastroenterol Hepatol 6:442–449
9. Soll AH, Weinstein WM, Kurata J, McCarthy D (1991) Nonsteroidal anti-inflammatory drugs and peptic ulcer disease. Ann Intern Med 114:307–319
10. Graham DY (1989) Campylobacter pylori and peptic ulcer disease. Gastroenterology 96:615–625
11. Ormand JE, Talley NJ (1990) H. pylori: controversies and an approach to management. Mayo Clin Proc 65:414–426
12. Peterson WL (1991) H. pylori and peptic ulcer disease. N Engl J Med 324:1043–1048
13. Blaser MJ (1992) Hypotheses on the pathogenesis and natural history of H. pylori-induced inflammation. Gastroenterology 102:720–727
14. Spicer CC, Stewart DN, Winser DM (1944) Perforated peptic ulcer during the period of heavy air-raids. Lancet 1:14
15. Peters MN, Richardson CT (1983) Stressful life events, acid hypersecretion, and ulcer disease. Gastroenterology 84:114–119
16. Doll R, Kellock TD (1951) The separate inheritance of gastric and duodenal ulcers. Ann Eugen 16:231–240
17. McConnell RB (1966) The genetics of gastro-intestinal disorders. Oxford University Press, London, pp 76–111
18. Fiddian-Green RG, Bank S, Marks IN, Louw JH (1976) Maximum acid output and risk of peptic ulcer. Lancet 2:1367–1369
19. Samloff IM, Liebman WM, Panitch NM (1975) Serum group I pepsinogens by radioimmunoassay in control subjects and patients with peptic ulcer. Gastroenterology 69:83–90
20. Rotter JI, Petersen G, Samloff IM, McConnell RB, Ellis A, Spence MA, Rimoin DL (1979) Genetic heterogeneity of hyperpepsinogenemic I and normopepsinogenemic I duodenal ulcer disease. Ann Intern Med 91:372–377
21. Fraser AG, Prewett EJ, Pounder RE, Samloff IM (1992) Short report: twenty-four-hour hyperpepsinogenemia in H. pylori-positive subjects is abolished by eradication of the infection. Aliment Pharmacol Ther 6:389–394
22. Sonnenberg A (1988) Concordant occurrence of gastric and hypertensive diseases. Gastroenterology 95:42–48
23. Sonnenberg A, Müller-Lissner SA, Vogel E, Schmid P, Gonvers JJ, Peter P, Strohmeyer G, Blum AL (1981) Predictors of duodenal ulcer healing and relapse. Gastroenterology 81:1061–1067

24. Østensen H, Gudmundsen TE, Østensen P, Burhol PG, Bonnevie O (1985) Smoking, alcohol, coffee, and familial factors: any association with peptic ulcer disease? A clinically and radiologically prospective study. Scand J Gastroenterol 20:1227–1235.
25. Jennings D (1940) Perforated peptic ulcer. Changes in age-incidence and sex-distribution in the last 150 years. Lancet 1:395–398, 444–447
26. Ivy AC, Grossman MI, Bachrach WH (1950) Peptic ulcer. Blakiston, New York
27. Clarke M, Halil T, Salmon N (1976) Peptic ulceration in men. Epidemiology and medical care. Br J Prev Soc Med 30:115–122
28. Susser M, Stein Z (1962) Civilization and peptic ulcer. Lancet 1:115–119
29. Sonnenberg A (1984) Occurrence of a cohort phenomenon in peptic ulcer mortality from Switzerland. Gastroenterology 86:398–401
30. Sonnenberg A, Müller H, Pace F (1985) Birth-cohort analysis of peptic ulcer mortality in Europe. J Chron Dis 38:309–317
31. Sonnenberg A (1987) Changes in physician visits for gastric and duodenal ulcer in the United States during 1958–1984 as shown by National Disease and Therapeutic Index (NDTI). Dig Dis Sci 32:1–7
32. Pulvertaft CN (1968) Comments on the incidence and natural history of gastric and duodenal ulcers. Postgrad Med J 44:597–602
33. Litton A, Murdoch WR (1963) Peptic ulcer in south-west Scotland. Gut 4:360–366
34. Nasiry R, Piper DW (1983) Social aspects of chronic duodenal ulcer. A case control study. Digestion 27:196–202
35. Sonnenberg A (1985) Disability pensions due to peptic ulcer in Germany between 1953 and 1983. Am J Epidemiol 122:106–111
36. Sonnenberg A, Sonnenberg GS (1986) Occupational mortality from gastric and duodenal ulcer. Br J Ind Med 43:50–55
37. Sonnenberg A, Sonnenberg GS (1986) Occupational factors in disability pensions for gastric and duodenal ulcer. J Occup Med 28:87–90
38. Sonnenberg A, Haas J (1986) The joint effect of occupation and nationality on the prevalence of peptic ulcer in German workers. Br J Ind Med 43:490–493
39. Würsch TG, Hess H, Walser R, Koelz HR, Pelloni S, Vogel E, Schmid P, Blum AL (1978) Die Epidemiologie des Ulcus duodeni. Untersuchungen an 1105 Patienten in Zürich. Dtsch Med Wochenschr 103:613–619
40. Sonnenberg A (1986) Smoking and mortality from peptic ulcer in the United Kingdom. Gut 27:1369–1372
41. Graham DY (1991) H. pylori: its epidemiology and its role in duodenal ulcer disease. J Gastroenterol Hepatol 6:105–113
42. Graham DY, Klein PD, Evans DG, Fiedorek SC, Evans Jr DJ, Adam E, Malaty HM (1992) H. pylori: epidemiology, relationship to gastric cancer and the role of infants in transmission. Eur J Gastroenterol Hepatol 4 (Suppl 1) :S1–S6
43. Howsen CP, Hiyama T, Wynder EL (1986) The decline in gastric cancer: epidemiology of an unplanned triumph. Epidemiol Rev 8, 1–27
44. Fry J (1964) Peptic ulcer: a profile. Br Med J 2:809–812
45. Greibe J. Bugge P, Gjørup T, Lauritzen T, Bonnevie O, Wulff HR (1977). Long-term prognosis of duodenal ulcer: follow-up study and survey of doctors' estimates. Br Med J 2:1572–1574
46. Achord JL (1981) Gastric pepsin and acid secretion in patients with acute and healed duodenal ulcer. Gastroenterology 81:15–18
47. Sonnenberg A (1988) Factors which influence the incidence and the course of peptic ulcer. Scand J Gastroenterol 23 (Suppl 155):119–140
48. Markiewicz K, Cholewa M, Gorski L, Chmura J (1977) Effect of physical exercise on gastric basal secretion in healthy men. Hepatogastroenterology 24:377–380
49. Markiewicz K, Cholewa M, Lukin M (1979) Gastric basal secretion during exercise and restitution in patients with chronic duodenal ulcer. Hepatogastroenterology 26:160–165
50. Øktedalen O, Guldvog I, Opstad PK, Berstad A, Gedde-Dahl E, Jorde R (1984) The effect of physical stress on gastric secretion and pancreatic polypeptide levels in man. Scand J Gastroenterol 19:770–778
51. Katschinski BD, Logan RFA, Edmond M, Langman MJS (1991) Physical activity at work and duodenal ulcer risk. Gut 32:983–986

52. Sonnenberg A, Sonnenberg GS (1986) Occupational factors in disability pensions for gastric and duodenal ulcer. J Occup Med 28:87–90
53. Sonnenberg A, Sonnenberg GS, Wirths W (1987) Historic changes of occupational work load and mortality from peptic ulcer in Germany. J Occup Med 28:756–761
54. Sato T, Fukuyama T, Suzuki T, Takayanagi J, Murakami T, Shiotsuki N, Tanaka R, Tsuji R (1959) Studies of the causation of gastric cancer. 2. The relation between gastric cancer mortality rate and salted food intake in several places in Japan. Bull Inst Publ Health 8:187–198
55. Hirayama T (1963) A study of epidemiology of stomach cancer, with special reference to the effect of diet factor. Bull Inst Publ Health 12:85–96
56. Joossens JV, Geboers J (1981) Nutrition and gastric cancer. Nutr Cancer 2:250–261
57. Sonnenberg A (1986) Dietary salt and gastric ulcer. Gut 27:1138–1142
58. Lu JB, Qin YM (1987) Correlation between high salt intake and mortality rates for oesophageal and gastric cancers in Henan province, China. Int J Epidemiol 16:171–176
59. Seidel H, Woller R (1980) Das Geschenk der Erde. Vom Salz zur modernen Chemie. Econ, Düsseldorf

NSAIDs and Gastroduodenal Lesions: How Big a Problem and How to Prevent?

D. Rachmilewitz

Introduction

Non-steroidal anti-inflammatory drugs (NSAIDs) are widely prescribed worldwide and gastrointestinal side effects are the most common known adverse reaction. The gastrointestinal side effects vary from mild symptoms such as indigestion, heartburn, and abdominal discomfort to serious events such as gastrointestinal bleeding, peptic ulcer disease, and its complications–bleeding and perforation.

Aspirin and NSAIDs damage the mucosa of the gastrointestinal tract. Initially NSAIDs were considered to damage the stomach and mainly the antrum, but now it is apparent that they also induce mucosal damage in the duodenum [1]. The incidence and severity of the damage in the duodenum are similar to those in the stomach [2], and the complications associated with NSAIDs result from duodenal ulcers as often as from gastric ulcers [3].

Acute and Chronic Injury

NSAID-induced mucosal injury has to be divided into the effects of acute versus chronic ingestion. Between 70% and 100% of healthy subjects taking NSAIDs on a daily basis for up to 16 days develop some kind of endoscopic mucosal injury [4]. The types of injury include erythema, hemorrhage, erosions, and, rarely, even an ulcer.

It is important to clearly define the endoscopic findings. Whereas the definitions of erythema and hemorrhage are obvious, the definition of an ulcer versus an erosion is not well established. An erosion is a superficial defect that involves only the mucosa, and since it is difficult to assess depth at endoscopy one has to rely on the size of the lesion. Small lesions, less than 3 mm in diameter, are more likely to be erosions rather than an ulcer. The wide range of reported NSAID-induced gastric ulcers is due to the various criteria used for the definition of an ulcer.

There is no direct correlation between acute endoscopic findings and risk of developing potential life-threatening complications such as bleeding and perforation [5]. Acute ulcers that have existed only for a short time, usually less than 2 weeks from previous endoscopy or initiation of NSAID treatment, tend to heal more rapidly than chronic ulcers. The later are usually deep and persistent and tend to induce the life-threatening complications. However, complications are possible also within days of initiation of NSAID treatment, not excluding bleeding from widespread mucosal erosions induced by NSAIDs although this is definitely not common.

Lack of Correlation Between Symptoms and Signs

Unfortunately there is no correlation between the presence of mucosal damage, ulcers, included, and the presence of upper gastrointestinal symptoms such as pain, heartburn, nausea, or vomiting [5]. This observation, known for years in duodenal ulcer patients, and not necessarily NSAID-induced, has also been verified in big trials and surveys among NSAID users [6]. The dissociation between symptoms and signs also holds in the development of severe ulcer complications [7].

Estimated Risk

Estimates of the risk of developing gastroduodenal damage and its complications as a consequence of NSAID treatment vary according to the designs used in the different studies. Estimates of the incidence of peptic ulcer disease among chronic NSAID users based on prevalence studies in which NSAID users undergo endoscopy for assessment of the presence or absence of mucosal damage range from 14% [8] to 31% [9]. The estimate of the risk of complications or death from ulcer disease related to NSAID treatment range between 1.1 [10] and 13.6 [11]. Similar figures were also reported for aspirin users. The estimated risk of developing ulcer complications and death related to NSAID treatment, on the basis of cohort studies, is between 1.4 [12] and 5.3 [13].

An association between chronic aspirin use and hospitalization for peptic ulcer disease was also found among 6524 subjects treated for 3 years with aspirin 1g/day. In this double-blind, randomized, placebo-controlled study [14] the risk of gastric ulcer was 9.1 and the risk of duodenal ulcer 10.7. It is also apparent that elderly NSAID users and patients with a previous history of ulcer disease are at increased risk [7].

In spite of the objective problems that characterize most of the studies addressing the issue, there is clearly a consistent association between NSAIDs and both upper gastrointestinal bleeding and peptic ulcer disease and its complications.

One objective in itself is to assess the gastrointestinal toxicity of the different NSAIDs available. This may have important clinical implications, especially if one drug is found to be safer and to induce less side effects than others. However, the data available are not consistent. In one study, for example [16], sulindac was suggested to have the higher risk of upper gastrointestinal bleeding but another study [17] indicated similar risk associated with sulindac and other NSAIDs. However, with respect to each of the available NSAIDs it seems that there is direct correlation between the incidence of side effects and the dose: the higher the dose, the higher the incidence of side-effects.

Prevention of NSAID-Associated Gastrointestinal Damage

It is important to differentiate between the prevention of acute damage induced by short-term NSAID treatment (1–2 weeks), and prevention of the damage induced by chronic NSAIDs use. In the latter group the lack of unified definition of endoscopic lesions and, particularly, of what constitutes an ulcer make the evaluation of the protective effects of the various drugs very difficult.

Prevention of Acute Damage

Most of the studies on this subject have been conducted in normal healthy volunteers, only few in patients – usually with musculoskeletal disorders. In most studies aspirin was used as the damaging NSAID. Since aspirin effects are pH-dependent and topical, prevention of aspirin-induced damage may not necessarily be relevant to other NSAIDs. In general, in all the acute studies gastric injury was more severe than duodenal injury. However, in one study, after 5–7 days of indomethacin treatment duodenal injury was similar to that found in the stomach [6]. Cimetidine was found to reduce dose-dependently both gastric and duodenal damage due to aspirin [18]. Doses of 200–300 mg cimetidine taken together with the aspirin induce immediate reduction of the acute injury. Cimetidine effectively reduces injury induced by indomethacin [6] and also protect against damage induced by tolmetin [19]. Sucralfate does not seem to provide significant protection against acute damage and its protection is inferior to that afforded by misoprostol or H_2-antagonists [20]. Lately the efficacy of omeprazole was also evaluated. Omeprazole in antisecretory doses was found to diminish aspirin-induced gastric mucosal lesions but to have less effect on mucosal lesions induced by other NDAIDs such as naproxen and diclofenac [21].

Prevention of Chronic Damage

H_2-blockers, sucralfate, and misoprostol were assessed for their efficacy in the prevention of gastroduodenal damage in patients who use NSAIDs for long periods of time. Whereas the incidence of gastric lesions was similar in rheumatic patients either treated for 4 weeks with ranitidine 150 mg b.i.d or given placebo [22], ranitidine given at the same dose for 8 weeks was found to provide significant protection to the duodenum [7]. Cimetidine treatment for 8 weeks did not provide mucosal protection to the stomach either [23]. These studies therefore suggest that H_2-antagonists protect the duodenum but have no significant effect in prophylaxis of NSAID-induced gastric ulceration. None of the studies evaluated the possible prevention of life-threatening complications such as bleeding and perforation.

In one placebo-controlled trial the prevention of gastroduodenal ulceration during 3 months of therapy with one of three non-aspirin NSAIDs by misoprostol, a prostaglandin E_1 analogue, was evaluated [24]. Misoprostol at doses of 100 or 200 μg four times daily suppressed the formation of gastric ulcers as defined in that study (lesions at least 3 mm in diameter). Unfortunately, the extrapolation of data from this trial to clinical ulcer disease is difficult. It is not clear whether the lesions which develop in 4 weeks of treatment – the interval after which endoscopy was performed – reflect the real incidence of chronic peptic ulcer, not to mention the diameter taken to define an ulcer in this study. Lesions with a diameter of 3–5mm have a greater chance of being an erosion rather than an ulcer. The trial also did not establish the possible prevention of serious side effects, since none of the 293 patients included had an ulcer-related complication. Clinical studies enrolling thousands of chronic NSAIDs users are needed to evaluate the validity of any treatment on the reduction of ulcer complications.

Most probably, patients with previous peptic ulcer disease are those who will benefit most from prophylactic treatment. Unfortunately, patients with recurrent gastric ulcer were excluded from the misprostol study and so this possible benefit was not evaluated. It should also be noted that misoprostol may induce diarrhea as a side effect, which may be a problem in its long term use as co-treatment to prevent NSAID-induced mucosal damage.

Attempts at prevention of NSAID-induced gastroduodenal damage during long term co-treatment with sucralfate are not encouraging. Sucralfate was found to be inferior to misoprostol [25]. Recently a novel approach to the prevention of NSAID-induced mucosal damage was advocated. Ketotifen, which is used in the long term in the management of asthma and allergic reactions, was found to protect the stomach against damage induced by indomethacin [26]. The effects of Ketotifen are ascribed to its prevention of the release of inflammatory mediators form mast cells and/or other inflammatory cells or to blocking of their action on target organs. The efficacy of ketotifen in the prevention of gastroduodenal mucosal damage in normal volunteers taking indomethacin for 1 week [27] suggests that it deserves also to be evaluated in patients undergoing long-term treatment with NSAIDs.

Summary

It has been shown without doubt that NSAIDs induce damage to the stomach and duodenum when taken for either short or long periods of time. However, since most of the information on the extent of damage is based on endoscopic evaluations whose clinical significance is not clear, it is rather difficult to recommend strategies to prevent this damage and its implications. All will agree that the initial preventive approach is to avoid the use of NSAIDs or to reduce their dosage. Of the drugs available, misoprostol is the only one shown to prevent acute gastric ulcers, while H_2-blockers seem to reduce the prevalence of NSAID-associated duodenal ulcers. Prevention is a special challenge in high-risk patients, although this population is not well defined. Subjects with a previous history of peptic ulcer and patients in generally poor health will benefit from co-administration of NSAIDs and an H_2-antagonist or misoprostol. Further studies are essential to improve our understanding and to justify more firm recommendations.

References

1. Eliakim R, Ophir M, Rachmilewitz D (1987) Duodenal mucosal injury with non-steroidal anti-inflammatory damage. J Clin Gastroenterol 9:395–399
2. Osnes M, Larsen S, Eidsaunet W, et al. (1979) Effect of diclofenac and naproxen on gastroduodenal mucosa. Clin Pharmacol Ther 26:399
3. Armstrong CP, Blower AL (1987) Non-steroidal anti-inflammatory drugs and life threatening complication of peptic ulceration. Gut 28:527–532
4. Llewelyn JG, Pritchard MH (1983) Acute gastric hemorrhage and its relationship to the use of anti-inflammatory analgesics (NSAIDs). Ann Rheum Dis 42:228
5. Langman MJS (1988) Drug-induced mucosal damage. In: Rees WWD (ed) Advances in peptic ulcer pathogenesis. MTP Press, Lancaster
6. Stalnikowicz R, Pollak D, Eliakim A, Wengrower D, Fich A, Goldin E, Ligumsky M, Rachmilewitz D (1988) Cimetidine decreases indomethacin induced mucosal damage in patients with acute musculoskeletal disorders. Gut 29:1578–1582
7. Ehsanullah RS, Page MC, Tildesley G, Wood JR (1988) Prevention of gastroduodenal damage induced by non-steroidal anti-inflammatory drugs: controlled trial of ranitidine. Br Med J 297:1017–21
8. Roth SH, Bennett RE, Mitchell CS, Hartman RJ (1987) Cimetidine therapy in nonsteroidal anti-inflammatory drug gastropathy. Double-blind long-term evaluation. Arch Intern Med 147:1798–801
9. Farah D, Sturrock RD, Russell RI (1988) Peptic ulcer in rheumatoid arthritis. Ann Rheum Dis 47:478–80
10. Duggan JM, Dobson AJ, Johnson H, Fahey P (1986) Peptic ulcer and non-steroidal anti-inflammatory agents. Gut 27:929–33
11. McIntosh JH, Byth K, Piper DW (1985) Environmental factors in aetiology of chronic gastric ulcer: a case control study of exposure variables before the first symptoms. Gut 26:789–798
12. Beard K, Walker AM, Perera DR, Jick H (1987) Nonsteroidal anti-inflammatory drugs and hospitalization for gastroesophageal bleeding in the elderly. Arch Intern Med 147:1621–1623.
13. Guess HA, West R, Strand LM, et al. (1988) Fatal upper gastrointestinal hemorrhage or perforation among users and nonusers of nonsteroidal anti-inflammatory drugs in Saskatchewan, Canada 1983. J Clon Epidemiol 41:35–45
14. Kurata JH, Abbey DE (1990) The effect of chronic aspirin use on duodenal gastric ulcer hospitalizations. J Clin Gastroenterol 12:260–266
15. Jicks SS, Perera DR, Walker AM, Jick H (1987) Non-steroidal anti-inflammatory drugs and hospital admission for perforated peptic ulcer. Lancet 2:380–382
16. Carson JL, Strom BL, Morse ML, et al. (1987) The relative gastrointestinal toxicity of the nonsteroidal anti-inflammatory drugs. Arch Intern Med 147:1054–1059

17. Griffin MR, Piper JM, Daugherty JR, Snowden M, Ray W (1991) Nonsteroidal anti-inflammatory drug use and increased risk for peptic ulcer disease in elderly persons. Ann Intern Med 116:257–263
18. Kimmey MB, Silverstein FE, Saunders DR, Chapman RC (1987) Reduction of endoscopically assessed acute aspirin-induced gastric mucosal injury with cimetidine. Dig Dis Sci 32:851–856
19. Lanza FL, Aspinal RL, Swabb EA, Davis RE, Rack MF, Rubin A (1988) Double-blind placebo-controlled endoscopic comparison of the mucosal protective effects of misoprostol versus cimetidine on tolmetin-induced mucosal injury to stomach and duodenum. Gastroenterology 95:289–294
20. Graham DY, Smith JL, Dobbs SM (1983) Gastric adaptation occurs with aspirin administration in man. Dig Dis Sci 28:1–6
21. Daneshamend TK, Stern AE, Bhaskar HK, Hawkey CJ (1990) Abolition by omeprazol of aspirin induced gastric mucosal injury in man. Gut 31:514–517
22. Bianchi Porro G, Pace F, Caruso I (1987) Why are non-steroidal anti-inflammatory drugs important in peptic ulceration. Alim Pharmacol Ther 1:5405–5475
23. Roth SH, Bennet RE, Mitchell CS, Hartman RJ (1987) Cimetidine therapy in non-steroidal anti-inflammatory drug gastropathy. Double-blind long term evaluation. Ann Intern Med 147:1798–1801
24. Graham DY, Agrawal NM, Roth SH (1988) Prevention of NSAID-induced gastric ulcer with misoprostol: multicenter, double-blind, placebo-controlled trial. Lancet 2:1277–1280
25. Lanza FL, Peace KE, Gustitis L et al. (1987) A blinded endoscopic comparative study of misoprostol versus sucralfate and placebo in the prevention of aspirin induced gastric and duodenal ulceration. Am J Med 83:14, 37–40
26. Karmeli F, Eliakim R, Okon E, Rachmilewitz D (1991) Gastric mucosal damage is mediated by substance P and prevented by ketotifen. Gastroenterology 100:1206–1216
27. Eliakim R, Karmeli F, Rachmilewitz D (1992) Prophylactic administration of ketotifen protects gastric mucosa from indomethacin induced damage in healthy volunteers. Gastroenterology 102, A63

Therapeutic Strategy in Gastro-oesophageal Reflux Disease

J.P. Galmiche, S. Bruley des Varannes, and C. Scarpignato

Introduction

Gastro-oesophageal reflux disease (GORD) encompasses a wide spectrum of disorders in which gastric refluxate causes symptoms and/or damage to the oesophageal mucosa (Fig. 1). It is a very common disorder, epidemiological surveys in Europe and USA having shown that 5%–15% of the general population suffer from frequent heartburn or regurgitation [1, 2]. Most subjects, however, have mild, intermittent symptoms. They do not seek medical help or are managed by primary care physicians. At the other end of the spectrum of the disease are patients with long-standing recurrent disease, persistent symptoms, severe oesophagitis lesions and complications such as strictures, bleeding, columnar-lined (Barrett's) oesophagus or extra-oesophageal complications (e.g. asthma, acid laryngitis or non-cardiac chest pain).

The pathogenesis of GORD is multifactorial [3] and several mechanisms are involved, including: (i) an incompetent anti-reflux barrier, (ii) abnormal acid clearance of the refluxed material, (iii) the composition of the refluxate, (iv) the resistance of the oesophageal mucosa, and (v), in some cases, slowed gastric emptying. In contrast to animal studies, there is now some evidence that in human beings GORD is primarily a motility disorder. The basic physiological abnormality is a mechanically defective lower oesophageal sphincter (LOS), resulting in increased oesophageal exposure to acid. Physiological reflux nearly always follows transient relaxation of the LOS, while in patients with oesophagitis this mechanism is responsible for only two-thirds of the episodes of reflux. A transient increase in intra-abdominal pressure and spontaneous reflux through a permanently hypotonic sphincter are responsible for the last one-third of reflux episodes in patients with oesophagitis. The majority of human studies do not support the hypothesis of secondary and therefore reversible impairment as suggested by animal experiments. This means that no medical treatment is actually curative and that no single drug can really address all the aspects of the pathogenetic mechanisms potentially involved. However, although gastric acid and pepsin output are normal in the large majority of patients with reflux [4], once reflux has occurred the composition of the refluxate plays a central role and determines whether or not reflux damages the oesophageal mucosa [5, 6]. Despite the fact that pancreatic enzymes and bile salts are noxious agents for oesophageal and gastric mucosa, their role in the pathogenesis of reflux oesophagitis is far less important than that of acid and pepsin [5].

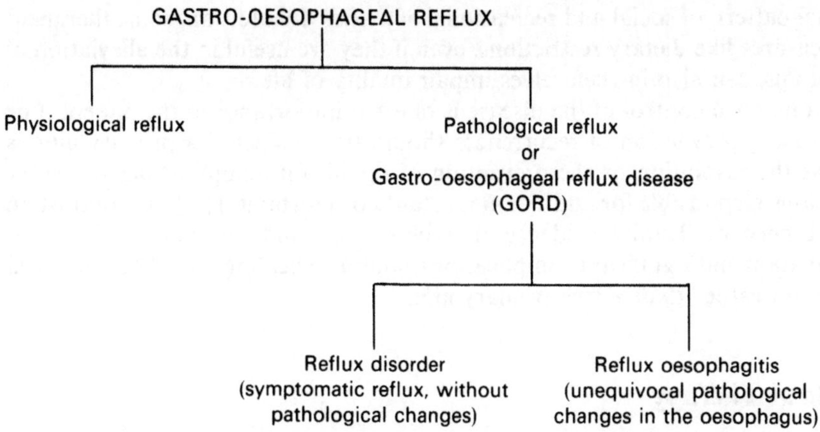

Fig. 1. The wide spectrum of gastro-oesophageal reflux, from physiological reflux to complicated gastro-oesophageal reflux disease

During the last decade many drugs have been introduced on the market, including very potent acid suppressors and more effective prokinetic agents. However, most of the trials have been limited primarily to short-term evaluation of individual drugs. Although these new drugs have dramatically extended our therapeutic armamentarium, in clinical practice it is frequently difficult to make rational choices. One reason for this is that the natural history of GORD remains insufficiently known. Also important is the fact that the safety profile of several drugs, especially of proton pump inhibitors, is not fully established, at least in the very long term.

The purpose of this article is to review briefly the different medical and surgical options now available and to provide practical guidelines for the management of GORD. It is therefore clinically relevant to first define what the aims of treatment are.

Aims of Treatment

It is generally accepted that treatment of GORD aims at (i) the control of symptoms, (ii) the healing of oesophageal lesions, and (iii) the prevention of relapses and complications. However, there is some confusion about the relative priority of these different goals and about how the success of therapy should be judged [7]. In the opinion of many gastroenterologists and in most of the published trials, the main criterion of judgement is the healing of oesophageal lesions after an acute treatment. However, for the patient, a primary concern is the relief of symptoms which interfere with daily activities and quality of life. If frequent and severe, symptoms can impair concentration and performance at work, and some patients may feel that they are no longer able to maintain their normal pattern of social and recreational activities. In addition, some therapeutic measures like dietary restrictions, even if they are useful in the alleviation of symptoms, can also in themselves impair quality of life.

Long-term control of the disease is of great importance to the patient. For this reason, prevention of recurrences should be considered a primary aim as well as the resolution or the prevention of significant complications (i.e. complications responsible for additional mortality or morbidity) [7]. By contrast, in the absence of definite evidence that persisting mild oesophagitis leads to aggravation and significant complications, complete healing is probably an ideal end-point rather than a true primary aim.

Medical Therapy

Life Style and Dietary Recommendations

This traditional component of GORD management includes elevation of the head of the bed, dietary modifications, weight loss, cessation of alcohol and nicotine consumption, and avoidance of tight garments. These measures are always recommended whatever the drug prescribed and the severity of the disease. As showed by pH-metric studies, at least some of them are actually effective in reducing oesophageal acid exposure or improving clearance time [8]. They can also enhance the efficacy of drugs, as showed for ranitidine in patients with erosive oesophagitis. However, the *compliance* of patients towards these conservative measures has not been really assessed in the long term. For instance, no clinical trial of the effect of stopping smoking has been performed, even if the negative effects of cigarette smoking on reflux are now better understood [9]. Clinical experience strongly suggests that many patients are unable or unwilling to follow tedious recommendations for long periods of time.

Many drugs can lower LOS tone and/or impair oesophageal motility (e.g. calcium channel blockers, tricyclic antidepressants, theophylline). However, the findings of pharmacological studies do not always correlate with clinical findings. For instance, a pH-metric study [10] of asthmatic refluxers showed no difference in acid oesophageal exposure or oesophageal motility parameters between one group of patients treated with bronchodilators and another group who did not receive these drugs. In any given reflux patient, before stopping a drug indicated because of a concurrent illness but which may adversely affect LOS pressure, a pragmatic approach weighing advantages and inconveniences should be preferred to dogmatic recommendations.

Drugs Used in the Treatment of GORD

Several reviews dealing with anti-reflux drugs and therapeutic trials in GORD have been published during the last few years (see [11–15]). We shall limit the discussion to an overview of the most effective drugs and/or to those which are

Table 1. Classification of drugs currently used in gastro-oesophageal reflux disease according to their efficacy in the short term and in the long term

	Acute treatment		Prevention of recurrences
	Symptoms	Oesophagitis	
Old drugs			
Antacids	±	–	–
Alginates/antacids	+	–	–
Metoclopramide and domperidone	+	–	–
H_2-receptor antagonists	+ +	+	±
Sucralfate	+	+	–
New drugs			
Cisapride	+ +	+	+
More potent or high doses of H_2-receptor antagonists	+ +	+ +	+
Proton pump inhibitors	+ + +	+ + +	+ + +

+ Drug of proved value (controlled trials)
– Not established (negative trial or untested)

currently used in routine practice. Table 1 provides a synoptic view of the efficacy of "old" and "new" drugs with regard to the various criteria previously described.

Antacids and Alginate/Antacid Compounds

Most patients with reflux symptoms initially use over-the-counter medications, mainly antacids or alginates, and in community practice recent surveys showed that 80% of patients who were consulting a general practitioner about their symptoms were self-medicating.

Antacids neutralize hydrogen ions present in gastric secretion, thereby reducing their concentration in the refluxed material. However the increase in gastric pH is of short duration. Alginates (Gaviscon) and alginate/antacid compounds are special preparations designed to float as a raft at the surface of the gastric content and to improve the defective anti-reflux barrier. Their composition and raft strength vary from country to country and sometimes with-in the same formulation [16].

Despite their wide use, very few studies have shown a statistically significant benefit of antacids even in the relief of symptoms. All trials failed to establish the superiority of antacids over placebo on the healing of lesions. Results are more encouraging with alginate/antacids. On the whole, clinical experience suggests that Gaviscon is effective in the relief of heartburn, but not in the healing of oesophagitis. In some countries, an association of carbenoxolone and alginate/-antacid compound (Pyrogastrone) is available as a chewable tablet. It seems that addition of carbenoxolone enhanced symptomatic relief and increased end-oscopic healing of reflux oesophagitis. However, side effects may occasionally occur with carbenoxolone, and the palatability of Pyrogastrone tablets is far from good.

No long-term controlled study of antacids or alginate/antacids given alone has yet been carried out. However, Behar et al. [17] reported the long-term results of medical management of patients with severe disease, including lifestyle modifications and antacids, compared with surgical treatment. After 5 years, results were rated good in only 27% of patients in the medically treated group, compared with 100% in the surgical group.

Sucralfate

Little is known of the resistant properties of the oesophageal mucosa and even less of its protective mechanisms, but there is a potential for the use of mucosal coating agents in GORD [14]. Sucralfate, a basic aluminum salt of sucrose sulfate, forms an adherent complex with proteins at the ulcer crater, protecting the underlying tissues against the noxious effects of acid and pepsin. It also binds and protects the oesophageal mucosa against bile salts. However, alkaline reflux does not seem to play any role in most cases. Several controlled trials have shown the efficacy of sucralfate (1 g suspension q.i.d.) in the acute treatment of reflux oesophagitis. In our experience, maintenance treatment with sucralfate (2 g/day) is not effective in the prevention of recurrences of oesophagitis (unpublished data). A trial also failed to show any benefit of combined treatment with sucralfate and ranitidine compared to sucralfate alone [18].

Prokinetic Drugs

Since GORD is a primary motility disorder and "dysmotility-like" dyspepsia (nausea, bloating, early satiety, fullness, etc.) is frequently associated with typical reflux symptoms in the same patient, there is a good rationale to use prokinetic compounds, either alone or combined with antisecretory drugs.

With the advent of new effective prokinetics some ancillary drugs have been relegated to a minor role, if any at all, in the management of GORD. For instance, bethanechol, a cholinergic agent effective against symptoms and lesions of oesophagitis, stimulates gastric acid secretion and causes adverse effects. Similarly, metoclopramide, although effective on reflux symptoms at quite high doses (at least 40 mg/day), frequently causes adverse effects (drowsiness, bowel disturbance, dizziness, etc.). It therefore seems now time to abandon bethanechol and metoclopramide in the treatment of GORD.

Domperidone is a more recently developed dopamine antagonist, related to the butyrophenones, which has nearly the same pharmacodynamic actions as metoclopramide on oesophageal and gastric motility. However, domperidone does not cross the blood-brain barrier and seldom causes extrapyramidal effects; it may, however produces symptoms related to hyperprolactinemia (galactorrhea, amenorrhea). Results similar to those obtained with metoclopramide would be expected in GORD, with an advantage for domperidone in terms of tolerance.

Cisapride is a new prokinetic drug without antidopaminergic effect. Its mechanism of action is thought to involve enhancement of acetylcholine release in the myenteric plexus of the gut [19]. There is also some evidence that cisapride acts both as an agonist (5-HT_4) and as an antagonist (5-HT_3) of serotonin receptors. Cisapride strengthens the amplitude of oesophageal body contractions, increases LOS pressure (especially in reflux patients with low baseline tone [20]) and accelerates gastric emptying. Although cisapride has indirect cholinomimetic effects, it does not affect gastric acid secretion. Cisapride has a good safety profile. The side effects most often reported are transient abdominal pain and diarrhea, rarely necessitating withdrawal of treatment.

The efficacy of cisapride (10 mg q.i.d.) in patients with various grades of oesophagitis has been established beyond doubt, both in adults and children, in many controlled trials [19, 21–25]. Cisapride compares well with cimetidine [21] and ranitidine [23] in terms of symptom relief and healing of lesions. In patients with severe reflux oesophagitis, two studies [24, 25] showed cisapride to be an effective add-on treatment with H_2-receptor antagonists. Recently, large placebo-controlled trials [26, 27] showed that maintenance treatment with cisapride (10 or 20 mg b.i.d or 20 mg nocte) significantly reduces the 6- and 12-month relapse rates in oesophagitis. However, the therapeutic gain was quite modest and mainly restricted to patients with mild or moderate oesophagitis.

Antisecretory Drugs

Although pirenzepine, a selective muscarinic compound, has been shown to be effective in GORD [28], only H_2-blockers and proton pump inhibitors are usually prescribed in routine practice.

H_2-receptor antagonists (cimetidine, ranitidine, famotidine and nizatidine) dose-dependently inhibit gastric acid secretion and reduce pepsin secretion. Their slight effect on oesophageal interdigestive motility is probably of no clinical relevance and, in contrast to anticholinergic drugs, they do not affect salivary secretion. Finally, treatment results in a reduction of acidity and volume available for reflux.

Although the efficacy and safety of H_2-blockers are well established, results are less satisfactory in reflux oesophagitis than in peptic ulcer disease [11–13]. Approximately 50% of patients with erosive or ulcerative oesophagitis are healed after 6 weeks, and 70% after 12 weeks [29]. The initial severity of oesophagitis is probably the major prognostic factor which negatively influences healing, but comparisons between different studies are sometimes difficult due to the lack of agreement between endoscopic classifications of lesions. Since both daytime and night-time reflux seem of importance in the pathogenesis of oesophagitis, the time and schedule for dose administration also differ from those recommended in peptic ulcer disease. Thus, recent studies with ranitidine [30], nizatidine [31], and famotidine [32] showed better symptomatic relief and healing rates with the twice-daily regimen than with a regimen giving a single evening dose. These results are in agreement with pH monitoring studies showing that a twice-daily regimen of famotidine is necessary to bring oesophageal acid exposure into the normal range in patients with severe GORD [33].

Also in contrast with peptic ulcer disease is the fact that low-dose maintenance treatment with H_2-blockers is ineffective in the prevention of relapse of oesophagitis [29]. In several studies with ranitidine, benefit of even a full-dose maintenance treatment was not established. However, effective prophylaxis of recurrences [32] was recently reported with a regimen of famotidine (20 mg b.i.d).

There is now some evidence to show that patients who do not respond to antisecretory treatment experience less reduction in gastric acidity and more prolonged acid exposure [34–36]. In these patients, who frequently present with Barrett's oesophagus, stronger acid suppression is usually required to achieve symptom relief and healing of lesions [36, 37]. In this connection, pH monitoring studies [38] have demonstrated that increasing doses of H_2-receptor antagonists result in dose-dependent reduction of oesophageal acid exposure. These studies provide an excellent rationale for using larger daily doses of H_2-blockers for treatment of patients with unresponsive GORD [39]. This has been confirmed by a trial [40] showing the superiority of ranitidine 300 mg q.d.s. over a standard twice daily regimen (150 mg b.i.d.). However, the uncertainties about the safety of potent acid suppression as well as the cost of this high-dose H_2-blocker treatment make the practical interest of this approach very questionable.

Finally, because they are more effective on symptoms [41] than on lesions, H_2-receptor antagonists may still continue to be useful drugs in the treatment of patients with intermittent symptoms of GORD and no or mild oesophagitis at endoscopy. The reason for the discrepancy between the effect on symptoms and on lesions may be related to the lower sensitivity threshold to acid of the oesophageal mucosa for pain perception than for promoting healing of oesophagitis [42].

Substituted benzimidazoles (omeprazole, lansoprazole) interact with gastric H^+K^+, ATPase, the enzyme constituting the final step in the formation of gastric acid. This specific inhibitory action on the proton pump offers a highly selective mean of controlling acid secretion [43].

The effects on healing and symptom relief have been of a magnitude never seen before. In clinical trials omeprazole always appeared superior to ranitidine and cimetidine [43], given as a single daily dose varying from 20 to 60 mg and with healing rates ranging from about 70% to 90% after 4–8 weeks of treatment. Healing did not seem influenced by factors other than initial severity of oesophagitis. The 40-mg dosage produced relief of heartburn and healing slightly more rapidly than the 20-mg dosage [44, 45]. Quite similar results were recently reported for lansoprazole (30 mg od). Omeprazole 40 mg also induced healing within 4–12 weeks in patients who were resistant to treatment with cimetidine or ranitidine for at least 12 weeks [46]. Unfortunately, relapse occurs quickly when treatment is stopped [44]. Results of maintenance treatment with omeprazole 20 mg are clearly superior to those achieved with ranitidine or cisapride [43, 47]. Weekend therapy with omeprazole 20 mg 3 days a week is not effective, but omeprazole 10 mg daily may be sufficient in a proportion of patients [47].

In fact, the problem with proton pump inhibitors or any other form of potent acid inhibition is not efficacy but safety. The potential risks include the consequences of prolonged hypergastrinemia (enterochromaffin-like cell hyperplasia and gastric carcinoids), the possibility of bacterial overgrowth and enteric infections and, more incidentally, some degree of impairment in nutrient absorption. Data on long-term treatment with omeprazole indicate that such treatment usually results in moderate hypergastrinemia, comparable to that in patients with parietal cell vagotomy. However, a small group of patients with high basal serum gastrin levels before treatment may develop very high gastrin levels while on omeprazole [47]. To date, however, no signs of dysplasia or neoplasia have been found in the surveillance programme of patients treated for more than 4 years with omeprazole at recommended doses. Similarly there is no convincing evidence that omeprazole is genotoxic. In conclusion, proton pump inhibitors represent a major advance in the treatment of patients with moderate and severe oesophagitis, especially in those who are refractory to H_2-blockade. Their place in treatment of the milder forms of oesophagitis and in non-erosive GORD has not yet been definitely determined.

Surgery

An effective operation can obviate the expense, inconvenience and risks of long-term medical therapy. Excellent surgical results have been reported by surgeons skilled in various techniques of fundoplication (e.g. Nissen, Belsey, Toupet fundoplications) [48]. Recently, Spechler et al. [49] conducted a long-term randomized trial of medical therapy and surgery in patients with severe complicated GORD (i.e. Barrett's oesophagus, peptic oesophageal ulcer, stricture, and/or erosive oesophagitis). Patients were randomly allocated either to continuous medical therapy (lifestyle modifications and up to four medications), medical therapy for symptoms only, or surgery (Nissen fundoplication). The mean activity index score and the grade of oesophagitis were significantly better in the surgical group than in medical groups during the 2 years of follow-up. There were no operative deaths. This trial clearly demonstrates the superiority of surgery to conventional medical therapy (antacids + ranitidine 150 mg b.i.d. and in some cases metoclopramide and sucralfate).

The scope of laparoscopic surgery is being expanded and it is likely to be applicable to the majority of functional gastrointestinal disorders [50]. Different techniques consisting of either laparoscopic reduction, crural repair and total fundoplication of large symptomatic hiatal hernia [50] or round ligament cardiopexy [51] have been recently described. At the moment experience is still limited, but the feasibility of laparoscopic treatment has been established and all the recognized important components of conventional surgery have been reproduced by this endoscopic approach. However, follow-up is at present too short for any definite conclusions on the long-term efficacy to be drawn. It is therefore of the utmost importance that these laparoscopic techniques remain in the hands of surgeons skilled in conventional surgery. They should be performed in a few reference centres and prospectively assessed according to rigorous protocols aimed at evaluating safety and long-term results.

Therapeutic Strategy

Since GORD is a wide-spectrum disorder which causes a range of symptoms and complications, it is crucial to identify prognostic criteria which can help the clinician in selecting patients with regard to the different investigations and therapeutic options now available. Unfortunately, despite the plethora of diagnostic tests and functional investigations now routinely performed, it is often difficult to predict the evolution of the disease in a given patient or to clearly identify the groups of subjects who are at risk of developing significant complications. Indeed, although the initial severity of the oesophagitis is probably one of the best prognostic factors in patients with objective mucosal breaks at endoscopy, one must remember that severe oesophagitis has a low prevalence and that there is frequently a poor correlation between symptoms and lesions in GORD (7). Among other factors predictive of recurrences, the presence of persistent symptoms at the time of healing and the duration of the acute treatment required to heal lesions have been inconsistently reported by some authors [29]. Similarly, low LOS tone or severe peristaltic dysfunction are frequently associated with a profile of severe lesions and chronic relapsing disease [52]. In a recent 3-year follow-up study of patients with reflux oesophagitis, supine reflux at initial 24-h pH monitoring was found to be an unfavourable prognostic factor for the long-term evolution [53], but in contrast to this, the pH profile was not found to be of any predictive value in other studies [54]. Finally, the prognostic value of other factors such as age, gender, smoking, alcohol consumption or the use of NSAIDs remains insufficiently documented.

It has been usual until recently to employ a *stepwise strategy*, starting with life style modifications and the safest and least expensive drugs (Fig. 2). However, recently Fraser et al. [55] presented arguments against this staged therapy and proposed using the most effective therapy (i.e. proton pump inhibitors) as the first approach in any individual patient. Although there is no doubt that omeprazole is the most effective drug both for acute and maintenance treatment of reflux oesophagitis, it has not been fully licensed, especially for long-term use in patients with non-erosive or mild oesophagitis. Until the safety of prolonged acid suppression has been more fully documented and the potential of omeprazole in the milder forms of the disease has been more completely explored, the majority of gastroenterologists and regulation authorities will probably continue to recommend the former stepwise approach.

In clinical practice, indications for treatment depend on age, severity of symptoms and lesions, response to medical therapy, presence or absence of complications, and on the individual course of the disease (relapses rare or frequent).

Since predominant heartburn and/or regurgitations have good specificity [56], young patients presenting with these typical symptoms of reflux can be

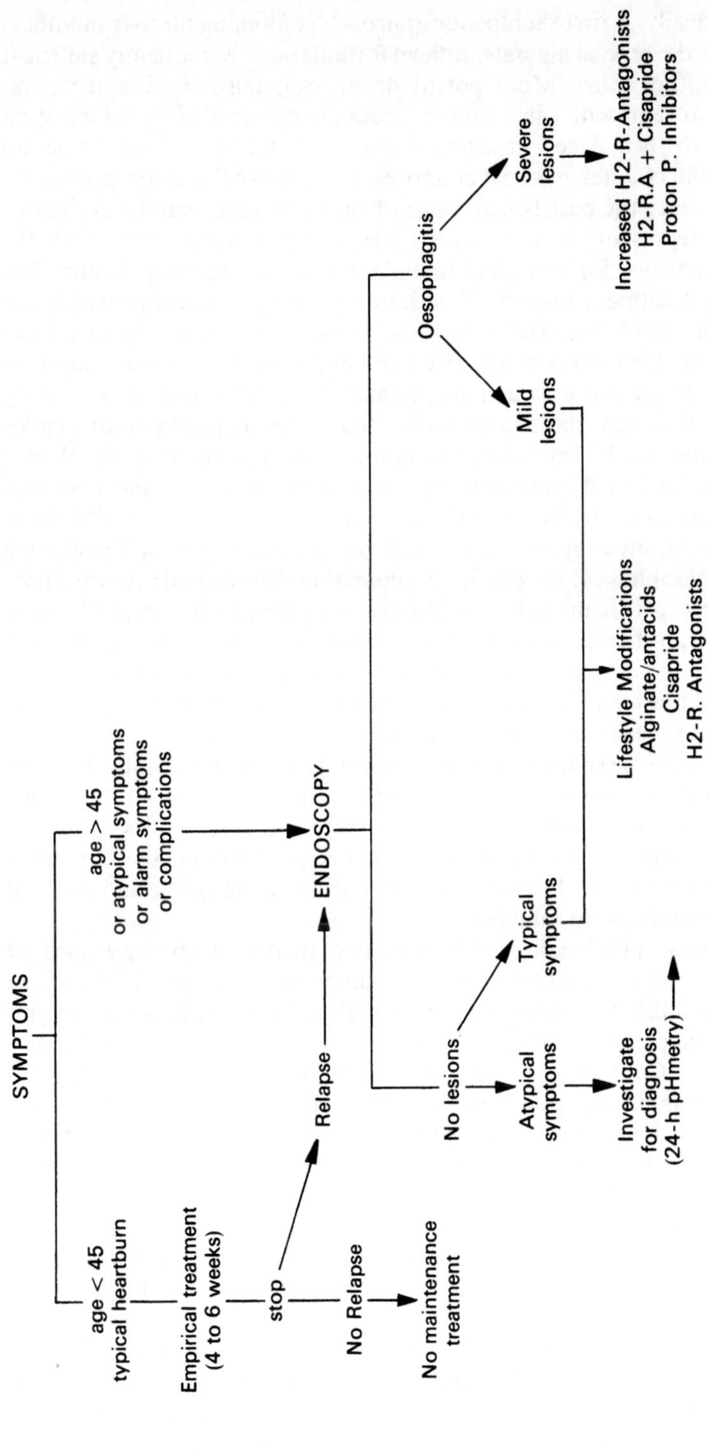

Fig. 2. Suggested flowchart for the initial management of a patient with symptoms (typical or atypical) suggestive of gastro-oesophageal reflux disease

managed empirically. A first therapeutic approach combining lifestyle modifications and one of the several alginate/antacid formulations is frequently sufficient to achieve symptom relief. More potent drugs, especially H_2-receptor antagonists, may also represent a first-choice treatment due to their good effect on symptoms and to their excellent safety profile. Cimetidine and ranitidine are now sold over the counter in some countries, but a surveillance programme is still necessary before the cost/benefit ratio of such a strategy can be evaluated. Cisapride may represent an alternative to H_2-receptor antagonists, with the possible inconvenience for empirical treatment of high-frequency dosing. The duration of any treatment prescribed without endoscopy should probably not exceed a maximum of 4–6 weeks. Studies of patients in primary care have showed that some 75%–90% experienced an improvement in reflux symptoms after 2 weeks of treatment with alginate/antacids [57] or ranitidine twice daily [58]. However, it is important to underline that, even in young adults, endoscopy is indicated each time alarm symptoms are present (e.g. dysphagia, anaemia, weight loss) or if symptoms are not relieved or recur a short interval after discontinuation of treatment. Patients over 45 years and those with alarm symptoms must be investigated to rule out the presence of a life-threatening condition (e.g. oesophageal or gastric carcinoma) and to provide reassurance.

If endoscopy reveals no objective lesions in a patient with atypical symptoms, it is important to demonstrate the oesophageal origin of the pain by 24-h pH-metry. Once the diagnosis is established, in patients in whom endoscopy shows no or mild lesions the treatment should be based on H_2-antagonists or cisapride for 6–12 weeks, as described above.

In patients with resistant symptoms and/or more severe lesions at endoscopy (i.e. confluent erosions or ulcerations) different medical strategies are available: (i) increased doses or improved therapeutic schedules with H_2-antagonists or change to a more potent H_2-blocker, (ii) combined therapy with a prokinetic drug (ranitidine 150 mg b.i.d + cisapride 10 mg q.i.d), and (iii), last but not least, proton pump inhibitors.

In most cases, after healing of lesions two treatment strategies can be proposed: no (or intermittent) treatment or maintenance treatment (Tables 2, 3). The former is suitable for younger patients with mild or moderate symptoms and infrequent relapses; they should be treated in the same way as the first time if symptoms return. Conversely, if symptoms recur shortly after treatment has been stopped, maintenance treatment with cisapride (10 mg b.i.d or 20 mg h.s.) may be proposed. Once again, although proton pump inhibitors are highly effective against both symptoms and lesions, long-term therapy cannot be presently recommended in young patients until their safety has been more extensively established. Surgery is certainly preferable to a life-time of medical therapy in young patients with uncomplicated GORD but with persistent or recurrent symptoms despite appropriate medical treatment. Careful preoperative evaluation including manometry must be performed in all these patients because surgery is contraindicated in those with severe peristaltic disturbances of the oesophageal body [48]. Conversely, in patients who are at high risk for surgery and/or in those with severe lesions refractory to other drugs, maintenance treatment with omeprazole keeps most in remission [46]. This mainten-

Table 2. Intermittent treatment in gastro-oesophageal reflux disease: criteria for patient selection. (Adapted from Bardhan in [12])

Age < 60 years
Relapse infrequent (< 3 per year)
Symptoms mild or moderate
Long-term NSAIDs not needed
No other major illness
No or mild erosive oesophagitis

NB: Intermittent treatment is used in patients who continue to meet *all* criteria on each occasion such therapy is considered (i.e. on relapse)

Table 3. Maintenance treatment in gastro-oesophageal reflux disease: criteria for patient selection. (Adapted from Bardhan in [12])

Age ≥ 60 years
Relapses frequent (≥ 3 per year)
Symptoms moderate or severe; continue despite healing
Long-term NSAIDs needed
Other major illness (e.g. cardiopulmonary)
Other systemic disease affecting oesophageal motility
Reflux contributes to other troublesome problems (e.g. non-cardiac chest pain)
Refractory disease or failure of intermittent treatment
Severe lesions at endoscopy (grades 3/4; stricture; Barrett's oesophagus)

ance treatment with proton pump inhibitors is probably the best option for older patients and/or those with complicated disease (e.g. stenosis or Barrett' oesophagus).

Conclusions and Priorities for Future Research

Despite the existence of a large number of publications and trials, there are still many unanswered questions about the efficacy and practical usefulness of the different forms of medical therapy.

Although proton pump inhibitors are very useful in the treatment of moderate and severe reflux oesophagitis, especially in patients who are refractory to treatment with H_2-receptor antagonists, the role of potent acid suppression in the management of mild oesophagitis and non-erosive GORD has not yet been exactly determined. Many practical issues concerning the minimum effective and safest doses, the place of combined treatments, and ways of monitoring patients need to be addressed in future studies.

There is also a need to develop accurate and reliable tools for measuring specifically the impact of GORD on quality of life and comparing the cost and effectiveness of different medical and surgical strategies. Although surgery has been proved superior to conventional medical therapy in the long-term treatment of patients with severe or complicated GORD, it is impossible to extrapolate from these data to the result of a comparison of surgery with potent acid suppression. It is therefore an appropriate time to consider a trial comparing omeprazole and fundoplication. The advent of laparoscopic surgery certainly deserves careful evaluation, but definitive conclusions will not be possible for several years yet.

References

1. Heading RC (1989) Epidemiology of oesophageal reflux disease. Scand J Gastroenterol 24 (suppl 168):33–37
2. Bruley des Varannes S, Galmiche JP, Bernades P, Bader JP (1988) Douleurs épigastriques et régurgitations: épidémiologie descriptive dans un échantillon représentatif de la population française. Gastroenterol Clin Biol 12:721–728
3. Janssens J, Galmiche JP (1990) Pathophysiology of gastro-oesophageal reflux. In: Vantrappen G, Mainguet P (eds) Peptic oesophagitis. Diagnosis and treatment. Excerpta Medica, Amsterdam, pp 9–18
4. Hirschowitz BI (1991) A critical analysis, with appropriate controls, of gastric acid and pepsin secretion in clinical esophagitis. Gastroenterology 95:37–43
5. Gotley DC, Morgan AP, Ball D, Owen RW, Cooper MJ (1991) Composition of gastro-oesophageal refluxate. Gut 32:1093–1099
6. Zaninotto G, Di Mario F, Costantini M et al. (1992) Oesophagitis and pH of refluxate: an experimental and clinical study. Br J Surg 79:161–164
7. Heading RC, Eaves NR (1992) Aims of treatment in gastroesophageal reflux disease. In: Scarpignato C (ed) Advances in drug therapy of gastroesophageal reflux disease. Frontiers of gastrointestinal research, vol 20. Karger, Basel, pp 1–10
8. Kitchin LI, Castell DO (1991) Rationale and efficacy of conservative therapy for gastroesophageal reflux disease. Arch Intern Med 151:448–454
9. Kahrilas PJ (1992) Cigarette smoking and gastroesophageal reflux disease. Dig Dis 10:61–71
10. Sontag SJ, O'Connell S, Khandelwal S et al. (1990) Most asthmatics have gastroesophageal reflux with or without bronchodilator therapy. Gastroenterology 99:613–620
11. Bell NJV, Hunt RH (1992) Role of gastric acid suppression in the treatment of gastro-oesophageal reflux disease. Gut 33:118–124
12. Scarpignato C (1992) Advances in drug therapy of gastroesophageal reflux disease. Frontiers of gastrointestinal research, vol 20. Karger Basel
13. Koelz HR (1989) Treatment of reflux esophagitis with H_2-blockers, antacids and prokinetic drugs. An analysis of randomized clinical trials. Scand J Gastroenterol 24 (suppl. 156):25–36
14. Scarpignato C, Galmiche JP (1988) Mucosal coating agents: pharmacology and clinical use. In Bianchi-Porro G (ed) Topics in digestive disease. Raven, New York, pp 73–133
15. Thomson ABR (1992) Medical treatment of gastroesophageal reflux disease: options and priorities. Hepato-Gastroenterol 39 (suppl 1):14–23
16. Scarpignato C, Galmiche JP (1992) Antacids and alginates in the treatment of gastroesophageal reflux disease: how do they work and how much are they clinically useful? In: Scarpignato C (ed) advances in drug therapy of gastroesophageal reflux disease. Frontiers of gastrointestinal Research. Basel, Karger, pp 153–181
17. Behar J, Sheahan DG, Biancani P, Spiro HM, Storer EH (1975) Medical and surgical

management of reflux esophagitis. A 38-month report on a prospective clinical trial. N Engl J Med 293:263–268
18. Vermeijden JR, Tytgat GNJ, Schotborgh RH et al. (1992) Combination therapy of sucralfate and ranitidine, compared with sucralfate monotherapy, in patients with peptic reflux esophagitis. Scand J Gastroenterol 27:81–84
19. McCallum RW, Prakash C, Campoli-Richards DM, Goa KL (1988) Cisapride. A preliminary review of its pharmacodynamic and pharmacokinetic properties, and therapeutic use as a prokinetic agent in gastrointestinal motility disorders. Drugs 36:652–681
20. Ceccatelli P, Janssens J, Vantrappen G, Cucchiara S (1988) Cisapride restores the decreased lower oesophageal sphincter pressure in reflux patients. Gut 29:631–635
21. Galmiche JP, Fraitag B, Filoche B et al. (1990) Double-blind comparison of cisapride and cimetidine in treatment of reflux esophagitis. Dig Dis Sci 35:649–655
22. Rode H, Stunden RJ, Mikllar AJW, Cywes S (1987) Esophageal pH assessment of gastroesophageal reflux in 18 patients and the effect of two prokinetic agents: cisapride and metoclopramide. J Pediat Surg 22:931–934
23. Janisch HD, Hutteman W, Bouzo MH (1988) Cisapride versus ranitidine in the treatment of reflux esophagitis. Hepato-Gastroenterol 35:125–127
24. Galmiche JP, Brandstatter G, Evreux M et al. (1988) Combined therapy with cisapride and cimetidine in severe reflux esophagitis. Gut 29:675–681
25. Wienbeck M (1986) Therapeutic effect of cisapride added on to ranitidine in patients with reflux esophagitis. Dig Dis Sci 31:275A
26. Toussaint J, Gossuin A, Deruyttere M, Hublé F, Devis G (1991) Healing and prevention of relapse of reflux oesophagitis by cisapride. Gut 32:1280–1285
27. Tytgat GNJ, Hansen OJA, Carling L et al. (1992) Effect of cisapride on relapse of reflux oesophagitis healed with an antisecretory drug. Scand J Gastroenterol 27:175–183
28. Sato TL, Wu WC, Castell DO (1992) Randomized, double-blind, placebo-controlled crossover trial of pirenzepine in patients with gastroesophageal reflux. Dig Dis Sci 37:297–302
29. Koelz HR, Birchler R, Bretholz A et al. (1986) Healing and relapse of reflux esophagitis during treatment with ranitidine. Gastroenterology 91:1198–1205
30. Johnson NJ, Laws S, Mills JG, Wood JR (1991) Effect of three ranitidine dosage regimens in the treatment of reflux oesophagitis: results of a multicentre trial. Eur J Gastroenterol Hepatol 3:769–774
31. Quick RPF, Cooper MJ, Gleeson M et al. (1990) A comparison of two doses of nizatidine versus placebo in the treatment of reflux oesophagitis. Aliment Pharmacol Therap 4:201–211
32. Wesdorp ICE (1992) Famotidine in gastroesophageal reflux disease (GERD). Hepato-Gastroenterol 39 (suppl 1):24–26
33. Orr WC, Robinson MG, Humphries TJ, Antonello J, Caglioola A (1988) Dose-response effect of famotidine on patterns of gastro-oesophageal reflux. Aliment Pharmacol Therap 2:229–235
34. Johansson KE, Tibbling L (1986) Gastric secretion and reflux pattern in reflux oesophagitis before and during ranitidine treatment. Scand J Gastroenterol, 21:487–492
35. Robertson DAF, Aldersley MA, Shepherd H, Lloyd RS, Smith CL (1987) H2 antagonists in the treatment of reflux oesophagitis: can physiological studies predict the response? Gut 28:946–949
36. Collen J, Lewis JH, Benjamin SB (1990) Gastric acid hypersecretion in refractory gastroesophageal reflux disease. Gastroenterology 98:654–661
37. Collen MJ, Johnson DA (1992) Correlation between basal acid output and daily ranitidine dose required for therapy in Barrett's esophagus. Dig Dis Sci 37:570–576
38. Jansen JBMJ, Baak LC, Lamers CBHW (1988) Effect of increasing doses of ranitidine on exposure of the esophagus to gastric acid in patients with reflux esophagitis. Scand J Gastroenterol 23 (suppl. 154):2–5
39. Castell DO (1991) Rationale for high-dose H_2-receptor blockade in the treatment of gastro-oesophageal reflux disease. Aliment Pharmacol Therap, 5 (suppl 1):59–67
40. Johnson NJ, Boyd EJS, Mills JG, Wood JR (1989) Acute treatment of reflux esophagitis: a multicentre trial to compare 150 mg ranitidine b.d with 300 mg ranitidine q.d.s. Aliment Pharmacol Therap 3:259–266
41. Tytgat GNJ, Nicolai JJ, Reman FC (1990) Efficacy of different doses of cimetidine in the

treatment of reflux esophagitis. A review of three large, double-blind, controlled trials. Gastroenterology 99:629–634
42. Smith JL, Opekun AR, Larkai E, Graham DY (1989) Sensitivity of the esophageal mucosa to pH in gastroesophageal reflux disease. Gastroenterology 96: 683–689
43. Maton PN (1991) Drug therapy: omeprazole. N Engl J Med 324:965–975
44. Hetzel DJ, Dent J, Reed WD et al. (1988) Healing and relapse of severe peptic esophagitis after treatment with omeprazole: a dose response study. Gastroenterology 95:903–912
45. Sontag SJ, Hirschowitz BI, Holt S et al. (1992) Two doses of omeprazole versus placebo in symptomatic erosive esophagitis: the U.S. multicenter study. Gastroenterology 102:109–118
46. Koop H, Arnold R (1991) Long-term maintenance treatment of reflux esophagitis with omeprazole. Prospective study in patients with H_2-blocker-resistant esophagitis. Dig Dis Sci 36:552–557
47. Klinkenberg-Knol EC (1992) The role of omeprazole in healing and prevention of reflux disease. Hepato-Gastroenterol 39 (Suppl 1):27–30
48. Stein HJ, Demeester TR (1992) Who benefits from antireflux surgery? World J Surg 16:313–319
49. Spechler SJ et al. (1992) Comparison of medical and surgical therapy for complicated gastroesophageal reflux disease in veterans. N Engl J Med 326:786–792
50. Cuschieri A, Shimi S, Nathanson LK (1992) Laparoscopic reduction, crural repair, and fundoplication of large hiatal hernia. Am J Surg 163:425–430
51. Nathanson LK, Shimi S, Cuschieri A (1991) Laparoscopic ligamentum teres (round ligament) cardiopexy. Br J Surg 78:947–951
52. Lieberman DA (1987) Medical therapy for chronic reflux esophagitis. Long-term follow-up. Arch Intern Med 147:1717–1720
53. Schindlbeck NE, Klauser AG, Berghammer G, Londong W, Muller-Lissner SA (1992) Three year follow up of patients with gastrooesophageal reflux disease. Gut 33:1016–1019
54. Olden K, Triadafilopoulos G (1991) Failure of initial 24-hour esophageal pH monitoring to predict refractoriness and intractability in reflux esophagitis. Am J Gastroenterol 86:1142–1146
55. Fraser R, Verdu E, Armstrong D, Blum A (1992) Gastroesophageal reflux disease, pH monitoring, and treatment. Current Opinion Gastroenterol 8:562–572
56. Klauser AG, Shindlbeck NE, Muller-Lissner SA (1990) Symptoms in gastrooesophageal reflux disease. Lancet 335:205–208
57. Bigard MA, Colin R, Galmiche JP, Rampal P, De Meynard C (1990) Evolution des symptômes de reflux gastro-œsophagien (RGO) après 2 semaines de traitement par alginate-antiacide. Facteurs prédictifs et données endoscopiques chez les non-répondeurs. Gastroenterol Clin Biol 14:A110 (abstr.)
58. Bennett JR (1992) A practical approach to patient management. First united European Congress, Athens, 28 Sept 1992

The Management of Zollinger-Ellison Syndrome

P.N. MATON

Diagnosis

The most difficult step in making the diagnosis of Zollinger-Ellison syndrome (ZES) is to think of the possibility. The typical presentation is no longer that of severe peptic ulceration in unusual sites, as originally described (Ellison and Wilson 1964). Patients often have a typical peptic ulcer, or they may have persistent, recurrent, or complicated peptic ulcer disease, severe esophagitis, or watery diarrhea or malabsorption with or without peptic ulcer disease (Jensen et al. 1986, Wolfe and Jensen 1987). Some patients may have renal stones and a family history of ulcers or other complaints (Eberle and Grun 1981). The diagnosis of ZES should also be entertained in any patient undergoing gastric surgery. The best screening test for ZES is measurement of the fasting serum gastrin (normal < 100 pg/ml). For the initial screen the patient can continue to take antisecretory medication, but if the gastrin result in the range 110–500 pg/ml with H_2-antagonists or 110–3000 pg/ml with omeprazole, the test should be repeated after the patient has stopped taking H_2-antagonists for 24 h or omeprazole for 6 days (Wolfe and Jensen 1987).

The commonest cause of hypergastrinemia is achlorhydria with or without pernicious anemia. Thus, if hypergastrinemia is found, the next step is to measure basal gastric acid output, which in patients with ZES is > 15 mEq/h (or > 5 mEq/h if the patient has had previous gastric surgery). Normal acid outputs are below 11 mEq/h in men and below 6 mEq/h in women (Feldman 1983). The combination of hypergastrinemia and acid hypersecretion occurs in ZES and in three rare conditions, chronic gastric outlet obstruction, retained gastric antrum, a complication of an improperly performed Billroth 2 gastrectomy, and antral gastrin cell hyperplasia. However, the very existence of this latter syndrome is in question. If acid output cannot be measured, gastric juice should be obtained by nasogastric tube and the pH determined. If the pH is > 3.5, the diagnosis is achlorhydria, but if the pH is lower a secretin test should be performed (Wolfe and Jensen 1987; Frucht et al. 1989). After blood samples for basal gastrins are taken at -15 and 0 min, 2 IU/kg secretin are given as a bolus intravenously and blood samples taken at 2, 5, 10, and 20 min. A rise in gastrin of more than 200 pg/ml, usually occuring at 2 or 5 min after injection, is highly suggestive of ZES. A secretin test, however, does not discriminate completely between ZES and other hypergastrinemic states. The secretin test is positive in 90% of patients with ZES, and occasional false positive results have been described in patients with hypochlorhydria.

When the diagnosis of ZES has been made, it is important to define which type of disease the patient is suffering from. About 80% of patients with ZES have the sporadic form, which occurs as an isolated disease. However, the other 20% have ZES as part of the autosomal dominant condition multiple endocrine neoplasia type 1 (MEN-1). The majority of but not all patients with MEN-1 have a family history, 95% have hyperparathyroidism, and about 10% have pituitary tumors (Eberle and Grun 1981). When the manifestations of ZES become apparent in a patient with MEN-1, typically in the fourth decade, most, but not all, will already have had kidney stones due to hyperparathyroidism. Therefore, in patients with ZES a history of renal stones should be sought, plasma calcium and parathormone should be measured, but the sella should be examined by CT scan or MRI. Nevertheless, on occasion it can be difficult to establish a diagnosis of MEN-1.

General Approach to the Patient

The management of patients with ZES is concerned with two distinct problems, control of acid hypersecretion and its manifestations, and preventing or delaying tumor growth and spread. It is important to control acid quickly and effectively, whilst the approach to the tumor can be more leisurely. Even if a patient with ZES has extensive metastatic disease, most symptoms are due to the consequences of gastric acid hypersecretion, and if this is controlled, the patient feels well. In the past, acid hypersecretion and its consequences were the major determinant of survival (Ellison and Wilson 1964), but since the advent of means of controlling acid output safely, tumor growth and spread has taken on increasing importance (Jensen et al. 1986, Wolfe and Jensen 1987).

Control of Acid Hypersecretion

Because patients with ZES can suffer perforation or bleeding from ulcers without any prior warning symptoms, adequate control of acid hypersecretion is the first and most important step. As soon as the diagnosis is suspected and a plasma gastrin sample drawn, antisecretory medication should be started and gastric acid output measured whether or not the patient is taking medication. Definitive measurement of unsuppressed acid output can be delayed and performed under controlled conditions if necessary. Acid output should be reduced to below 10 mEq/h as many studies have shown that reduction of acid output to such levels allows healing of ulcers and prevents complications in most patients (Jensen et al. 1986; Jensen et al. 1983; Collen et al. 1984; Vinayek et al. 1983; Raufman et al. 1983; McArthur et al. 1985).

Emergency Control of Acid Hypersecretion

Immediate control of gastric acid secretion may sometimes be required, for example, if patient has a huge nasogastric output after an operation for presumed idiopathic peptic ulceration. Continuous intravenous cimetidine and ranitidine in large doses are equally effective at reducing acid outputs to within safe limits (Saeed et al. 1989, Fraker et al. 1988). Presumably famotidine is also effective, but no tolerability studies of the high doses required have been performed. Because ranitidine is more potent than cimetidine on a weight basis, the dose of cimetidine required is three times the dose of ranitidine (Howard et al. 1985). An appropriate regime is to give 100 mg ranitidine i.v. as a bolus and then follow this immediately with a continuous infusion of 0.5 mg/kg ranitidine per hour. Acid output should be measured 4 h later and if it is above 10 mEq/h the ranitidine dose should be increased to 1 mg/kg per hour. Acid output should be rechecked every 4 h and the dose increased until the acid output is below 10 mEq/h. A dose of 1 mg/kg ranitidine per hour will control acid output in 70% of patients with ZES (Saeed et al. 1989; Fraker et al. 1988), but doses as high as 4 mg/kg per hour have been used with no serious side effects. If the patient is switched to an oral H_2-antagonist, the dose required can be estimated by multiplying the total daily intravenous dose by 1.5, dividing by 4, and giving that dose of oral drug every 6 h. Nevertheless, the adequacy of the dose of oral medication should be checked by measuring acid output in the last hour before the next dose of drug (see below).

It is likely that in time intravenous omeprazole will replace intravenous H_2-antagonists for the immediate control of acid output in patients with ZES. Omeprazole has been shown to be effective in these patients (Vinayek et al. 1990), but the formulation is not available at the time of writing.

Long-Term Control of Acid Hypersecretion with Histamine H_2-Receptor Antagonists

Although acid hypersecretion can be controlled safely and effectively by oral cimetidine, ranitidine, or famotidine (Jensen et al. 1986; Jensen et al. 1983; Collen et al. 1984; Vinayek et al. 1983; Raufman et al. 1983; McArthur et al. 1985), these drugs have largely been superseded by omeprazole. However, no matter which drug is used, it is essential that, as with intravenous therapy, acid output be measured, because symptoms are not a reliable guide to the presence of mucosal disease. The dose of antisecretory drug required is not related to the patient's basal acid output, maximal acid output, plasma gastrin concentration, or extent of tumor, and thus the dose required has to be determined in each patient individually (Jensen et al. 1986; Wolfe and Jensen 1987). Acid output can be controlled in nearly every patient if sufficient medication is given. However, most patients with ZES will require drug administration every 6 h and some every 4 h, whilst a few will also need an anticholinergic. Each of the H_2-antagonists can be used. However, because cimetidine can cause gynecomastia and impotence in men and there are few toxicity data on high-dose regimens of famotidine, ranitidine is probably the drug of choice. The mean daily dose of ranitine required in the National Institutes of Health study was 1200 mg, with a range of 450–9200 mg/day. No serious toxicity was seen even at these high doses. With each of the H_2-antagonists drug requirements tend to increase with time, and thus acid output should be remeasured at least every 12 months.

Long-Term Control of Acid Hypersecretion with H^+K^+ATPase Inhibitors

The use of the potent, long-acting H^+K^+ATPase inhibitor omeprazole (Olbe et al. 1982; Clissold and Campoli-Richards 1986; Maton 1991; Frucht et al. 1991) has simplified the control of acid secretion in patients with ZES. Omeprazole given once or twice per day can safely and effectively control acid secretion in all patients (McArthur et al. 1985; Maton et al. 1989; Lamers et al. 1984; Lloyd-Davies et al. 1988; Delchier et al. 1986). As with H_2-antagonists, the dose of omeprazole required has to be determined empirically. A reasonable dose to start with is 60 mg/day and then measure acid output in the last hour before the next dose of drug. The dose should be increased and acid checked daily until acid output is below 10 mEq/h. The dose can be increased up to 120 mg once per day, but if this does not reduce acid output to below 10 mEq/h the dose should be split and given as 60 mg every 12 h. This dose is sufficient to control acid output even in patients who require more than 9000 mg ranitidine per day. Unlike H_2-antagonists, does not have its full omeprazole effect for several days, and it may be possible subsequently to reduce the dose. There has been no significant toxicity with omeprazole even with the high doses used. Patients prefer omeprazole to the H_2-antagonists because of the dosing interval and numbers of tablets, and most patients say they feel better on omeprazole.

One concern over the long-term use of omeprazole (and other powerful antisecretory drugs) is the risk of development of gastric carcinoid tumors. Omeprazole produces gastric carcinoids in rats as a consequence of achlorhydria and hypergastrinemia (Maton 1991). Patients with ZES are already hypergastrinemic, and these patients, particularly those with MEN-1 (Solcia et al. 1990), are at increased risk of developing carcinoids. Because patients with ZES are hypersecretors of acid, even large doses of omeprazole do not usually produce the marked hypochlorhydria that triggers hypergastrinemia in normal subjects. Furthermore, unlike patients with idiopathic acid peptic disease, the plasma gastrin in patients with ZES is produced by the tumor and is not under physiological control. Therefore omeprazole does not cause increased hypergastrinemia in patients with ZES (Maton et al. 1990). Follow-up studies of patients with ZES given omeprazole have shown no increase in ECL cells (enterochromaffin-like cells, the precursor cells of gastric carcinoids) (Maton et al. 1990; Lehy et al. 1989), and there have been no unexpected gastric carcinoid tumors. Patients with ZES and MEN-1 taking omeprazole have been described with gastric carcinoid tumors, but these were probably a preexisting condition (Lehy et al. 1989). Further long-term studies are required to establish the magnitude of the risk of carcinoid tumors in patients with ZES on long-term antisecretory medicine.

Lansoprazole, a second H^+K^+ATPase inhibitor, has also been used in patients with ZES. With respect to its pharmacology, tolerability, efficacy, and potency, lansoprazole appears to be very similar to omeprazole (Hochlaf et al. 1991; Metz et al. 1992). More experience with this drug, which is not yet available, will be required to compare it fully to omeprazole.

Control of Acid Hypersecretion in Special Circumstances

Patients with ZES who have had a previous Billroth 1 or 2 gastrectomy (usually for presumed idiopathic peptic ulcer disease) require particular care in the control of acid secretion. These patients, unlike those with an intact stomach, can develop complications of their ulcer disease when acid outputs are below 10 mEq/h. In these patients drug dosage should be increased until acid output is below 5 mEq/h and then the appearance of the mucosa should be checked by endoscopy (Maton et al. 1988). The dose should be increased until the upper intestinal mucosa is normal. Most of these patients will require omeprazole.

About 60% of patients with ZES not taking medication have esophagitis (Miller et al. 1990), and even when therapy reduces acid output to below 10 mEq/h, 20% will still have symptoms. Indeed, 5% of patients have recurrent dysphagia and stricture formation despite acid outputs beings below 10 mEq/h. When these patients are given sufficient omeprazole to reduce acid output to below 1 mEq/h (usually with omeprazole 60 mg every 12 h) symptoms resolve and the need for esophageal dilatation declines markedly (Miller et al. 1990).

Patients who require surgery, or patients who for whatever reason are unable to tolerate oral medication even for a few hours, require intravenous antisecretory medication. Intravenous ranitidine or another H_2-antagonist can be given as outlined under "Emergency control of acid secretion." Care must be taken in the postoperative period to re-check acid outputs, as 50% of patients will require an increase in dose in the first few days after surgery (Saeed et al. 1989; Fraker et al. 1988). In the future intravenous omeprazole, probably at a dosage of 60 mg every 12 h, may well become the drug of choice, as it is highly effective and does not seem to require dosage adjustment in the postoperative period (Vinayek et al. 1990).

Most patients with ZES and MEN-1 develop hyperparathyroidism and hypercalcemia at some stage. In these patients acid outputs and drug requirements increase if the hypercalcemia increases (Norton et al. 1987). Therefore, these patients need regular monitoring of their plasma calcium and adjustment of their antisecretory drug dose if measurement of acid output shows that to be necessary. In addition, in such patients, a parathyroidectomy may be indicated (Norton et al. 1987) (see below).

Patients who are cured of ZES as judged by a normal fasting plasma gastrin concentration and a negative secretin test, may still have abnormally high acid outputs for months after surgery (Fraker et al. 1988; Pisegna et al. 1992). Such patients should be considered for antisecretory medication, although the doses required are usually small.

Control of Acid Hypersecretion by Surgery

Because acid output can be controlled in all patients by medical means, and because total gastrectomy carries a significant mortality (Fox et al. 1974; Thompson et al. 1983) and morbidity, including cholelithiasis (Cattey and Wilson 1989). Total gastrectomy should be reserved for the rare patient who is unable to tolerate oral medication. A partial gastrectomy is never indicated as it does not prevent further peptic ulceration, and may even render the stomach more sensitive to the effects of acid (Maton et al. 1988).

A parietal cell vagotomy reduces acid output and drug requirements in patients with ZES (Richardson et al. 1985), but the patients still require antisecretory medication. In patients with ZES as part of MEN-1 who have hyperparathyroidism, a parathyroidectomy which renders the patient normocalcemic will reduce acid output and drug requirements (Norton et al. 1987), and occasionally results in normal plasma gastrins and acid output.

Control of the Gastrinoma

General Approach

The management of the tumor in patients with ZES has undergone changes in the last few years because of increasing knowledge of the pathology of gastrinomas. Gastrinomas were thought to be islet cell tumors (although gastrin-containing cells are not present in the adult human pancreas), and therefore thought to be all pancreatic in origin. However, it has become clear that these tumors arise in a number of different areas, which has implications for therapy. The behavior of gastrinomas vary considerably. About 30% of patients have hepatic metastases at presentation, 30% have identifiable localized tumor, and about 30% have no evident tumor (probably small intraduodenal tumors, see below). In fact, patients with short histories usually have metastatic tumor and those with long histories have no identifiable tumor (Howard and Passaro 1989; P.N. Maton, unpublished observations), suggesting that tumors differ in their aggressiveness from their inception, rather than progressing through a benign stage to a frankly malignant one.

Sporadic ZES

Pathology

Patients with sporadic ZES were initially thought to have a single pancreatic tumor but unlike insulinomas, which occur principally in the pancreatic body and tail, gastrinomas tend to occur in the pancreatic head region (Wolfe and Jensen 1987; Vinayek et al. 1990). Nevertheless, even early studies suggested that not all gastrinomas were pancreatic. Reports describe patients with tumors that were in the duodenum, lymph nodes, liver, and other sites. Indeed, this distribution of primary tumors was described as the "gastrinoma triangle," an area bordered by the hilum of the liver, the second part of the duodenum, and the pancreatic head (Howard and Passaro 1989). More recent studies both of the results of exploratory laparotomy (Norton et al. 1992, Thompson 1989) and of pathology specimens (Dunow et al. 1991) have provided further evidence for the existence of primary extrapancreatic gastrinomas. Indeed, recent operative series suggest that in sporadic ZES approximately 40% of primary tumors are duodenal, 40% pancreatic, and 10%–20% arise in lymph nodes (Norton et al. 1992; Thom et al. 1991; Dunow et al. 1991). Wherever these tumors arise they usually metastasize first to local lymph nodes, then to liver, and subsequently throughout the body.

Preoperative Imaging

Preoperative imaging is helpful in two ways; to demonstrate which patients have metastatic disease, and to identify the site of the primary tumor. The sensitivity and specificity of various imaging modalities for identifying hepatic metastases have been determined in careful prospective studies. Of ultrasound, magnetic resonance imaging (MRI), computed tomographic (CT) scan, and angiography, CT scan with intravenous contrast provides the best single screening test, but detects only about 80% of metastases. Angiography is more sensitive but more technically demanding and difficult for the patient. However, the combination of CT scan plus angiography detects virtually all hepatic metastases. Therefore, every patient should undergo selective angiography to identify small hepatic metastases missed by CT, and thus avoid an unnecessary laparotomy.

With respect to the primary tumor, imaging methods have been less successful. Ultrasound and MRI are less useful than CT scan, but even CT scan detects only 60% of those tumors found subsequently by the surgeon (Wank et al. 1987, who in these studies found tumors in about 70% of patients). Angiography is little better, the combination of CT and angiography identifying only about 60% of primary tumors (Maton et al. 1987). Venous sampling of portal vein radicals for gastrin (Cherner et al. 1986; Miller et al. 1992), or measurement of gastrin after intra-arterial secretin (Imamura et al. 1989; Doppman et al. 1990) have not proved generally beneficial, although when a gastrin gradient is identified, only the general region of the gastrinoma, not its specific location, can be identified.

Intraoperative Imaging

Intraoperative techniques undertaken by surgeons experienced in operating on patients with ZES have led to major improvements in identifying primary gastrinomas. Intraoperative ultrasonography has proved helpful in identifying pancreatic tumors (Norton et al. 1988), and transillumination of the duodenum using an endoscope has led to the identification of many small duodenal tumors missed by preoperative imaging, intraoperative ultrasonography and palpation (Frucht et al. 1989). In addition, it may be that a duodenotomy may lead to detection of yet further duodenal tumors, though probably with an increase in operative morbidity (Norton and Jensen 1991).

Results of Surgery for Localized Tumors

The increasing knowledge of pathology has modified surgery for ZES. Initially exploration of the pancreas was performed, and if no tumor was found, a blind resection of the body and tail was performed. Although this approach was fairly successful for insulinomas it was not effective for gastrinomas because of their distribution in the region of the pancreatic head. Subsequent careful prospective studies of preoperative imaging (Wank et al. 1987; Frucht et al. 1989; London et al. 1989; Maton et al. 1987; Cherner et al. 1986; Miller et al. 1992) and exploratory led to an approach of detailed pre-operative imaging followed by a detailed exploratory laparatomy with Kocherization of the duodenum, and intraoperative ultrasonography of the pancreas (Norton et al. 1986; Norton et al. 1988). Even with this approach tumors were found in only about 60% of patients. With the realization that tumors can arise in the submucosa of the proximal duodenum, intraoperative endoscopic transillumination and duodenectomy were added to the surgical approach as a means of identifying resectable tumors. These approaches have changed the perception and potential curability of these tumors. Whereas early series cured only 5% of patients (Wolfe and Jensen 1987). Recent studies indicate that tumors can be found in 90% and cure achieved in around 50% (Norton et al. 1992). Currently therefore the recommendation is that every patient with sporadic ZES undergo detailed preoperative imaging, and then have an exploratory laparotomy by a surgeon with extensive experience with the disease and who can perform intraoperative ultrasound, trans-illumination of the duodenum and a duodenotomy.

Follow-Up After Cure

If all visible tumor is removed after surgery, it is safest to continue the patient on an antisecretory drug regimen and reassess 3 months later when acid outputs may have declined. A patient who has normal gastrin levels, a negative secretin test, and no visible tumor on imaging tests can be considered cured. Such patients should still be seen annually and fasting plasma gastrin measurements, secretin tests, and acid measurements performed. As mentioned above, many of these patients remain mild gastric acid secretors and need small doses of medication (Pisegna et al. 1991). Furthermore, of those patients who are cured at a 6-month postoperative assessment, about 50% will have a recurrence by 5 years (Norton et al. 1992)

Long-term follow-up studies suggest that most patients, even if they are not cured, will live for many years with gastrinoma unless the tumor has metastasized to the liver (Norton et al. 1992; Howard and Passaro 1989; Malagelada 1983). Some authors have argued, therefore, that little is achieved by operating on these patients, but the balance are generally in favor of surgery (Norton and Jensen 1991).

Metastatic Tumor

Although gastrinoma metastatic to local lymph nodes should be treated surgically, no firm recommendations can be made currently as to the management of hepatic metastases. In a few carefully selected patients in whom the distribution of metastases is favorable, extensive surgery with resection of metastases may prolong life (Norton et al. 1986), and occasionally resection of a single hepatic tumor that might be thought of as metastatic and thus incurable has led to complete cure (Goletti et al. 1992). In the majority of patients who are not surgical candidates, other therapeutic options are not very efficacious. Furthermore, patients with extensive gastrinoma in liver and elsewhere are often asymptomatic if acid output is under satisfactory control. Therefore the potential benefit of any anti-tumor therapy needs to be balanced against side effects. There are no data to suggest that hepatic arterial embolization prolongs life (Carasco et al. 1983), possibly because bone metastases are not affected (Barton et al. 1986). Chemotherapy (typically with streptozotocin, 5 fluorouracil, and doxorubicin) may lead to a reduction in quality of life with little or no prolongation of life (Moertel et al. 1980; von Schrenck et al. 1988). Trials of the long-acting somatostatin analogue octreotide do not seem to have led to an overall increase in survival (Maton 1989; Trautman et al. 1990), while interferon has significant toxicity and has produced no clearcut benefit (Erickson et al. 1986; Slimak et al. 1991). At present, management of patients with metastatic disease should be tailored to the patient, though with the knowledge that none of the available approaches is very efficacious.

ZES as Part of MEN-1

Pathology

The gastrinomas in patients with MEN-1 differ from those in patients with sporadic ZES and from other pancreatic tumors in patients with MEN-1. Most islet cell tumors in patients with MEN-1 that give rise to clinical syndromes (i.e., insulinoma, VIPoma, glucagonoma, growth-hormone-releasing-hormone-producing tumors) are curable by resection of a single tumor, even though there may be many other tiny tumors in the pancreas (Sheppard et al. 1989). That is not true of patients with ZES. Such patients have undergone 90% pancreatic resections with unchanged serum gastrins. It has recently become clear that there are not only multiple gastrin-producing tumors throughout the pancreas, but also multiple small submucosal duodenal gastrinomas (Dunow et al. 1991; Thomson et al. 1983; Thompson et al. 1984). Thus, these patients are generally regarded as not being curable by any procedure other than a total pancreatectomy and duodenectomy. Clearly this has influenced the approach to these patients.

Imaging and the Role of Surgery

Imaging studies are important for the identification of those patients with metastases. However, identification of localized tumors in ZES as part of MEN-I has not been as useful as in sporadic ZES, as even in those patients in whom tumors are imaged or who have positive venous gastrin gradients, resection of localized tumors does not cure the patient, for reasons mentioned above [although occasional exceptions have been observed (Cherner and Sawers 1992)]. Because the only operation likely to lead to cure (total pancreatic and duodenal resection) has an unacceptable morbidity for a relatively nonaggressive tumor, the role of surgery in these patients remains uncertain. At some centers, patients are not operated on (Malagelada et al. 1983), in others patients with large (> 1.5 cm) primary tumors in the pancreas undergo resection of the tumor with removal of the pancreatic body and tail, not to produce a cure, but in an attempt to prevent metastases (Norton et al. 1986), whilst in others surgery is undertaken only if there is a gastrin gradient indicating a localized source of gastrin (Thomson et al. 1983, 1989), or if there is a gradient of pancreatic polypeptide (Freisen et al. 1983). The efficacy of these approaches has not been established, and thus the risk-benefit ratio cannot be estimated.

Metastatic Gastrinoma

In general the gastrinomas in patients with ZES and MEN-1 have been regarded as being less malignant than those in sporadic ZES. However, this may be simply a reflection of selection of patients. Certainly, some patients with MEN-1 and ZES develop metastatic gastrinoma which may kill them. Metastatic gastrinoma in ZES associated with MEN-1 and in sporadic ZES is treated identically.

References

1. Barton, JC, Hirschowitz BI, Maton PN, Jensen RT (1986) Bone metastases in malignant gastrinoma. Gastroenterology 91:915–925
2. Carrasco CH, Chuang VP, Wallace S (1983) Apudoma metastatic to the liver: treatment by hepatic artery embolization. Radiology 149:79–83
3. Cattey R, Wilson S (1989) Cholelithiasis follows total gastrectomy in Zollinger-Ellison syndrome. Surgery 106:1070–1073
4. Cherner JA, Doppman JL, Norton JA, et al. (1986) Prospective assessment of selective venous sampling for gastrin to localize gastrinomas. Ann Intern Med 105:841–847
5. Cherner J, Sawyers JL (1992) Benefit of resection of metastatic gastrinoma in multiple endocrine neoplasia type I. Gastroenterology 102:1049–1053
6. Clissold SP, Campoli-Richards DM (1986) Omeprazole. Drugs 32:15–47
7. Collen MJ, Howard JM, McArthur KE, et al. (1984) Comparison of ranitidine and cimetidine in the treatment of gastric hypersecretion. Ann Intern Med 100:52–58
8. Delchier JC, Soule JC, Mignon M, et al. (1986) Effectiveness of omeprazole in seven patients with Zollinger-Ellison syndrome resistant to histamine H_2-receptor antagonists. Dig Dis Sci 31:693–699

9. Donow C, Pipeleers-Marichal M, Schoder S, Stamm B, Heitz P, Kloppel G (1991) Surgical pathology of gastrinoma: site, size, multicentricity, association with multiple endocrine neoplasia type 1, and malignancy. Cancer 68:1329–1334
10. Doppman JI, Miller DL, Chang R, Maton PN, London JF, Gardner JD, Jensen RT, Norton JD. (1990) Gastrinoma: localization by means of selective intraarterial injection of secretin. Radiology 174:25–29
11. Eberle F, Grun R (1981) Multiple endocrine neoplasia, type I (MEN 1). Ergeb Inn Med Kinderheilkd 46:75–150
12. Ellison EH, Wilson SD (1964) The Zollinger-Ellison syndrome: reappraisal and evaluation of 260 registered cases. Ann Surg 160:512–53
13. Erickson B, Oberg K, Alm G, et al. (1986) Treatment of malignant endocrine pancreatic tumours with human leucocyte interferon. Lancet 2:1307–1308
14. Feldman M (1983) Gastric secretion. In: Sleisenger MH, Fordtran JS (eds). Gastrointestinal disease 3rd edn. Saunders, Philadelphia, pp 541–558
15. Fox PS, Hofman JW, Wilson SD, DeCosse JJ (1974) Surgical management of Zollinger-Ellison syndrome. Surg Clin North Am 54:395–407
16. Fraker D, Norton JA, Saeed ZA, Maton PN, Gardner JD, Jensen RT (1988) A prospective study of pre-and post operative control of acid hypersecretion in patients with Zollinger-Ellison syndrome. Surgery 104:1054–1063
17. Freisen SR, Tomita T, Kimmel MJR (1983) Pancreatic polypeptide update: its role in detection of trait for multiple endocrine adenopathy syndrome type 1 and pancreatic polypeptide-secreting tumors. Surgery 104:1028
18. Frucht H, Doppman JL, Norton JA, et al. (1989) MRI imaging of gastrinomas: comparison with computed tomography, angiography and ultrasound. Radiology 171:713–717
19. Frucht H, Howard JM, Slaff JI, McCarthy DM, Maton PN, Wank SA, Vinayek R, Gardner JD, Jensen RT (1989) Secretin and calcium provocative tests in Zollinger-Ellison syndrome: a prospective study. Ann Intern Med111:713–722
20. Frucht H, Maton PN, Jensen RT (1991) Use of omeprazole on patients with Zollinger-Ellison syndrome. Dig Dis Sci 36:394–404
21. Frucht H, Norton JA, London JF, Vinayek R, Doppman JL, Gardner JD, Jensen RT, Maton PN (1990) Detection of duodenal gastrinomas by operative endoscopic transillumination: a prospective study. Gastroenterology 99:1622–1627
22. Goletti O, Chiarugi M, Buccianti P, Tortora A, Castagna M, Guerra P, Viacava P, Cavina E (1992) Resection of liver gastrinoma leading to persistent eugastrinemia. Eur J Surg 158:55–57
23. Hochlaf S, Vatier J, Ruszniewski P, Poitevan MJM, Lewin M, Mignon M (1991) Is lansoprazole as effective as omeprazole in patients with Zollinger-Ellison syndrome (ZES). Gastroenterology 100; A84
24. Howard JM, Chremos AN, Collen MJ, et al. (1985) Famotidine, a new, potent, long-acting histamine H_2-receptor antagonist: comparison with cimetidine and ranitidine in the treatment of Zollinger-Ellison syndrome. Gastroenterology 88:1026–1033
25. Howard T, Passaro E (1989) Gastrinoma: New medical and surgical approaches. Surg Clin N Amer 69:3:667–681
26. Imamura M, Takahashi K, Isobe Y, Hattori Y, Satomura K, Tobe T (1989) Curative resection of multiple gastrinomas aided by selective arterial secretin injection test and intraoperative secretin test. Ann Surg 210:710–718
27. Jensen RT, Doppman JL, Gardner JD (1986) Gastrinoma. In: Go VLW et al. (eds) The exocrine pancreas: biology, pathobiology and diseases. New York, pp 727–745
28 Jensen RT, Gardner JD, Raufman JP, Pandol SJ, Doppman JL, Collen MJ (1983) Zollinger-Ellison syndrome: current concepts and management. Ann Intern Med 98:59–75
29. Lamers CBHW, Lind T, Moberg S, Jansen JBM, Olbe L (1984) Omeprazole in Zollinger-Ellison syndrome: effects of a single dose and a of long-term treatment in patients resistant to histamine H_2-receptor antagonists. N Engl J Med 310:758–776
30. Lehy T, Mignon M, Cadiot G et al. (1989) Gastric endocrine cell behavior in Zollinger-Ellison patients upon long term potent antisecretory treatment. Gastroenterology 96:1029–1040
31. Lloyd-Davies KA, Rutgersson K, Solvell L (1988) Omeprazole in Zollinger-Ellison syndrome: four year international study. Aliment Pharmacol Ther 2:13–37

32. London JF, Vinayek R, Frucht H, et al. (1989) Prospective assessment of abdominal ultrasound in patients with Zollinger-Ellison syndrome. Radiology 178:763–767
33. McArthur KE, Collen MJ, Maton PN, et al. (1985) Omeprazole: effective convenient therapy for Zollinger-Ellison syndrome. Gastroenterology 88:939–944
34. Malagelada JR, Edis AJ, Adson MA, von Heerden JA, Go VLW (1983) Medical and surgical options in the management of patients with gastrinoma. Gastroenterology 84:1524
35. Maton PN (1989) The use of the long-acting somatostatin analogue, octerotide in patients with islet cell tumors. Gastroenterol Clin North AM 18:897–922
36. Maton PN (1991) Omeprazole. N Engl J Med 324:965–975
37. Maton PN, Frucht H, Vinayek R, Wank SA, Gardner JD, Jensen RT (1988) Medical management of patients with Zollinger-Ellison syndrome who have had previous gastric surgery: a prospective study. Gastroenterology 94:294–299
38. Maton PN, Lack EE, Collen MJ, Cornelius MJ, David E, Gardner JD, Jensen RT (1990) The effect of Zollinger-Ellison syndrome and omeprazole therapy on gastric oxyntic endocrine cells. Gastroenterology 99:943–950
39. Maton PN, Miller DL, Doppman JL, et al. (1987) The role of selective angiography in the management of patients with Zollinger-Ellison syndrome. Gastroenterology 92:913–918
40. Maton PN, Vinayek R, Frucht H, et al. (1989) Long-term efficacy and safety of omeprazole in patients with Zollinger-Ellison syndrome: a prospective study. Gastroenterology 97:827–836
41. Metz DC, Pisegna JR, Ringham GL, Fishbeyn VA, Benya RV, Gardner JD, Jensen RT (1992) Efficacy and safety of lansoprazole in patients with Zollinger-Ellison syndrome (ZES). Gastroenterology 102:A125
42. Miller DL, Doppman JL, Metz DC, Maton PN, Norton JA, Jensen RT (1992) Zollinger-Ellison syndrome: technique, results, and complications of portal venous sampling. Radiology 182:235–241
43. Miller LS, Vinayek R, Frucht H, Gardner JD, Jensen RT, Maton PN (1990) Reflux esophagitis in Zollinger-Ellison syndrome. Gastroenterology: 341–346
44. Moertel CG, Hanley JA, Johnson LA (1980) Streptozotocin alone compared with streptozotocin plus fluorouracil in the treatment of advanced islet-cell carcinoma. N Engl J Med 303:1189–1192
45. Norton JA, Collen MJ, Gardner JD, et al (1986) Prospective study of gastrinoma localization and resection in patients with Zollinger-Ellison syndrome. Ann Surg 204:468–478
46. Norton JA, Cornelius MJ, Doppman JL, Maton PN, Gardner JD, Jensen RT (1987) Effect of parathyroidectomy in patients with hyperparathyroidism and Zollinger-Ellison syndrome and multiple endocrine neoplasia type I: a prospective study. Surgery 102:958–966
47. Norton JA, Cromack DT, Shawker TH, et al. (1988) Intraoperative ultrasonographic localization of islet cell tumors: a prospective comparison to palpation. Ann Surg 207:160–168
48. Norton J, Doppman J, Jensen R (1992) Curative resection in Zollinger-Ellison syndrome: results of a 10-year prospective study. Ann Surg 215: 8–18.
49. Norton J, Jensen R (1991) Unresolved surgical issues in the management of patients with Zollinger-Ellison syndrome. World J Surg 15:151–159
50. Norton JA, Sugarbaker PH, Doppman JL, et al. (1986) Aggressive resection of metastatic disease in selected patients with malignant gastrinoma. Ann Surg 203:352–359
51. Olbe L, Haglund U, Leth R, et al. (1982) Effects of substituted benzimidazole (H 149/94) on gastric acid secretion in humans. Gastroenterology 83:193–198
52. Pisegna J, Norton J, Slimak G, Metz D, Maton P, Gardner J, Jensen R (1992) Effects of curative gastrinoma resection on gastric secretory function and antisecretory drug requirement in the Zollinger-Ellison syndrome. Gastroenterology 102:767–778
53. Raufman JP, Collins SM, Pandol SJ, et al. (1983) Reliability of symptoms in assessing control of gastric acid secretion in patients with Zollinger-Ellison syndrome. Gastroenterology 84:108–113
54. Richardson CT, Peters MN, Feldman M, et al. (1985) Treatment of Zollinger-Ellison syndrome with exploratory laparotomy, proximal gastric vagotomy, and H_2-receptor antagonists: a prospective study. Gastroenterology 89:357–367
55. Saeed ZA, Norton JA, Frank WO, et al. (1989) Parenteral antisecretory drug therapy in patients with Zollinger-Ellison syndrome. Gastroenterology 96:1393–1402

56. Sheppard BC, Norton JA, Doppman JL, Maton PN, Gardner JD, Jensen RT (1989) Management of islet cell tumors in patients with multiple endocrine neoplasia: a prospective study. Surgery 106:1108–1118
57. Slimak GC, Pisegna J, Metz DC, Gardner JD, Jensen RT, Maton PN (1991) Use of alpha interferon in patients with metastatic gastrinoma. Gastroenterology 100:A299.
58. Solcia E, Capella C, Fiocca R, Rindi G, Rosai J (1990) Gastric argyrophil carcinoidosis in patients with Zollinger-Ellison syndrome due to type 1 multiple endocrine neoplasia. A newly recognised association. Am J Surg Path 14:503–513
59. Thom A, Norton J, Axiotis C, Jensen R (1991) Location, incidence, and malignant potential of duodenal gastrinomas. Surgery 110:1086–1093
60. Thompson JC, Lewis BG, Wiener I, Townsend CM, Jr (1983) The role of surgery in the Zollinger-Ellison syndrome. Ann Surg 197:594–607
61. Thompson NW, Bondeson AG, Bondeson L, Vinik A (1989) The surgical treatment of Zollinger-Ellison syndrome in patients with multiple endocrine neoplasia type 1. Surgery 106:1081
62. Thompson NW, Lloyd RU, NIshiyama RH, et al. (1984) MEN-I pancreas: a histological and immunohistochemical study. World J Surg 8:561–568
63. Thompson N, Vinik A, Eckhauser F (1989) Microgastrinomas of the duodenum. Ann Surg 209:396–404.
64. Trautmann ME, Neuhaus C, Bruns C, Hugens-Penzel M, Schwerk WV, Koop H, Arnold R (1990) Secondary failure of growth inhibition by SMS 201–995 if accompanied by increased hormone levels without loss of SMS receptors. Digestion 46 (Suppl 1):115–116
65. Vinayek R. Frucht H, Chiang H-CV, Maton PN, Gardner JD, Jensen RT (1990) Zollinger-Ellison syndrome: recent advances in the management of the gastrinoma. Gastroenterol Clin North Am 19:197–218
66. Vinayek R, Howard JM, Maton PN, et al. (1983) Famotidine in the therapy of gastric hypersecretory states. Am J Med 81 (suppl 4B):49–59
67. Vinayek R, Frucht H, London JF, Miller LS, Stark HA, Norton JA, Cedeberg C, Jensen RT, Gardner JD, Maton PN (1990) The use of intravenous omeprazole in patients with Zollinger-Ellison syndrome undergoing surgery. Gastroenterology 99:10–16
68. von Schrenck T, Howard JM, Doppman JL, et al. (1988) Prospective study of chemotherapy in patients with metastatic gastrinoma. Gastroenterology 94:1326–1334
69. Wank SA, Doppman JL, Miller DL, et al. (1987) Prospective study of the ability of computerized axial tomography to localize gastrinomas in patients with Zollinger-Ellison syndrome. Gastroenterology 92:905–912
70. Wolfe MM, Jensen RT (1987) Zollinger-Ellison syndrome. N Engl J Med 317:1200–1209

Medical Treatment of Acute Peptic Ulceration

W. Domschke

Introduction

The natural history of peptic ulcers of the stomach and duodenum is one of repeated recurrence. Accordingly, management should aim not only at treating the episodes of active ulceration, but at preventing the next recurrence. From time to time, with innovations in treatment, the borders between indications for conservative or operative treatment may shift. While in earlier days about every fifth patient with a gastric ulcer and every third patient with a duodenal ulcer had to undergo surgery at some point during the course of the illness, the introduction of histamine H_2-receptor antagonists seems to have altered the natural history of ulcers to the extent that the overall number of ulcer operations carried out in recent years has gone down. This drop has been mainly in elective operations; the incidence of emergency ulcer operations has remained more or less constant. Of course, it remains to be seen whether this state of affairs is permanent.

Close interdisciplinary cooperation between physician and surgeon is essential for correct decisions in the management of both normal and complicated peptic ulcers. In some cases a psychosomatic approach may also be necessary.

The place for conservative treatment of ulcers is in the area between spontaneous ulcer healing and the absolute indication for surgery on the grounds of perforation, penetration or conservatively uncontrollable haemorrhage. The decision for medical treatment of a peptic ulcer must be based on:

1. The proven efficacy of the drug in question compared to placebo (in Germany, Switzerland and the United States the rate of spontaneous healing is over 50%, whereas in England it is only about 20%–30%)
2. Knowledge and a weighing up of the risks and costs of treatment

Medical treatment of the active ulceration episode has two basic goals:

1. Relieving the patient of pain
2. Accelerating healing of the ulcer and preventing complications

How well the drug is tolerated, how it is administered and, of course, what it costs must also be taken into consideration.

Therapy

General Treatment Principles

Uncomplicated ulcers can be treated on an outpatient basis. This avoids the high costs of a hospital stay, in addition to which the patient can remain in his or her familiar environment at home and at work. Patients with complications – penetrating, perforating or bleeding ulcers, stenosis, excessive pain or particular difficulties at home – should of course be hospitalized.

Special diets no longer play any major part in ulcer management. Nevertheless, discussion of this subject is felt to be part of the physician's general contribution. Patients with ulcers should eat little and often and avoid too much spiciness, too much fried food, and food that is very hot or very cold. (Real) coffee, sweets and citrus fruits are usually poorly tolerated. The basic rule is that patients can eat what they like as long as it agrees with them.

Moderate alcohol consumption (less than 20 ml ethanol per day, and no strong spirits) can be allowed; it may even promote healing of the ulcer.

Smoking has been statistically proven to delay healing and promote relapse, and should definitely be stopped.

If possible, potentially ulcerogenic drugs (e.g. antirheumatic drugs, non-steroidal anti-phlogistics) should be stopped. If maintenance of anti-rheumatic treatment is necessary, the patient should be transferred onto corticosteroid treatment.

Principles of Medical Treatment

Conservative treatment of peptic ulcers is governed by two principles: reduction of factors that attack the mucosa, and reinforcement of those that protect it. Table 1 lists the mechanisms of effect of preparations that follow these two therapeutic lines. Effective medical treatment of active ulceration can be equally well done with acid- and pepsin-inhibiting "anti-aggressive" drugs (H_2-blockers, antacids, pirenzepine, benzimidazoles) or with "cytoprotective" drugs (sucralfate, colloidal bismuth, prostaglandin analogues). However, there are differences in the incidence and severity of side effects, convenience of administration, and cost. Not least importantly, the speed of healing varies from regime to regime (Fig. 1).

Commonly Used Ulcer Drugs

This section will discuss individually the most important drugs for the treatment of ulcers.

Table 1. Principles of medical treatment of peptic ulcers

I. *Inhibition of aggressive factors*

1. Inhibition of acid and pepsin

   Neutralization of acid by:
      nutritional buffers or antacids in the stomach
      pancreatic bicarbonate in the duodenum

   Inhibition of acid and pepsinogen secretion by:
      anticholinergics, H_2-receptor antagonists, prostaglandins, somatostatin, secretin, blockers of the parietal cell H^+/K^+ – ATPase (benzimidazoles), psychiatric drugs (trimipramine, tritiozine), gastrin receptor antagonists (proglumide)?

   Inhibition of peptic activity by:
      inhibition of the conversion of pepsinogen to pepsin
         antacids (pH effect), carbenoxolone
      adsorption of pepsin
         aluminium hydroxide-containing antacids, carbenoxolone, colloidal bismuth
      inhibition of the pepsin-substrate interaction
         sulphated disaccharides (sucralfate)
      alteration of the gastric pH
         acid inhibitors, antacids
   Elimination of acid and pepsin by accelerated emptying of the stomach
      motility regulators: metoclopramide, bromopride, domperidone, sulpiride, cisapride

2. Elimination of potentially cytotoxic elements of the duodenal fluid (bile acids, lysolecithin)

   Adsorption by:
      aluminium hydroxide-containing antacids, cholestyramine, sulphated disaccharides (sucralfate)

   Accelerated emptying of the stomach by:
      motility regulators (see above)

3. Elimination of *H. pylori* by:
   colloidal bismuth, acid suppression, antibiotics?

II. *Reinforcement of protective factors*

1. Normalization of the gastric epithelial layer (strengthening of the gastric mucosal barrier) by:
   carbenoxolone

2. Stimulation of gastric mucus and alkaline secretions (strengthening of the gastric mucous barrier) by:
   carbenoxolone, prostaglandins

3. Increasing the gastric mucosal blood flow by:
   prostaglandins, secretin

4. Formation of a film on the gastric mucosa and stimulation of endogenous prostaglandin synthesis by:

   colloidal bismuth, sulphated disaccharides (sucralfate), sulphated polysaccharides (amylopectin sulphate)?

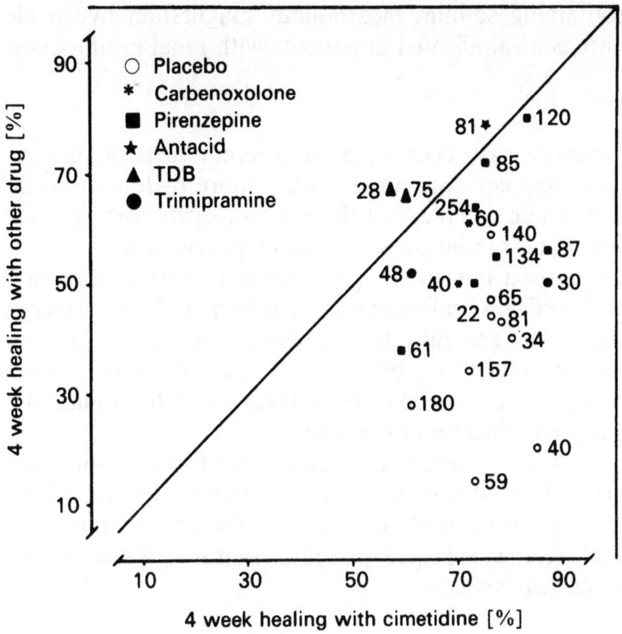

Fig. 1. Comparison of 4-week healing rates of duodenal ulcers treated with cimetidine (*x*-axis) and other drugs (*y*-axis). Data from double-blind studies. The figures by each symbol refer to the number of patients studied. From [1]

Antacids [2–5]

The following chemical compounds are commonly used as antacids: aluminium magnesium hydroxide, aluminium magnesium silicate hydrate, aluminium magnesium hydroxide plus calcium carbonate, etc.

Ulcer patients take antacids alone or in combination with other drugs to alleviate the pain caused by the ulcer. Moreover, gastric and duodenal ulcers heal more quickly with antacid treatment than when placebo is given. However, the mode of administration (doses taken 4–7 times a day) is inconvenient and does not easily fit into every kind of working day.

In cases of gastric ulcer, a dosage of 100–200 mmol neutralization capacity per day is enough to achieve healing; for duodenal ulcers, 200–300 mmol is required. Doses are taken 1 h after main meals and before retiring, and if necessary additionally 3 h after main meals.

Interactions with other drugs are in the main caused by the adsorptive capacity of the antacids and may hinder or even entirely prevent intestinal absorption of concurrent medication. This applies, for instance, to corticosteroids, digitalis preparations and antibiotics. Antacids should therefore be taken at a different time from other medicines.

Antacids containing aluminium may cause constipation and those containing magnesium diarrhoea. For this reason, most drugs combine both these substances. Antacids containing sodium bicarbonate, magnesium hydroxide and calcium carbonate are contraindicated in patients with renal insufficiency.

Anticholinergics [6–8]

The traditional anticholinergics have been replaced in recent years by pirenzepine and its successor, telenzepine – substances with a more or less stomach-specific effect via the muscarinic receptors of the mucosa of the gastric body (antimuscarinic substances) and inhibit the secretion of gastric acid.

According to studies carried out so far, pirenzepine (2×50 mg/day) and telenzepine (3 mg at night) speed up healing of both duodenal and gastric ulcers, although for gastric ulcers they generally have to be taken for 12 weeks to achieve a comparable healing rate to H_2-blockers. In cases of poorly healing peptic ulcers antimuscarinics can be added to a regimen of histamine H_2-receptor antagonists as an intensification of treatment.

At dosages above 100 mg/day, pirenzepine usually leads to the familiar side effects of anticholinergics: visual disturbances, photophobia, dryness of the mouth, and disturbances of micturition. Antimuscarinic therapy is contraindicated in patients with glaucoma, enlarged prostate, stenosis of the pyloric sphincter or gastro-oesophageal reflux.

Histamine H_2-Receptor Antagonists [9–17]

H_2-Antagonists (cimetidine, ranitidine, famotidine, nizatidine, roxatidine) are the most commonly used drugs for ulcer treatment all over the world, and are those against which all other future ulcer drugs will be measured. Numerous studies have proved beyond doubt the therapeutic efficacy of H_2-blockers for duodenal and gastric ulcers, both in relation to the active ulceration episodes and to prevention or recurrence.

During active ulceration episodes, 800 mg cimetidine, 300 mg ranitidine, 40 famotidine, 300 mg nizatidine, or 150 mg roxatidine should be taken with the evening meal. In the treatment of an acute duodenal ulcer, 300 mg ranitidine/day for 4 weeks is still regarded as the gold standard.

Although anti-androgenous effects and inhibition of the phase I metabolism of other drugs have been described in association with cimetidine, these side effects largely disappeared in the later generations of H_2-blockers. Confusional states may occasionally arise. Of course, less clinical experience has been accumulated with the newest preparations (nizatidine, roxatidine) than with the older ones.

H^+/K^+-ATPase Inhibitors: Proton Pump Inhibitors [18–26]

Substituted benzimidazole compounds of the omeprazole type can inhibit gastric secretions even better than histamine H_2-receptor antagonists, by inhibiting the K^+-dependent ATPase located in the parietal cell membrane, which has a crucial influence on acid secretion.

Omeprazole given in a single dose of 40 mg inhibits gastric acid for over 24 h and produces an alkaline environment. Pathophysiologically, however, there is no reason why such a massively acid-suppressive effect should be required in normal peptic ulcers, and it may even be harmful. We ourselves therefore reserve omeprazole treatment for ulcers that are refractory to H_2-blockers, for Zollinger-Ellison syndrome, and the severer forms of oesophageal reflux.

At a dosage of 20 mg/day omeprazole heals gastric and duodenal ulcers as fast as H_2-blockers. At higher dosages (e.g. 40 mg/day) omeprazole succeeds faster than the H_2-antagonists.

As a result of the drastically reduced gastric secretion caused by omeprazole, serum gastrin concentrations rise to two or three times the norm – an increase comparable to that seen after proximal selective vagotomy. This moderate hypergastrinaemia is probably harmless in humans, even if it continues long term. Nevertheless, since enterochromaffin-like cell hyperplasia and carcinoid tumours have been observed in rats receiving long-term treatment with higher than therapeutic doses of omeprazole, the use of omeprazole for long-term therapy of ulcer patients is still regarded with understandable caution. Consequently, treatment of peptic ulcers with omeprazole is restricted to 8 weeks at the most (except in patients with Zollinger-Ellison syndrome).

Recently a new benzimidazole derivative, lansoprazole, has become available. In the first studies [28, 29] this proton pump blocker, given to patients with duodenal ulcers at a dosage of 30 mg/day, brought about healing within 4 weeks, which corresponds to the healing rates with ranitidine or famotidine.

Prostaglandin Analogues [30–35]

So far, prostaglandin analogues have failed to become established in the treatment of ulcers, because of their considerable side effects at therapeutic doses (e.g. misoprostol 2×400 μg/day or 4×200 μg/day), even though various studies have shown that they achieve healing rates comparable to H_2-blockers in gastric and duodenal ulcers. The same applies to the other prostaglandin derivatives – enprostil, arbaprostil, trimoprostil and rioprostil. All these drugs have to be taken twice or four times a day, which naturally has a negative effect on patient compliance. Possible side effects of prostaglandin analogues include diarrhoea, abdominal cramps and uterine contractions, for which reason these drugs are contraindicated in women of child-bearing age because of the danger of a miscarriage.

On the other hand, one indication for the use of prostaglandin derivatives — at lower than therapeutic dosages – seems to be prophylaxis of gastric lesions caused by non-steroidal anti-inflammatory drugs. At any rate, preventive effects have been described in patients predisposed to such lesions when treated prophylactically with, e.g., 2×200 μg/day misoprostol [36].

Sulphated Disaccharides [37–39]

Sucralfate, an aluminium salt of saccharose sulphate, has been shown in several studies of the treatment of gastric and duodenal ulcers to have a positive effect, better than placebo, and has in some cases even proved comparable to H_2-blockers in regard to healing rate. Sucralfate has to be given for 12 weeks for the H_2-blocker-type therapeutic effects to appear, however.

During active ulceration episodes, sucralfate is given at a dosage of 4×1 g/day or 2×2 g/day. The four times daily regimen in particular is experienced by patients as disruptive at work and is therefore not always regularly observed.

Since sucralfate is hardly absorbed at all intestinally, no systemic side effects are to be anticipated. Care should be taken with patients with renal insufficiency, however, in whom even the smallest amounts of absorbed aluminium can accumulate over time.

Occasional reports of constipation are ascribed to the aluminium content of sucralfate.

Sucralfate appears to be particularly effective in the prophylaxis of gastroduodenal stress lesions in high-risk patients [40–42]. Various studies have shown equality between sucralfate and H_2-blockers in this respect. Especially in patients maintained on long-term ventilation, who are at risk of pneumonia, it can be argued that treatment with sucralfate should be preferred.

Colloidal Bismuth [43–45]

The following bismuth compounds are in use: bismuth dicitrate, bismuth subsalicylate, bismuth subgallate, bismuth subnitrate and bismuth subcarbonate. The healing rates in both gastric and duodenal ulcers are the same as with H_2-blockers. In addition, the natural course of an ulcer in a patient who has been treated with bismuth appears to show a reduced incidence of recurrences. This prophylactic effect against recurrences appears only to hold for the first year after successful acute-episode treatment, after which the recurrence patterns become comparable to those associated with other methods of ulcer therapy. It is under discussion whether this prophylactic effect of bismuth preparations is related to the fact that bismuth is intestinally absorbed in small quantities, stored, and then, like a slow-release drug preparation, gradually released again over a period of months [46].

Bismuth preparations are taken half an hour before each of three main meals and before going to bed. Alternatively, the regime can be concentrated into double the dose taken twice daily.

Of the possible side effects, black coloration of the tongue, gums and dental prostheses can have cosmetic significance. The black coloration of the faeces of course makes melaena difficult to recognize.

Since bismuth is partially absorbed intestinally and then eliminated according to renal function [47], bismuth preparations are contraindicated in patients with severe renal insufficiency. Different bismuth preparations appear to have different pharmacokinetics: bismuth subcarbonate is intestinally absorbed only to a very small extent, whereas the rate of absorption of bismuth dicitrate is about ten times higher [48]. Overall, however, the plasma concentrations reached with normal therapeutic dosages of bismuth are low enough to make the occurrence of bismuth encephalopathy very unlikely.

Bismuth preparations have often been mentioned and used in connection with the eradication of *H. pylori*, which some authors have implicated in the pathogenesis of peptic ulcers. In the hope of more effective recurrence prophylaxis, several suggestions have been made to attempt elimination of the bacteria in a *H. pylori*-positive ulcer even during the acute treatment phase [49–53]. To this end, bismuth preparations have been given in combination with antibiotics – e.g. amoxicillin, tetracyclines, metronidazole. The efficacy of these extremely complicated therapy schemes has yet to be studied in double-blind trials, however, before they can be recommended for use on the large scale.

Active Ulceration Episodes: Individualized Recommendations

In a recently reported study [54] it was shown that the patient's compliance with drug therapy in an episode of active ulceration depends in the first instance on the simplicity/complexity of the drug regimen, i.e. medication that has to be taken once a day will be more reliably taken correctly than one that has to be taken four times a day.

On the question of how far the gastric secretion of acid has to be reduced for a duodenal ulcer to heal, a comprehensive review [55] of clinical studies has shown that ulcer healing increased with duration of acid suppression and with rising gastric pH. Raising the pH above 3.0 gained no additional effect, however.

The recommendations below take these two points into account.

1. *"Normal" peptic ulcers* (gastric or duodenal) should be treated with an H_2-blocker, the last daily dose to be taken with the last meal of the day. Generally, treatment of duodenal ulcers should continue for 4 weeks and treatment of gastric ulcers for 8 weeks. In the case of gastric ulcers, the lesion should be checked for healing and non-malignancy by endoscopy and biopsy.
2. *Ulcers refractory to treatment by H_2-blockers* should be managed according to the scheme in Fig. 2. As a rule, 95% of peptic ulcers heal within 2 months when treated with H_2-blockers. In about 5% of patients, conventional therapy fails to achieve remission. The first step with these patients is to check by suitable means (radio-immunological determination of plasma gastrin concentration before and after secretin stimulation) that they are not suffering from Zollinger-Ellison syndrome. If there is no sign of this syndrome, procedure should follow this sequence:

- Double the usual daily dose of the H_2-blocker given initially [56, 57].
- Change to combination therapy with H_2-blockers and an anti-muscarinic or antacid.
- Change to a cytoprotective drug such as colloidal bismuth [52, 58, 59], sucralfate or a prostaglandin analogue.
- Change (the therapeutic last resort) to a proton pump inhibitor. Controlled studies have shown that for this purpose omeprazole must be given at a dosage of 40 mg/day, as at a dosage of 20 mg/day its effects were not superior to those of continued H_2-blocker treatment [60, 61].

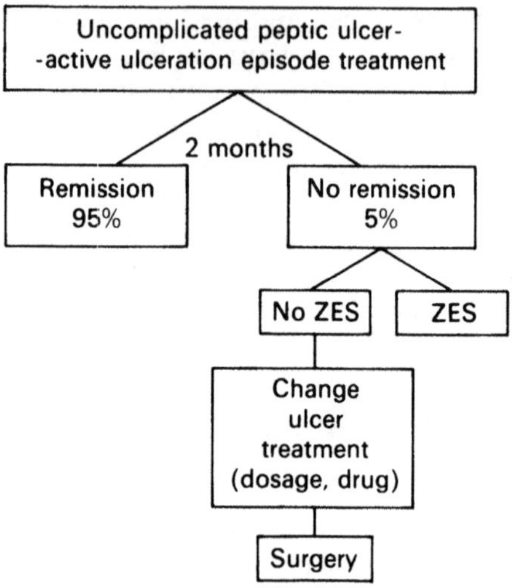

Fig. 2. Management procedure for peptic ulcers that have failed to heal after 2 months' conventional therapy (refractory ulcers). *ZES*, Zollinger-Ellison syndrome

Whether elimination of *H. pylori* has a positive effect in the treatment of refractory peptic ulcers is still a matter of debate. That giving up smoking contributes to healing, on the other hand, is beyond any doubt.

If even these intensive therapeutic regimens fail to produce healing within about 12 weeks, the patients should be operated on. Because of the inherent risk of malignity, the indication for surgery of a gastric ulcer should be taken as broader than for a duodenal ulcer.

3. *Anastomotic ulcers* should be treated right from the start with double the normal daily dose of H_2-blocker or with 40 mg/day omeprazole.
4. Treatment of *ulcers in Zollinger-Ellison syndrome* is covered in detail elsewhere in this book.

References

1. Bauerfeind P, Popien J, Traber M et al. (1986) Clinical perspectives of drugs inhibiting acid secretion: histamine H_2 antagonists. Scand J Gastroenterol 21 (suppl 125):42–48
2. Bianchi Porro G, Parente F, Lazzaroni M et al. (1986) Medium-dose antacids versus cimetidine in the short-term treatment of duodenal ulcer. J Clin Gastroenterol 8:141–145
3. Lux G, Hentschel H, Rohner HG et al. (1986) Treatment of duodenal ulcer with low-dose antacids. Scand J Gastroenterol 21:1064–1068
4. Becker U, Linkorff K, Andersen C, Ranlov PJ (1987) Antacid treatment of duodenal ulcer. Acta Med Scand 221:95–101
5. Pace F, Bianchi Porro G, Bode Ch, Bröker HJ, Caspary W, Domschke W, Blum AL (1989) Presenting characteristics of benign gastric ulcer and outcome of medical treatment. Eur J Gastroent Hepatol 1:175–185
6. Jaup BH, Cronstedt J, Dotevall G et al. (1985) Pirenzepine versus cimetidine in duodenal ulcer treatment. Scand J Gastroenterol 20:183–188
7. Hüttemann W, Schneider A (1989) Dose finding study of telenzepine in acute treatment of

duodenal ulcer. A double-blind, randomized, multicentre parallel group comparison. Med Klin 84:574–577

8. Simon B, Reinicke HG, Dammann HG, Müller P (1990) 3 mg telenzepine nocte in the treatment of benign stomach ulcer disease: a double-blind comparative study with 300 mg ranitidine nocte. Z Gastroenterol 28:90–93
9. Di Mario F, Battaglia G, Naccarato R et al. (1990) Comparison of 150 mg nizatidine bid or 300 mg at bedtime, and 150 mg ranitidine bid in the treatment of gastric ulcer – an 8-week randomized, double-blind multicentre study. Hepato-Gastroenterol 37 (Suppl II): 62–65
10. Merki HS, Halter F, Wilder Smith C et al. (1990) Effect of food on H_2-receptor blockade in normal subjects and duodenal ulcer patients. Gut 31: 148–150
11. Bianchi Porro G, Lazzaroni M, Barbara L et al. (1991) Famotidine versus ranitidine in acute duodenal ulcer. A multicentre endoscopic trial. Ital J Gastroenterol 23:65–69
12. Glise H, Martinson J, Solhang J et al. (1991) Two and four weeks' treatment for duodenal ulcer. Scand J Gastroenterol 26:137–145
13. Katchinsky B, Goebell H, Arnold R et al. (1991) Smoking as a risk factor for slow duodenal ulcer healing. Eur J Gastroenterol Hepatol 3:443–447
14. Feldman M, Burton ME (1991) Histamine-H_2-receptor antagonists: standard therapy for acid-peptic diseases (First of two Parts). N Engl J Med 323:1673–1680
15. Feldman M, Burton ME (1991) Histamine-H_2-receptor antagonists: standard therapy for acid-peptic diseases (Second of two Parts). N Engl J Med 323:1749–1755
16. Walt RP, Logan R, Hawkey C et al. (1991) A comparison of roxatidine and ranitidine for the acute treatment of duodenal ulcer. Aliment Pharmacol Therap 5:301–307
17. Patel N, Ward U, Rogers MJ, Primrose JN (1992) Night-time or morning dosing with H_2-receptor antagonists: studies on acid inhibition in normal subjects. Aliment Pharmacol Therap 6:381–387
18. Classen M, Dammann HG, Domschke W et al. (1985) Abheilungsraten nach Omeprazol und Ranitidin-Behandlung des Ulcus ventriculi. Dtsch Med Wochenschr 110:628–633
19. Walan A, Bader JP, Classen M et al. (1989) Effect of omeprazole and ranitidine on ulcer healing and relapse in patients with benign gastric ulcer. N Engl J Med 320:69–75
20. Cooperative Study Group (1990) Double blind comparative study of omeprazole and ranitidine in patients with duodenal or gastric ulcer: a multicentre trial. Gut 31:653–656
21. Davis RH, Scott NC, Barber JH et al. (1990) Treatment of peptic ulcer in general practice and in hospital: a comparison of omeprazole and cimetidine. Br J Clin Pract 44:13–16
22. Lind T, Cederburg C, Olansson M, Olbe L (1990) 24-hour intragastric acidity and plasma gastrin after omeprazole treatment and after proximal gastric vagotomy in duodenal ulcer patients. Gut 99:1593–1598
23. McFarland RJ, Bateson MC, Green JR et al. (1990) Omeprazole provides quicker symptom relief and duodenal ulcer healing than ranitidine. Gastroenterology 98:278–283
24. Gloria V, Domingo E, Makalinao A et al. (1991) Comparison of omeprazole and ranitidine in the management of patients with duodenal ulcer. Eur J Gastroenterol Hepatol 3:215–221
25. Lind T, Cederberg C, Idström JP et al. (1991) 24-hour intragastric acidity and plasma gastrin during long-term treatment with omeprazole or ranitidine in patients with reflux esophagitis. Scand J Gastroenterol 26:620–626
26. Valenzuela J, Berlin R, Snape W et al. (1991) US experience with omeprazole in duodenal ulcer. Dig Dis Sci 36:761–768
27. Koop H, Eissele R (1991) Gastrale Säurereduktion: Pathophysiologische und klinisch relevante Folgen. Z Gastroenterol 29:613–617
28. Londong W, Barth H, Dammann HG et al. (1991) Dose-related healing of duodenal ulcer with the proton pump inhibitor lansoprazole. Aliment Pharmacol Therap 5:245–254
29. Hotz J, Kleinert R, Grymbowski T et al. (1992) Lansoprazole versus famotidine: efficacy and tolerance in the acute management of duodenal ulceration. Aliment Pharmacol Therap 6:87–95
30. Bright-Asare P, Sontag, SJ, Gould RJ et al. (1986) Efficacy of misoprostol (twice daily dosage) in acute healing of duodenal ulcer. A multicenter double-blind controlled trial. Dig Dis Sci 31:63S–67S
31. Lam SK, Lam WY, Chai TK et al. (1986) Prostaglandin E_1 (misoprostol) overcomes the adverse effects of chronic cigarette-smoking on duodenal ulcer. Dig Dis Sci 31:68S–74S

32. Carling L, Unge P, Almostrom C et al. (1987) Enprostil and cimetidine: comparative efficacy and safety in patients with duodenal ulcer. Scand J Gastroenterol 22:325–331
33. Coremans G, Vantrappen G, Businger JA, Demol P (1989) Efficacy and safety of rioprostil, 300 micrograms b.d., in the treatment of duodenal ulcer. A double-blind, controlled multicentre clinical study vs. ranitidine. Scand J Gastroenterol 24 (suppl 164): 198–205
34. Corsing C, Demol P (1989) Drug safety of rioprostil in patients with active gastric or duodenal ulcer. Scand J Gastroenterol 24 (suppl 164):232–237
35. Euler AR, Krawiec J, Odes H et al. (1990) An evaluation of arbaprostil at multiple doses for the treatment of acute duodenal ulcer: a randomized double-blind placebo-controlled international trial. Am J Gastroenterol 85:145–149
36. Graham DY, Agrawal N, Roth SH (1988) Prevention of gastroduodenal damage induced by NSAIDs: a multicenter, double-blind, placebo-controlled trial. Lancet 2:1277–1281
37. Bendtsen F, Ebbeho N, Fallingborg J et al. (1990) Duodenal ulcer healing on 2 g of sucralfate daily at bedtime compared to 1 g four times daily. Aliment Pharmacol Therap 4:97–99
38. Blum AL, Bethge H, Bode J Ch, Domschke W (1990) Sucralfate in the treatment and prevention of gastric ulcer: multicentre double blind placebo controlled study. Gut 31:825–830
39. Dobrilla G, Amplatz S, Andreoli R, Vallaparta PA (1990) First randomized controlled trial with sucralfate versus H_2-antagonists in the treatment of duodenal ulcer non-responders to initial treatment with sucralfate. Hepato-Gastroenterol 37:239–241
40. Vor der Bruegge WF, Peura DA (1990) Stress-related mucosal damage: review of drug therapy. J Clin Gastroenterol 12 (suppl 2):35–40
41. Lamothe PH, Rao E, Serra AJ et al. (1991) Comparative efficacy of cimetidine, famotidine, ranitidine and mylanta in postoperative stress ulcers. Gastroenterology 100:1515–1520
42. Tryba M (1991) Sucralfate vs. antacids or H_2-antagonists for stress ulcer prophylaxis – a metaanalysis on the efficacy and pneumonia rate. Crit Care Med 19:942–947
43. Glover SC, Cantley JS, Weir MB et al. (1983) Oral tripotassium dicitrato bismuthate in gastric and duodenal ulceration. A double blind controlled trial. Dig Dis Sci 28:13–17
44. Lee FI, Samloff IM, Hardman M (1985) Comparison of tripotassium dicitrato bismuthate tablets with ranitidine in healing and relapse of duodenal ulcers. Lancet 1:1299–1301
45. Hamilton I, O'Connor JH, Wood NC et al. (1986) Healing and recurrence of duodenal ulcer after treatment with tripotassium dicitrato bismuthate tablets and cimetidine. Gut 27:106–110
46. Gavey CJ, Szeto ML, Nwokolo CU et al. (1989) Bismuth accumulates in the body during treatment with tripotassium dicitrato bismuthate. Aliment Pharmacol Therap 3:21–28
47. Treiber G, Gladziwa U, Ittel TH et al. (1991) Tripotassium dicitrato bismuthate: absorption and urinary excretion of bismuth in patients with normal and impaired renal function. Aliment Pharmacol Therap 5:491–502
48. Madaus S, Schulte-Frohlinde E, Scherer C et al. (1992) Comparison of plasma bismuth levels after oral dosing with basic bismuth carbonate or tripotassium dicitrato bismuthate. Aliment Pharmacol Therap 6:241–249
49. Collins R, Keane C, O'Morain C (1991) Omeprazole and colloidal bismuth subcitrate +/− adjuvant antibiotics in the treatment of Helicobacter pylori associated duodenal ulcer. Gastroenterology 100:A48
50. De Koster E, Burette A, Nyst J et al. (1991) HP treatment: bismuth, omeprazole, antibiotics. Gastroenterology 100:A52
51. Lamonliatte H, Bernard P, Boulard A et al. (1991) Controlled study of omeprazole-amoxicilline-tinidazole vs ranitidine-amoxicilline-tinidazole in Helicobacter pylori associated duodenal ulcer. Gastroenterology 100: A104
52. Wagner S, Gebel M, Haruma K et al. (1992) Bismuth subsalicylate in the treatment of H_2-blocker resistant duodenal ulcers: role of Helicobacter pylori. Gut 33:179–183
53. Patchett S, Beattie S, Keane C, O'Morain C (1992) Short report: short-term triple therapy for H. pylori-associated duodenal ulcer disease. Aliment Pharmacol Therap 6:113–117
54. Farup PG (1992) Compliance with anti-ulcer medication during short-term healing phase clinical trials. Aliment Pharmacol Therap 6:179–186
55. Burget DW, Chiverton SG, Hunt RH (1990) Is there an optimal degree of acid suppression for healing of duodenal ulcers? Gastroenterology 99:345–351
56. Butruk E, Gabryelewicz A, Hasik J et al. (1989) Ranitidine 300 mg twice daily compared with

ranitidine 300 mg at night in the treatment of duodenal ulcer: a multicentre trial. Eur J Gastroenterol Hepatol 1:63–67
57. Dobrilla G, De Pretis G, Arcidiacono R et al. (1989) Comparison of ranitidine 300 mg nocte with ranitidine 300 mg bid morning and bedtime. A randomized double-blind Italian multicentre trial. Clin Trial J 26:153–162
58. Lam SK, Lee NW, Koo J et al. (1984) Randomised, crossover trial of tripotassium dicitrato bismuthate versus high dose cimetidine for duodenal ulcers resistant to standard dose of cimetidine. Gut 25:703–706
59. Bianchi Porro G, Parente F, Lazzaroni M (1987) Tripotassium dicitrato bismuthate versus two different dosages of cimetidine in the treatment of resistant duodenal ulcers. Gut 28:907–911
60. Delchier JC, Isal JP, Erikssosn S, Soule JC (1989) Double blind multicentre comparison of omeprazole 20 mg once daily versus ranitidine 150 mg twice daily in the treatment of cimetidine or ranitidine resistant ulcers. Gut 30:1173–1178
61. Bardhan KD, Naesdal J, Bianchi Porro G et al. (1991) Treatment of refractory peptic ulcer with omeprazole or continued H_2 receptor antagonists: a controlled clinical trial. Gut 32:435–438

Rational Long-Term Therapy of Peptic Ulcer Disease

G. Bianchi Porro and F. Parente

Introduction

Peptic ulcer is a chronic disease characterized by spontaneous remissions and relapses which may lead to potentially lethal complications such as haemorrhage and perforation. The duration of this relapsing tendency is unpredictable in any individual patient but may last for many years, if not the entire lifetime, thus making a long-term treatment strategy a necessity. In recent years, various therapeutic opinions to maintain the disease in remission have become available, each one with a number of advantages and disadvantages. The present paper aims to review the different therapeutic options for the long-term management of peptic ulcer disease, with particular reference to their ability to prevent recurrences and complications.

Natural History of Peptic Ulcer Disease

Apart from subjects developing acute ulceration during stress conditions or induced by drugs, virtually all patients with duodenal ulcer, and the majority of those with gastric ulcer, will experience recurrences after the first episode of the disease if they are not given any form of long-term treatment. This was first shown in pre-endoscopic studies based on symptomatic diagnosis of peptic ulcer recurrences and more recently confirmed by the endoscopic follow-up of patients taking long-term placebo in controlled clinical trials.

Most of the information about the tendency towards recurrences prior to the introduction of histamine$_2$-blockers was provided by the follow-up studies conducted in patients selected from general and hospital practice. Krause [17] followed the clinical course of 624 patients with peptic ulcer for more than 25 years after the initial diagnosis; he showed that in 89% of male and 82% of female patients with duodenal ulcer the disease took a serious course during this period, the corresponding figures in patients with gastric ulcers were 70% and 62%. To establish the proportion of patients with still active disease over the years following the initial diagnosis, Krause examined each 5-year period separately and found that the proportion of patients with recurrent disease was 50% during the first 5 years but declined to 25% – 30% 20 – 25 years after the initial diagnosis. Fry [11], in his follow-up of 265 ulcer patients from suburban

London for up to 15 years, observed that the severity of ulcer symptoms was maximal over a period of approximately 8 years from the onset of the disease and declined thereafter: after 10 years 59% of patients still being followed up were free of symptoms, whereas after 15 years, the percentage had risen to 76%. Similar results were found by Greibe et al. [13], who followed 227 duodenal ulcer patients for 13 years after the initial diagnosis: they showed that at the end of follow-up, 37% of the surviving patients had no symptoms, 29% had mild symptoms and 12% severe symptoms.

Very different conclusions emerged in the study by Viskum [29], who followed 1679 patients with peptic ulcer for a mean period of 18 years. He showed that as many as 50% of the male and 33% of the female patients underwent surgical treatment for their disease, and only 20% of all patients were free of symptoms at the end of follow-up.

In the endoscopic era, controlled clinical trials conducted to ascertain the therapeutic efficacy of new anti-ulcer agents have confirmed that the natural tendency of peptic ulcer is to recur in most patients after initial healing. For example, Bardhan [2] conducted a 12-month follow-up in duodenal ulcer patients not receiving any form of long-term therapy after the initial healing (ascertained by endoscopy) and showed that 17% suffered three or more relapses, 24% had two relapses and 33% had one relapse during that time; only 26% of patients remained free of symptoms. In addition, the numerous clinical studies comparing H_2-antagonists against placebo in long-term maintenance of duodenal ulcer patients have documented that 80%–90% of duodenal ulcers in patients receiving placebo recur within 1–2 years from healing [6].

In conclusion, the available information supports the view that peptic ulcer disease is a long-lasting disease, with periodic recurrences, although this tendency to relapse may decrease with time.

Risk of Complications

The proportion of patients with peptic ulcer not receiving long-term treatment who develop haemorrhage in the years following the initial diagnosis of ulcer has been evaluated in a number of studies. Viskum [29] reported that 39% of male and 36% of female patients with duodenal ulcer suffered haemorrhage during a follow-up period of 15 years, whereas the corresponding figures for gastric ulcer were 42% in male and 47% in female patients. Fry [11] reported that 14% of patients with peptic ulcer developed gastrointestinal haemorrhage during a follow-up period of 15 years, while Krag [16] found that 25% of patients with duodenal ulcer and 27% of patients with gastric ulcer suffered haemorrhage during a follow-up period ranging from 17 to 27 years.

Pulvertaft [25] established that the average risk of haemorrhage was 18% in the 10 years following the diagnosis of duodenal ulcer and the established risk per year of follow-up was 2.7% in male and 2.5% in female patients.

Combining the results of various studies [24], it emerges that approximately 15% of patients with peptic ulcer develop digestive haemorrhage within 10 years from the initial diagnosis of ulcer, and this proportion tends to increase progressively with time. In addition, the peptic ulcer patient who has already suffered haemorrhage once has an increased risk of developing a further episode of gastrointestinal bleeding.

As far as the risk of perforation in patients with peptic ulcer is concerned, the available information is scarce, partly due to the relatively low frequency of such a complication. The reported frequency of perforation in three different studies ranged from 5.6% to 11% within 5–27 years of follow-up [11, 16, 21]. The most complete data on this topic were reported by Pulvertaft [25], who estimated that the risk of perforation of duodenal ulcer was 0.8% and 0.3% per year in male and female patients respectively after the initial diagnosis. As in the case of bleeding from peptic ulcer, the risk of perforation is higher in ulcer patients who have already suffered from this complication.

Impact of Short-Term Anti-Ulcer Therapy on Relapse

A single short-term course of treatment with any anti-ulcer agent is unable to alter the long-term course of peptic ulcer. Indeed, in a recent prospective study on 562 patients with duodenal ulcer, healed with a variety of antiulcer agents and subsequently receiving no further therapy, there was no difference in the cumulative rates of recurrence after 4 years of follow-up among groups treated with H_2-antagonists, sucralfate, colloidal bismuth subcitrate and pirenzepine [19] (Fig. 1). However, the recurrence rates within 1 year from ulcer healing may vary according to the drug used in the acute phase: the proportion of recurrent ulcers 12 months after cessation of H_2-antagonists does not differ significantly from that observed after discontinuation of pirenzepine, omeprazole, synthetic analogues of prostaglandin E [6], or sucralfate nor does the length of the acute therapy (4, 8 or more weeks) influence the risk of subsequent relapse [3]; by contrast, patients initially healed on colloidal bismuth subcitrate are less prone

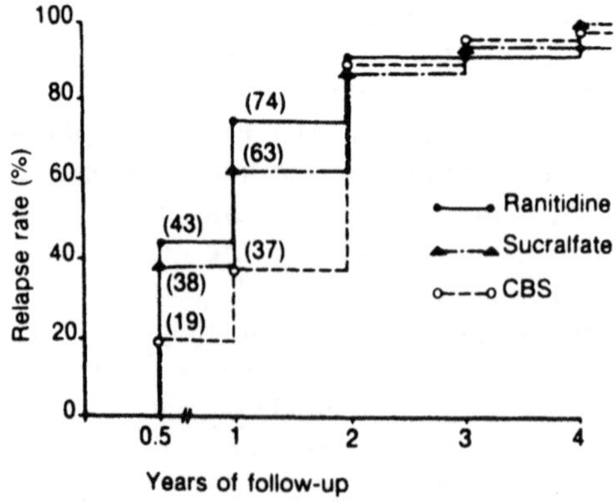

Fig. 1. Relapse rates in duodenal ulcer patients over 4 years after initial healing with ranitidine, sucralfate or colloidal bismuth subcitrate (CBS) treatment. (Adapted from Lane and Lee [19])

to recurrence within 12 months from treatment than those treated with any other anti-ulcer agent [10]. Whether this fact should influence our current anti-ulcer prescribing policy still remains a matter of debate (see anti-infective therapy).

Current Options for Long-Term Treatment of Peptic Ulcer

Various therapeutic options can be used to keep a peptic ulcer in remission after initial healing. They include: (a) continuous maintenance treatment with low-dose anti-ulcer agents (namely H_2-blockers); (b) intermittent treatment with an anti-ulcer agent (on demand or prescribed as a prophylactic regimen seasonally or at week-ends); (c) anti-infective therapy against *Helicobacter pylori*; (d) surgery. Each option has a number of advantages and disadvantages which will be briefly discussed herewith, except for surgery which has been examined elsewhere in this volume.

Continuous Maintenance Treatment

It is now widely accepted that continuous administration of low-dose H_2-antagonists is highly effective in reducing the spontaneous recurrence rates of duodenal ulcer at one year from initial healing. Numerous studies, indeed, have shown that maintenance treatment with H_2-antagonists significantly reduces the rate of ulcer recurrence compared with that observed during the administration of placebo (Table 1). Approximately one-third of patients receiving placebo remain free of symptomatic recurrence, in comparison with two-thirds of those

Table 1. Recurrence rates in the main placebo-controlled studies concerning the continuous long-term treatment of duodenal ulcer with H_2-blockers

Drug	Daily dosage (mg)	Recurrence rate at 12 months (% range)
Cimetidine	400 nocte	7 – 63
Placebo		53 – 83
Cimetidine	800 nocte	5 – 25
Placebo		48 – 100
Ranitidine	150 nocte	11 – 35
Placebo		39 – 87
Famotidine	20 nocte	19 – 30
Placebo		57 – 73
Nizatidine	150 nocte	34
Placebo		64

treated with H_2-blockers, with some difference in efficacy between different compounds.

For instance, a meta-analysis of studies comparing cimetidine against ranitidine in the prevention of duodenal ulcer relapse indicated a greater efficacy of ranitidine [18]. By contrast, no significant advantages of the new H_2-antagonists (famotidine, nizatidine, roxatidine) over ranitidine have emerged in terms of prophylactic activity.

Low-dose cimetidine and ranitidine are also significantly effective in preventing recurrences of gastric ulcer as compared to placebo, although the spontaneous recurrence rate of gastric ulcer after initial healing is less than that for duodenal ulcer. The proportion of patients whose gastric ulcer remains in remission after 12-month maintenance with cimetidine 400–800 mg ranges from 83% to 100%, and with ranitidine 150 mg it is greater than 80% [24].

Stopping continuous maintenance treatment after 1 year results in a prompt recurrence of duodenal ulcer disease. This became evident in our study which compared the recurrence rates in patients who stopped cimetidine 400 mg after 1 year with those in patients continuing the drug for a 2nd year: at the end of the 2nd year almost all patients who had come off cimetidine experienced relapse, whereas recurrences were very few among those who had continued maintenance treatment [7]. It appears, therefore, that 1 year of continuous maintenance therapy with H_2-antagonists is not sufficient to alter the natural tendency of duodenal ulcer to relapse, but extending therapy for a second year maintains a prophylactic effect comparable to that observed during the first year.

A number of recent studies have followed up duodenal ulcer patients for 4–6 years on continuous maintenance therapy with cimetidine or ranitidine after the initial healing and show that this regimen remains effective and safe for such long periods as well. In addition, all these studies confirmed that the rate of recurrence progressively decreases with the duration of treatment.

Long-term continuous maintenance appears to be able to reduce the risk of complications of both duodenal and gastric ulcer. Indeed, in a large multicentre European study including more than 1800 patients with duodenal ulcer maintained on cimetidine 400 mg/nocte for up to 4 years, the overall rate of complications was 1.7% with an estimated annual risk of 0.95 [30]. A similar rate of complications was reported by the Anglo-Irish cimetidine study group who followed up 402 duodenal ulcer patients maintained on cimetidine 400 mg for up to 6 years. The prevalences of haemorrhage and perforation were 0.7% and 0.5% respectively [1]. In another study evaluating the efficacy of continuing maintenance with ranitidine 150 mg/nocte for up to 5 years, the cumulative risk of haemorrhage from duodenal ulcer was 1.8% after 5 years in the ranitidine group compared with 15.2% after 3 years in patients without anti-ulcer therapy [22].

Long-term maintenance with H_2-blockers appears to be effective in reducing the risk of complications in gastric ulcer as well; indeed, none of the 120 patients with gastric ulcer maintained on ranitidine for up to 7 years suffered from haemorrhage or perforation [23].

As far as the safety of such a long-term therapy with H_2-antagonists is concerned, it should be stated that the incidence of adverse effects during continuous maintenance treatment is very low, and tends to decrease the longer treatment goes on. In 1423 patients on continuous maintenance with cimetidine 400 mg/nocte for up to 5 years, the incidence of possible or probable drug-related adverse effects declined from 8% during the 1st year to only 1% in the 4th year and beyond [5]. A recent 6-year study with cimetidine confirmed this low incidence of side effects and failed to give evidence of any significant modification in haematological or serum biochemical parameters over such a long period [3].

Intermittent Treatment

Intermittent therapy of peptic ulcer consists of repeated short courses of full-dose anti-ulcer agents (namely H_2-blockers or proton pump inhibitors), to be started under medical supervision in the case of the recurrence of ulcer symptoms or to be taken during a previously fixed period of the year (seasonal therapy). The hypothetical rationale for this therapy lies in the fact that the severity and the frequency of peptic ulcer relapse may vary considerably from patient to patient; such an approach may be more advantageous than continuous maintenance for those who present spontaneous long periods of remission, especially in terms of cost. The great disadvantage of this form of treatment is that it does not really prevent relapses and consequently ulcer complications, which should be the aim of a prophylactic therapy; on the other hand, it should be emphasized that the development of dyspeptic symptoms does not necessarily mean the reappearance of ulcer, and patients risk being "overtreated".

With regard to the efficacy of this therapy in clinical trials, by pooling the results of available studies, it emerges that an average of 70% of patients have at least one symptomatic relapse, nearly 40% have two relapses and approximately 20% three recurrences within 1 year of follow-up. In addition, in contrast to the earliest studies, the most recent experiences indicate a consistent risk of ulcer complications with this treatment. For example, Gustavsson et al. [14], registering complications in a group of 490 patients with duodenal ulcer treated with intermittent courses of H_2-antagonists over a period of 7 years, estimated the annual risks of haemorrhage, perforation and death at 2.1%, 0.2% and 0.2%, respectively.

Seasonal therapy with H_2-blockers was also found to be significantly inferior to continuous maintenance in terms of relapse rates in two recent controlled trials [9, 26]; no data on the risks of ulcer complications during such treatment are at present available.

A special form of intermittent therapy (weekend therapy) consists in the administration of full-dose omeprazole for 3 days a week (usually Friday, Saturday and Sunday), which theoretically permits adequate control of gastric secretion without inducing profound acid suppression and consequent sustained hypergastrinaemia. A recent study comparing the effect of omeprazole 10 mg/day or 20 mg at weekends with placebo in duodenal ulcer patients [20] showed that recurrence rates at 6 months were similar in both omeprazole regimens (29% and 26% respectively) and significantly lower than with placebo

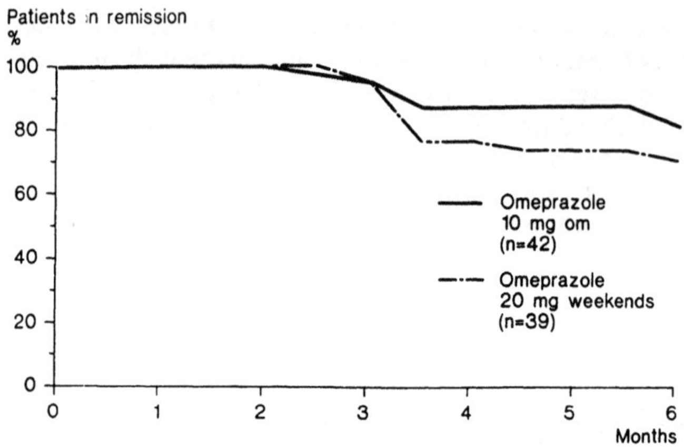

Fig. 2. Omeprazole 20 mg at weekends versus omeprazole 10 mg/day in the long-term treatment of duodenal ulcer. (From Bianchi Porro et al., 1993, in press)

(83%). These data have been confirmed by our study showing that omeprazole 20 mg at weekends was as effective as omeprazole 10 mg/day in preventing duodenal ulcer relapse within 6 months of healing (Fig. 2), with a significant advantage for the weekend regimen concerning the increase in gastrin levels (lower than that observed with the continuous regimen). These preliminary reports suggest that weekend therapy with omeprazole may become an effective alternative to continuous maintenance in reducing recurrence rates of duodenal ulcer; however, the impact of this form of treatment on ulcer complications has still to be evaluated in further studies, since at present no data exist on this topic.

Anti-infective Treatment

There is now a huge amount of clinical evidence suggesting that it is worth attempting the eradication of *Helicobacter pylori* in duodenal ulcer patients in whom this organism is present. Indeed, several studies have shown that the relapse rate of duodenal ulcer is markedly reduced (approximately 10% – 20% at 12 months) if *H. pylori* has been eradicated at the time of ulcer healing [27]. In addition, preliminary data show that patients who remain free from *H. pylori* colonization for longer periods (4 years) also remain free from ulcer recurrence, which suggests the possibility of a real "cure" for duodenal ulcer disease [12] (Fig. 3).

However, regimens designed to eradicate *H. pylori* infections are still at an early stage of development and not completely satisfactory in terms of efficacy, compliance and side effects. Indeed, the most effective regimen, which consists of a combination of bismuth salts, metronidazole and amoxicillin or tetracycline for 2 weeks, eradicates *H. pylori* from approximately 80% of patients [15] but can give rise to troublesome adverse effects in 20% – 30% of cases; in addition,

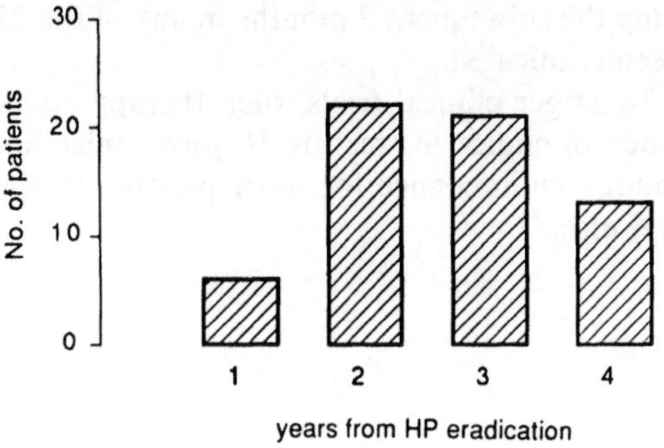

Fig. 3. Long-term follow-up (up to 4 years) of 62 duodenal ulcer patients after *Helicobacter pylori* eradication. The vertical bars represent the number of patients still in remission

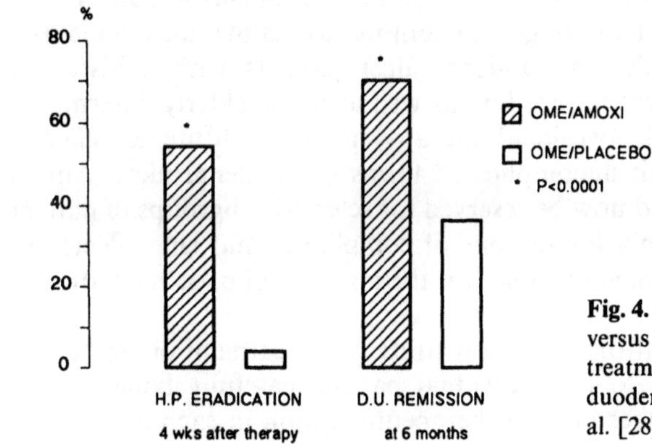

Fig. 4. Omeprazole plus amoxicillin versus omeprazole plus placebo in the treatment of *Helicobacter pylori*-positive duodenal ulcers. (Adapted from Unge et al. [28])

patient compliance appears to be uncertain and resistance to antibiotics (particularly to metronidazole) develops rapidly.

To overcome these problems, simpler anti-infective regimens are under study. An interesting possibility seems to be constituted by the association of proton pump inhibitors and amoxicillin. Omeprazole has a weak suppressive effect on *H. pylori*; preliminary reports suggest that when it is given in combination with amoxicillin, this leads to a strong synergistic effect, producing eradication rates comparable to those obtained with the classic triple therapy and minimal side-effects. Unge et al. [28] treated 157 patients with *H. pylori*-positive duodenal ulcer with a combination of omeprazole 40 mg/day for 4 weeks with amoxicillin 750 mg b.i.d. in the last 2 weeks, and obtained eradication of *H. pylori* in 54% of the cases; at 6 months the recurrence rate in the 72 *H. pylori*-negative patients was 16%, as compared to 45% in the *H. pylori*-positive patients (Fig. 4). Bayerdörffer et al. [4] treated 27 patients with *H. pylori*-positive duodenal ulcer with omeprazole 40 mg b.i.d. and amoxicillin 1 g b.i.d. for 10 days followed by omeprazole 20 mg/day for a total duration of 6 weeks, obtaining eradication of *H. pylori* in 22 cases (82%). No relevant side effects were observed among patients treated with such an association and no ulcer recurrence was observed during the subsequent 9 months in any of the 22 patients in whom *H. pylori* had been eradicated.

If these results are confirmed by larger clinical trials, such therapy could become the pharmacological regimen of choice in treating *H. pylori* infection and a useful alternative to continuous maintenance for most patients in the long-term management of duodenal ulcer.

Conclusions

After a decade in which the long-term medical therapy of peptic ulcer has been based mainly upon the use of H_2-antagonists, a number of effective alternatives are now potentially available. If long-term continuous maintenance remains at present the option of choice in duodenal ulcer patients with a history of complications (haemorrhage, perforation) as well as in the elderly, intermittent treatment with omeprazole (weekend therapy) may constitute an effective alternative for patients with uncomplicated forms of duodenal ulcer. Anti-*H. pylori* therapy, which should now be reserved for selected subgroups of patients with duodenal ulcers, mainly for reasons of compliance and side effects, will probably become the treatment of choice for the majority of patients in the next few years.

It is time, therefore, that the long-term strategy of treatment of peptic ulcer disease should be tailored to the individual patient, carefully balancing the advantages and disadvantages of each therapeutic option in each case.

References

1. Bardhan KD (1988) Six years of continuous cimetidine treatment in peptic ulcer disease: efficacy and safety. Aliment Pharmacol Therap 2:395–405
2. Bardhan KD (1988) Intermittent treatment of duodenal ulcer for long-term medical management: a review. Postgrad Med J 64 (Suppl. 1):40–46
3. Bardhan KD, Cole DS, Hawkins BW, Franks CR (1982) Does treatment with cimetidine extended beyond initial healing of duodenal ulcer reduce the subsequent relapse rate? Brit Med J 284:621–624
4. Bayerdörffer E, Mannes GA, Sommer A et al. (1992) High-dose omeprazole treatment combined with amoxicillin eradicates Helicobacter pylori. Eur J Hepatol Gastroenterol, 1992, 4, 697–702
5. Bianchi Porro G (1985) Symposium proceedings. XII International Congress of Gastroenterology, Lisbon, pp. 33–38, Universitetsfor-laget, Oslo, 1985
6. Bianchi Porro G, Parente F (1991) Long-term treatment of duodenal ulcer. A review of management options. Drugs 1991; 41:38–51
7. Bianchi Porro G, Petrillo M, Lazzaroni M, Sangaletti O (1982) The longer-term treatment of duodenal ulceration with cimetidine. In Bianchi Porro & Bardhan (Eds) Peptic ulcer disease: advances in pathogenesis and treatment, pp. 107–113, Cortina International, Verona, 1982
8. Bianchi Porro G, Bolling E, Barbara L et al. (1990) Maintenance treatment with omeprazole in the prevention of duodenal ulcer relapse: a double-blind comparative trial. Digestive Disease Week, S. Antonio, May 13–16, 1990, 213-A

9. Blasi A, Magiameli A, Castelli G et al. (1987) Long-term (24 month) ranitidine in prevention of duodenal ulcer relapse: comparison of continuous and seasonal treatment. Ital J Gastroenterol 19:141–144
10. Dobrilla G, Vallaperta P, Amplatz S (1988) Influence of ulcer healing agents on ulcer relapse after discontinuation of acute treatment: a pooled estimate of controlled clinical trials. Gut 29:181–187
11. Fry J (1964). Peptic ulcer: a profile. Br Med J 2:808–812
12. George L, Hyland L, Morgan A et al. (1990) Smoking does not contribute to duodenal ulcer relapse after eradication. Gastroenterology 98:A48 (Abstract.)
13. Greibe J, Bugge P, Gjorup T, Lauritsen T, Bonnevie O, Wulff HR (1977) Long-term prognosis of duodenal ulcer; follow-up study and survey of doctor's estimates. Br Med J 2:1572–1574
14. Gustavsson S, Holmberg L, Nyren O, Dhrvall U, Wells L (1990) Risk of serious complications in patients with duodenal or prepyloric ulcers, Gastroenterology 98, 54A
15. Heatley RV (1992) Review article: the treatment of Helicobacter pylori infection. Aliment Pharmacol Ther 6:291–303
16. Krag E (1966) Long-term prognosis in medically treated peptic ulcer. Acta Med. Scand 180, 657–668
17. Krause U (1963) Long-term results of medical and surgical treatment of peptic ulcer. Acta Chir Scand 125 (Suppl. 310):5–111
18. Kurata JH, Koch GG, Nogawa AN (1987) Comparison of ranitidine and cimetidine ulcer maintenance therapy. J Clin Gastroenterol 9:644–650
19. Lane MR, Lee SP (1988) Recurrence of duodenal ulcer after medical treatment. Lancet 1:1147–1149
20. Lauritsen K, Andersen BN, Laurse LS et al. (1991) Omeprazole 20 mg three days a week and 10 mg daily in the prevention of duodenal ulcer relapse. Double-blind comparative trial. Gastroenterology 100:663–669
21. Martin L, Lewis N (1949) Peptic ulcer cases reviewed after 10 years. Lancet ii:1115–1120
22. Penston J, Wormsley KG (1989) Efficacy and safety of long-term maintenance therapy of duodenal ulcers. Scand J Gasterentol 24:1145–1152
23. Penston JG, Wormsley KG (1990) Long-term maintenance treatment of gastric ulcers with ranitidine. Aliment Pharmacol Therap 4:339–355
24. Penston JG, Wormsley KG (1992) Review article: maintenance treatment with H_2-receptor antagonists for peptic ulcer disease. Aliment Pharmacol Therap 6:3–29
25. Pulvertaft CN (1968) Incidence of natural history of gastric and duodenal ulcer. Postgrad Med J 44:597–602
26. Susi D, Ianetti G, Di Pietro AM (1987) Long-term therapy of peptic ulcer: our experience with ranitidine after 4 years. Ital J Gastroenterol 19:69S
27. Tytgat GNJ, Noach LA, Rauws E (1992) Helicobacter pylori. Eur J Gastroenterol Hepatol 4 (suppl. 1):57–515
28. Unge P, Eriksson K, Bergman B et al. (1992) Omeprazole and amoxicillin in patients with duodenal ulcer: helicobacter pylori eradication and remission of ulcers and symptoms during a 6-month follow-up. Digestive Disease Week, S. Francisco, May 10–13, 1992, A163
29. Viskum A (1976) A comparison of the course of the disease among patients with gastric ulcer, duodenal ulcer, and ulcer dyspepsia without ulcer demonstrable by X-ray. Dan Med Bull 23:129–136
30. Walan A, Bianchi Porro G, Hentschel E, Bardhan KD, Delattre M. Maintenance treatment with cimetidine in peptic ulcer disease for up to 4 years. Scand J Gastroenterol 1987; 22:397–405

Endoscopic Diagnosis and Treatment of Bleeding Gastroduodenal Ulcers

P. Rutgeerts

Introduction

The search for safe, effective, and inexpensive endoscopic methods to control severe peptic ulcer bleeding continues. Upper gastro-intestinal bleeding in this era of high medical technology still has an overall mortality of about 10%. The incidence of this often dramatic emergency is estimated at 1/1000 per year. Prognostic factors for outcome have been clearly defined and have somewhat changed over the last decades, as bleeding occurs more now in elderly and critically ill patients [1–4]. About 70%–80% of the patients have already stopped bleeding when admitted to hospital. No transfusion or only a few units of blood are required. Endoscopy in these patients visualizes a nonbleeding lesion, mostly without stigmata of recent hemorrhage. The evolution will be uneventful and any aggressive therapy may harm the patient. Twenty to thirty percent of the patients are admitted with arterial hypotension and continue to bleed or rebleed while in the hospital. These patients have high transfusion requirements and are at high risk.

Severe bleeding almost always originates from peptic ulcers or from esophageal or fundic varices. In patients with severe bleeding upper gastrointestinal endoscopy should be performed as soon as possible after resuscitation. There is no doubt that the diagnostic yield of early endoscopy in upper gastrointestinal hemorrhage is superior to that of a barium meal. The timing of endoscopy influence the frequency of active bleeding present at endoscopy [4]. If performed within 12 h of admission, 41% of the patients will have active bleeding. When endoscopy is performed more than 12 h after admission, the incidence of active bleeding is about 30%. In a survey by the American Society for Gastrointestinal Endoscopy [4], active bleeding at endoscopy was associated with a mortality rate of 16.1%; if there was no active bleeding the mortality dropped to 6.7%.

The nature of the bleeding lesion has prognostic importance. Therapeutic efforts should be directed to those patients who continue to bleed or are likely to rebleed. It is critical to identify these high-risk groups.

Bleeding from esophagitis, Mallory-Weiss tears, neoplasms, gastric erosions, erosive duodenitis, and vascular malformations is usually mild. When peptic ulcers or varices are diagnosed at endoscopy the finding of stigmata of recent hemorrhage predicts further bleeding.

In 1978 Foster et al. [5] identified three endoscopic stigmata of recent hemorrhage as predictors of continuing or recurrent bleeding: fresh bleeding from the lesion, fresh or altered clot or black slough adherent to the lesion, and, thirdly, a vessel protruding from the base or the margin of an ulcer. Griffiths [6] confirmed the prognostic importance of the visible vessel. Accurate prospective data were obtained by Storey and Swain [7, 8]. It is easy to identify a spurting hemorrhage or a pulsating pseudoaneurysm as arterial in origin. Identification of a nonbleeding artery is more subjective. According to Storey [7] and Swain [8], a nonbleeding artery appears on endoscopy as an elevated red or blue spot, resistent to gentle washing, often associated with a red clot and almost always unique in the ulcer crater. Overall recurrent bleeding occurred in 85% of ulcers presenting with spurting hemorrhage at endoscopy, in 51% of ulcers with a nonbleeding visible vessel, in 5% of ulcers with other stigmata of recent hemorrhage, and in 0% of ulcers without stigmata.

These data were challenged recently by Wara [9], who found a lower rebleeding rate (32%) of ulcers with nonbleeding visible vessel. He suggested that a visible vessel carries a high rebleeding risk only when oozing hemorrhage or an overlying clot is present at endoscopy. Another recent study by Bornman [10] showed that the association of shock with important endoscopic signs is a stronger predictor of rebleeding than either shock or important signs alone.

One decade ago patients with severe upper gastrointestinal hemorrhage were candidates for emergency surgery, carrying a mortality of approximately 25% in contrast with the 3% mortality of elective surgery for upper gastrointestinal hemorrhage.

Several methods of hemostasis in upper gastrointestinal bleeding have been developed and evaluated in animal experiments, human pilot studies, controlled clinical trials, and randomized comparative studies. The ultimate benefit of endoscopic hemostasis for the patient with upper gastrointestinal hemorrhage is reduction of mortality, but benefits might also encompass lowered morbidity and reduced cost of patient care. Efficacious endoscopic hemostasis would reduce mortality due to bleeding; by avoiding emergency surgery it would also decrease the often lethal postoperative complications.

We will discuss those methods of endoscopic hemostasis for which clinical data and, especially, controlled trials are available. These include thermal methods, i.e., laser photocoagulation, monopolar and bipolar electrocoagulation, heater probe, and various injection methods. Therapy modalities for thermal methods are summarized in Table 1 and various injection modalities in Table 2.

Table 1. Thermal methods: treatment modalities

	Neodymium-YAG laser	Bipolar electrocoagulation (Bicap)	Heater probe
Power	70–90 W	50 W output 5–7 25 W output 10	30 J
Pulse duration	0.5–1 s	1–2 s	± 4 s
Number of pulses	Unlimited	Unlimited	> 3, Unlimited
Repeated therapy	Yes	Yes	Yes

Table 2. Injection therapy: agents, volumes, techniques

Sclerosant	Volume per injection (ml)	Total volume (ml)	Injection site
Epinephrine 1‰	1–2	10–20	Ulcer rim, Vessel
Polidocanol 1%	1	5–10	Vessel
Absolulte ethanol	0.1	1–2	Vessel
Ethanolamine oleate	0.5	2–5	Vessel
100 IU thrombin/normal saline	2–3	10–15	Vessel
Fibrin glue	0.5	2–6 Clots	Vessel

Neodymium-YAG Laser Photocoagulation

The controversy that existed as to which of the gastrointestinal lasers, the argon or the neodymium: yttrium-aluminium-garnet (neodymium-YAG) laser, should be used, has been solved by clinical use. The 1.06 μm YAG laser is preferred because its beam is not absorbed by overlying blood and because its greater depth of penetration makes it more efficacious than the argon laser in the treatment of large bleeding vessels. The fear of excessive transmural injury by the YAG laser beam causing gut perforation proved to be unwarranted; this laser has proved to be quite safe in clinical setting.

The modalities of power and exposure setting for YAG photocoagulation and the mechanism of hemostasis have been studied experimentally in dogs [11–13]. Hemostasis is achieved by protein coagulation, denaturation of collagen, formation of platelet thrombi, and vessel constriction. These features occur at tissue temperatures between 60° and 80°C. A temperature plateau of about 70° C at the tissue level is best achieved by repeated short (0.5–1 s) pulses of high power (70–90 W). At higher temperatures, e.g., 100°C, vaporization occurs and an ulcer is created. When hemostasis is being attempted, this is dangerous for two reasons: (1) ulcer formation increases the risk of transmural injury and perforation, and (2) the cutting of the laser may incise the vessel and cause severe bleeding.

In the clinical setting most gastroenterologists use high power and short pulses, although some prefer continuous photocoagulation. When severe bleeding is present it may be necessary to use longer exposure times, because some energy is carried away by blood flow. The working distance varies between 0.5 and 1.5 cm. The output of the laser beam at the fiber tip should be checked regularly. Visible tissue erosion should always be avoided. Most endoscopists now use the flexible transmission fibre with CO_2 gas.

When treating a visible vessel with YAG laser alone, photocoagulation should be started circumferentially to the vessel, followed by photocoagulation of the vessel itself. At the end of the session the vessel of "sentinel clot" should always be completely destroyed, leaving a flat lesion in order to ensure complete closure of the vessel. Direct application of high energy to the vessel may induce dramatic hemorrhage, especially when a branch of the gastroduodenal artery is involved.

Following the pioneering work of P. Kiefhaber [14] in Germany and R. Dwyer in the United States [15], a number of centers have gained an extensive experience with YAG laser hemostasis of gastrointestinal bleeding lesions. Kiefhaber [14] reported successful results in 94% of 692 unselected patients with upper gastrointestinal bleeding due to various causes. Sander [16] and Shönekäs [17] have also reported excellent results, with hemostasis rates exceeding 90% using neodymium-YAG laser photocoagulation in large series of patients with gastrointestinal bleeding. However, as shown by our own pilot studies [18], overall results have to be interpreted with care, as these tend to overestimate the efficacy of the technique because a number of the lesions treated, e.g., erosions, Mallory-Weiss tears, tumors, and postpolypectomy hemorrhages, have low bleeding potential and in most cases stop bleeding spontaneously. In severe bleeding from ulcers with visible vessels, initial hemostasis is readily achieved, but recurrent bleeding occurs frequently. Therefore, the true benefit of endoscopic hemostasis can only be determined by randomized controlled studies. These studies are, however difficult to carry out.

Three out of six controlled trials [19–24] using neodymium-YAG laser photocoagulation for hemostasis showed significant benefit. The trial of McLeod et al. [22] showed significant reduction of rebleeding and emergency surgery in severe bleeders. Our trial [23] also showed significant reduction of rebleeding and emergency surgery rate when actively bleeding ulcers and ulcers with stigmata of recent hemorrhage were combined. The trial of Swain [24] showed, besides a significant reduction of the rebleeding and emergency surgery rate, a significant reduction in mortality as well.

The trials with negative results have some methodological drawbacks. In the trial of Ihre [20] only a small number of patients were included. Escourrou [19] included in his series "endoscopic failures," i.e., patients in whom the lesions could not be reached by the endoscope, while Krejs [21] excluded severe bleeders from the trial.

The success rate of YAG laser hemostasis in patients with severe bleeding from visible vessels in ulcers was rather disappointing in our hands. Although an initial hemostasis rate of more than 80% was obtained, recurrence of bleeding occurred frequently, and up to 50% of these patients had to undergo surgery. We therefore tried to improve the success rate of YAG laser therapy in two ways. The first [25] was based on the combination of local epinephrine injection (to stop or reduce the bleeding at least temporarily) followed by YAG laser photocoagulation (to obliterate and completely destroy the vessel that caused the bleeding). For small ulcers 2 ml epinephrine solution 1‰ was injected through a sclerotherapy needle submucosally in each quadrant of the ulcer rim. For large ulcers with a central vessel the solution was injected in the ulcer base around the vessel. After injection the lesion was treated by neodymium-YAG laser photocoagulation. When bleeding was not controlled by laser, a second injection was given to arrest or slow down the bleeding in order to facilitate further YAG laser therapy.

The second way consisted of repeated therapy sessions. In the early years of laser therapy this was only rarely done because of the penetration depth of the laser and the fear for perforation. Using pretreatment with injection of epinephrine 1‰ and repeated YAG laser therapy upon recurrence, the definite success rate of YAG hemostasis increased from 62% to 89% in ulcers with bleeding and nonbleeding visible vessels.

The complication rate of endoscopic YAG laser therapy is surprisingly low. Preforation has been reported in 1.2% of treated patients.

Perforation with free abdominal gas occurred in 2 of 344 patients treated in our department (0.6%). The most common complication is probably aspiration pneumonia, which occurs in about 10% of the patients with severe bleeding. The exact incidence is difficult to assess. Although this complication is seen after diagnostic endoscopy in patient with upper gastrointestinal bleeding, the risk of aspiration is probably increased when the duration of the procedure is increased due to endoscopic hemostasis. Laser-induced massive hemorrhage occurs rarely but could be controlled by continuing therapy. Damage to the endoscope by laser carried a high cost. The frequency of fiber burn depends on the gas flow used. Cut and polish of the fiber has to be performed routinely.

Electrocoagulation Techniques

Heating and desiccating by electrical current flowing through the tissue results in vessel shrinkage and thrombosis. With monopolar electrocoagulation the current goes from the ball electrode through the patient to the ground plate. A number of uncontrolled [26–31] studies have reported success rates of 70%–95%. The depth of injury, however, is a problem with this monopolar technique and perforation rates are as high as 1%–20%. One controlled trial by Papp [32] showed significant benefit of monopolar electrocoagulation in preventing hemorrhage from ulcer with nonbleeding visible vessels. The disadvantages of monopolar electrocoagulation, however, preclude its general use. These are the unpredictable current flow, occasionally resulting in transmural injury and clinical perforation, sticking of the electrode to the tissue, and possible acute vessel damage resulting in severe bleeding.

Electrohydrothermal therapy has been proposed [33–35] by German groups as a modification of monopolar electrocoagulation, but does not seem to have advantages over bipolar electrocoagulation, which is easier to use. Reports on two controlled randomized trials using this technique have been published. Freitas et al. [34] and Boix et al. [35] both reported on significant reduction of rebleeding rate.

Bipolar electrocoagulation is characterized by flow of current between two different parts of one electrode or two electrodes close to each other. A modification of the bipolar electrode is the multipolar electrode, which consists of spaced electrode stripes along the side and over the tip of the probe. Water can be pumped through a central opening to wash blood away. Large (10 F:

3.2 mm) and small (7 F: 2.4 mm) probes are available. The large probe can only be passed through a large channel endoscope. Uncontrolled trials [36–41] with bicap, using the small electrode, have reported a high efficacy in controlling active hemorrhage (86%–98%) but high rebleeding rates (15%–29%).

Although the experimental and these pilot data on bipolar electrocoagulation are encouraging, few controlled trials have been carried out thus far. Two controlled trials [42, 43] showed no benefit of multipolar electrocoagulation using the 7 F (2.3 mm) bicap probe. The controlled trial of O'Brien (44) showed benefit of the bicap, although not significant. A controlled trial by Laine [45] showed a significant reduction in continued bleeding, transfusion requirements, hospital stay and mortality for patients treated with bicap electrocoagulation. In this study the 10 F bicap was used (3.2 mm).

Comparative experimental studies of YAG laser and bicap suggest that both modalities area equally effective. In a small randomized clinical trial by Goff [46], bicap seemed somewhat more efficacious than YAG laser (no rebleeding in 3/8 after YAG, 6/11 after bicap; $P < 0.1$). In that study the results of either treatment were poor.

In a large randomized comparison carried out in our department [47], we showed that in patients presenting at endoscopy with peptic ulcer and a spurting or oozing vessel or with a nonbleeding visible vessel, YAG laser and bicap were equally effective and resulted in definitive hemostasis in about 72% after one session and 86%–88% after two sessions. It should be stressed that in that study we always used pretreatment with epinephrine 1‰ injection in both groups. The bicap probe diameter (10 F versus 7 F) seems to be very important for the efficacy of multipolar electrocoagulation of bleeding ulcers. Consequently, the application of bicap always necessitates the use of large-channel endoscopes, while the laser fiber can be introduced through the channel of any standard gastroscope. The output of the bicap unit seems less critical. We obtained very good results with the 25 W bicap unit at about 10. With the 50 W bicap, unit 5–7 is the output to be used. The risk of transmural injury and perforation seems definitely lower than for YAG laser therapy, although at least one perforation with bicap has been reported [47]. Coaptation of the vessel by appositional pressure also avoids initiation of severe bleeding. Procedure-related complications, e.g., aspiration, occur with bicap as well as with laser therapy. Sticking of the multipolar to the tissue does not occur.

Heater Probe

Another thermal modality, the heater probe, has been studied experimentally and seems to be very effective for hemostasis. The probe is an aluminum cylinder with an inner heater coil insulated from the cylinder. The whole is coated with Teflon. Although the probe has been modified sticking still occurs, although to a lesser degree. Broad clinical data are lacking. Johnston [48] compared the heater probe in a nonrandomized study with the YAG laser and found the heater probe to be more effective than the YAG laser. Nonrandomized comparisons, however, need to be interpreted with care. One controlled randomized comparison with the YAG laser showed that the YAG laser was superior to the heat probe for ulcer hemostasis [49].

Injection Therapy

Injection therapy has become the most widely used method for controlling active peptic ulcer bleeding and preventing rebleeding from peptic ulcers with visible vessels. Data are accumulating to indicate that injection therapy is at least as effective as thermal modalities for endoscopic hemostasis.

Early uncontrolled studies [50–61] have shown that endoscopic hemostasis may be accomplished by local injection at the bleeding site. Various solutions have been used, as well as combinations of agents. Almost every source of bleeding has been treated by this method, including benign and malignant tumors, vascular malformations, Mallory-Weiss tears, and ulcers. In recent years a number of well-designed studies have been completed on the use of injection techniques for treatment .of bleeding from visible vessels in peptic ulcers.

Experimental Studies in Animals

Experimental use of injection therapy in animals did not reproduce the efficacy seen in clinical practice. Three experimental studies of injection therapy for bleeding peptic ulcer have been carried out. Two studies [62, 63] in which the effect of injection was compared with thermal effects showed that in the experimental ulcer model and in the mesenteric vessel model injection therapy was far less efficacious than thermal methods in controlling bleeding. These studies however, have to be interpreted with caution. The experimental ulcer does not really mimic the bleeding peptic ulcer with central vessel and bleeds profusely from its edges. Exposed serosal vessels lack the surrounding submucosal tissue. It is clear that hemostasis by injection results from compression and sclerosis. Randall et al. [64] found ethanol and TES, (1% tetradecyl sulfate, 32% ethanol, and 0.3 normal saline) to be the most effective agents for arterial coagulation, while polidocanol was somewhat less effective.

A striking result was the serious necrosis induced by the injection of sclerosing agents. Absolute ethanol and 1% polidocanol cause tissue necrosis with ulceration besides vessel thrombosis. Absolute ethanol fixes the tissue, whereas polidocanol 1% causes acute edema, with subsequent inflammation and sclerosis.

Injection Techniques and Solutions Used (Table 2)

A disposable Teflon sclerotherapy catheter with a 23-gauge retractable needle is used that can be passed through the biopsy channel of a standard panendoscope. The volumes and injection sites further depend on the solution used for injection.

Epinephrine 1‰

One milliliter of epinephrine 1‰ is diluted in 9 ml saline. This solution is first injected submucosally in the rim of a small or medium-sized ulcer with a central bleeding or non-bleeding vessel. The injection of 2 ml of this solution will immediately induces marked swelling and whitening of the treated area. The injection is then repeated in the three other quadrants of the rim of the ulcer. It is important to inject first the rim of the ulcer that is furthest away from the scope. In this way small ulcers will raise towards the scope. If the nearest border is injected first, the swelling will impair vision of the ulcer and render further treatment more difficult. If the ulcer is large, submucosal injection of epinephrine 1‰ in the rim of the ulcer will not be efficacious and injection near the vessel site or in the vessel is necessary, but we feel that in this case epinephrine is not the appropriate solution to use. A sclerosant is necessary in this clinical situation. The total volume of epinephrine 1‰ injected is not critical. Usually 8–10 ml is injected, but volumes as high as 20–30 ml can be used safely.

Polidoconol 1% (Aethoxysclerol 1%)

Polidacanol 1%. is seldom used as sole injection solution. Mostly it is used after pretreatment with epinephrine. After submucosal epinephrine injection in the rim of the ulcer, polidocanol is injected at the vessel site or in the vessel. Wördehoff [60], the only author who uses polidocanol 1% as sole solution, injects up to 10–15 ml of this solution. Most other authors inject 3–5 ml directly at the vessel after epinephrine pretreatment. This treatment may be repeated, but in contrast to epinephrine 1‰ the marked necrosis induced by polidocanol may predispose to perforation.

Absolute Ethanol (98%–99.5% Pure Dehydrated Ethanol)

For the injection of alcohol 98% a 1-ml plastic disposable tuberculin syringe is used. Before introduction the needle is filled with the solution to be injected, to allow careful quantitation of the injected volume. When a bleeding or non-bleeding vessel is exposed, 98% ethanol is slowly injected in amounts of 0.1–0.2 ml per injection at three or four sites close to the vessel or in the vessel. The volume injected usually does not exceed 1 ml because of the marked necrosis induced by ethanol.

Ethanolamine Oleate 5%

Pretreatment with epinephrine 1‰ is usually carried out. Subsequently, 0.5 ml aliquots of ethanolamine oleate 5% are injected around and directly to the vessel, up to a total of 2 ml. When ethanolamine oleate 5% is used without epinephrine pretreatment, up to 5 ml is injected.

Thrombin

Pretreatment is usually carried out with epinephrine 1‰ injection. One hundred international units of thrombin in 3 ml 0.9% salt solution are used. Usually 10–15 ml solution is necessary.

Fibrin Glue

Injection of fibrin glue is carried out using a twin-lumen probe. Thrombin/calcium choride is injected via one inlet and fibrinogen/aprotinin through the other inlet. Both substances are injected simultaneously and both syringes are flushed with saline. When the two substances mix in the tissue a nice clot is formed. Two to six clots are usually injected near the vessel. Preparation of the substances and the injection itself are somewhat more difficult and time-consuming than in other injection techniques. To obtain a clear endoscopy field when there is active bleeding, the lesion can be pretreated with epinephrine 1‰ injection.

Sham-Controlled Trials of Injection Therapy

In recent years a number of excellent sham-controlled trials of injection therapy have been carried out using the different injection solutions.

Epinephrine

Chung et al. [65] studied in a controlled trial the efficacy of epinephrine injections for peptic ulcer hemostasis. Five of 34 patients in the injection group underwent emergency operation, vs 14 of 34 patients in the control group ($p < 0.02$).

Epinephrine-Polidocanol

Panes et al. [66] showed that injection with epinephrine-polidocanol was associated with significantly less severe rebleeding (5.5% versus 43%) and less surgery (5% versus 34%) than no treatment in patients with peptic ulcers with visible vessels with active bleeding, visible vessels without bleeding, and ulcers with oozing hemorrhage or clot adherence to the ulcer base. Another trial by Balanzo et al. [67] showed also benefit for epinephrine-polidocanol injection as compared to medical therapy only in regard to rebleeding (7 of 36 patients 15/36 patients; $p < 0.05$) and transfusion needs (1.63 units vs 2.86 units; $p < 0.05$), but the data are less impressive.

Absolute Ethanol

Pascu et al. [68] reported on a randomized controlled trial of injection therapy with absolute ethanol for hemostasis for ulcer bleeding. They had a 36% surgery rate in the control patients as compared to a 15% surgery rate ($p < 0.02$) in the patients treated with ethanol injection. Mortality was 12.8% in the control group and 3% in the injection therapy group ($p < 0.05$).

Ethanolamine Oleate 5%

Two controlled studies have been published on injection therapy with ethanolamine oleate 5% for peptic ulcer bleeding. In both studies pretreatment was carried out with epinephrine injection. Rajgopal et al. [69] reported on a significantly reduced rebleeding rate in the treated group (12.5% vs 47%; $p < 0.001$). The results were quite similar in the study of Oxner et al. (70) with rebleeding of 16.7% in the injection group as compared to 46.7% in the control group ($p = 0.011$).

Trials Comparing Different Injection Methods or Injection with Thermal Therapy

In a controlled randomized comparative trial [71] we have shown that injection therapy with epinephrine followed by polidocanol is more effective in preventing rebleeding from ulcers with bleeding and nonbleeding visible vessels than injection of epinephrine alone, and at least as effective as injection of epinephrine followed by YAG laser therapy. In a subsequent trial [72] we found injection of absolute ethanol to be comparable to injection of epinephrine-pollidocanol for prevention of rebleeding from ulcers with nonbleeding visible vessels.

In a prospective randomized trial involving 64 patients with bleeding ulcers Balanzo et al. [73] compared injection therapy using epinephrine with injection of epinephrine plus thrombin. The addition of thrombin to epinephrine did not improve the results of therapy.

Laine [74] in a trial comparing injection therapy with absolute ethanol with multipolar electrocoagulation (MPEC), found both methods to be equally effective and safe for controlling active bleeding from peptic ulcers or preventing rebleeding from ulcers with a nonbleeding visible vessel.

In a prospective randomized trial, Chung et al. [75], compared the efficacy of endoscopic epinephrine injection and heater probe in actively bleeding peptic ulcers. Bleeding was initially better controlled with epinephrine injection (96%) than with heater probe (83%; $p < 0.05$), but outcome was more comparable in both groups. In the heater probe group there were two perforations.

In a randomized controlled trial comparing absolute alcohol injection with heater probe for the treatment of bleeding and nonbleeding vessels from peptic ulcers, Lin et al. [76] found the heater probe to be more effective than injection. In this trial emergency both techniques reduced surgery and mortality rates compared to controls.

Injection Therapy Prior to Thermal Modalities

Thermal modalities, especially laser photocoagulation, are difficult to use in the presence of active bleeding. Therefore, temporary hemostasis can be achieved by pretreatment with epinephrine. Pretreatment with epinephrine greatly improves the efficacy of YAG laser therapy [25, 77]. However, a recent comparative trial by Loizou and Bown [78] has shown that epinephrine injection alone is as effective as epinephrine followed by YAG laser photocoagulation.

Complications

The experimental studies have shown that most of the sclerosants used may cause important stomach wall injury. Clinical experience has also shown that injection therapy is associated with about the same complication rate as thermal therapy. Induction of active bleeding is rare and is usually the consequence of touching the visible vessel when the needle is advanced through the biopsy channel. Perforations have been described with injection of absolute ethanol, polidocanol, and ethanolamine oleate [52, 79–81].

Conclusions

Data on the efficacy of injection therapy for hemostasis of peptic ulcer bleeding are growing rapidly. The available studies show clearly that the method is simple and efficacious and probably as effective as thermal treatment modalities. The main therapeutic problem remains the 10%–20% treatment failures, mostly due to the large size of arteries in the ulcer. More studies are necessary to identify modalities or combinations of modalities that will allow a reduction in failure rates.

References

1. Allan R, Dykes P (1976) A study of the factors influencing mortality rates from gastrointestinal hemorrhage. Q J Med (NS) 180:533–538
2. Avery-Jones F (1956) Hematemesis and melaena with special reference to causation and to factors influencing the mortality from bleeding peptic ulcers. Gastroenterology 30:166–169
3. Schiller KFR, Truelove SG, Williams DG (1970) Haematemesis and melaena, with special reference to factors influencing outcome. Br Med J 2:7–14
4. Silverstein FE, Gilbert DA, Tedesco FJ et al. (1981) The national ASGE survey on upper gastrointestinal bleeding. Parts 1–3. Gastrointest Endosc 27:73–102
5. Foster DN, Miloszewski KJA, Losowsky MS (1978) Stigmata of recent haemorrhage in diagnosis and prognosis of upper gastrointestinal bleeding. Br Med J 1:1173–1177
6. Griffiths WJ, Neumann DA, Welsh JD (1979) The visible vessel as an indicator of uncontrolled or recurrent gastrointestinal haemorrhage. N Engl. J Med 300 (1): 411–413
7. Storey DW, Bown SG, Swain CP (1981) Endoscopic prediction of recurrent bleeding of peptic ulcers. N Engl J Med 305:915–916
8. Swain CP, Storey DW, Bown SG, Heath J, Mills TN, Salmon PR, Northfield TC, Kirkham JS, O'Sullivan JP (1986) Nature of the bleeding vessel in recurrently bleeding gastric ulcers. Gastroenterology 90:595–608

9. Wara P (1985) Endoscopic prediction of major rebleeding – a prospective study of stigmata of hemorrhage in bleeding ulcers. Gastroenterology 88:1209–1214
10. Bornman PC, Theodorou NA, Shuttleworth RD, Essel HP, Marks IN (1985) Importance of hypovolemic shock and endoscopic signs in predicting recurrent hemorrhage from peptic ulceration: a prospective evaluation. BMJ 291:245–247
11. Bown SG, Salmon PR, Storey DW (1980) Neodymium-YAG laser photocoagulation in the dog stomach. Gut 21:818–825
12. Geboes K, Rutgeerts P, Vantrappen G (1980) A microscopic and ultrastructural study of hemostasis after laser photocoagulation. Gastrointest Endosc 26:131–133
13. Rutgeerts P, Vantrappen G, Geboes K (1981) Safety and efficacy of Neodymium-YAG laser photocoagulation – an experimental study in dogs. Gut 22:38–44
14. Kiefhaber P, Nath G, Moritz K (1977) Endoscopic control of irradiation with a high power neodymium YAG laser. Prog. Surg. 15:140–145
15. Dwyer RM, Yellin AE, Craig J (1976) Gastric hemostasis by laser phototherapy in man. J Am Med Assoc 236:1383–1386
16. Sander R, Pösl H, Spuhler A, Hitzler H (1981) Der Neodymium-YAG-Laser: Ein effectives Instrument für die Stillung lebensbedrohlicher Gastrointestinalbutungen. Leber Magen Darm 11 (1):31–36
17. Shönekäs: personal communication
18. Rutgeerts P, Vantrappen G, Geboes K, Broeckaert L (1983) Neodymium-YAG laser photocoagulation for hemostasis of gastrointestinal non-variceal hemorrhage. Z Gastroenterol 21:263–267
19. Escourrou J. Frexinos J, Bommelaer G et al. (1981) Prospective randomized study of YAG photocoagulation in gastrointestinal bleeding. In: Atsumi, Nimsakul N (eds) Proceedings of laser Tokyo, pp 5–30
20. Ihre T, Johansson C, Seligson U et al. (1981) Endoscopic YAG laser treatment in massive upper gastrointestinal bleeding. Scan J Gastroenterol 16:633–640
21. Kreis GJ, Little KH, Westergaard H et al. (1985) Laser photocoagulation for the treatment of acute peptic ulcer bleeding: a randomized controlled clinical trial. Gastroenterology 88:1457
22. McLeod I, Mills PR, MacKenzie JF et al. (1983) Neodymium YAG laser photocoagulation for major hemorrhage from peptic ulcers and single vessels. Br Med J 286:345–348
23. Rutgeerts P, Vantrappen G, Broeckaert L, Janssens J, Coremans G, Geboes K, Schurmans P (1992) Controlled trial of YAG laser treatment of upper digestive hemorrhage. Gastroenterology 83:410–4216
24. Swain CP, Bown SG, Salmon PR et al. (1986) Controlled trial of neodymium YAG laser photocoagulation in bleeding peptic ulcers. Lancet 1: 1113–1117
25. Rutgeerts P, Vantrappen G, Broeckaert L (1984) A new and effective technique of YAG laser photocoagulation for severe upper gastrointestinal bleeding. Endoscopy 16:115–117
26. Papp JP (1982) Endoscopic electrocoagulation in the management of upper gastrointestinal tract bleeding. Surg Clin North Am 62:797–806
27. Gaisford WD (1979) Endoscopic electro-haemostasis with active upper gastrointestinal bleeding. Am J Surg 137:47–53
28. Volpicelli NA, McCarthy JD, Bartlett JD, Badger WE (1978) Endoscopic electrocoagulation. An alternative to operative therapy in bleeding peptic ulcers. Arch Surg 113:483–486
29. Sugawa C, Shier M, Lucas CE, Walt AJ (1975) Electrocoagulation of bleeding in the upper part of the gastrointestinal tract. Arch Surg 110:975–979
30. Wara P, Hojsgaard A, Amdrup E (1980) Endoscopic electrocoagulation – An alternative to operative hemostasis in active gastroduodenal bleeding? Endoscopy 12:237–240
31. Koch M, Pesche MJ, Bauerla M (1972) Erste experimentelle Untersuchungen und klinische Erfahrungen zur Elektrocoagulation blutenden Läsionen im oberen Gastrointestinaltrakt. Fortschr Endoscop 67:10
32. Papp JP (1979) Endoscopic electrocoagulation of the non bleeding visible ulcer vessel. Gastrointest Endosc 28:45–46
33. Matek W, Fruhmorgen P, Kaduk P, Reidenbach HD, Bodem F, Demling L (1979) Modified electrocoagulation and its possibilities in the control of gastrointestinal bleeding. Endoscopy 11:253–258

34. Freitas D, Donato A, Monteiro JG (1985) Controlled trial of liquid monopolar electrocoagulation in bleeding peptic ulcers. Am J Gastroenterol 80:853–857
35. Boix J. Planas R, Humbert C, Fabrega C, Villagrassa M (1987) Endoscopic hemostasis by injection therapy and electro-hydro-coagulation in high-risk patients with active gastroduodenal bleeding ulcer. Endoscopy 19:225–227
36. Gilbert DA, Verhoeven T, Jessen K, Bown G, Bowers JM, Papp JP (1982) Endoscopy in upper gastrointestinal bleeding. Gastrointest Endosc 27:94–102
37. Jensen DM, Machicado GA, Silpa ML (1984) Argon laser versus heater probe or bicap for control of severe ulcer bleeding. Gastrointest Endosc 30:134
38. Jessen K (1983) Bicap control of UGI bleeding. Gastroenterology 21:68A
39. Hajiro K, Yamamoto H, Matsui H (1984) Endoscopic bipolar electrocoagulation in upper gastrointestinal bleeding. Endoscopy 16:6–9
40. Donahue PE, Morbarhan S, Layden TJ, Nyhus LM (1984) Endoscopic control of upper gastrointestinal hemorrhage with a bipolar coagulation device. Surg Gynecol Obstet 159:113–118
41. Winkler WP, Comer G, McCray RS (1983) Initial experience with bicap multipolar electrocautery in the control of upper gastrointestinal hemorrhage. Gastrointest Endosc 29:169A
42. Goudie BM, Mitchell KG, Birnie GG, Mackey C (1984) Controlled trial of endoscopic bipolar electrocoagulation in the treatment of bleeding peptic ulcers. Gut 25:A1185
43. Kernohan RM, Anderson JR, McKelvey STD, Kennedy TL (1984) A controlled trial of bipolar electrocoagulation in patients with upper gastrointestinal bleeding. Br J Surg 71:889–891
44. O'Brien J, Day SJ, Burnham W (1986) Controlled trial of small bipolar probe in bleeding peptic ulcers. Lancet 1:464–467
45. Laine L (1987) A controlled trial of multipolar electrocoagulation in the treatment of the upper gastrointestinal hemorrhage. N Engl J Med 316:1613–1617
46. Goff JS (1986) Bipolar coagulation versus Neodymium-YAG laser photocoagulation for upper gastrointestinal bleeding lesions. Dig Dis Sci 31:906–910
47. Rutgeerts P, Vantrappen G, Van Hootegem Ph, Broeckaert L, Janssens J, Coremans G, Geboes K (1987) Neodymium-YAG laser photocoagulation versus multipolar electrocoagulation for the treatment of severely bleeding peptic ulcers: a randomized comparison. Gastrointest Endosc 33:199–202
48. Johnston J, Stones J, Long B (1984) Heater probe is superior to YAG laser in clinical endoscopic treatment of major bleeding from peptic ulcers. Gastrointest Endosc 30:154–156
49. Matthewson K, Swain CP, Bland M, Kirkham JS, Bown SG, Northfield TC (1990) Randomized comparison of Nd YAG laser, heater probe and no endoscopic therapy for bleeding peptic ulcers. Gastroenterology 98:1239–1244
50. Soehendra N, Grimm H, Stenzel M (1985) Injection of non-variceal bleeding lesions of the upper gastrointestinal tract. Endoscopy 17:129–132
51. Kortan P, Haber G, Marcon N (1986) Endoscopic injection for non variceal bleeding lesions of the upper gastrointestinal tract. Gastrointest Endosc 32:145
52. Asaki S, Nishimura T, Iwai S (1981) Tissue solidification in coping with digestive tract bleeding – hemostatic effect of local injection of 99.5% ethanol. Gastrointest Endosc 23:792–799
53. Asaki S, Nishimura T, Saloh A (1983) Endoscopic control of gastrointestinal hemorrhage by local injection of absolute ethanol: a basic assessment of the procedure. Tohoku J Exp Med 141:373–383
54. Chen P, Wu, CS, Liaw YF (1986) Hemostatic effect of endoscopic local injection with hypertonic saline-epinephrine solution and pure ethanol for digestive tract bleeding. Gastrointest Endosc 32:319–323
55. Fuchs KH, Wintz HJ, Schaube H (1986) Initial experience with thrombin as injection agent for bleeding gastroduodenal lesions. Endoscopy 18:146–148
56. Naka H, Matsuura K (1983) Hemostatic effect on endoscopic local injection of hypertonic saline epinephrine (HS-E) solution to arrest hemorrhage from the digestive tract. Gastrointest Endosc 25:1612–1616
57. Hirao M, Kobayaski T, Masuda K (1985) Endoscopic local injection of hypertonic saline-epinephrine solution to arrest hemorrhage from the upper gastrointestinal tract. Gastrointest Endosc 31:313–317

58. Hirao M, Yamazaki H, Masuda K (1980) Hemostatic procedure by endoscope for gastrointestinal bleeding: clinical practice of endoscopic local injection of hypertonic epinephrine (HS-E) solution. Stomach Intestin 7:751–755
59. Sugawa C, Fujita Y, Ikeda T (1986) Endoscopic hemostasis of bleeding of the upper gastrointestinal tract by local injection of ninety-eight per cent dehydrated ethanol. Surg Gynec Obstet 162:159–163
60. Wördehoff D, Gros H (1982) Endoscopic haemostasis by injection therapy in high-risk patients. Endoscopy 14:196–199
61. Friederichs O, Beecu L, Knieriem HJ, Papen J, Sabinasz A (1990) Submuköse Fibrinklebung bei peptischen Blutungen. In: Harüng R (ed) Gastrointestinale Blutung. Blackwell Ueberreuter, 101–108
62. Rutgeerts P, Geboes K, Vantrappen G (1989) Experimental studies of injection therapy for severe nonvariceal bleeding in dogs. Gastroenterology 97:610–621
63. Swain CP, Kalabakas A (1991) A randomized controlled comparison of injection of epinephrine, polidocanol, alcohol, hypertonic saline, normal saline and bipolar electrocoagulation in treatment of standard experimental ulcers and bleeding mesenteric vessels. Gastroenterology 100:A170
64. Randall GM, Jensen DM, Hirabayashi K, Machicado GA (1989) Controlled study of different sclerosing agents for coagulation of canine gut arteries. Gastroenterology 96:1274–1281
65. Chung SCS, Leung JWC, Steele RJC, Crofts TJ, Li AKG (1988) Endoscopic injection of adrenaline for actively bleeding ulcers: a randomized trial. Br Med J 296:1631–1633
66. Panes J, Forné M, Marco C, Viver J, Garcia-Olicones E, Garau J (1987) Controlled trial of endoscopic sclerosis in bleeding peptic ulcers. Lancet ii:1292–1294
67. Balanzo J, Sainz S, Such J, Espinos JC, Guarner G, Casso X, Mones J, Villardel F (1988) Endoscopic hemostasis by local injection of epinephrine and polidocanol in bleeding ulcer. A prospective randomized trial. Endoscopy 20:289–291.
68. Pascu O, Drãghici A, Acalovehi I (1989) The effect of endoscopic hemostasis with alcohol on the mortality rate of non variceal upper GI hemorrhage. A randomized prospective study. Endoscopy 21:53–55
69. Rajgopal C, Palmer KR (1991) Endoscopic injection sclerosis: effective treatment for peptic ulcer. Gut 32:727–729
70. Oxner RBG, Simmonds NJ, Gertner DJ, Nightingale JMD, Burnham WR (1992) Controlled trial of endoscopic injection treatment for bleeding from peptic ulcers with visible vessels. Lancet 339:966–968.
71. Rutgeerts P, Broeckaert L, Janssens J, Vantrappen G, Coremans G, Hiele M (1989) Comparison of endoscopic polidocanol injection and YAG laser therapy for bleeding peptic ulcers. Lancet I:1164–1167
72. Rutgeerts P, Gevers AM, Hiele M, Broeckaert L, Coremans G, Janssens J, Vantrappen G (1990) Injection therapy for prevention of rebleeding from peptic ulcers with protruding vessel: which method is best? Gastroenterology 98:A115
73. Balanzo J, Villanueva C, Sainz S, Espinos JC, Mendez C, Guarner C, Vilardell F (1990) Injection therapy of bleeding peptic ulcer. A prospective randomized trial using epinephrine and thrombin. Endoscopy 22:157–159
74. Laine L (1990) Multipolar electrocoagulation versus injection therapy in the treatment of bleeding peptic ulcers. A prospective randomized trial. Gastroenterology 99:1303–1306.
75. Chung CSC, Leung JWC, Sung JY, Lo KK, Li AKC (1991) Injection or heat probe for bleeding ulcer. Gastroenterology 100:33–37.
76. Lin HJ, Lee FY, Kang WM, Tsai YT, Lee SD, Lee CH (1990) Heat probe thermocoagulation and purealcohol injection in massive peptic ulcer haemorrhage: a prospective randomized controlled trial. Gut 31:753–757.
77. Heldwein W, Lehnert P, Martinoff S, Loeschke K (1988) Local epinephrine injection improves the therapeutic effect of Nd-YAG laser treatment of arterial peptic ulcer bleeding. Endoscopy 20:2–4
78. Loizou LA, Bown SG (1991) Endoscopic treatment for bleeding peptic ulcers: randomized comparison of adrenaline injection and adrenaline injection + Nd:YAG laser. Gut 12:1100–1103

79. Levy J, Khakoo S, Barton R, Vicary R (1991) Fatal injection sclerotherapy of a bleeding ulcer. Lancet 337:504
80. Chester JF, Hurley PR (1990) Gastric necrosis: a complication of endoscopic sclerosis for bleeding peptic ulcer. Endoscopy 22:287–288
81. Loperfido S, Patelli G, La Torre L (1990) Extensive necrosis of gastric mucosa following injection therapy of bleeding peptic ulcer. Endoscopy 22:285–286

Are There Any Indications for Surgery in Peptic Ulcers Today?

B. Reers and H. Bünte

Introduction

One hundred and eleven years after it began, the operative treatment of ulcers is once again–or, rather, still–under discussion. Even the first gastric resection for ulcer disease, performed by Rydygiér [13], met with not unmixed criticism. In the past few decades, it has been repeatedly asserted that operative ulcer treatment has reached the peak of its development [1]. Every time, however, further improvements proved to be possible. The most decisive turn in the development of operative treatment for ulcer disease was no doubt the arrival of the potent stomach drugs of the histamine H_2-receptor blocker type. The question in the title of the present chapter refers to this event.

Operative Treatment of Ulcers in Münster

Between 1973 and 1991, 1279 patients were operated on for peptic ulcer in the General Surgery Department of the Münster University Hospital (Fig. 1). Sixty-five percent of the patients were undergoing first operations, while in 35% repeat operations were being carried out.

Professor Bünte took over as head of department in the middle of 1973; in the remaining months of the year 30 patients were operated on. Up until 1977 the number of operations increased annually up to about 120 a year. With the advent of H_2-receptor blockers, the number of ulcer operations in our hospital dropped sharply from 1979 onwards. In the past few years, they have levelled out at about a quarter of the number performed every year in the "heyday" of ulcer surgery. At present, only about 30 operations a year are performed in our hospital for gastroduodenal ulcers.

Over the course of the past 18 years, 34% of all operative ulcer patients underwent surgery for acute ulcer complication. Chronic complications were the indication in 30%. Twenty percent of the patients underwent surgery because they did not respond to medical therapy, while in the remaining 16% the indications were complicated and related to particular problems of the individual patients (Fig. 2). This last group includes patients from abroad who were completely free of complaints under conservative treatment here, but whose further treatment when they returned to their countries of origin could not be

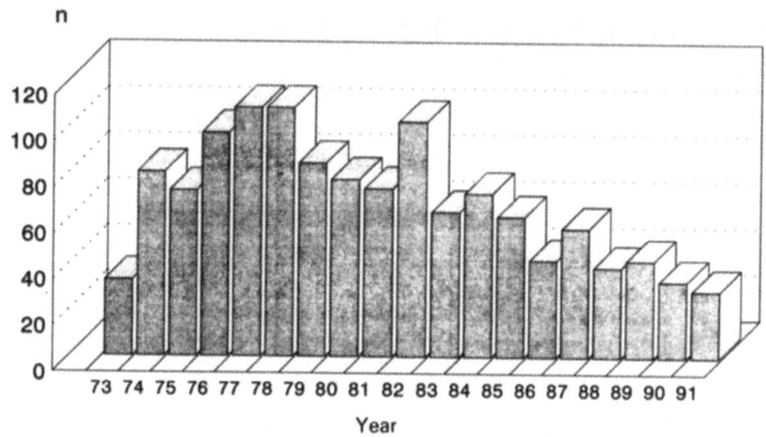

Fig. 1. Evolution of surgical operations for gastroduodenal ulcer at Münster University Hospital: number of operations per year (n = 1279)

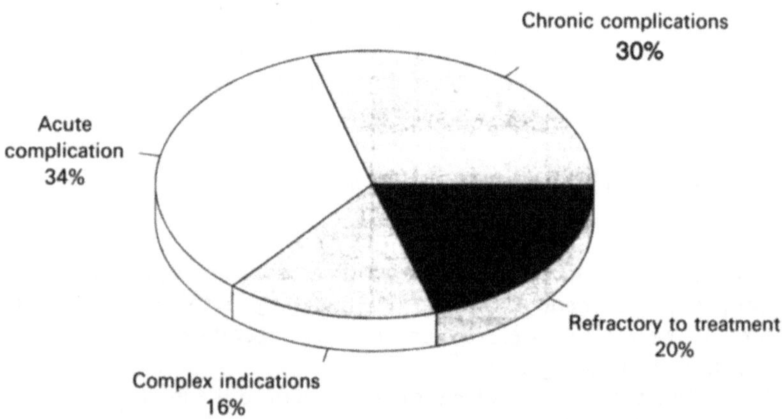

Fig. 2. Distribution of indications for surgery for gastroduodenal ulcer from 1973 to 1991

guaranteed. This can always constitute an indication for surgery in individual cases.

Regressional analysis carried out by computer shows a clear drop in the number of gastroduodenal ulcer operations (Fig. 3). The line of regression calculated by the computer tends towards zero, although it will never quite reach it. This is a tendency that has been seen the world over in recent years [4, 9, 11, 14, 16, 18].

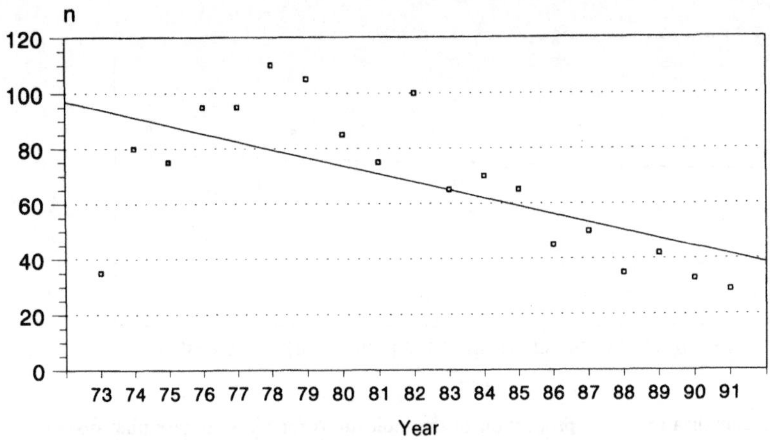

Fig. 3. Analysis of evolution of number of operations for gastroduodenal ulcer 1973–1991: regressional analysis using a computer ($n = 1279$)

Acute Complications

In absolute figures, the number of operations undertaken by us for acute complications of ulcers (haemorrhage, perforation) is also decreasing, but the proportion they represent of all ulcer operations is increasing (Fig. 4). Continuous and even increasing incidences of acute ulcer complications requiring surgery are reported by many centres [4, 11, 14, 18].

About two-thirds of the acute complications of ulcers are haemorrhage. This complication, in which up until about 8 years ago surgical control was bringing about ever better results, has more recently been associated with as high mortality. One reason for this is that such complications occur more among older patients [14, 18], but another is that in the past few years conservative treatment has become more widespread and increasingly uncritically employed, resulting in considerable worsening of the prognosis of surgical treatment. Here we can only support the concept put forward in the previous chapter, that of course at first conservative treatment is indicated, in which emergency endoscopy should aim to locate the source of the bleeding as well as stop it. This is just how we manage bleeding ulcers primarily admitted to our care. In our department, as in the Department of Internal Medicine, there is a round-the-clock endoscopy service, so that we too can perform emergency endoscopy immediately on the patient's admission. If one keeps to the principle that two endoscopic attempts at arresting haemorrhage are the maximum allowed, the serious consequence of continuing a conservative therapy that is no longer adequate to the circumstances will be avoided. In some years we found that in more than half the patients mass transfusions had already led to extremely severe pulmonary damage, and that their coagulation systems were

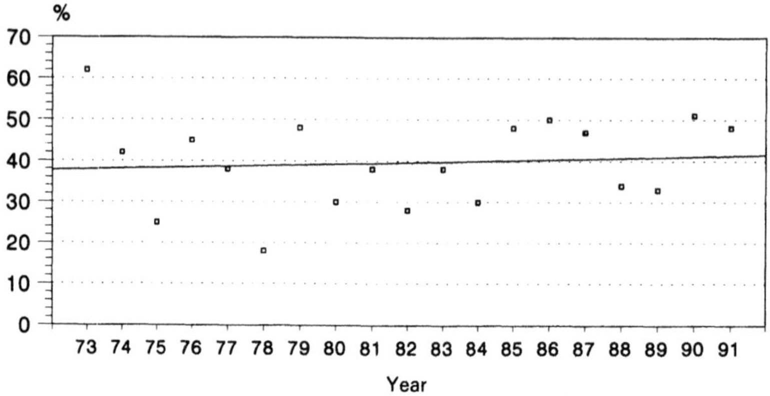

Fig. 4. Acute complications as a proportion of the indications for ulcer surgery (first operation) 1973–1991

irreparably damaged by the continuous bleeding. In such situations, surgery is usually not more than a last desperate effort and associated with an enormously increased mortality. These bad experiences have led us to recommend a relatively aggressive approach to bleeding ulcers, requiring close cooperation between the internist or intensive care specialist and the surgeon [12]. Even among patients whose haemorrhage has been successfully arrested endoscopically, those with a Forrest type Ia haemorrhage or with a visible vascular stump not bleeding at present (Forrest type II) should undergo definitive elective surgery at once.

Perforation of the ulcer is a classical indication for surgery, and will probably remain so. Completely conservative treatment without opening the abdomen is still indicated in only a few exceptional cases. An alternative to the classical surgical operation that has arisen in the past few years is the laparoscopy procedure, whereby the perforated ulcer is sewn or stapled together and the abdominal cavity can at the same time be given a thorough lavage [10]. Definitive surgical treatment is not possible with this method, however, despite the fact that in many places laparoscopic vagotomy using Taylor's procedure is offered for this indication.

Chronic Complications

The proportion of cases in which chronic complications (penetration and pyloric stenosis) are given as reasons for peptic ulcer surgery has increased continuously in the past few years. At present, about 60% of all operations are carried out for this reason (Fig. 5).

Looking at this group of cases in detail, it can be seen that as far as numbers are concerned, the rise in frequency of this indication for operation is clearly due to the increased incidence of pyloric stenosis (Fig. 6). On the other hand, the

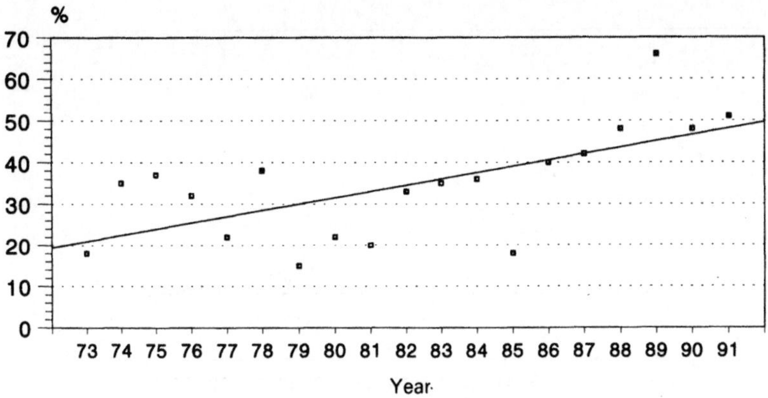

Fig. 5. Chronic complications as a proportion of the indications for ulcer surgery (first operation) 1973–1991

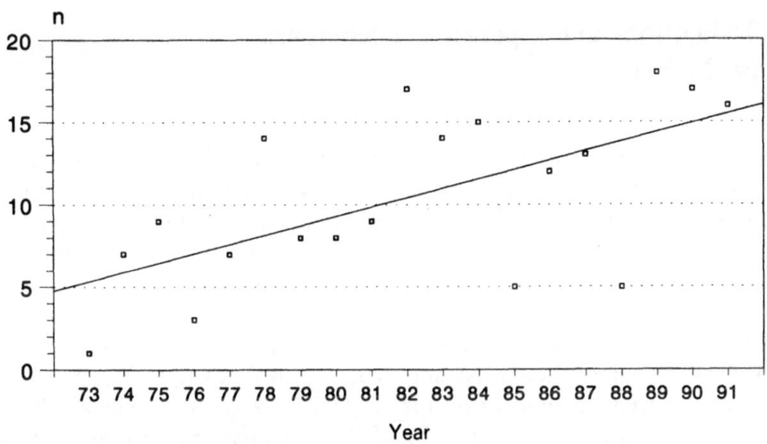

Fig. 6. Numbers of cases of pyloric stenosis due to scarring 1973–1991

numbers of cases of ulcer penetration have dropped very considerably in the past 10 years (Fig. 7). Quite obviously, modern ulcer therapy is capable of bringing about the healing of practically all ulcers, so that penetration as a manifestation of failed conservative treatment has become virtually unknown. However, conservative treatment has no control over the scarring that takes place during healing, and for this reason scar stenosis of the pylorus repeatedly occurs in patients with recurrent gastroduodenal ulcers. For this condition, resection alone seems to promise success. Vagotomy with pyloroplasty creates an unphysiological environment with duodenogastric reflux, while conservative dilatation of the pyloric stenosis cannot prevent later ulcers from forming new scars.

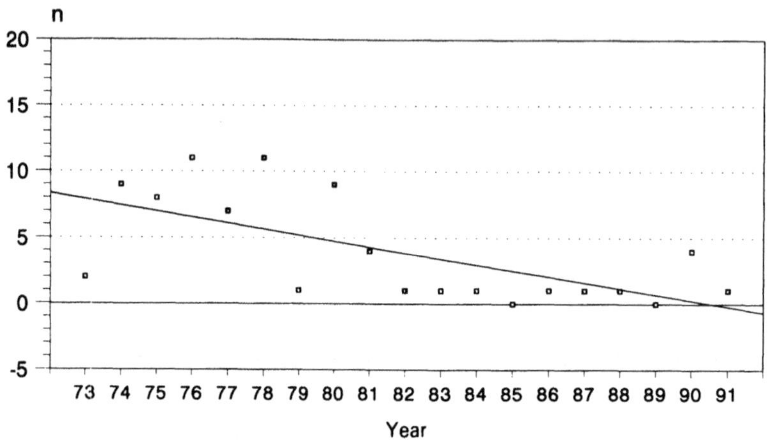

Fig. 7. Numbers of cases of ulcer penetration as indication for ulcer surgery 1973–1991

Surgical Indications and Operative Techniques in the Past 20 Years

Looking at the changes over time in our own patient population, we find that from 1973 to 1988, acute complications (haemorrhage and perforation) made up 40% of all operative indications. This figure has not changed much in the past 3 years, although the reduction in the overall number of ulcer operations means that the percentage represents a smaller actual number. Haemorrhages make up two-thirds of the acute complications.

Up until 1988, chronic complications represented only about 30% of the operative indications; since then it has doubled, so that today pyloric stenosis is definitely the most frequent indication for surgery on a gastroduodenal ulcer. Refractory ulcers represented about 36% of the operative indications overall over the last 20 years. For the past 3–4 years alone, however, it is impossible to calculate a meaningful percentage, since refractoriness to treatment was seen only in very unusual cases, and only one patient or at most two per year were operated on for this reason. We can hardly remember when we last operated for uncomplicated, treatment-refractory gastroduodenal ulcer (Table 1).

The tendencies we describe here largely match the findings of a survey carried out by the German Surgeons' Association in 1989. In university surgical departments, distal gastric resection for ulcer treatment is no longer listed under the ten most common operations (Fig. 8). The enthusiastically fêted vagotomy as operative procedure of choice in gastroduodenal ulcers had a temporary boom at the end of the 1970s, but has now lost significance and has become a rarely performed procedure. The incidence of operations for ulcer complications dropped considerably around 1979; however, the success of conservative treatment is obviously leading to another rise in these complications, so that these procedures are now carried out as often as they were in 1969.

Table 1. Comparison of cases of peptic ulcer undergoing surgery at the Münster University Hospital 1973–1988 and 1988–1991

		%
1989–1991	Acute haemorrhage	28
	Perforation	15
	Total	43
1973–1988	Acute complications	40
1989–1991	Chronic complications	57
1973–1988	Chronic complications	30
1973–1991	Uncomplicated ulcers	36
1992	Uncomplicated ulcers	0

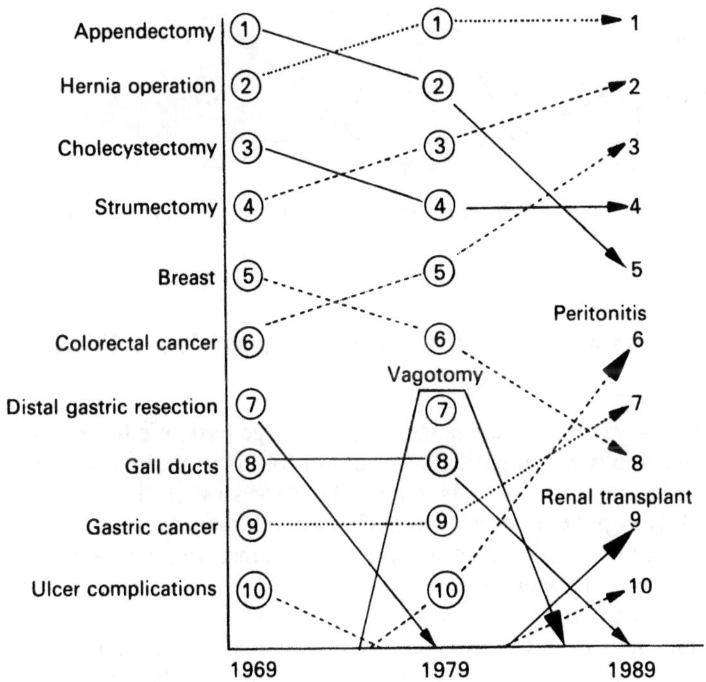

Fig. 8. Changes in the rank order of the ten most common operations in university hospitals 1969–1989. (From [16])

A similar picture is seen in the large municipal hospitals (Fig. 9). Here too, distal resection of the stomach is much less often performed, even though it is still among the ten most common procedures in these hospitals. Distal gastric resection as an elective procedure has, however, been far overtaken by operations for ulcer complications. After a heyday around 1979, vagotomy has also fallen into comparative disuse.

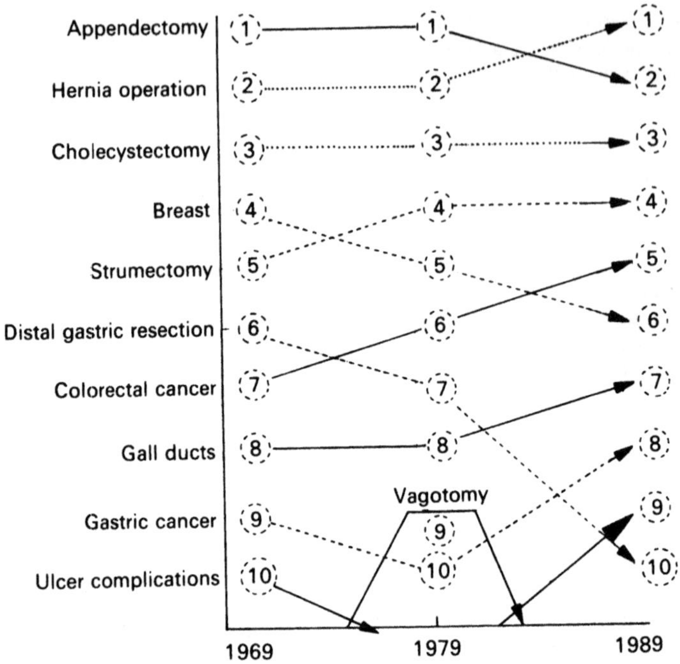

Fig. 9. Changes in the rank order of the ten most common operations in municipal hospitals 1969–1989. (From [16])

The Münster Treatment Plan for Gastroduodenal Ulcer Disease

Among our patients, vagotomy has never played a large part. We have always been very selective about which patients we submit to this procedure, and were very critical of the euphoric reports about the successes of this operative technique [2]. Only in patients whose stomach was undamaged and who either had a duodenal ulcer that really was unresponsive to conservative treatment or in whom conservative treatment was not possible did we carry out proximal selective vagotomy. In patients with ulcer complications, a long, chronic ulcer history or organic changes in the stomach, we always performed resection [6]. Now as before, the various forms of vagotomy are still regarded as standard therapy for duodenal ulcer in many hospitals [3, 7–9, 11, 14, 18], but it seems that even the greatest afficionados of the technique have to accept recurrence rates of up to 40%. Even if recurrence after vagotomy is less symptomatic [9], it must be asked whether this operative technique is still justified given the possibilities of medical treatment today. Despite the introduction of modernizations such as laparoscopic vagotomy [5], we tend to agree with Alexander-Williams [1], who sees this technique as dying out.

On the strength of experimental and clinical studies, since the mid-1970s we have progressively introduced high gastric resection with gastroenterostomy

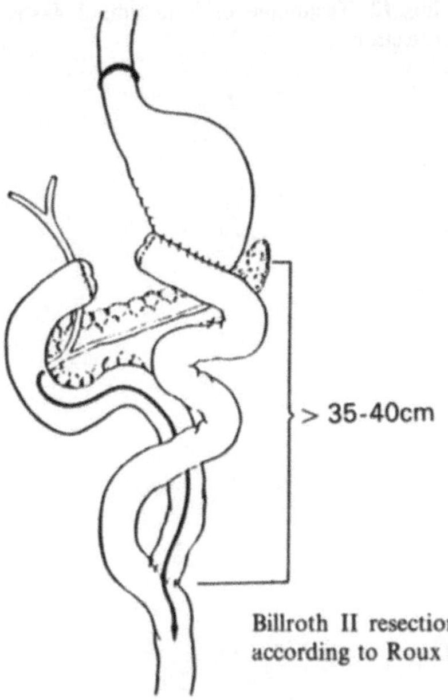

Fig. 10. Diagram of the operative technique together with the technical advantages of high gastric resection with Roux' gastroenterostomy

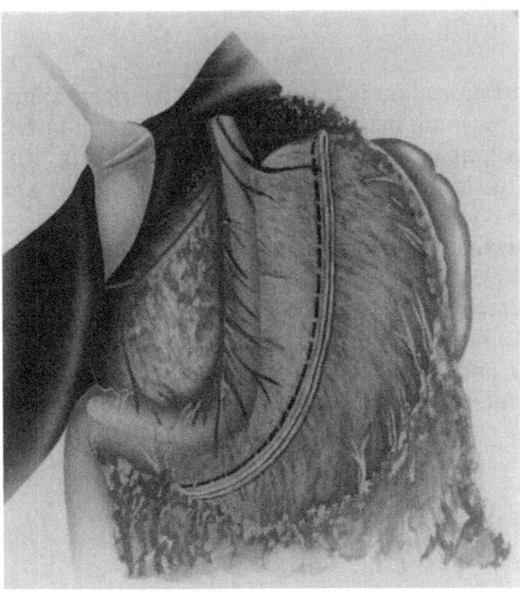

Fig. 11. Longitudinal gastric resection

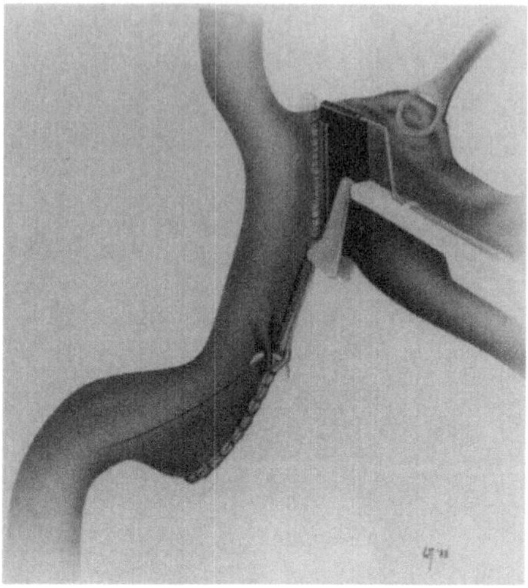

Fig. 12. Technique of longitudinal gastric resection

Table 2. Our results after high gastric resection with Roux' gastroenterostomy

Mortality	2.2%
Duodenal stump insufficiency	0.8%
Ulcer recurrence (clinical)	2.5%

according to Roux as the standard procedure in operative ulcer treatment. This has many advantages over other resection methods, and leads to a much lower recurrence rate than vagotomy as long as it is competently performed (Fig. 10). If the resection is too small and the loop is of the wrong length then ulcers are likely to recur after this operation.

Our experiences with this technique in our own patients have been extremely good (Table 2). Mortality is comparable to if not lower than that associated with other operative techniques, and the rate of duodenal stump insufficiency is remarkably low. Clinical symptoms of recurrence have occurred in 2.5% of our patients. Probably, endoscopic follow-up of all operated patients would show a higher rate of recurrent ulcers, but the patients obviously feel untroubled by them.

Conclusion

We see the answer to the question contained in the title of this chapter as follows:

1. Surgery continues to have a firm place in the treatment of gastroduodenal ulcers.
2. Uncomplicated ulcers are unquestionably candidates for conservative treatment. Refractory ulcer as an indication for surgery no longer exists.
3. The place for surgery is in acute and chronic complications of peptic ulcer. Close collaboration with the internists is particularly important in this area.
4. Vagotomy will continue to fade out as a treatment for peptic ulcer. This operative method can only achieve part of what can be done by successful conservative treatment, and will probably soon be of no more than historical interest.
5. A properly performed gastric resection results, with very few exceptions, in ulcer healing, and is accompanied by a very low mortality rate.

Perspectives

There have been many stocktakings in the history of surgery that have ended with the conclusion that the peak of perfection has currently been reached [1]. Despite of the decreasing significance of surgical ulcer treatment, it should be pointed out that here are many promising new areas of research too.

As early as in 1940, Wangensteen [19] introduced the method of longitudinal gastric resection. This concept was extended on the basis of theoretical considerations, and was further developed by Saegesser [15] up to 1966 as possibly the "ideal" gastric resection.

We took up this method and analysed it in large-scale animal experiments [17]. Results were excellent. This technique allowed the area of acid- and enzyme-producing gastric mucosa to be dramatically reduced without greatly impairing the physiological functions. No anastomoses had to be sewn, both baseline and maximally stimulated acid production were reduced by 70%, and there were almost no postoperative complications (Figs. 11, 12).

Encouraged by these superb experimental results, we employed the method in treating two patients with duodenal ulcers. As far as the ulcer was concerned, healing was complete and long-lasting. Unfortunately, both patients developed reflux oesophagitis due to hiatal insufficiency, which was obviously caused by the fundus resection. We are at present trying to get this sequela of the operative method under control.

It remains to be seen whether, given the overall development of peptic ulcer, indications will continue to exist for longitudinal gastric surgery. At all events, it should be remembered that development, in ulcer surgery as elsewhere, has by no means come to an end.

References

1. Alexander-Williams J (1991) A requiem for vagotomy – despite the last ditch efforts of surgeons. Br Med J 302:547–548
2. Bünte H (1971) Vagotomie: ein neuer Irrweg in der Ulkus-Chirurgie? Dtsch Med Wochenschr 96:633–640
3. Hildebrandt J, Herrmann U (1992) Die selektiv proximale Vagotomie mit und ohne Pyloroplastik beim unkomplizierten chronischen Ulcus duodeni. Zentralbl Chir 117:36–40
4. Jordan PH (1991) Surgery for peptic ulcer disease. Curr Probl Surg 28:265–330
5. Katkhouda N, Mouiel J (1991) A new technique of surgical treatment of chronic duodenal ulcer without laparotomy by videocoelioscopy. Am J Surg 161:361–364
6. Langhans P, Bünte H (1987) Operationsindikation und Verfahrenswahl beim Gastro-Duodenalulkus. In: Bünte H, Demling L, Domschke S, Langhans P (eds) Folgeerkrankungen in der Ulkuschirurgie. Edition Medizin, Weinheim, pp 27–45
7. Macintyre IM, Millar A (1991) Highly selective vagotomy – a safe operation for duodenal ulcer. Immediate and long-term complications and sequelae in 500 patients. Eur J Surg 157:261–265
8. Maddern GJ, Vauthey JN, Devitt P, Britten-Jones R, Hetzel DJ, Gamieson GG (1991) Recurrent peptic ulceration after highly selective vagotomy: long-term outcome. Br J Surg 78:940–941
9. McEntee G, Ryan W, Peel ALG, Rosenberg IL, Devlin HB (1988) A district general hospital experience of surgical treatment of gastric and duodenal ulcer from 1970 to 1982. Surg Gynecol Obstet 167:53–60
10. Mouret P, Francois Y, Vignal J, Barth X, Lombard-Platet R (1990) Laparoscopic treatment of perforated peptic ulcer. Br J Surg 77:1006
11. Paquet KJ (1986) Das Ulcus ventriculi, Ulcus duodeni und Anastomosenulkus aus chirurgischer Sicht. Therapiewoche 36:628–641
12. Reers B, Kautz G, Winde G (1991) Die Ulkusblutung–Therapiekonzept aus chirurgischer Sicht. Medwelt 42:198–206
13. Rydygiér L (1882) Die erste Magenresektion beim Magengeschwür. Zentralbl Chir 12:198–199
14. Sachdeva AK, Zaren HA, Sigel B (1991) Surgical treatment of peptic ulcer disease. Med Clin North Am 75:999–1012
15. Saegesser M (1966) Die operativen Maßnahmen bei Ulcus pepticum–die "ideale" Magenresektion. In: Saegesser M (ed) Der Ulkus-Magen. Pathologische und chirurgische Probleme. Huber, Bern
16. Siewert JR, Bollschweiler E, Hempel K (1990) Wandel der Eingriffshäufigkeit in der Allgemeinchirurgie. Chirurg 61:855–863
17. Spiegel HU (1992) Die Magenlängsresektion als alternatives chirurgisches Therapieverfahren zur Ulkusbehandlung?–Eine funktionelle und morphologische Studie. Thesis, Münster University
18. Taylor TV, Lythgoe JP, McFarland JB, Gilmore T, Thomas PE, Ferguson GH (1990) Anterior lesser curve seromyotomy and posterior truncal vagotomy versus truncal vagotomy and pyloroplasty in the treatment of chronic duodenal ulcer. Br J Surg 77:1007–1009
19. Wangensteen OH (1940) Aseptic gastric resection. I. A method of aseptic anastomosis adaptable to any segment of the alimentary canal (esophagus, stomach, small or large intestine). II. Including preliminary description of subtotal excision of the acid secreting area of ulcer. Surg Gynecol Obstet 70:59–70

Nonulcer Dyspepsia: A Diagnostic and Therapeutic Challenge

A. Berstad and T. Hausken

Introduction

Dyspepsia is a common complaint. When asked, about one in three to four of the population at large admits to suffering from dyspepsia [58, 66]. This high prevalence of dyspepsia is reflected in the general practitioner's consulting room. A Danish study reports that, in 1 year, 12% of the district's population went to see their doctor for dyspeptic complaint [30]. In Sweden, Adami et al. [1] found "gastritis" (clinically assessed) to be the fourth commonest diagnosis in general practice and the seventh commonest in outpatient clinics, accounting for 2% of all outpatient consultations, and for 31% of consultations for gastrointestinal disorders. On investigation, evidence of peptic ulcer disease may be found in only 20%–30% of dyspeptic patients, whilst in 20%–50% no definite pathology can be found to explain the symptoms [6, 15, 39, 47, 52, 53, 57].

The constellation of dyspeptic symptoms in the absence of demonstrable organic disease has been denoted "X-ray negative dyspepsia", "gastritis", "pseudo-ulcer syndrome", "functional dyspepsia", "non-organic dyspepsia", "nervous dyspepsia", and other names. The expression "pseudo-ulcer" [29] clearly reflects the previously dominant viewpoint that dyspepsia without ulcer probably represented a special, more peaceful, course of "ulcer disease", with subsequent development of ulcer in a large proportion of the patients [29, 62]. However, repeated observations have shown a low propensity to ulcer development in this patient group [17, 27, 51], which suggests that dyspepsia without ulcer is not merely a form of "ulcer disease" (Moynihan's disease) [48] but an entity on its own.

Recent discoveries have contributed considerably to progress in this area. It is now generally recognised that true ulcer disease is strongly associated with gastric infection with *H. pylori* [37, 60], whereas non-ulcer dyspepsia may be causally related to mental stress and abnormal filling of the gastric antrum [19, 46]. The latter stress-related type of dyspepsia is in this paper denoted *functional dyspepsia*. The condition seems unrelated to *H. pylori* infection. It appears, however, that gastric *H. pylori*, possibly by way of the induced *gastritis*, may in some cases cause dyspepsia and thus constitute a second subtype of non-ulcer dyspepsia. A third subgroup of non-ulcer dyspepsia patients may be those who present symptoms of *gastro-oesophageal reflux* (*GER*) in the absence of endoscopic oesophagitis. How large a percentage each of these subgroups makes up of the total non-ulcer dyspepsia population is at present unknown. Our personal guesses are that the dysmotility type comprises 80%, *H. pylori*-induced gastritis 10%, and GER without oesophagitis 10%, but, of course, great overlaps may exist.

Diagnosis

Non-ulcer dyspepsia is defined as symptoms indicative of ulcer, in the absence of ulcer, cancer, and oesophagitis as examined by upper alimentary endoscopy. Consequently, gastroscopy is obligatory for diagnosis. Attempts at distinguishing between organic and non-organic disease on the basis of symptoms alone greatly overdiagnose organic disease [26]. In our hospital, abdominal ultrasonography is also regularly performed as a primary diagnostic aid to exclude organic disease. As ultrasonographic equipment becomes more readily available, this practice will probably gain wider acceptance.

Classification of subgroups of dyspeptic patients according to symptoms has proved largely useless [56]. In the following, therefore, we will refer to the subgroups of non-ulcer dyspepsia alluded to above.

Functional Dyspepsia

Non-ulcer dyspepsia often does not respond to treatments that reduce gastric acidity [32, 41, 44, 64], which supports the view that the condition is not an "ulcer disease". Several studies indicate that disturbances of upper gastrointestinal motility are important. Such dysmotility can be induced by mental stress, and it is a widely held view that mental stress is an important cause of non-ulcer dyspepsia. The condition is, therefore, now often called "functional dyspepsia". The new thing is that the wish is to focus on the functional disturbance and get away from the old view that this type of dyspepsia is a weaker form of ulcer disease. Recent knowledge has taught us that functional dyspepsia is a distinct, stress-related disease without any clear relationship to ulcer disease [9]. Peptic ulcer disease is associated primarily with gastric *H. pyloric* infection — not with stress. The relationship between ulcer and stress is less clear than formerly believed [2]. It appears as if it is functional dyspepsia, not ulcer, that is the stress disease.

Stress

In a previous study Nesland et al. [40] noted that as many as 82% of their 101 patients with functional dyspepsia felt mental stress to be a considerable problem. At follow-up approximately 4 years later, 77% of the patients still complained of stress and none of the patients had developed active ulcer disease [51]. Nyren et al. [43] found that patients with functional dyspepsia had visited a psychiatrist, changed work, and had financial and additional non-abdominal complaints more often than healthy persons. Talley et al. [54, 55] found that increasing age, male gender, being unmarried, and having social class incongruity were associated with increased frequency and severity of non-ulcer dyspepsia. Hui et al. [23] found that these patients saw "major life events" more negatively than controls. These studies indicated, first, that psychological factors are strongly associated with functional dyspepsia, and, secondly, that functional dyspepsia is not a forerunner or a weaker form of the ulcer disease.

Recent studies have suggested mechanisms by which mental stress may play a causal role in functional dyspepsia. During exposure to stress a series of reactions are activated in the central nervous systems giving rise to efferent impulses to peripheral organs where stress reactions may become manifested. The stomach is one such organ where stress reactions easily become apparent, not by changes in acid production, but by quick changes in motility.

Dysmotility

Antral hypomotility [28, 36, 49], impaired antroduodenal coordination [31], disturbed intestinal motility [28, 36, 49], and delayed gastric emptying [24] are common findings in functional dyspepsia. Malagelada and Stanghellini [36] studied pressure activity in the stomach and upper intestine in 104 patients referred for evaluation of functional symptoms (nausea, vomiting, upper abdominal pain, or other dyspeptic symptoms in the absence of structural gut abnormalities). Manometric abnormalities were found in 75 patients. Forty-three of these had gastric abnormalities and 32 patients had both gastric and intestinal abnormalities. The hypomotility of the antrum was either due to decreased amplitude of the pressure waves, or lower frequency, or in most cases, a combination of both.

It appears that gastric emptying is delayed in a substantial proportion of patients with dyspepsia, but certainly not in all. The percentage of patients with abnormal gastric emptying varies between 30 and 44 [24, 63, 65]. Jian et al. [24] utilized a dual-isotope technique to measure simultaneously liquid and solid emptying in patients with idiopathic dyspepsia, and found that delayed emptying of liquids was more common than delayed emptying of solids. In contrast, Urbain et al. [61], also using a dual-radionuclide technique, found delayed emptying of solids, but not of liquids among patients with idiopathic dyspepsia.

Marked and quick changes of antral motility in response to stress can easily be visualized by conventional ultrasonography. The ultrasonographic sections we have used in our studies on antral motility are shown in Figs. 1 and 2. When a healthy person is fed 500 ml liquid meat soup (20 kcal), a fed motility pattern, i.e., approximately three antral contractions per minute, is elicited. Stress in the form of a video game where the test person is driving a car on a screen trying to

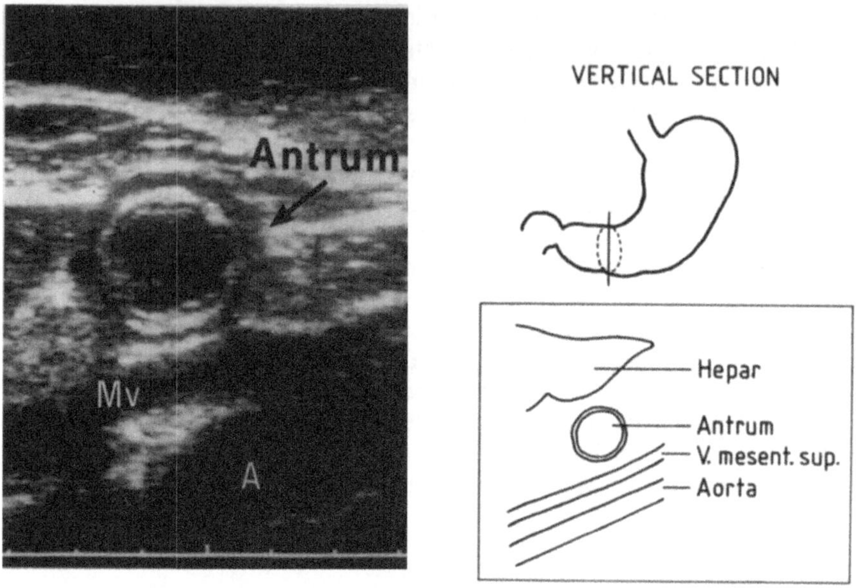

Fig. 1. Vertical ultrasonographic scan (*left*) and diagram of scan (*right*) though antrum, superior mesenteric vein (*Mv*), and aorta (*A*). *Calibration bars* indicate centimetres. This scan is used for monitoring numbers and amplitudes of antral contractions, and for calculating width of antral area. (From Hausken and Berstad [22])

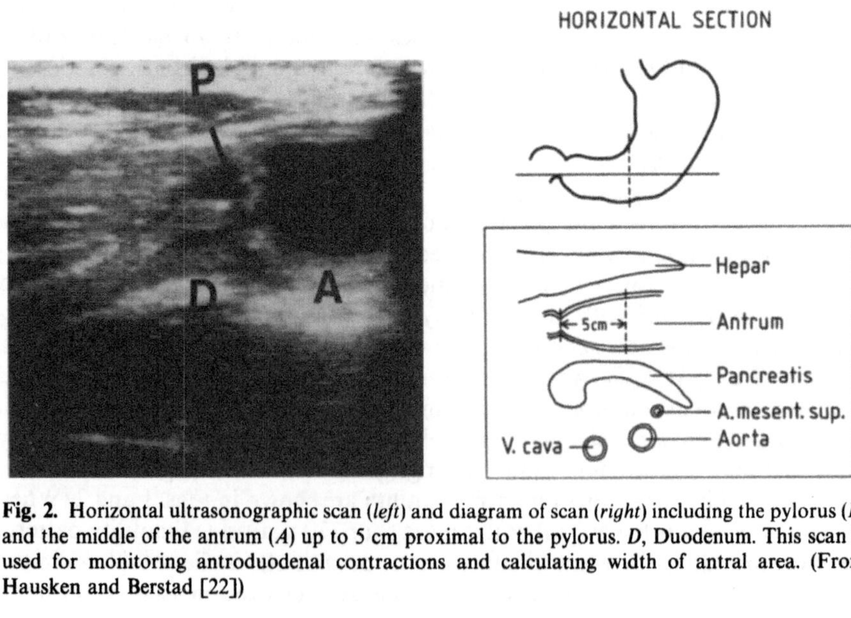

Fig. 2. Horizontal ultrasonographic scan (*left*) and diagram of scan (*right*) including the pylorus (*P*) and the middle of the antrum (*A*) up to 5 cm proximal to the pylorus. *D*, Duodenum. This scan is used for monitoring antroduodenal contractions and calculating width of antral area. (From Hausken and Berstad [22])

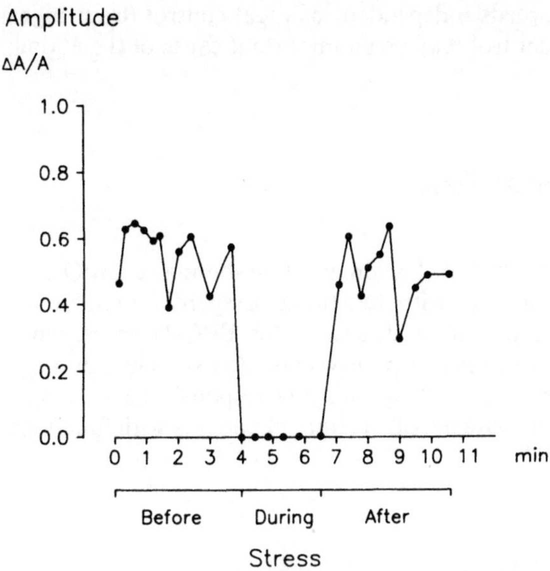

Fig. 3. Amplitude of antral contrations before, during and after acute mental stress induced by a video game in a healthy person. Note the rapid changes (diminution and restitution of amplitudes) in response to stress

avoid collision on a highway, is enough to virtually abolish the motility within seconds. Immediately after cessation of the stress exposure normal motility is resumed (Fig. 3). It is mainly the force (amplitude) and to a lesser extent the frequency of the constructions that are reduced. The speed of the changes suggest that neural impulses are involved.

Many patients with functional dyspepsia have weak antral motility at baseline and do not exhibit this normal inhibition of antral motility in response to stress [8, 21].

Low Vagal Tone

Vagal tone can be measured by the variations in frequency of the heart rate with respiration. Normally, the heart rate decreases during inspiration and increases during expiration. This variation in heart rate with respiration is dependent on and a quantitative estimate of the vagal tone. [22]. Our recent studies have shown that, in general, patients with functional dyspepsia have a considerably reduced vagal tone [22]. Although the method employed measures the vagal influence on the heart, there is good reasons to suppose a similar vagal effect on the stomach [22]. The low vagal tone may be responsible for the poor antral motility and failing inhibition in response to stress. It appears as if antral motility in these patients proceeds independent of vagal control (from higher centres). The defective vagal control may be an important cause of the abdominal discomfort.

Neuroticism and Low Vagal Tone

The neuroticism score on the Eysenck Personality Questionnaire (EPQ-N) is significantly higher among patients with functional dyspepsia than among controls (and patients with peptic ulcer disease). This EPQ-N score, which reflects a general disposition to hyper-responsiveness, was significantly negatively correlated to vagal tone, i.e. psychological hyper-responsiveness is associated with low vagal tone and a characteristic feature of patients with functional dyspepsia [18].

Wide Gastric Antrum

Recent ultrasonographic studies have revealed that patients with functional dyspepsia on an average have a wider antrum, both fasting and post-prandially, than healthy controls (Fig. 4) [22]. Most of the patients with a wide antrum also have weak antral motility, and 19 out of 25 patients had upper abdominal discomfort (mainly a feeling of fullness and nausea) after drinking 500 ml meat soup in 4 min, while, only one out of 23 healthy control persons complained of discomfort after drinking the soup. The patients who had the widest antral areas

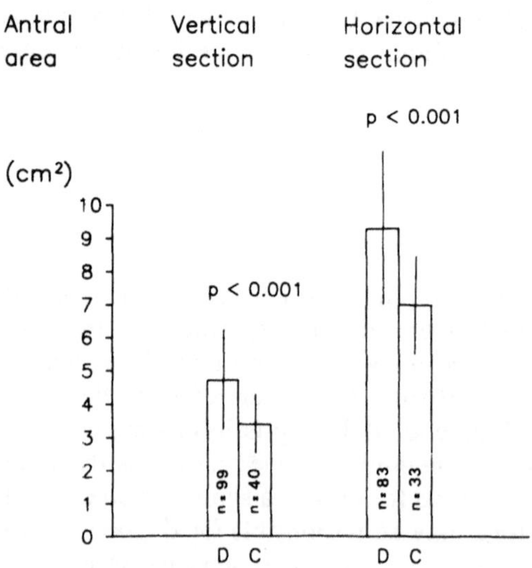

Fig. 4. SD Antral area (mean ± SD in healthy control subjects (*C*) and in patients with non-ulcer dyspepsia and erosive pre-pyloric changes (*D*). Vertical and horizontal section. (From Hausken and Berstad [22])

also had most discomfort following ingestion of the soup (Fig. 5) [19, 21, 22]. Theoretically, the weak vagal control of gastroduodenal motor function may be the main cause of both the dysmotility and the meal-related discomfort in these patients.

Adaptive Relaxation

When the stomach is filled, the fundic part dilates by a physiological vago-vagal reflex known as adaptive relaxation [11, 12]. This reflex makes it possible to eat a big meal without increasing intragastric pressure. Such gastric adaptation is reported to be impaired after vagotomy [3]. Seeing that low vagal tone is a characteristic feature of patients with functional dyspepsia, a similar disturbance would be expected in these patients. However, intragastric pressure-volume curves were similar in patients with functional dyspepsia and in controls [7, 33], and clear indications of disturbed gastric adaptation have been difficult to find. Experiments by Coffin et al. [10] indicate, though, that a similar reflex (i.e. gastric relaxation) is elicited by dilatation of the proximal duodenum, and that this reflex may be weakened in patients with functional dyspepsia.

Recent observations support the notion that something is wrong with gastric adaptation in functional dyspepsia. Both scintigraphic [35, 59] and ultrasonographic [21] studies have shown abnormal intragastric distribution of food in patients with functional dyspepsia: relatively more of the ingested food is pooled in the antrum in these patients than in healthy controls (Fig. 6). The reason for this is not known. The abnormal antral filling is due either to defective accommodation of the proximal stomach or to delayed emptying of the distal stomach; the disturbance may be a consequence of the low vagal tone.

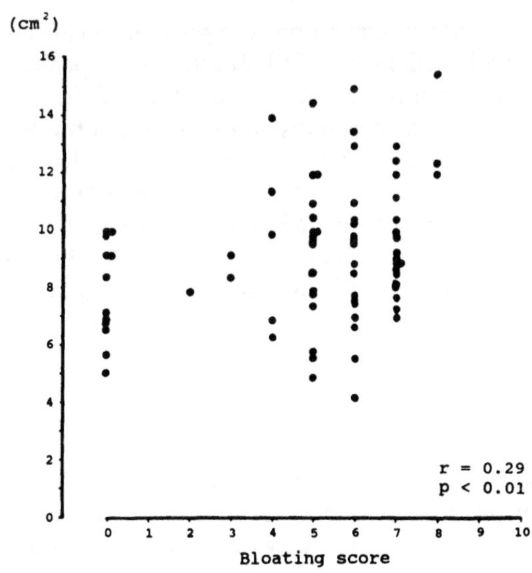

Fig. 5. Correlation between bloating score and width of antral area (horizontal section) in patients with non-ulcer dyspepsia and erosive pre-pyloric changes. (From Hausken and Berstad [22])

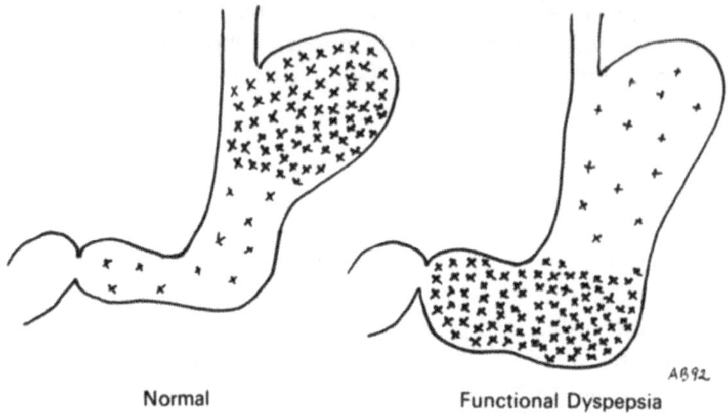

Fig. 6. Schematic representation of the abnormal intragastric distribution of food in patients with functional dyspepsia. Note the abnormally filled gastric antrum

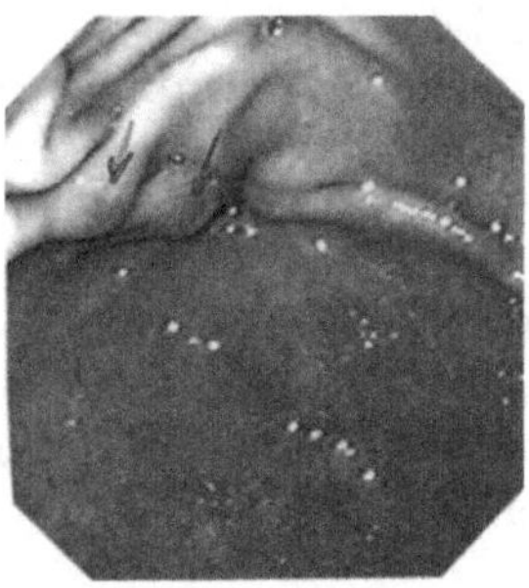

Fig. 7. Endoscopic picture of the pre-pyloric area in a patient with erosive pre-pyloric changes grade 2, i.e. standing, coarse prepyloric folds (*arrows*) with red spots (shown as light spots here) on top of the folds

Several observations suggest that antral distention is important in causing functional dyspepsia. Two studies by Hausken et al. [19, 21] indicate a positive correlation between degree of antral filling and degree of discomfort. The discomfort may not necessarily be due to *abnormal* distention: several observations suggest that, instead, the threshold for visceral perception is low in functional dyspepsia [10, 38]. Our hypothesis is that chronic mental stress (beyond the individual's ability to cope) renders the individual hypersensitive to both visceral and psychological stimuli. By similar mechanisms the vagal tone is suppressed. The latter is in turn responsible for disturbances in gastric adaptation to ingested food and thereby for localising symptoms to the stomach.

Erosive Pre-pyloric Changes

Erosive pre-pyloric changes, (EPC) constitute a well-defined endoscopic picture often seen in patients with non-ulcer dyspepsia (Fig. 7) [40]. Functional dyspepsia patients with EPC may represent a subgroup within the heterogenous non-ulcer dyspepsia group. Usually, the spectrum of symptoms does not include pain [5], but rather epigastric discomfort, bloating and nausea [20], i.e. the typical symptoms in functional dyspepsia. The fact that functional dyspepsia patients with EPC have a wider gastric antrum [19] and higher stress scores than healthy controls [22], and that stress aggravates EPC [42] and disturbs antral motility [22], suggest a relationship between mental stress on one hand and antral dysmotility, with functional dyspepsia and EPC, on the other. This is not to say that EPC is causally related to functional dyspepsia. It may rather represent a co-phenomenon and a marker of the motility disturbance.

H. pylori Gastritis

The reported increased prevalence of *H. pylori* in patients with non-ulcer dyspepsia compared with controls suggests a possible causative role in at least a subset of patients with non-ulcer dyspepsia. Accordingly, some clinicians believe that *H. pylori* causes non-ulcer dyspepsia and treat these patients for *H. pylori* infection. However, the data supporting this practice are poor [13, 14]. Patchett et al. [45] concluded that antral infection with the organism does not seem to have an important aetiological role in short-term non-ulcer dyspepsia. On the other hand, Goh et al. [16] reported that patients with non-ulcer dyspepsia improved significantly more than controls during treatment with colloidal bismuth subcitrate. Clearly, further studies of patients with non-ulcer dyspepsia are needed to clarify the conflicting results.

GER without Oesophagitis

GER (gastro-oesophageal reflux) associated with a drop in oesophageal pH (as measured by continuous pH-metry) is sometimes felt as heartburn even in the absence of endoscopic signs of oesophagitis. Although it may be possible to demonstrate a plausible cause (the acid reflux), such symptoms are commonly classified as non-ulcer dyspepsia. The main reason for not excluding patients with such symptoms is that heartburn often constitutes just a minor part of the patients' dyspeptic symptom complex (bloating, discomfort, nausea, early satiety, etc). In our opinion the term "GER without oesophagitis" should be used in adults only when heartburn is the main symptom.

Small children may have serious GER problems (vomiting, aspiration, etc.) without endoscopic signs of oesophagitis. In older patients, the resistance of the oesophageal mucosa may be poorer than in younger patients because in older age groups heartburn is regularly associated with oesophagitis. How often GER without visible lesions is a problem in adults, is a matter of debate. Clearly, it depends on the criteria of endoscopic oesophagitis. The first endoscopic signs of oesophagitis are red streaks extending upwards from the ora serrata [50]. When this grade I oesophagitis (which is the most prevalent form of oesophagitis) was not excluded, Johannessen et al. [25] classified about 30% of patients with non-ulcer dyspepsia as "responders" to cimetidine. These "responders" were characterised by having symptoms of GER. It is reasonable to assume that if all patients with grade I oesophagitis had been excluded, the percentage of "responders" in the study of Johannessen et al. [25] would have been considerably lower than 30%. GER without oesophagitis, therefore, probably affects only a minor subgroup of patients with non-ulcer dyspepsia. Moreover, because GER is a physiological phenomenon, patients with non-ulcer dyspepsia may have occasional GER (and thus "respond" to an H_2-receptor antagonist) without having a reflux disease.

Treatment

Because psychological factors are thought to play an important role in the pathogenesis of functional dyspepsia, non-drug treatment is important. Moreover, functional dyspepsia is characterised by discomfort rather than pain. The discomfort is not unbearable when the cause is explained and the patient assured that it is not dangerous. Many patients consult the doctor because of uncertainty about the cause of the discomfort [34]. Two Norwegian studies indicate that around 40% of the patients fear they may have cancer [26, 64]. Therefore, merely taking the patients seriously and offering them a thorough examination may help. Rational treatment would also be to try to support the vagal function by drugs or, possibly, by cognitive psychotheraphy. Prokinetic drugs as cisapride should be tried if non-drug treatment fails [20]. Oral administration of glyceryl trinitrate (which acts by releasing nitric oxide) decreased the width of the gastric antrum, but did not significantly relieve postprandial discomfort in a small group of patients with functional dyspepsia [21]. Because nitric oxide is involved in the reflex relaxation of the stomach to accommodate food [12], further studies with nitric oxide are warranted.

Patients with GER may benefit from treatment with H_2-receptor antagonists, but this concerns just a small subgroup and does not justify treating all patients with functional dyspepsia primarily with such drugs. A "therapeutic challenge" is, therefore, not merely to find the right medicine, but more often to withhold medicine and care for the patient by other means. Seeing that functional dyspepsia is not an ulcer disease, drugs for ulcer treatment especially should be withheld. It is also a "challenge" with therapeutic implications to work for more insight into the pathophysiology of this prevalent and annoying disease.

Conclusion

Non-ulcer dyspepsia and peptic ulcer disease evoke similar symptoms, but are pathophysiologically different disease entities and should be treated accordingly. The diagnosis of non-ulcer dyspepsia is still based on negative criteria, i.e.

it depends on our ability to exclude organic diseases. The majority of patients with non-ulcer dyspepsia have a functional disorder, possibly as a consequence of psychological stress which, by activating processes within the central nervous system, may evoke a sequence of reactions: due to suppression of vagal tone, fundic adaptation to ingested food may be impaired and the gastric antrum thereby abnormally filled. The latter may constitute an important and hitherto largely unrecognised cause of dyspeptic symptoms. Increased responsiveness or hypersensitivity to visceral (gastric distention) and psychological (mental stress) stimuli may constitute important contributing factors. The treatment of such a complex condition is difficult and may not be solved by medical intervention alone.

References

1. Adami H-O, Agenas I, Gustavsson S, Lööf S, Nyberg A, Nyren O, Tyllström J (1984) The clinical diagnosis of "gastritis". Aspects of demographic epidemiology and health care consumption based on a nationwide sample survey. Scand J Gastroenterol 19:216–219
2. Adami H-O, Bergström O, Nyrén O et al. (1987) Is duodenal ulcer really a psychosomatic disease? A population based case control study. Scand J Gastroenterol 22:889–896
3. Aune S (1969) Intragastric pressure after vagotomy. Scand J gastroenterol 4:447–452
4. Azpiroz F, Malagelada J-R (1990) Perception and reflex relaxation of the stomach in response to gut distention. Gastroenterology 98:1193–1198
5. Bernersen B, Johnsen R, Straume B, Burhol PG (1992) Erosive prepyloric changes in dyspeptics and non-dyspeptics in a defined population. The Sørreisa Gastrointestinal Disorder Study. Scand J Gastroenterol 27:233–237
6. Bonnevie O, Kallehauge HE, Wulff HR, Wulff MR (1971) Prognostic value of the augmented histamine test in ulcer disease and X-ray negative dyspepsia. Scand J Gastroenterol 6:732–729
7. Bradette M, Pare P, Douville P, Morin A (1991) Visceral perception in health and functional dyspepsia. Crossover study of gastric distention with placebo and domperidone. Dig Dis Sci 36:52–58
8. Camilleri M, Malagelada J-R, Kao PC, Zinsmeister AR (1986) Gastric autonomic responses to stress in functional dyspepsia. Dig Dis Sci 31:1169–1177
9. Cederberg A, Varis K, Salmi HA, Sipponen P, Harkonen M, Sarna S (1991) Young onset peptic ulcer disease and non-ulcer dyspepsia are separate entities. Scand J Gastroenterol 186:33–44
10. Coffin B, Azpiroz F, Malagelada J-R (1991) Elective gastric hypersensitivity and reflex hyporeactivity in functional dyspepsia. Gastroenterology 100:A431
11. De Ponti F, Azpiroz F, Malagelada JR (1989) Relaxatory responses of the canine proximal stomach to esophageal and duodenal distention: importance of vagal pathways. Dig Dis Sci 34:873–881
12. Desai KM, Sessa WC, Vane JR (1991) Involvement of nitric oxide in the reflex relaxation of the stomach to accommodate food or fluid. Nature 351: 477–478
13. Dooley CP (1991) Helicobacter pylori: review of research findings. Aliment Pharmacol Ther 5, Suppl 1:129–143
14. Elta GH (1991) Helicobacter pylori in patients with non-ulcer dyspepsia. Rev Infect Dis 13, Supply 8:S696–S699
15. Gear MWL, Barnes RJ (1980) Endoscopic studies of dyspepsia in a general practice. Br Med J 58:437–443
16. Goh KL, Parasakthi N, Peh SC, Wong NW, Lo YL, Puthucheary SD (1991) Helicobacter pylori infection and non-ulcer dyspepsia: the effect of treatment with colloidal bismuth subcitrate. Scand J Gastroenterol 26:1123–1131
17. Gregory DW, Davies GT, Evans KT, Rhodes J (1972) Natural history of patients with X-ray negative dyspepsia in general practice. Br Med J 4:519–520

18. Haug TT, Svebak S, Hausken T, Wilhelmsen I, Berstad A (1992) Personality factors as predictors of stress-related antral motility, vagal activation and symptoms in functional dyspepsia patients. Scand J Gastroenterol 27, suppl 190:106
19. Hausken T, Berstad A (1992) Wide gastric antrum in patients with non-ulcer dyspepsia. Effect of cisapride. Scand J Gastroenterol 27:427–432
20. Hausken T, Berstad A (1992) Cisapride treatment of patients with non-ulcer dyspepsia and erosive prepyloric changes. A double-blind, placebo-controlled trial. Scand J Gastroenterol 27:213–217
21. Hausken T, Berstad A (1992) Effect of glyceryl trinitrate on symptoms and antral size and motility in patients with functional dyspepsia. Scand J Gastroenterol 27, Suppl 190:106
22. Hausken T, Svebak S, Wilhelmsen I, Tangen Haug T, Pettersson E, Olavsen K, Hveem K, Berstad A (1993) Low vagal tone and antral dysmotility in patients with functional dyspepsia. Psychosomatic Medicine. 55:12–22.
23. Hui WM, Shiu LP, Lam SK (1991) The perception of life events and daily stress in nonulcer dyspepsia. Am J Gastroenterol 86:292–296
24. Jian R, Ducrot F, Piedeloup C, May JY, Najean Y, Bernier JJ (1985) Measurement of gastric emptying in dyspeptic patients. Effect of a new gastrokinetic agent (cisapride). Gut 26:352–358
25. Johannessen T, Fjøsne U, Kleveland PM, Halvorsen T, Kristensen P, Løge I, Hafstad PE, Sandbakken P, Petersen H (1988) Cimetidine responders in non-ulcer dyspepsia. Scand J Gastroenterol 23:327–336
26. Johannessen T, Petersen H, Kleveland PM, Dybdahl JH, Sandvik AK, Brenna E et al. (1990) The predictive value of history in dyspepsia. Scand J Gastroenterol 27;689–697
27. Karvonen A-L, Lehtola J (1984) Outcome of gastric mucosal erosions. A follow-up study of elective gastroscopic patients. Scand J Gastroenterol 19:228–234
28. Kerlin P (1989) Postprandial antral hypomotility in patients with idiopathic nausea and vomiting. Gut 30, 54–59
29. Krag E (1965) Pseudo-ulcer and true peptic ulcer. A clinical, radiographic and statistical follow-up study. Acta Med Scand 178:713–728
30. Krag E (1982) Non-ulcer dyspepsia. Introduction: Epidemiological data. Scand J Gastroenterol 17, Suppl 79:6–8
31. Labo G, Bortolotti M, Vezzadini P, Bonora G, Bersoni G (1986) Interdigestive gastroduodenal motility and serum motilin in patients with idiopathic delay in gastric emptying. Gastroenterology 90:20–26
32. Lance, P, Wastell C, Schiller KFR (1986) A controlled trial of cimetidine for the treatment of non-ulcer dyspepsia. J Clin Gastroenterol 8:414–418
33. Lehmann M, Dederding JP, Flourie B, Franchisseur C, Rambaud JC, Rian R (1991) Abnormal perception of visceral pain in response to gastric distention in chronic idiopathic dyspepsia. The irritable stomach syndrome. Dig Dis Sci 36:1249–1254
34. Lydeard S, Jones R (1989) Factors affecting the decision to consult with dyspepsia: comparison of consulters and non-consulters. J R Coll Gen Pract 39:495–498
35. Magnall YF, Houghton LA, Bread NW, Johnsen AG (1991) Non-ulcer dyspepsia: Pattern of emptying of fatty liquids from the proximal and distal stomach. Eur J Gastroenterol Hepatol 3, Suppl 1, 9 (abstract)
36. Malagelada JR, Stanghellini V (1985) Manometric evaluation of functional upper gut symptoms. Gastroenterology 88:1223–1231
37. Marshall BJ, McGechie DB, Roger PA, Glancy RJ (1985) Pyloric Campylobacter infection and gastroduodenal disease. Med J Aus 142:439–444
38. Mearin F, Cucala M, Azpiroz F, Malagelada J-R (1991) The origin of symptoms on the brain-gut axis in functional dyspepsia. Gastroenterology 101:999–1006
39. Møllmann K-M, Bonnevie O, Gudmand-Høyer E, Wulff HR (1975) A diagnostic study of patients with upper abdominal pain. Scand J Gastroenterol 10:805–809
40. Nesland Aa, Berstad A (1985) Erosive prepyloric changes in persons with and without dyspepsia. Scand J Gastroenterol 20:222–228
41. Nesland Aa, Berstad A (1985) Effect of cimetidine in patients with non-ulcer dyspepsia and erosive prepyloric changes. Scand J Gastroenterol 20:629–635
42. Nesland Aa, Øktedalen O, Opstad PK, Serck-Hanssen A, Aase S, Berstad A (1989) Erosive prepyloric changes—a manifestation of stress? Scand J Gastroenterol 24:522–528

43. Nyrén O, Adami HO, Bergström R, Gustavsson S, Lööf L (1985) Psychological factors are crucial in the etiology of non-ulcer dyspepsia. A population based case-control study. In: Nyrén O. Non-ulcer dyspepsia. Acta Univ Upsal 527, 1–34 (thesis)
44. Nyrén O, Adami HO, Bergström R, Gustavasson S, Lööf L, Nyberg A (1986) Absence of therapeutic benefit from antacids or cimetidine in non-ulcer dypepsia. N Engl J Med 314:339–343
45. Patchett S, Beattie S, Leen E, Keane C, O'Morain C (1991) Eradicating Helicobacter pylori and symptoms of non-ulcer dyspepsia. BMJ 303:1238–40
46. Ricci R (1987) Are dyspeptic symptoms related to distension of the gastric antrum? Dig Dis Sci 32, 924
47. Saunders JHB, Oliver RJ, Higson DL (1986) Dyspepsia. Incidence of non-ulcer disease in a controlled trial of ranitidine in general practice. Br med J 292: 665–668
48. Spiro HM (1974) Visceral viewpoints. Moynihan's disease? The diagnosis of duodenal ulcer. N Engl J Med 290:567–569
49. Stanghellini V, Ghidini C, Maccarini MR, Paparo GF, Corinaldesi R, Barbara L (1992) Fasting and postprandial gastrointestinal motility in ulcer and non-ulcer dyspepsia. Gut 33:184–190
50. Stene-Larsen G, Weberg R, Frøyshov Larsen I, Bjørtuft Ø, Hoel B, Berstad A (1988) Relationship of overweight to hiatus hernia and reflux oesophagitis. Scand J Gastroenterol 23:427–432
51. Stene-Larsen G, Nesland Aa, Berstad A (1989) Follow-up study of erosive prepyloric changes. Scand J Gastroenterol 24:430–433
52. Switz DM (1976) What the gastroenterologist does all day: a survey of a state society's practice. Gastroenterology 70:1048–1050
53. Talley NJ, Piper DW (1985) The association between non-ulcer dyspepsia and other gastrointestinal disorders. Scand J Gastroenterol 20:896–900
54. Talley NJ, Piper DW (1987) A prospective study of social factors and major life stress in patients with dyspepsia of unknown cause. Scand J Gastroenterol 22, 268–272
55. Talley NJ, Jones M, Piper DW (1988) Psychological and childhood factors in essential dyspepsia. Scand J Gastroenterol 23, 341–346
56. Talley NJ, Zinsmeister AR, Schleck CD, Melton III, LJ (1992) Dyspepsia and dyspepsia subgroups: A population based study. Gastroenterology 102:1259–1268
57. Thompson WG (1984) Non-ulcer dyspepsia. Can Med Assoc J 130:565–569
58. Tibblin G (1985) Introduction to the epidemiology and dyspepsia. Scand J Gastroenterol 20, Suppl 109:29–33
59. Troncon LEA, Bennett RJM, Ahluwalia NK, Thompson DG (1992) Abnormal intragastric distribution of food during gastric emptying in functional dyspepsia. Gut 33, Suppl 1, 22
60. Tytgat GN, Graham DY, Lee A, Marshall BJ, Dixon MF, Axon ATR (1991) Helicobacter pylori: causal agent in peptic ulcer disease? J Gastroenterol Hepatol 6:103–140
61. Urbain JC, Siegel J, Debie NC, Pauwels SP (1988) Effect of cisapride on gastric emptying in dyspeptic patients. Dig Dis Sci 33, 779–783
62. Viskum K (1977) Ulcer disease. A comparison of some clinical and genetic aspects in patients suffering from duodenal ulcer, gastric ulcer and pseudo-ulcer syndrome. Dan Med Bull 24:213–235
63. Waldron B, Cullen PT, Kumar R, Smith D, Jankowski J, Hopwood D, Sutton D, Kennedy N, Campbell FC (1991) Evidence for hypomotility in non-ulcer dyspepsia: a prospective multifactorial study. Gut 32, 246–251
64. Weberg R, Berstad A (1988) Low-dose antacids and pirenzepine in the treatment of patients with non-ulcer dyspepsia and erosive prepyloric changes. A randomized, double-blind, placebo-controlled trial. Scand J Gastroenterol 23:237–243
65. Wegener M, Borsch G, Schaffstein J, Schulz-Flake C, Mai U, Leverkus F (1988) Are dyspeptic symptoms in patients with Campylobacter pylori-associated type B gastritis linked to delayed gastric emptying? Am J Gastroenterol 83, 737–740
66. Weir RD, Backett EM (1968) Studies of the epidemiology of peptic ulcer in a rural community: Prevalence and natural history of dyspepsia and peptic ulcer. Gut 9:75–83

Endosonography of the Stomach and Its Disorders

T.L. Tio

Introduction

Transcutaneous ultrasound (US) has been established as a standard diagnostic imaging modality in gastroenterology. The ultrasound energy must travel through the subcutaneous tissues, air-containing bowel and, in special cases, also the ribs, which leads to the loss of US energy and the quality of images. Endoscopy has also been established as a valuable diagnostic and therapeutic procedure due to its excellent image quality and the possibility to perform an endoscopically guided biopsy procedure. Endoscopic ultrasonography (EUS), also called endosonography, was developed at the end of 1970 to overcome the limiting factors of conventional US and to improve the image quality of US. In the last few years, EUS has been increasingly reported to accurately diagnose gastrointestinal lesions, which cannot accurately be diagnosed with conventional US and endoscopy. The aim of this study was to review the usefulness of EUS in the diagnosis of gastric abnormalities.

Instruments and Techniques of Investigation

At present, there are three types of EUS instruments, which differ in the manner of application:

1. Echoendoscope consisting of a lateral-view or forward-view endoscope
2. Nonoptic flexible or rigid US instrument
3. Endoscopically guided catheter echoprobe (radial or linear array)

In general, an echoprobe is placed at the tip of the instrument, which must be positioned to the target lesion to achieve ultrasonic images. To achieve optimal images, an acoustic window must be produced by filling the balloon with water attached at the transducer or by filling the gastrointestinal lumen with water.

The investigation technique is similar to gastroscopy. Oral oropharyngeal anaesthesia and intravenous sedation are necessary due to the discomfort caused by insertion of the rigid tip of the instrument into the pharynx and by filling the balloon and/or the gastric lumen with water. The instrument should be carefully introduced into the esophagus because the lateral optics do not allow accurate endoscopic visualization of the esophagus. Lesions in the stomach, however, can be localized endoscopically and the transducer should be positioned close to the target of interest. Thereafter, the balloon and/or the stomach can be filled with water. To standardize images, cross sectional images comparable with CT scans and sagittal or oblique sections comparable with those of conventional US can be used. At the termination of the procedure, water in the stomach should be removed endoscopically to avoid any aspiration complication.

Interpretation of EUS Images

At the beginning of 1985, the interpretation of EUS images of the gastrointestinal wall architecture was controversial among many investigators [1–3]. The dilemma, however, has recently been resolved and each individual layer defined. Border echos created by the passage of ultrasound through various layers of the gastrointestinal wall appear to be responsible for the increased thickness on US as compared with that found by histology [4]. The first hyperechoic (echogenic) layer and the second hypoechoic (echopoor) layer correspond with the mucosa (lamina propria plus muscularis mucosae) and the border echo. The third hyperechoic layer corresponds with the submucosa and the border echo. The fourth hypoechoic layer corresponds with the muscularis propria minus the border echo because the border echo between the muscularis propria and the submucosa and the muscularis propria with the subserosa are added to the connective tissue and not the muscle tissue.

The fifth echogenic layer corresponds to the subserosa and serosa plus the border echo as mentioned previously. Abnormalities are defined as partial or total destruction of the five distinct echo patterns of the wall or changes of the surrounding tissues or organs.

Indications for EUS

The logical indications for EUS are diagnosing, staging and follow-up of patients in whom endoscopy and other imaging modalities such as conventional US or CT are not sufficient to give an accurate diagnosis. In general, the following indications are accepted in most centers:

1. Gastric cancer staging and follow-up
2. Gastric non-Hodgkin lymphoma (NHL) staging and follow-up
3. Diagnosing, staging and follow-up of submucosal tumors
4. Diagnosing and staging of gastric varices
5. Diagnosing of splenic artery aneurysms
6. Diffuse submucosal gastric wall abnormalities

Results

Diagnosis, Staging and Follow-up of Gastric Cancer

The recently modified TNM classification is based on the depth of tumor infiltration. Gastric carcinoma is imaged as a hypoechoic tumor with partial or total destruction of the gastric wall architecture. Early gastric cancer is visualized as a hypoechoic tumor located in the mucosa (T1, mucosal type) and/or submucosa (T1, submucosal type). Advanced gastric cancer is seen as a hypoechoic tumor with penetration into the muscularis propria, subserosa (T2) and/or serosa (T3) or into adjacent structures such as major blood vessels, liver, spleen, pancreas or the crus of the diaphragm (T4).

In our previous series involving 72 patients who underwent surgery, the accuracy of EUS in predicting T1 carcinomas was 76.1%, T2 carcinomas 93.3%, T3 81.8%, and T4 carcinomas 87.5%. The overall accuracy of EUS was 83.8% [5]. The relatively low accuracy of EUS in diagnosing early gastric cancers was due to peritumoral inflammation, which led to overstaging of tumor. In diagnosing regional lymph nodes, the accuracy of EUS was 50.5%, 61.3% and 89.7% for N0, N1 and N2, respectively. The overall accuracy was only 68.1% [5]. Other studies have reported a high accuracy of EUS [6, 7]. Lightdale et al. at the Sloan-Kettering Cancer Institute reported an accuracy of EUS in staging gastric cancer of 92% for tumor classification and 88% in diagnosing regional lymph nodes [8]. Aibe et al. in Japan reported a series of 67 patients with gastric cancer with a 67% accuracy of EUS in diagnosing early gastric cancer and 81% in staging advanced cancers [9]. Recently, Akahoshi reported a 81% accuracy of EUS for tumor staging in a series of 74 cases [10].

Gastric Non-Hodgkin Lymphoma Staging and Follow-up

In our initial studies involving eight patients with gastric non-Hodgkin lymphoma (NHL), EUS findings consisted of intramural infiltration and mucosal alteration together with perigastric abnormalities. Lymph node involvement was suggested by the presence of inhomogeneous hypoechoic patterns with sharply demarcated boundaries. EUS was more accurate than CT in detecting mural abnormalities and adjacent lymph node involvement. EUS was also helpful in assessing the resectability. In a follow-up study of 24 cases, staging was carried out with the Ann Arbor system. EUS findings were also correlated with the endoscopic feature for the initial staging and follow-up. EUS was more accurate in staging and follow-up due to its ability to image submucosal abnormalities and perigastric lymph node involvement. However, it is difficult to distinguish between irradiation related fibrosis and malignant infiltration. Interestingly, we found an early gastric cancer in a patient who successfully underwent irradiation for gastric NHL, which has been described elsewhere. The carcinoma was accurately staged with EUS and confirmed by the histology of resected specimen. A remnant of NHL infiltration was not found. In an ongoing study involving 40 cases of gastric NHL, we have found that EUS is more accurate than CT and endoscopy in staging and follow-up. The recently modified TNM staging system has been incorporated, which appears to be more suitable than the Ann Arbor system. Calletti et al. reported the role of EUS in detecting, staging and planning the strategy of treatment of 10 patients with gastric NHL. Bolondi et al. described the use of EUS in distinguishing gastric NHL from gastric cancers using the echo pattern as the criterion. However, no objective criteria were described comparing the echogenicity of both malignant diseases [11–14].

Diagnosis and Follow-up of Submucosal Tumors

Endoscopy is not accurate in diagnosing submucosal tumors because the underlying disease cannot be seen. EUS allows seeing through the mucosa and identifying the extent and nature of the disease.

The most common submucosal tumors are leiomyoma and lipoma. Leiomyoma is visualized as local thickening of the muscularis propria or a hypoechoic, clearly defined pattern without penetration into adjacent structures. The size of the tumor is often less than 4 cm in diameter. Extensive tumor size may result in reduction of the blood supply, which may lead to ulceration. Lipoma is diagnosed when a hyperechoic (echogenic) tumor presents with echogenicity similar to that of fat tissue. Leiomyosarcoma or leiomyoblastoma is visualized as a hypoechoic tumor mass often penetrating into adjacent structures or associated with suspicious lymph nodes, central ulcer or a fistulous tract. Carcinoid of the stomach is often seen as a relatively small hypoechoic tumor in the submucosa without adjacent lymph node involvement. Endoscopic removal of the tumor may be adequate when EUS is carried out prior to the treatment in order to exclude extramural spreading of carcinoid. Pancreatic tail carcinoma involving the gastric wall may simulate the presence of smooth muscle tumor. In a case report, we found a submucosal tumor in the fundus of the stomach, which was confirmed by CT. EUS, however, identified a pancreatic tail tumor penetrating into the submucosa of the stomach. EUS guided cytology through the mucosa confirmed the diagnosis of pancreatic carcinoma. Hepatoma may cause compression of the stomach, which may lead to an incorrect diagnosis of submucosal tumor. Liver, spleen and splenic vessels at the splenic hilum protruding into the lumen may also lead to a diagnosis of smooth muscle tumor at endoscopy. Recently, there have been many reports concerning the use of EUS in the diagnosis of submucosal tumors [15, 16].

Diagnosis and Staging of Gastric Varices

The diagnosis of fundic varices can be difficult endoscopically because the overlying mucosa may be normal. Distinguishing between leiomyomas and gastric varices is often not possible. Endoscopic biopsy may be associated with a high risk of bleeding. On EUS, gastric varices can be seen as an anechoic blood vessel in the submucosa often associated with perigastric collateral veins. In the case of pancreatic carcinoma or chronic pancreatitis, segmental portal hypertension with or without gastric varices can be found. Cessation of gastric variceal bleeding can be difficult endoscopically or even surgically. EUS may be helpful in the detection and staging of fundic varices in planning the strategy of treatment. Using the information gathered with EUS, the surgeon may ligate the varices or endoscopic cessation with histoacryl can be performed. There are some publications concerning the use of EUS in diagnosing and staging gastric varices. Follow-up with EUS after endoscopic treatment has also been reported [16–18].

Splenic Artery Aneurysm

Aneurysms of the splenic artery adjacent to the splenic hilum may protrude into the gastric lumen. Calcification of the splenic artery adjacent to the aneurysm can often be found. EUS can readily visualize aneurysmatic dilation of the splenic artery with its calcification of the aortic wall. In such cases, color Doppler US will be very helpful in the imaging of the turbulent blood stream. Resection of such aneurysms should be recommended because of the high risk of fatal bleeding. In some cases, fatal bleeding during pregnancy due to splenic artery aneurysm has been reported [19].

Diffuse Gastric Wall Abnormalities

Diffuse gastric wall abnormalities may be seen as diffuse thickening of gastric folds. Endoscopically, hypertrophic gastritis, or Ménétrier's disease, cannot be distinguished from gastric linitis. Hypertrophic gastritis can be visualized as diffuse hypoechoic thickening of the mucosa without involvement of the submucosa and muscularis propria. Gastric linitis is imaged as diffuse hypoechoic abnormality in the submucosa with or without penetration into the deeper layers of the gastric wall. The muscularis propria is often thickened up to 2–4 times as compared to its normal thickness. The overlying mucosa may be normal. Endoscopic biopsy may also be negative because the target lesion may not be reached with the biopsy forceps. In such cases, EUS may be helpful in localizing the optimal site of biopsy, and EUS guided aspiration biopsy may be helpful in ascertaining the diagnosis of malignancy [20].

Conclusions

EUS has been established as a diagnostic procedure in many centers. Endoscopy is highly accurate in diagnosing mucosal abnormalities. EUS, however, allows seeing through the mucosa. Combination of these modalities has proven effective in the field of gastroenterology. In the near future, the routine use of

EUS-guided aspiration cytology will become an important step in achieving a tissue diagnosis similar to that of endoscopic biopsy in the past decades. Recently, some Japanese authors have reported the use of EUS in the staging of early gastric cancer. In the case of mucosal type carcinoma found by EUS, endoscopic mucosectomy after submucosal injection with saline can be performed instead of invasive surgical treatment. The incidence of lymph node metastases in T1-mucosal type carcinoma has been reported to be less than 5%. The use of EUS in selecting the appropriate patient for minimally invasive surgery will become the trend in the future.

References

1. Tytgat GNJ, Tio TL (1986) Endoscopic ultrasonography: The 5th international symposium on endoscopic ultrasonography. Scand J Gastroenterol
2. Tio TL, Tytgat GNJ (1986) Atlas of transintestinal ultrasonography. Mur-Kostverloren, Aalsmeer
3. Tio TL, Tytgat GNJ (1984) Endoscopic ultrasonography in the diagnosis of tumors in the oesophagus, stomach and papilla of Vater and in the detection of extraesophageal lesions. Endoscopy 4:220–225
4. Kimmey MB, Martin RW, Haggitt RC, Wang KY, Franklin DW, Silverstein F (1989) Histologic correlates of gastrointestinal ultrasound images. Gastroenterology 96:433–441
5. Tio TL, Schouwink MH, Cikot RJLM, Tytgat GNJ (1989) Preoperative TNM classification of gastric carcinoma by endosonography in comparison with the pathological TNM system: a prospective study of 72 cases. Hepato-gastroenterology 36:51–56
6. Heyder N (1987) Endoscopic ultrasonography of tumors of the oesophagus and stomach. Surg Endosc 1:17–23
7. Yasuda K, Kiyoshi K, Kakayima M, Kawai K (1987) Fundamentals of endoscopic laser therapy for Gi-tumors; new aspects with endoscopic ultrasonography. 19:2–6
8. Lightdale CJ, Botet JF, Kelsen DP, Turnbull AD, Brennan MF (1989) Diagnosis of recurrent gastric cancer at the surgical anastomosis by endoscopic ultrasound. Gastrointest Endosc 35:407–412
9. Aibe T, Fujimura H, Noguchi T, Ohtani T, Nakata K, Ito T, Fuji T, Takemoto T (1987) Endosonographic detection and staging of early gastric cancer. In: Dancygier MM (ed) 5th international symposium on endoscopic ultrasonography. Demeter, Gräfelfing
10. Akahoshi K, Misawa T, Fujishima H, Chijiwa Y, Marouka A, Ohkuba A, Nawata H (1991) Preoperative evaluation of gastric cancer by endoscopic ultrasound. Gut 32:479–482
11. Tio TL, den Hartog Jager FCA, Tytgat GNJ (1986) Endoscopic ultrasonography of non-Hodgkin lymphoma of the stomach. Gastroenterology 91:401–408
12. Tio TL, den Hartog Jager FCA, Tytgat GNJ (1986) Endoscopic ultrasonography in detection and staging of gastric non-Hodgkin lymphoma. Comparison with gastroscopy, barium meal and computed tomography. Scand J Gastroenterol 21 (suppl 123):52–58
13. Tio TL, den Hartog Jager FCA, Tytgat GNJ (1987) Non-Hodgkin lymphoma of the stomach: endosonographic strategies in diagnosis and treatment. In: Dancygier H, Classen M (eds) 5th international symposium on endoscopic ultrasonography. Demeter, Gräfelfing
14. Fujishima H, Misawa T, Marouka A, Chijiwa Y, Sakai K, Nawata H (1991) Staging and follow-up of primary gastric lymphoma by endoscopic ultrasound. Am J Gastroenterol 86:719–724
15. Tio TL, Tytgat GNJ, den Hartog Jager FCA (1989) Endoscopic ultrasonography for the evaluation of smooth muscle tumors in the upper gastrointestinal tract: an experience with 42 cases. Gastrointest Endosc 36:342–350

16. Yasuda K, Nakajima M, Yoshida S, Kiyota K, Kawai K (1989) The diagnosis of submucosal tumors of the stomach by endoscopic ultrasonography. 35:10–15
17. Caletti G, Brochi E, Baraldini M, Ferrari A, Gilbidaro M, Barbara L (1990) Assessment of portal hypertension by endoscopic ultrasonography. Gastrointest Endosc 36 (suppl):21–27
18. Tio TL, Kimmings N, Rauws E, Jansen P, Tytgat GNJ (1993) Endosonography of gastroesophageal varices. Clinical staging and follow-up of 76 cases. Gastrointest Endosc (submitted for publication)
19. Busuttil RW, Briun J (1980) The diagnosis and management of visceral artery aneurysm. Surgery 88:619–624
20. Tio TL, Maas JJ, Collin EM, Tytgat GNJ (1992) Endosonography in diagnosing and staging diffuse gastric wall abnormalities. DDW, San Francisco, abstract 2520

Operative Endoscopy in the Stomach: Polypectomy

B. Högemann

Introduction

Gastric polyps are usually incidental findings at routine endoscopy, seen as well-circumscribed swellings in the gastric mucosa. Polyps are found in 0.2%–1.2% of patients undergoing endoscopic screening and in about 2.5% of patients undergoing endoscopy because of upper abdominal complaints. The surface of the polyps is usually smooth and their diameter in most cases less than 20 mm. In 40% of cases multiple polyps are present. The histological type can be various, but in more than 90% the polyps represent changes of epithelial origin [4]. The endoscopic/macroscopic appearance does not allow an estimation of the status of the polyps.

Most polyps cause no symptoms; occasionally they can cause haemorrhage or obstruction. Polyps are divided according to histomorphological criteria into focal hyperplasia, hyperplasiogenic polyps, body gland cysts, adenomas in various stages of differentiation, borderline lesions and early-stage carcinomas [4]. Only about 3%–4% of epithelial gastric polyps are malignant [13].

The most frequent localizations are the antrum and the corpus; only about 10% of polyps are found in the area of the fornix and the cardia [10]. Mesenchymal (non-epithelial) polyps constitute less than 10% of gastric polyps [7]. These are usually lipomas, leiomyomas, fibromas, haemangiomas or neurinomas growing submucosally. Heterotopic pancreatic tissue can also appear as a polypous space-occupying lesion. Rare findings include eosinophilic granuloma and polyposis ventriculi (multiple adenomatosis of the gastric mucosa). Gastric polyps seen as part of Peutz-Jeghers syndrome are hamartomas with a slight degenerative tendency.

Indications for Gastric Polypectomy

The procedure of choice is endoscopic polypectomy using the high-frequency diathermy loop [1,3]. This is unconditionally suitable for use on polyps of 10 mm diameter or more. Smaller polyps are first biopsied. If the polyp proves histologically to be an adenoma, it is completely removed by endoscopy [5]. Polyps with a diameter of more than 30 mm should be operated on because of the risk of haemorrhage.

Contraindications for Gastric Polypectomy

The following are contraindications for endoscopic polypectomy:

- Haemorrhagic diathesis (Quick value < 50%, thrombocyte count < 50 000/mm³)
- Diameter of polyps more than 30 mm
- Polyp cannot be reached by endoscopy
- Uncooperative patient

Technique of Polypectomy

The technique of polypectomy is well standardized and is similar to the technique for removing polyps in the colon. A high-frequency generator is connected to a large-surface electrode attached to the patient's thigh. The polypectomy loop constitutes the second (active) electrode. The polyp is brought into endoscopic view and the loop extended and placed around it. The loop is then retracted, the tube being simultaneously pushed forward, until the loop grips the base of the polyp. The polyp is then luxated into the lumen of the stomach in order to avoid undesired coagulation effects outside of the loop and polyp. Administration of electric impulses lasting 1–4 s using coagulation or undulatory current usually results in nearly bloodless detachment of the polyp. This can then easily be removed by suction at the endoscope. Another alternative is to use a Dormia basket, loop, or forceps. More details of the technique can be obtained from review articles [2, 5].

Results

When a polyp is removed from a healthy person, the further course of therapy depends on the histological classification and work-up of the removed polyp. Adenomas are rare in the stomach (5% of polyps) [12], while early gastric carcinomas and borderline lesions are found in about 2%–3% of cases (Table 1). In cases where an adenoma is found – assuming complete endoscopic removal – a follow-up programme of regular clinical, endoscopic, and histological check-ups can be planned [5]. In patients with polyps more than 3 cm in diameter, early-stage gastric carcinoma, polyposis ventriculi, non-epithelial and angiomatous tumours, operative treatment should be the first aim [7]. If this is impossible (e.g. the patient is not operable), endoscopic treatment using loop-assisted mucosectomy [6], electro- or laser coagulation, photodynamic therapy or injection therapy (polidocanol, 5-fluorouracil) can be considered for malignant lesion [8, 11, 14].

Table 1. Histological findings in gastric polyps removed by endoscopy ($n = 6243$) [12]

	n	%
Epithelial polyps	4941	79.1
hyperplasiogenic	2961	47.4
focal hyperplasia	1537	24.6
adenoma	337	5.4
other	96	1.5
Mesenchymal polyps	204	3.3
Body gland cysts	787	12.6
Early gastric cancer	119	1.9
type I	53	0.8
type IIa	63	1.0
other	3	0.05
Borderline lesion	192	3.0

Complications

The complications rate associated with endoscopic gastric polypectomy is low as long as the endoscopist has adequate mastery of the technique and does not remove polyps larger than 3 cm in diameter. Known complications include haemorrhage and perforation. The overall complications rate is 0.6% [9].

Conclusions

Endoscopic gastric polypectomy is a standardized, low-risk procedure for the diagnosis of polypous lesions of the gastric mucosa. Careful histological study allows follow-up or treatment programmes to be planned and is the decisive factor in the indication for surgery. In rare cases of adenoma with dysplasia of varying degree or gastric carcinoma, endoscopic treatment may be undertaken, especially in patients who cannot undergo operation.

References

1. Classen M, Demling L (1971) Operative Gastroskopie: fiberendoskopische Polypenabtragung im Magen. Dtsch Med Woschenschr 96: 1466–1467
2. Cotton PB, Williams CB (1985) Lehrbuch der praktischen gastrointestinalen Endoskopie. Perimed Erlangen, pp 100–101
3. Deyhle P, Seuberth K, Jenny S, Demling L (1971) Endoscopic polypectomy in the proximal colon. Endoscopy 3: 103–105
4. Elster K (1986) Klassifikation und Dignität gastrointestinaler Polypen. In: Mörl M (ed) Die endoskopisch-bioptische Untersuchung. Perimed, Erlangen, pp 105–115

5. Frühmorgen P (1991) Polypektomie. In: Frühmorgen P (ed) Diagnostische und therapeutische Endoskopie in der Gastroenterologie. Springer, Berlin Heidelberg New York, pp 297–305
6. Fujimori T, Nakamura T, Hirayama D, Satonaka K, Ajiki T, Kitazawa S, Maeda S, Nagasako K, Yamaguchi H, Yoshida S (1992) Endoscopic mucosectomy for early gastric cancer using modified strip biopsy. Endoscopy 24:187–189
7. Högemann B, Keferstein RD (1992) Benigne Magentumoren. In: Krück F, Kaufmann W, Wilmanns W, Bünte H, Gladtke E, Tölle R (eds) Therapie-Handbuch, 4th edn. Urban and Schwarzenberg, Munich
8. Lambert R (1992) Endoscopic therapy of esophago-gastric tumors. Endoscopy 24:24–33
9. Ottenjann R (1979) Esophageal and gastric polypectomy – indications and early results. In: Demling L, Koch H (eds) Operative endoscopy. Past and Future. Schattauer, Stuttgart
10. Riemann JF, Demling L (1986) Operative Endoskopie. In: Mörl M (ed) Die endoskopisch-bioptische Untersuchung. Perimed, Erlangen, pp 133–140
11. Salmon PR (1992) Endoscopic treatment of gastro-intestinal tumours: can surgery be avoided? Endoscopy 24:229–231
12. Seifert E, Gail K, Weismüller J (1983) Gastric polypectomy. Long-term results (survey of 23 centres in Germany). Endoscopy 15:8–11
13. Singer M, Busse R, Seib HJ, Elster K, Ottenjann R (1975) Endoskopische Polypektomie im oberen Verdauungstrakt. Ergebnisse und klinische Bedeutung. Dtsch Med Wochenschr 100:2313–2316
14. Takechi K, Mihara M, Saito Y, Endo J, Maekawa H, Usui T, Moriwaki H, Muto Y (1992) A modified technique for endoscopic mucosal resection of small early gastric carcinomas. Endoscopy 24:215–217

Operative Endoscopy in the Stomach: Percutaneous Endoscopic Gastrostomy

B. Högemann

Introduction

The long-term nutrition of patients who are unable to take food orally due to pharyngeal or oesophageal disease, neurological pathology or other disturbances gives rise to a number of technical and metabolic problems. Exclusively parenteral nutrition leads in a short time to clinically significant alterations in the metabolism and morphology of the digestive organs. Changes in the kinetics of the gall bladder with formation of sludge, disturbances of the bile acid metabolism and pancreatic secretion, villous atrophy and reduction in the activity of brush border enzymes of the small intestine, and catheter-related complications such as thrombosis and infection [1].

For these reasons, nowadays some form of enteral nutrition via a nasogastric or percutaneously implanted tube made out of some synthetic substance is generally favoured. Tubes that emerge through the nose are poorly tolerated by patients and also look cosmetically bad. Late complications such as dislocation of the tube, formation of loops in the stomach and occlusion occur frequently and lead to repeated changing of the tube, with all the stress for the patient that this involves [15].

Percutaneous endoscopically guided gastrostomy (PEG) is a minimally invasive alternative to the nasogastric tube and has come into widespread use in recent years. The technique was first described by Gauderer et al. [3] in 1980 and by Larsen et al. [10] in 1983.

Implantation Techniques

There are several different ways of pulling through the guidewire in PEG, either under endoscopic guidance or using direct puncture techniques under radiographic or ultrasonographic guidance [2, 6, 14].

The method employed by Keymling [7, 8] is used widely and is attractive for its simplicity and low complication rate. When the endoscope has been introduced, the stomach is inflated with air. Stenoses in the upper gastrointestinal tract are not generally a problem and can be treated by bougienage in the usual way. In the area where diaphanoscopy can be used, under sterile conditions and with local anaesthesia, the stomach is directly punctured in the left upper abdominal region and the puncture site in the stomach brought into endoscopic view. After the puncture needle, equipped with a mandrin, is withdrawn, a guidewire is advanced into the gastric lumen, caught in a biopsy forceps, or loop, and pulled out via the mouth by retraction of the endoscope. The end of the tube is attached to the wire and pulled into the stomach. A holding plate at the distal end of the tube ensures fixation against the inner gastric wall. The stomach wall is then gently pulled against the inside of the abdominal wall and the tube fixed in this position with a second holding plate applied on the outside. Within a few days, the outer gastric wall becomes affixed to the peritoneum. The usual catheter diameters are 9 and 15 French [Freka, PEG standard (gastric/duodenal); Freka, PEG universal (gastric/intestinal); Fresenius, Bad Homburg, Germany].

Modifications of this method have been described. Sometimes it can be useful to place the tube in the duodenum, the longer intragastric part of the tube being endoscopically guided into the duodenum or upper part of the small intestine. Double-lumen catheters allow intrajejunal nutrition with the risk of reflux largely eliminated, and when the bile ducts are obstructed, the bile can be simultaneously transported to the intestines via percutaneous transhepatic cholangiodrainage [8].

When the direct puncture technique is used, the stomach is distended without endoscopic guidance, the catheter introduction system (split canula, peel-away sheaths) removed, and the tube fixed in the stomach using a T-piece or a balloon [6, 14]. Using this system, however, difficulties with fixation and dislocation are not infrequent. The most recently described technique using a memory catheter (Memosond, Pfrimmer-Viggo, Erlangen) also requires distension of the stomach, which can be achieved using a narrow lumen catheter pushed past the obstruction. After puncture of the stomach under radiographic guidance, the tube is warmed with hot water ($>65°$); as it cools, it forms a spiral in the gastric lumen, allowing fixation to the gastric wall. This technique is associated with serious complications, however (dislocation into the free abdominal space, gastric perforation [4, 12]), and should therefore only be used when gastroscopy is impossible [2].

Accompanying Procedures

Tube implantation requires two operators. The patient receives light premedication; our preference here is pethidine 100 mg i.v. or pethidine 50 mg with midazolam 1–2.5 mg i.v.. The operative field is covered with sterile drapes. To clear as many bacteria from the stomach as possible, administration of histamine H_2-blockers should be stopped beforehand. Before nutrition is started, the position of the tube should be checked endoscopically; radiography is less reliable. Prophylactic antibiotic treatment for about 10 days with, for example, a cephalosporin, is recommended. The tube should not be changed within the first 10 days, as before this an adequately fibrous puncture canal will not have formed and the stomach will not yet adhere to the inner abdominal wall.

Table 1. Indications for percutaneous endoscopic gastrostomy

Reversible or irreversible dysphagia in patients with neurological disturbances (head injury, neurogenic or myogenic dysphagia)
Obstruction due to malignancy in the upper gastrointestinal tract or the region of the pharynx
Cancerous cachexia
Malabsorption syndrome, short-bowel syndrome
Radiation or cytostatic effects in the gut
PEG as adjuvant therapy in cancer treatment

Indications

PEG is always indicated when the patient is likely to be unable to swallow for a long time; if parenteral nutrition is likely to last for no more than 4 weeks, a nasogastric tube will answer the case. Further indications are temporary inaccessibility of the oral route after operations in the oropharynx or due to oesophageal erosion, rupture or fistula. After healing has taken place, the tube can easily be removed endoscopically. Table 1 summarizes the indications.

Contraindications are absence of diaphanoscopy or presence of coagulation disorders, ileus or peritonitis, ascites, acute pancreatitis, pathological alterations of the gastric wall, and, of course, patient refusal. Care is needed when placing a PEG in immune-suppressed patients or those who have just undergone gastric or oesophageal resection.

Results

As long as there are no obstructions that cannot be overcome endoscopically, a PEG can almost always be placed by the guidewire method. Obstructions in the oesophagus can be removed by bougienage in the usual way to allow the passage of the endoscope into the stomach. Only in the presence of an immovable obstruction should the direct puncture technique be used, if an operative catheter jejunostomy is ruled out. If the tube becomes blocked, it can easily be extracted endoscopically and reimplanted in the same procedure. In patients with neurological disease, the tube can remain in place for an average of 5 months (range 1–453 days); in those with malignant disease the average is 3.8 months (range 1–540 days) [6]. After numerous positive reports, it remains controversial whether implantation of a PEG is to be preferred to a surgical gastrostomy; however, in one prospective randomized study published recently, no difference in morbidity or mortality was found between the group of patients given PEG and those treated surgically [13]. Factors speaking in favour of PEG, however, are that it is cost-effective and well-tolerated by the patient.

Sometimes percutaneous endoscopic jejunostomy is suggested for patients who are unable to tolerate intragastric feeding, but no clear advantage of this over PEG has been shown even in large studies (for review see [11]).

PEG is generally well accepted among patients, staff and patients' relatives. There are no cosmetic problems and the tube is easy to maintain, so that after a little instruction even the relatives can take over the maintenance.

Complications

Complications with the guidewire method are few – about 3.3% (tearing of the wire, catheter breakage, obstruction) [8]. Slight complications such as pain, local infection, pneumoperitoneum, local bleeding, reflux oesophagitis and aspiration of gastric contents occur in up to 14% of patients, but are usually easy to treat. As prophylaxis against local wound infection, a short course of cephazolin is recommended [5]. The mortality associated with PEG is low, less than 1%, and in even these cases concurrent cardiopulmonary disease must usually be regarded as the cause of death rather than the PEG itself [7, 9, 11].

The reported incidence of metabolic complications varies and applies as much to nasogastric tubes as to the PEG systems. Hyperhydration, electrolyte disturbances, hyperglycaemia and even hyperosmolar coma have been described. However, these complications can be to a large extent prevented by properly adjusted nutrition combined with regular clinical examinations and laboratory tests [1]. It is extremely helpful if outpatients can be looked after by nurses specializing in nutrition in close cooperation with the hospital, and makes it much easier to maintain the tubes, obtain and administer the nutritional solutions, and keep up clinical surveillance. At about 1%, the incidence of metabolic complications is markedly lower than with total parenteral nutrition (5%) [1].

Conclusions

Percutaneous endoscopic gastrostomy is an established method of feeding patients who need to be fed partly or entirely by an enteral route for more than 4 weeks. Although it is an invasive procedure, PEG is technically simple and associated with very few serious complications. Associated mortality is below 1%. Among the various methods, the most widely used is the guidewire method. Direct puncture techniques should only be used if impassable stenosis is present in the upper gastrointestinal tract, and require extra care and surveillance. In the presence of certain pathological conditions (oesophagotracheal fistula, manifest reflux oesophagitis, long-term ventilated tracheotomized patients, patients who have just undergone gastric resection), specially modified tubes can be positioned in the upper small intestine under endoscopic guidance.

In critical cases, implantation of a PEG allows patients – many of them incurably ill – to receive adequate caloric, physio-logical nutrition without detracting from their general well-being.

References

1. Clement T, Lembcke B (1991) Enterale Sondenernährung und perkutane endoskopische Gastrostomie. Inn Med 18:48–53
2. Frühmorgen P (1991) Perkutane endoskopische Gastrostomie. In: Frühmorgen P (ed) Diagnostische und therapeutische Endoskopie in der Gastroenterologie. Springer, Berlin Heidelberg New York, pp 253–259
3. Gauderer MWL, Ponsky JL, Izant RJ Jr (1980) Gastrostomy without laparotomy: a percutaneous endoscopic technique. J Pediatr Surg 15:872–875
4. Hardegg G, Heller T, Frühmorgen P (1991) Sondendislokation nach perkutaner endoskopisch kontrollierter Gastrostomie – ein Fallbericht. Z Gastroenterol 29:655 – 658
5. Jain NK, Larson DE, Schroeder KW, Burton DD, Cannon KP, Thompson RL, DiMagno EP (1987) Antibiotic prophylaxis for percutaneous endoscopic gastrostomy. Ann Intern Med 107:824–828
6. Jung M, Harz C, Pimentel F (1991) Perkutane endoskopische Gastrostomie. Dtsch Med Wochenschr 116:1063–1068
7. Keymling M (1989) Perkutane endoskopisch kontrollierte Gastrostomie. Z Gastroenterologie 27 (Suppl 1):65–68
8. Keymling M, Schroeder M, Wörner W (1985) Erfahrungen mit der perkutan endoskopisch kontrollierten Gastrostomie (PEG). Med Welt 36:1297–1301
9. Larson DE, Burton DD, Schroeder KW, DiMagno EP (1987) Percutaneous endoscopic gastrostomy: indications, success, complications, and mortality in 314 patients. Gastroenterology 93:48–52
10. Larson DE, Fleming CR, Ott BJ, Schroeder KW (1983) Percutaneous endoscopic gastrostomy. Simplified access for enteral nutrition. Mayo Clin Proc 58:103-107
11. Mellinger JD, Ponsky JL (1992) Percutaneous endoscopic gastrostomy. Endoscopy 24:64–67
12. Nattermann C, Dancygier H (1991) Tödliche Komplikation bei perkutaner endoskopischer Gastrostomie. Dtsch Med Wochenschr 116:77
13. Steigmann GV, Goff JS, Silas D (1990) Endoscopic vs operative gastrostomy: final results of a prospective randomized trial. Gastrointest Endosc 36:1–5
14. Vestweber KH, Paul A, Becker A, Viell B (1992) Perkutane endoskopische Gastrotomie. In: Fuchs KH, Hamelmann H, Manegold BC (eds) Chirurgische Endoskopie im Abdomen. Blackwell, Berlin, pp 196–201
15. Wicks C, Gimson A, Vlavianos P, Lombard M, Panos M, Macmathuna P, Tudor M, Andrews K, Westaby D (1992) Assessment of the percutaneous endoscopic gastrostomy feeding tube as part of an integrated approach to enteral feeding. Gut 33:613–616

Operative Endoscopy in the Stomach: Cystogastric Pancreatic Drainage

E.C. Foerster and W. Domschke

Introduction

Cystogastric catheter drainage under endoscopic and ultrasonographic guidance as introduced by Hancke and Heriksen has developed into a minimally invasive alternative to percutaneous or operative drainage. In cystogastric drainage, a pigtail catheter (2.8 mm external diameter) is placed in the pancreatic pseudocyst via a percutaneous, transgastric cannula under percutaneous ultra sonographic guidance. When the metal guide-sleeve has been retracted, the two preformed ends of the catheter coil up into a double pigtail catheter with the distal end in the cyst and the proximal in the stomach (Figs. 1, 2). The catheter is usually 8 cm in length. The best way to remove the double pigtail catheter is endoscopically, either using a polypectomy noose or a forceps.

Evaluative Summary

Experience to date shows that, to undergo endoscopy-assisted percutaneous, ultrasonographic catheter drainage, the pancreatic pseudocyst should have a wide surface contact with the dorsal gastric wall and be adequately impressed into it. It should be not less than 6 cm in diameter. With cysts of this size or more, secondary disturbance of the bile flow or an incipient functional duodenal obstruction is present. Before carrying out this procedure on the pancreas, endoscopic retrograde pancreatography should be performed to rule out filling of the pseudocyst with contrast medium from the pancreatic duct, which would be a contraindication. It must be ensured that the drainage is not placed ventrally through intestinal loops; this can be checked by ultrasonography. Pseudocysts best suited to this treatment are those with adequately mature walls, i.e. with incipient induration due to scarring, under which conditions high intraluminal pressure can be expected to cause the pseudocyst to shrink. The very high amylase and lipase concentrations regularly found in pancreatic pseudocysts apparently prevent occlusion of the drainage catheter in many cases. However, pancreatic sequestra in the pseudocyst or contents that appear inhomogeneous on ultrasonography, such as sediments, are unsuited to internal drainage. Contraindications to intragastric drainage are fistulae between the

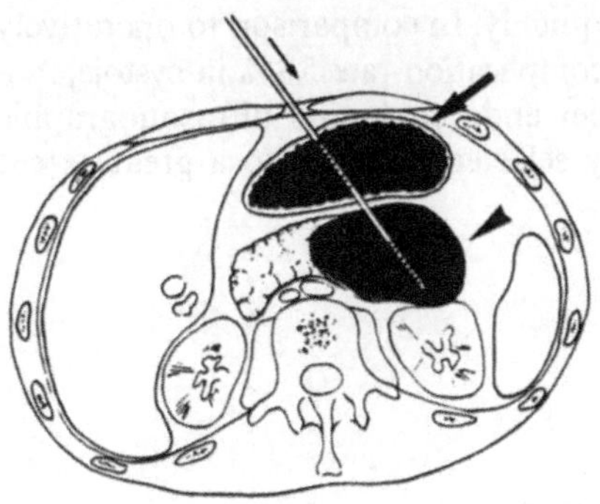

Fig. 1. Implantation of the pigtail catheter (*light arrow*; 2.8 mm external diameter) in the pancreatic pseudocyst via a percutaneous, transgastric cannula under percutaneous ultrasonographic guidance. *Heavy arrow*, stomach; *arrowhead*, pancreatic pseudocyst

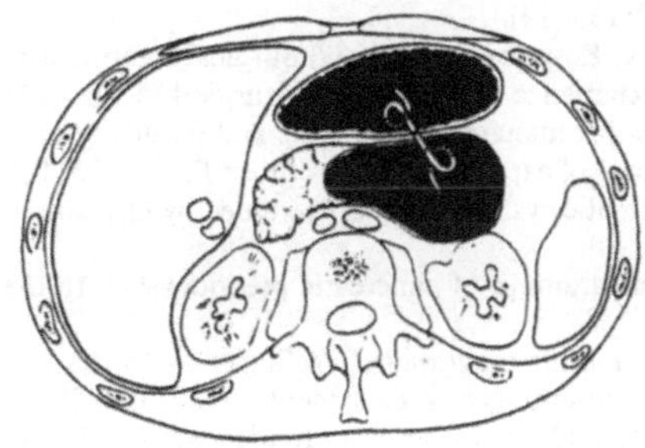

Fig. 2. When the metal guide-sleeve has been retracted, the two preformed ends of the catheter coil up into a double pigtail catheter with the distal end in the cyst and the proximal in the stomach

pancreatic duct and the pseudocyst, blood in the pancreatic juice and pseudocysts containing blood [2].

The best time to carry out combined endoscopic and ultrasonographic cystogastric drainage seems from experience to be about 6–8 weeks after acute formation of the pseudocyst; by this time both the cyst contents and the cyst wall have normally consolidated. Before puncture, endosonography should be carried out in the dorsal gastric wall in order to rule out the presence of any vascular malformation in the area of the puncture canal.

The complication rate associated with endoscopic cystoenterostomy is around 23.5%; one fatal haemorrhage has been reported [8]. In one case catheter breakage 4 months after implantation was reported, so that remaining drainage contents had to be operatively removed from the pseudocyst [7]. Superimposed bacterial infection of the cystogastric drainage must be expected in 2.5% of cases, usually colonization by *Candida albicans.* As leucocytosis has frequently been observed after drainage of pancreatic pseudocysts, prophylactic treatment with broad-spectrum antibiotics for 3 days (imipenem 3 × mg, tobramycin 2 × 80 mg, metronidazole 3 × 500 mg i.v.) is recommended.

The success rate in placing an intragastric drain is 60%–96% [4, 8]. Successful drainage, i.e. permanent drainage of the pancreatic pseudocyst, is achieved in about 75% of cases [7]. Experience has shown about 3–6 months to be the right length of time for drainage; with this drainage technique, of course, patients are not restricted in their movements as they are by external drainage and usually become fully mobilized quite quickly. In comparison to operatively treated patients (success rate 78%–100%, complication rate 5.8% in cystojejunostomies [1, 3]), intragastric drainage under endoscopic and ultrasonographic guidance is less invasive and, in carefully selected patients, to a great extent primarily successful.

References

1. Andersson R, Janzon M, Sundberg I, Bengmark S (1989) Management of pancreatic pseudocysts. Br J Surg 76:550–552
2. Bradley EL, Clements JL, Jr, Gonzales AC (1979) The natural history of pancreatic pseudocysts: a unified concept of management. Am J Surg 137:135–141
3. Campion JP, Baradxoglou E, Caillon P, Faroux R, Bourdonnec P (1989) Surgical treatment of chronic pancreatitis. Indications and results. An experience of 246 cases. Chirurgie 115:123–131
4. Cremer M, Deviere J, Engelholm L (1989) Endoscopic management of cysts and pseudocysts in chronic pancreatitis: long term follow-up after 7 years of experience. Gastrointest Endosc 35:1–9
5. Hancke S, Heriksen FW (1985) Percutaneous pancreatic cysto-gastrostomy guided by ultrasound scanning and gastroscopy. Br J Surg 72:916–917
6. Heyder N, Flügel H, Domschke W (1988) Catheter drainage of pancreatic pseudocysts into the stomach. Endoscopy 20:75–77
7. Heyder N, Günter E, Hahn EG (1992) Endoskopisch-sonographisch geführte zysto-gastrale Katheterdrainagen pankreatogener Flüssigkeitsansammlungen. Z Gastroenterol 30:553–557
8. Sahel J, Bastid C, Pellat B, Schurgers P, Sarles H (1987) Endoscopic cystoduodenostomy of cysts of chronic calcifying pancreatitis. A report of 20 cases. Pancreas 2:447–453
9. Van Sonnenberg E, Wittich GR, Casola G, Brannigan TC, Karnel F, Stabile BE, Varney RR, Christensen RR (1989) Percutaneous drainage of infected and noninfected pancreatic pseudocysts: experience in 101 cases. Radiology 170:757–761

Laser Treatment of Early Gastric Carcinoma in Japan: An Overview

Y. Oguro

Introduction

As is well known, the mortalities of both men and women from gastric cancer in Japan have been the highest in the world for years. Prevention, detection, and treatment of gastric cancer are therefore one of the biggest medical problems in our country. In 1962, the definition, criteria, and classification of early gastric cancer were proposed, and then its diagnosis was studied. With the rapid improvement and progress in endoscopy and the development of endoscopic treatment, it has been possible to treat some types of early gastric cancer recently by endoscopic methods, with successful results. For this purpose, early gastric cancers have to be divided at diagnosis into two groups: one to undergo curative endoscopic treatment and the other requiring surgery. After endoscopic treatment of the lesion, there is no decrease of quality of life and performance status, which are usually affected to some degree after surgery. Endoscopic treatment is the best method in as much as it is a minimally invasive treatment.

Endoscopic Methods for Treatment of Early Gastric Cancer

Some endoscopic methods have been developed for treatment of early gastric cancer. Of these, laser endoscopy and the high-frequency electric current technique are the most important and most frequently used. The latter is an endoscopic resection method (ER), which includes endoscopic polypectomy (EP) and endoscopic mucosal resection (EMR), strip biopsy (SB), etc. The former is a nonresectioning form of endoscopy (non-ER). As Table 1 shows, when ER is used, the curability of the lesion removed can be investigated by histological study, but there is a limit in the size of the lesion that can be treated; it must measure less than 1.5 cm. Of the non-ER methods, laser endoscopy is typical; some others are microwave coagulation therapy, heater probe coagulation, and endoscopic local injection. Although non-ER methods cannot remove the lesion and require a follow-up study with biopsy after the treatment, they can treat much larger lesions than those that are resectable and curable by EMR. Moreover, larger lesions suitable for non-ER methods are more frequently seen than smaller lesions.

Table 1. Endoscopic radical treatment for early gastric cancer

	Resection	No resection
Methods	Polypectomy Strip biopsy ER-HSE	Laser Microwave Heater probe Injection
Histology of total lesion	Possible	Impossible
Curable size	≤ 1.5 cm	> 1.5 cm
Patients	Any	High surgical risk

ER-HSE, Endoscopic resection high saline epinephrine

Development of Laser Endoscopic Treatment

In laser endoscopic treatment, there are three principal methods: vaporization, photodynamic therapy and laserthermia.

Vaporization Using Nd:YAG Laser

Laser endoscopy was first developed by Nath and Kiefhaber et al. [1], West Germany, in 1972, transmitting a laser beam through a specially devised quartz fiber. Through it, they transmitted first an argon laser into the stomach with success and then a Nd:YAG laser. At this stage, the fiber was too delicate and fragile, so that it could not project beyond the tip of the fiberscope without being destroyed by the burning of blood or mucus attached on it. This method was inconvenient for transmitting laser to a target lesion endoscopically. I have called this method "intrafiberscopic irradiation" (Fig. 1).

Research was directed to improving the durability of the tip of a quartz fiber, covering it with a special metal. This brought the better handling of "extrafiberscopic irradiation", which greatly improved the technique and the effectiveness of laser irradiation. Even with this improved quartz fiber, however, the tip could not touch the target lesion without being damaged. This method is called "non-contact irradiation".

In 1983 in Japan in collaboration with the USA a new probe made from a special ceramic was devised to protect the tip of the quartz fiber. This ceramic probe is highly tolerant of heat and burning and provides excellent transmission of the laser beam as well. With this probe, the quartz fiber became completely safe from burning of mucus or blood adhering to it, so that the new techniques of contact irradiation [2] and laserthermia (laser hyperthermia or local interstitial laser hyperthermia) were developed, in 1986 [3].

In the initial stages of laser endoscopy, the interest of almost all the laser endoscopists in the world was focused on hemostasis of gastrointestinal bleed-

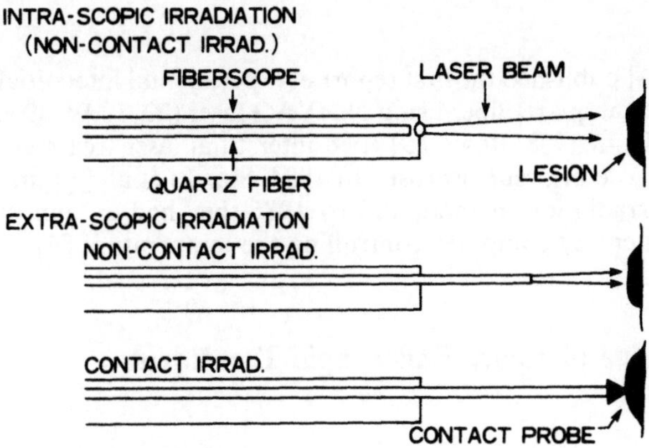

Fig. 1. The three stages in the development of laser endoscopic treatment

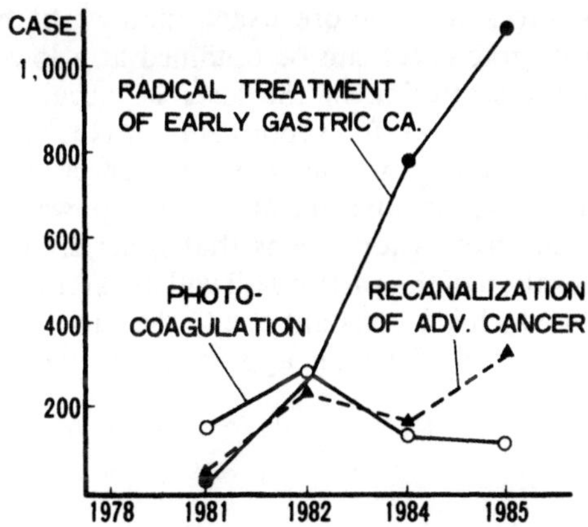

Fig. 2. Laser endoscopic treatment for gastrointestinal lesions in Japan

ing, by the method called photocoagulation. However, we thought that laser endoscopy should be employed in the treatment of cancer, and in 1976 we started experimental and then clinical studies of this problem, which has now become the main target of laser endoscopy (Fig. 2).

Photodynamic Therapy

In 1975, Dougherty et al. reported the treatment of animal tumors with hematoporphyrin derivative (HpD) and irradiation with a mercury lamp, and in 1979 discovered the effectiveness of an argon dye laser with a 630-nm wavelength on tumor. This is called photodynamic therapy (PDT) and is applied endoscopically in the treatment of gastrointestinal and bronchial cancer.

Laserthermia

In 1980, Fukutomi et al. [4] published the first report of experimental interstitial irradiation, inserting a special quartz fiber using Nd:YAG laser (20–30 W, 30 s) and causing tissue necrosis. In 1983, Bown [5] tried interstitial laser treatment and confirmed the occurrence of tissue necrosis. In 1984, Suzuki et al. [3] first reported on the contact irradiation method, and by 1986 they had an almost complete laserthermia system by computer-controlling the temperature [6].

Principles and Technique of Laser Endoscopic Treatment

Vaporization

Some types of early gastric cancer can be treated radically by vaporization (Fig. 3). For vaporization of cancerous tissue by laser, Nd:YAG laser is usually applied; occasionally the argon laser is used. With the contact method, the effectiveness of laser irradiation becomes much more exact than with the noncontact method, and a good vaporizing effect can be obtained at a lower laser power, because there is no back scattering of the laser as occurs in noncontact irradiation (Fig. 4). As Table 2 shows, for vaporization a Nd:YAG laser requires 60–100 W in noncontact irradiation, but the same effect – and more constant – can be obtained in contact irradiation at a lower power of 10–30 W. The constant effect of contact irradiation means that generally less cancerous tissue will remain and perforation of the gastric wall will be rarer than in noncontact irradiation, the effect of which is inconstant due to the variability of distance and direction (Fig. 5). The price of a laser apparatus for contact irradiation is much cheaper.

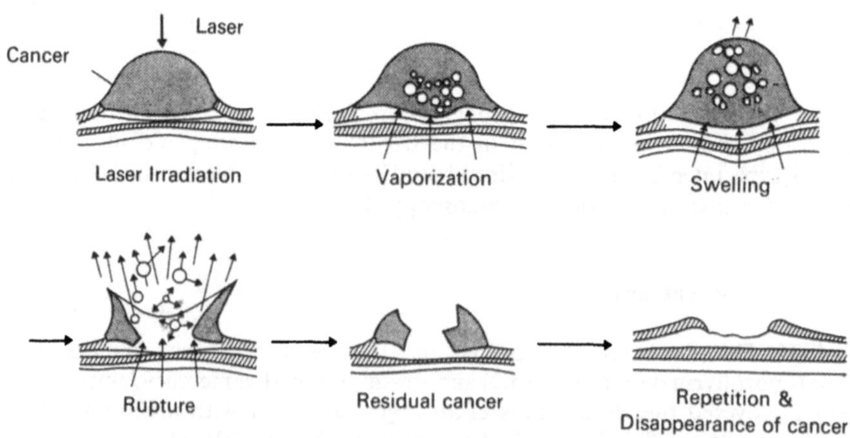

Fig. 3. Vaporization of early gastric cancer by high-power laser irradiation

Table 2. Noncontact and contact irradiation with Nd:YAG laser

	Noncontact	Contact
Distance	Irregular	Fixed (0 cm)
Power (W)	60 ~ 100	10 ~ 25
Effect	Irregular	Constant
Incomplete resection, perforation	Possible	Rare
Cost	Expensive	Cheaper

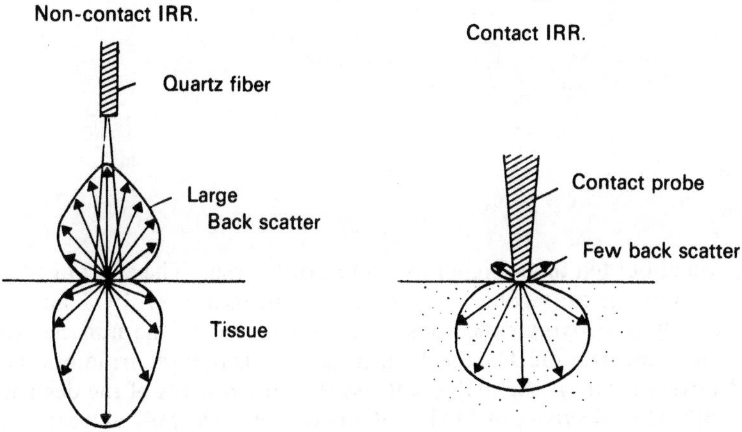

Fig. 4. Back scatter in noncontact and contact irradiation

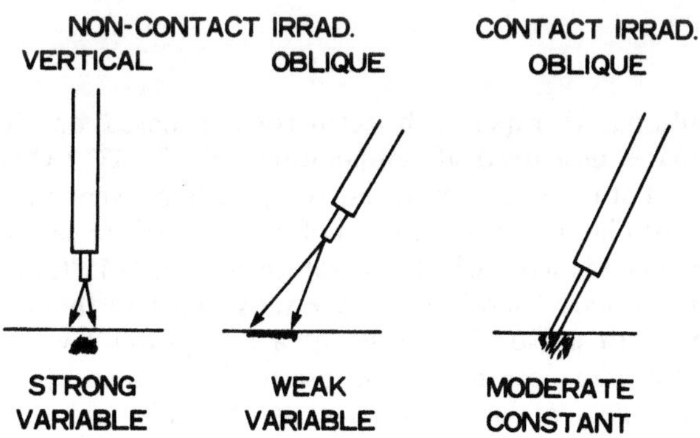

Fig. 5. The advantages of contact irradiation: distance and strength of effect are kept more constant throughout the procedure than in noncontact irradiation

Photodynamic Therapy

48 h after intravenous administration of a HpD at a dose of 2.5 mg/kg, an argon dye laser at a low power of 300–400 mW is transmitted to the lesion and its surroundings for 20–30 min. At this time, HpD is located in malignant tissue at

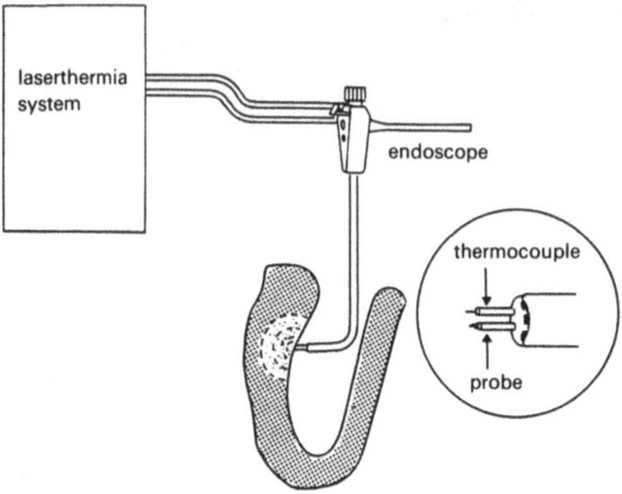

Fig. 6. Laser hyperthermia system using an endoscope

a concentration about ten times higher than in normal tissue. The effect of PDT then influences only the cancerous tissue to the submucosal layer. PDT has the effect of selectively destroying cancerous tissue, compared to the nonselective destruction with vaporization. The mechanism of PDT is that the irradiation of the laser selectively destroys the malignant tissue in the process of the destruction of the HpD. The selectivity of PDT is of advantage in the radical treatment of early gastric cancer of indistinct extent, especially superficial esophageal cancer.

Laserthermia

The mechanism of conventional therapeutic hyperthermia is based on the phenomenon that carcinoma is destroyed at temperatures of 42°–43°, while normal tissue is not so affected at these temperatures. With the improvement in contact irradiation by Nd:YAG laser, the ceramic tip of the quartz fiber can be inserted into a cancerous lesion and increase its temperature up to 42°–45°C at a low laser power level, causing destruction of the lesion. Endoscopic laserthermia is performed by irradiation with a Nd:YAG laser at a low power level of 1.5–3.0 W for about 20 min through a ceramic probe inserted into a tumor (Fig. 6). We confirmed the effectiveness of laserthermia experimentally and then clinically in a patient with inoperable, advanced gastric cancer, and found it resulted in marked tumor reduction [7]. As Fig. 7 shows, the viability of human pancreatic cancer cells decreased most remarkably by the combination of simple heating at 42°C and irradiation with a low-power Nd:YAG laser at 2 W continuously for 30 min, compared to simple heating or the combination of simple heating and microwave hyperthermia. As to the mechanism of laserthermia, it seems that the immediate effect is cellular damage caused by both heat

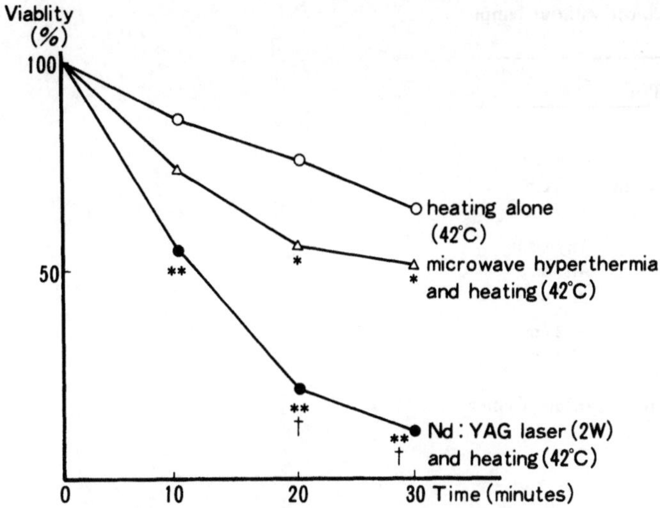

Fig. 7. Superiority of low-power Nd: YAG laser combined with simple heating (42° C) over both simple heating and simple heating combined with microwave hyperthermia in destroying the viability of human pancreatic cancer cells

and the Nd:YAG laser beam, followed by subsequent destruction of tumor vessels.

Indications for Laser Endoscopic Radical Treatment of Early Gastric Cancer

Radical endoscopic treatment by ER should be performed only in early gastric cancer without lymph node metastases, preferably limited to the mucosal layer and not too large. Treatment by laser endoscopy should be performed for the same kind of lesions and principally in patients with high surgical risk.

Early Gastric Cancer Without Lymph Node Metastases

In Japan, very many cases of early gastric cancer have been treated surgically and studied pathologically. In our study [8] on lymph node metastases in gastric cancer, the existence of metastases was closely related to the depth of cancerous invasion, type, and size, and it was confirmed that in some types of early gastric cancer, no lymph node metastases were present (Table 3). The following types are best suited to radical ER:

1. Type I (elevated type) early gastric cancer, limited to the mucosa (m) and especially with a stalk, not accompanied by lymph node metastases, regardless of carcinoma size. This type has to be treated by EP.

Table 3. Early gastric cancer without lymph node metastases

Cancer type	Depth	Size
Elevated		
I	m	Any size
IIa	m & sm	≤ 2 cm
Flat & depressed		
Ul(−)·IIb	m	Any size
IIc	m	Any size
IIc	sm	≤ 3 cm
Ul(+)·IIb	m	≤ 2 cm
IIc	m	≤ 2 cm

1430 cases, in National Cancer Center Hospital
m, sm: see text.

2. Type IIa (superficial elevated type) early gastric cancer less than 2.0 cm in size with invasion limited to the submucosa (sm), and with no lymph node metastases. This type has to be treated by EP or EMR.

3. Types IIb (superficial flat type) and IIc (superficial depressed type) with no disruption of the mucosal muscle (Ul(−)), carcinomatous tissue limited to m, and no lymph node metastasis, regardless of carcinoma size. These types less than 1.5 cm in size have to be treated by EMR.

4. Ul(+) IIc type early gastric cancer, which is usually accompanied by mucosal converging folds. Lymph node metastasis is recognized rather more frequently in this type than in Ul(−)IIc. Therefore, in Ul(+)IIc gastric cancer, only lesions less than 1.5 cm in size can be assigned to radical endoscopic treatment of EMR.

Selection of Radical Endoscopic Treatment by Laser or Another Method for Early Gastric Cancer (Table 4)

The general condition of the patient with high surgical risk is the other important indication for radical endoscopic treatment of early gastric cancer. In such patients, a lesion less than 1.5 cm in size and with Ul(−) is to be treated by EMR and a larger one by laser endoscopy (Table 5).

Current Review of Laser Endoscopic Treatment of Early Gastric Cancer in Japan

According to a nation-wide Japanese study [9] in 1987, 1436 cases of gastric cancer have been treated radically using a single endoscopic method. Laser endoscopic treatment was the most frequently performed (764 cases), especially

Table 4. Endoscopic treatments for gastric cancer

	HFC		LASER				
	POLPEC	SB	VAP	PDT	MCT	HPC	INJN
Early gastric cancer							
I: m, stalk	○						
IIa:							
≤ 2 cm, m, sm	○	○	○	○	○	○	
> 2 cm	○		○	○	○	○	
IIb, IIc (Ul −):							
m, sm: 1 cm		○	○	○	○	○	
~ 1.5 cm		○	○	○	○	○	
~ 3.0 cm			○	○			
IIb, IIc (Ul +):							
≤ 2 cm, m		○	○	○	○	○	
Advanced gastric cancer							
Hemostasis			○			○	○
Recanalization			○				
Tumor reduction			○				○

Table 5. Indications for and selection of endoscopic method to treat early gastric cancer

	Lesion size	
	≤ 1.5 cm	≥ 1.5 cm
No risk for surgery	EMR	Surgery
High risk for surgery	EMR	EMR + laser or laser alone

EMR, Endoscopic mucosal resection
Laser, Nd: YAG laser

by Nd:YAG laser, and then EP and EMR in 511 cases (Table 6). Two hundred and seventeen were treated by a combination of EP or EMR and laser (Table 7). Out of these, a combination of EP or EMR and laser was applied most often in 153 cases.

In 1984, we studied the nation-wide laser endoscopy results in Japan [10]. One thousand one hundred and fifty-eight cases of early and advanced gastric cancer were treated by laser endoscopy, out of a total of 1859 cases including other types of gastrointestinal cancer. Radical endoscopic laser irradiation had been performed in 824 patients with early gastric cancer, 736 patients were treated mostly by Nd:YAG laser, and then 55 by PDT and 33 by other lasers. Negative biopsy results were obtained in 218 out of 256 cases in the group with follow-up of less than 1 year, in 316 out of 411 with follow-up of 1–3 years, in 120 out of 139 with follow-up of 3–5 years, and in 16 out of 18 with follow-up of more than 5 years. According to the other nation-wide follow-up study on early gastric cancer with radical laser endoscopic treatment [11], out of the 893 cases treated with Nd:YAG laser, 69 cases were reported who had not been operated on and had no recurrence over a 5-year period.

Table 6. Endoscopic treatment of early gastric cancer: method and cases (single treatment) (1987)

	No. of cases
Laser	764
Nd:YAG	673
argon	10
PDT	81
High freq. current	511
polypectomy	317
strip biopsy	97
others	97
Microwave	101
Local injection	60
Total	1436 Cases

Table 7. Endoscopic treatment of gastric cancer (1987)

	No. of cases
Early cancer	1653
Single treatment	1436
Combined treatment	217
Advanced cancer	386
Recanalization	164
Tumor reduction	106
Hemostasis	116
Gastric adenoma	945

In the collective study [9] on negative biopsy results at final biopsy at follow-up more than 1 year after radical endoscopic treatment (single method) of early gastric cancer, 455 cases were reported after 1–3 years, 195 cases after 3–5 years, and 46 cases after more than 5 years – in total, 696 cases. The negative biopsy percentages more than 1 year after radical endoscopic treatment (single method) by laser were between 83% and 85%. This difference may be caused by selection of the cases with or without indications for radical endoscopic treatment. To increase the percentage of negative follow-up biopsies, it is important to select and carry out the most appropriate radical endoscopic treatment for each case on the basis of the absolute indication. For early gastric cancer in a patient with high surgical risk, however, laser endoscopic treatment has to be performed even when the indication is only relative, so it is difficult to get a higher negative biopsy rate.

Endoscopic treatment can be repeated on the same lesion and can be performed with a combination of more than two methods to improve results. In this study [9], the combination of ER and laser was the most often performed (115 cases), and negative biopsy was found after more than 1 year in 108 cases (94%).

According to the nation-wide collective follow-up study [11] in 1987 on cases of early gastric cancer treated by laser endoscopy, 126 out of 611 patients (20.6%) died of other causes and there were 0.58% direct deaths due to surgery (death within 30 days after surgery) among patients with early gastric cancer with invasion. Thus, surgery should not be performed in every patient with early gastric cancer.

Other Aspects of Laser Endoscopic Treatment of Early Gastric Cancer

Reasons for Selection of Radical Endoscopic Treatment

According to our nation-wide study in 1986 [10], the most frequent reason for selection of endoscopic treatment for early gastric cancer was "inoperability due to complications" (33/58 institutions). The next most frequent reasons were "advanced age of patient" and "patient refused surgery" (8 each), followed by "radical endoscopic treatment possible in patient without surgical risk" (2). According to the other collective study in 1987 [11], on the reasons for performing laser treatment, out of 2040 cases including early and advanced cancer, "high surgical risk" was the most frequent (967 cases), and then "preoperative treatment" (303 cases), "unresectable" (297 cases), "surgery rejected" (178 cases), "lesion curable by laser" (87 cases), and lastly "unclear" (208 cases). Notable points are that nearly half of the patients treated had high surgical risk, and that there were so many refusers of surgery and so many cases of curable early gastric cancer by laser treatment alone.

In the workshop "Problems in endoscopic treatment of early gastric cancer" at the 74th Congress of the Japanese Society of Gastroenterology, in 1988 [12], we studied the reasons for selecting endoscopic treatment for the lesion in a total of 698 patients. "High surgical risk due to complications or old age etc." was the most frequent reason (288 cases), followed by "radical endoscopic treatment possible, even though surgery possible" (260 cases), "preoperative irradiation" (57 cases), "surgery refused" (52 cases), and "other" (41 cases).

Quality of Life After Endoscopic Treatment and Surgery

At the Research Congress of Gastric Cancer in 1989 [13], it was agreed that radical endoscopic treatment for early gastric cancer with appropriate indication may be performed even in a patient without surgical risk. According to a study on the question of quality of life [14], patients' quality of life after radical endoscopic treatment for early gastric cancer was much better than after surgery, with no decrease in performance status. Radical endoscopic treatment, therefore, has recently become the first choice for early gastric cancer, with the appropriate indications, even if the patient is not a surgical risk, because of the worse quality of life after surgery. Therefore, from the point of view of quality of life in the old patient with early gastric cancer and a high surgical risk, endoscopic treatment including laser endoscopy should be performed instead of surgery.

Ratio of Radical Endoscopic Treatment to Surgery

According to our study in 1986 [10] in major hospitals where both endoscopic treatment and surgery were performed for early gastric cancer during a given period, the ratio of radical laser endoscopic treatment to surgery was 14.4:100 (824:5375). In our study in 1988 [12], the ratio had increased to 18.6:100 (636:3415). These results show that radical endoscopic treatment for this lesion with appropriate indications is establishing a foothold.

References

1. Nath G, Gerisch W, Kiefhaber P (1973) First laser endoscopy via transmission system. Endoscopy 5:208–213
2. Oguro Y, Tajiri H (1986) YAG laser treatment for stenosis due to advanced cancer of esophagus and stomach – non-contact and contact irradiation. In: Waidelich W, Kiefhaber P (eds) Laser-optoelectronics in medicine. Springer, Berlin Heidelberg New York, pp 338–343
3. Suzuki S, Shiina Y, Miura T et al. (1980) Effect of Nd: YAG laser radiation on the gastrointestinal mucosa. Gastroenterol Endosc 26:705–710 (in Japanese with English abstract)
4. Nakahara A, Takase Y, Fukutomi H et al. (1980) The fundamental and clinical studies on the endoscopic laser therapy for the protruding lesions. Gastroenterol Endosc 22:1360–1373 (in Japanese with English abstract)
5. Bown SG (1983) Tumor therapy with Nd:YAG laser. In: Joffe SN (ed) Neodymium YAG laser in medicine and surgery. New York, Elsevier, New York. pp 51–58
6. Suzuki S, Aoki J, Shiina Y, Nomiyama T, Miwa T, Daikuzono N (1986) Endoscopic local hyperthermia with Nd-YAG laser – experimental study and development of computed thermo-system. J Jpn Soc Laser Medicine 6:347–50 (in Japanese with English abstract)
7. Tajiri H, Shiotani H, Oguro Y et al. (1986) A study on photodynamic therapy and local interstitial hyperthermia using low power Nd: YAG laser, including experimental studies. Gastroenterol Endosc 28:2282–2288 (in Japanese with English abstract)
8. Oguro Y (1990) Recent advances in endoscopic treatment. In: Oguro Y, Takagi K (eds). Endoscopic approaches to cancer diagnosis and treatment, Gann monograph on cancer research, Japanese Scientific Societies Press, Tokyo, pp 89–99
9. Kasugai T (1987) Endoscopic treatment for gastric tumor and follow-up study. The 48th Japanese Research Meeting of Gastric Cancer (in Japanese)
10. Oguro Y, Tajiri H (1980) The present status of YAG laser medicine in Japan – endoscopic laser treatment for GI cancer. In: Oguro Y, Atsumi K, Joffe SN (eds) Nd: YAG laser in medicine and surgery. Professional Postgraduate Services, Tokyo, pp 3–9
11. Watanabe Y, Oguro Y, Takemoto T, Sakita T (1988) Present status of endoscopic laser therapy for cancers of the gastrointestinal tract. Prog Dig Endosc 33:121–125 (in Japanese with English abstract)
12. Oguro Y, Hiki Y (1988) Workshop: Problems in endoscopic treatment of early gastric cancer. The 74th Congress of the Japanese Society of Gastroenterology, Sendai, March 1988
13. Oshiba S, Oguro Y (1990) Discussion on endoscopic treatment for early gastric cancer. J Jpn Soc Cancer Ther 25:1376
14. Kasugai T, Ito Y, Kametani A, Kano T (1988) Curative endoscopic treatment of early gastric cancer, results, prognosis and quality of life. Geka Shinryo 30:1193–1199 (in Japanese)

Photodynamic Therapy of Gastric Malignancies: Current Status and Future Prospects

C.S. Loh and S.G. Bown

Introduction

Photodynamic therapy (PDT) is a new approach to the local treatment of cancers. A photosensitiser, non-toxic in the dark, is administered to a patient. The photosensitiser is retained with some degree of selectivity by tumour tissue. On exposure to light of the appropriate wavelength, highly reactive but very short lived chemical species are produced which cause cell death. The short half life of these toxic species ensures that the cytotoxic effect is confined to the tissue exposed to the therapeutic light, thus avoiding systemic toxicity.

Discovery of PDT

The discovery of photodynamic effects was accidental. In the winter of 1897–1898, Raab, while studying the toxicity of acridine on protozoan paramecia, came upon widely different results in two experiments using similar dilutions. The only difference in the conditions between these two studies was a great thunder storm during one. Raab was quick to see the possible role of light in affecting the outcome and subsequently confirmed this experimentally (Raab 1900). Later, von Tappeiner, Raab's professor, and Jesionek (1903), a dermatologist, described the first attempts to treat tumours using topically applied eosin (5% aqueous solution) as a photosensitiser, supplemented by fluorescein and anthracine disulphonate in some cases, together with either white light from an arc lamp or direct sunlight to treat skin cancers and they documented tumour responses. Von Tappeiner introduced the term "photodynamische Erscheinung" to describe this effect in 1907.

Haematoporphyrin Derivative

Later, Auler and Banzer (1942) in Berlin studied the photodynamic effect of haematoporphyrin on experimental tumours. Using Flicks-Jobling carcinomas and Jensen's sarcoma, they produced tumour necrosis using photodyn (haematoporphyrin) and a strong quartz lamp. They were the first to describe preferential tumour uptake of porphyrins. In 1948, Figge and his colleagues from Baltimore reported on tumour affinity of various porphyrins and first suggested exploiting this phenomenon to enhance tumour detection. They also suggested incorporating a radioactive metal into porphyrin for use in the treatment of tumours. In 1955, Rassmussen-Taxdal et al. reported visualising red fluorescence in human tumours after haematoporphyrin injection. In the mid 1950s, Schwartz and his colleagues in the University of Minnesota introduced a new acetic-sulphuric acid derivative of haematoporphyrin with better tumour affinity, which has come to be known as haematoporphyrin derivative, HpD. Later, Lipson and Baldes showed enhanced tumour localisation with improved photodynamic properties of this compound (1961–1967) and firmly established HpD as the most important and most studied photosensitising substance to date. The standard preparation of HpD has remained essentially the same since that described by Lipson and Baldes in details in 1960. Until quite recently, HpD and its related "purified" preparation, Photofrin (QLT, Vancouver) were the only photosensitisers to be used clinically.

The advent of laser technology offered the feasibility of delivering light at appropriate power levels down optic fibres. Internal organs became accessible to light illumination for PDT. Endoscopists were quick to see the potential, and endoscopic PDT of visceral tumours became possible. The first patient had a bronchial carcinoma and was treated with PDT through a bronchoscope by Hayata and Kato at the Tokyo Medical College in 1980. They subsequently reported their results in a series of 13 patients and showed that the best results were obtained treating early tumours (Hayata et al. 1982).

Mechanism of Photodynamic Effect

Upon photoactivation, a photosensitiser molecule becomes excited from its stable ground state into an unstable "energised" singlet state. It may then spontaneously return to its ground state, releasing the absorbed energy as heat (internal conversion) or light (fluorescence) or may alternatively become converted into a metastable excited state known as the triplet state (by intersystem crossing). Interaction of this triplet state with tissue components is thought to be mediated mainly by its reaction with molecular oxygen, generating an excited species known as singlet oxygen (Weishaupt et al. 1976). Singlet oxygen reacts avidly with various cell constituents causing damage to plasmal, mitochondrial, lysosomal, endoplasmic reticular and nuclear membranes, depending on the intracellular distribution of photosensitiser (Moan et al. 1989). Thus, PDT relies on the availability of oxygen for its toxic effect (Gomer and Razum 1984; Moan and Sommer 1985) and, rather like with ionising radiation, hypoxic tissue is less sensitive to damage.

In vitro studies have shown that cells with varying capacity for DNA repair appear to be universally sensitive to PDT damage (Gomer et al. 1988). More recently, Kessel and Erickson (1992) showed no difference in sensitivity to PDT damage between cell lines with and without multi-drug resistance phenotypes. These findings are consistent with the clinical observation that few tumours exhibit intrinsic resistance to PDT (Dougherty 1990), in contrast to chemotherapy and radiotherapy. This is pertinent as gastric malignancies are generally poor responders to both the latter treatment modalities.

Tissue damage is dependent on the rate of singlet oxygen generation, which in turn correlates with tissue sensitiser concentration and light dose as well as oxygenation. Given adequate tissue oxygenation, photodynamic action will occur wherever the product of tissue photosensitiser concentration and light dose exceed a certain threshold (Cowled and Forbes, 1985). The optical penetration of red light at 635 nm (as required for HpD) varies with the tissue type (Svaasand 1984) but it is possible to get PDT effects up to about 10 mm below the surface exposed to the therapeutic light. There had been very little study on the quantitative effect of PDT. Using endosonography, Barr et al. (1990) were able to show a mean depth of tumour destruction of only 6 mm in rectal carcinomas using HpD with red light. Such measurements have not yet been reported for gastric carcinomas. PDT is thus generally not suitable for treatment of advanced and bulky disease.

Histopathological and Functional Changes

It is surprising how little work has been done on the nature of PDT damage to normal and neoplastic areas in any tissue, although studies on normal rat stomach using aluminium sulphonated phthalocyanine as photosensitiser have recently been reported (Loh et al., 1992). These showed that apart from blanching of the treated tissue, no macroscopically discernible change was obvious immediately following PDT, although changes in the affected cells can be seen microscopically. Coagulative necrosis, predominantly of the mucosa, is apparent by 24 h, although the general structural architecture of the gastric wall, in particular the collagen rich submucosa, remains intact. However, by the end of 1 week, full-thickness necrosis has become apparent. The full-thickness defect in the gastric wall is bridged by scar tissue on the serosal aspect. Interestingly, the mechanical strength of the gastric wall as measured by bursting pressures is maintained at all times (Loh, unpublished observation). It would seem likely that mechanical strength is initially maintained by submucosal collagen fibres and later afforded by serosal scar tissue as full-thickness necrosis is established. Thus, unlike full-thickness thermal laser effects, PDT carries minimal risk of causing visceral perforation, as shown previously in the colon (Barr et al. 1991). Epithelial cells regenerate from adjacent healthy mucosa and complete re-epithelialisation is generally accomplished by the 6th week. The regenerated mucosa is initially non-specialised of mucous glandular type, although oxyntic cell repopulation becomes evident after 12 weeks (Loh, unpublished observations).

Selectivity

Most of the early interest in PDT centred on the possibility of selective tumour destruction. It is now clear that this aspect has been very much over-emphasised.

The real value of PDT is the nature of the tissue damage produced, as normal tissues heal so well with no risk of perforation even in hollow organs with full-thickness necrosis, so such damage to normal areas may be acceptable. Nevertheless, some selectivity is possible. Animal studies in a range of organs have shown that the photosensitiser is predominantly located in the vascular stroma rather than the parenchyma in both tumour and normal tissue (Bugelski et al. 1981; Chatlani et al. 1992). Disruption of this vascular region plays a major role in the tumoricidal effect of PDT in vivo (Nelson et al. 1987; Stern et al. 1990). The best ratio of photosensitiser concentration between tumour and normal areas is only 2 or 3 to 1 (Tralau et al. 1987). Truly selective tumour necrosis can only be achieved by judicious manipulation of treatment parameters, but the extent of tumour necrosis so achieved is only 1–2 mm, making such an approach impracticable in most cases (Barr et al. 1991).

Current Practice

PDT is still largely regarded as an experimental treatment modality, although phase III clinical trials in certain tumours using Porfimer sodium (Photofrin, QLT, Vancouver) as photosensitiser are near completion. Clinical experience until now has been built on rather selected groups of patients. These are either those with surgically treatable disease but who are unfit for surgery for other medical reasons, or patients who are unsuitable for surgical resection by virtue of the extent of their disease. Large clinical studies have emanated from Japan and China where gastric cancer is relatively common. In a report by Kato et al. (1986), 10 out of 17 patients with early carcinoma achieved complete remission, six of which were confirmed histologically following subsequent gastrectomy. On the other hand, all the 11 patients with advanced cancer treated only responded partially and residual tumour was confirmed histologically on cases undergoing subsequent resection. The authors cited insufficient light dosage as a likely cause of failure for some early cancers. Another group (Tajiri et al. 1987) treated 13 patients with superficial gastric cancers and reported no recurrence in 9 on follow-up for between 4 and 28 months. However, residual tumours were encountered histologically in 2 cases subsequently operated on. Ito and Kasugai (1987) also reported encouraging results, achieving successful treatment in 5 out of 14 patients with partial response in a further 5 patients. As the selection criteria and the definition of successful treatment differed very considerably in these studies, the widely varying results are not surprising, although good results were consistently achieved only in early and superficial lesions without metastases. Late in situ recurrence after initial tumour clearance has also been reported (Kato et al. 1985; Krasner, personal communication). In none of these series was any real attempt made to match the precise extent of the cancer being treated to the dose and distribution of therapeutic light.

From these data, the role of PDT in gastric cancer is by no means clear. Although complete eradication of early local disease has been achieved on a few occasions, until accurate staging of the disease locally and systemically can be established with confidence, surgery should remain the primary treatment for this group of patients. The real problem is assessing lymphatic spread. It may be possible to assess nodes immediately adjacent to the gastric wall with endoscopic ultrasound, but it is much more difficult for more distant nodes. However, PDT has potential for those patients in whom other medical conditions preclude surgery. The role of PDT in advanced gastric cancer is even more doubtful, particularly for palliation of obstructing gastric cancers. Combination therapy using the Nd: YAG laser initially to debulk the tumour before attempting eradication with PDT has been advocated (Ito and Kasugai 1987). However, unless distant metastasis can be excluded, the value of this approach for more advanced gastric tumours is questionable. We have found PDT useful for the treatment of anastomotic recurrences following surgical resection (Loh and Krasner, unpublished observation). These lesions are often small when detected and easier to eradicate locally, although unfortunately most patients later succumb to distant metastases.

Current Clinical Techniques

Most investigators to date have used HpD (2.5–5 mg/kg) or Photofrin (2–3 mg/kg) given intravenously 24–72 h prior to light exposure. The time interval between administration of sensitiser and light was chosen largely as animal studies showed the best differential distribution of photosensitiser between tumour and normal areas at these times, although these are not necessarily the optimum conditions. These photosensitisers work but have the major drawback that they leave patients sensitive to sunlight for 4–6 weeks. In one series of 180 patients, sunburn occurred in about 10% of all the patients despite their having been given verbal and written instructions on its prevention. All these patients had received either 3 mg/kg HpD or 2 mg/kg. Photofrin (Razum et al. 1987). Recently, antihistamines (H_1 and H_2) and thromboxane inhibitors (aspirin and indomethacin) have been shown to reduce cutaneous photosensitivity (Abulafi et al. 1992). Newer photosensitisers with less cutaneous phototoxicity are being developed (Roberts et al. 1989; Tralau et al. 1989) and should be available for clinical use relatively soon.

Suitable light sources include the gold vapour laser (628 nm) and the argon or copper vapour pumped tunable dye laser. All are satisfactory, although the tunable lasers offer more flexibility for choosing the best wavelength for new photosensitisers. Solid state diode technology holds the promise of low cost and reliability and powerful lasers of this class operating in the red part of the spectrum should be available in the near future. Light delivery to the tumour is generally by means of an optic fibre passed down the biopsy channel of a fibreoptic gastroscope. The side-viewing duodenoscope may be useful for high lesser curve lesions. Illumination of tumour can be achieved superficially using a fibre with a microlens tip (Fig. 1) or interstitially using bare cleaved fibres (Fig. 2) or cylindrical diffusors (Fig. 3). Much work remains to be done to optimise fibre design.

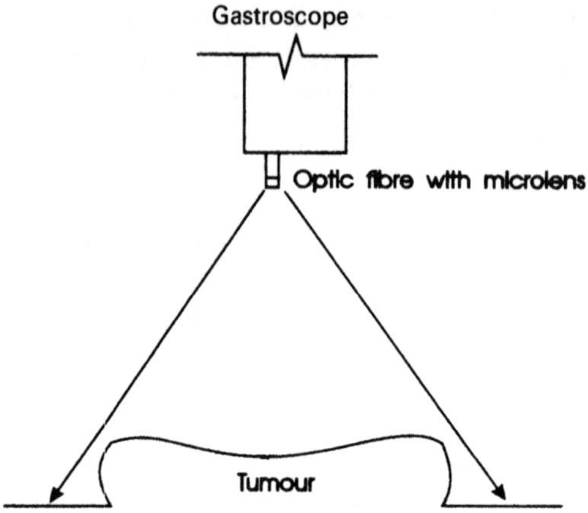

Fig. 1. Superficial illumination of tumour using a fibre with a microlens tip

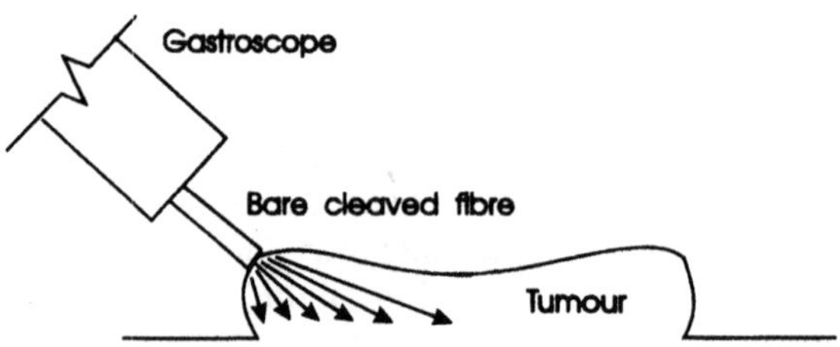

Fig. 2. Interstitial illumination of tumour using bare cleaved fibres

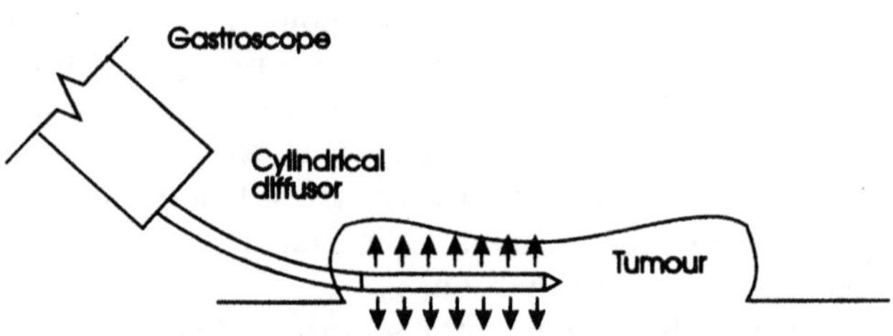

Fig. 3. Interstitial illumination of tumour using a cylindrical diffusor

A typical light dose is 100–300 J/cm^2 for surface illumination. The power at which this is delivered should be kept down to less than 100 mW/cm^2 to reduce the risk of producing thermal effects. This is especially important when irradiation is carried out using the bare fibre in contact with tissue, as too high an output power is likely to lead to charring of tissue and compromises light delivery.

At our centre, treatment is generally carried out under midazolam sedation. We favour the interstitial method of light delivery, as respiratory movement can make consistent surface illumination difficult. The treatment itself is painless and following treatment, patients are generally kept on omeprazole. H_2 antagonists have recently been shown to reduce photosensitivity (Abulafi et al. 1992) and should not be prescribed prior to PDT as they may compromise the efficacy of treatment.

Future Developments

Light

While the introduction of simpler, more reliable solid state diode lasers in the near future may make PDT a cheaper treatment modality, it is unlikely to significantly popularise the technique unless the major limitations are overcome. This will largely depend on the development of better photosensitisers and improved, more reliable light delivery systems.

Photosensitisers

Several photosensitisers with improved photochemical and biological characteristics are now available and currently undergoing preclinical and toxicological evaluation. This generation of agents includes many more porphyrin derivatives and particularly the phthalocyanines, which cause less cutaneous phototoxicity to sunlight as the only absorption peaks in the visible part of the spectrum are in the red (Tralau et al. 1989), where light penetration is better (MacRobert et al. 1989). However, the most important development of the last couple of years has been the realisation that 5-aminolaevulinic acid (ALA) can be used as a precursor for the photosensitiser protoporphyrin IX (PPIX).

ALA is a naturally occurring precursor in haem synthesis. Its biosynthesis is tightly regulated by end product inhibition (Rimington 1966; Marriott 1968). However, by administering a large quantity of exogenous ALA both to in vitro systems and to whole animals, it has been shown that the natural synthetic ability of cells can become saturated and, as a result, porphyrin intermediates of the biosynthetic pathway, particularly PPIX, accumulate (Malik and Djaldetti 1979; Sima et al 1981). This transient accumulation of PPIX can be exploited for PDT (Divaris et al. 1990). Exogenous ALA applied topically has been shown to be effective in the photodynamic treatment of various cutaneous cancers (Kennedy et al. 1990; Wolf and Kerl 1991). PPIX is cleared rapidly in the living system by ferrochelatase, which converts it to the non-photoactive haem, which is in turn broken down into bilirubin and excreted into bile.

We have found that following intravenous administration of ALA in rats, accumulation of photoactive PPIX occurs predominantly in mucosal epithelial cells of hollow viscera (Bedwell et al. 1992; Loh et al., 1992). In general, a differential of at least 10 times was achieved between normal mucosa and underlying muscularis propria. An even higher accumulation occurred in neoplastic epithelial cells and a sixfold differential was found by Bedwell et al. (1992) between neoplastic and normal colonic mucosa. Importantly, in all tissues examined, the accumulation of PPIX was transient, lasting approximately 8–12 h. The high differential between mucosa and muscularis has been exploited by us to produce selective mucosal ablation in the stomach with preservation of underlying muscularis, and this was followed by prompt and safe healing (Loh et al., 1992). It would seem that using this technique there is the potential to ablate dysplastic mucosa, although the safe healing of large mucosal defects still needs to be established. Nevertheless, ALA-induced photosensitisation still has the advantages of a short-lived action and improved selectivity between tumour tissue and underlying normal tissue. The short action and lack of drug accumulation should also permit multiple treatment sessions without fear of toxicity and photosensitivity. Such an approach may be useful for the treatment of bulky tumours which can not be photoirradiated all at once. Thus each treatment will result in removal of a certain depth of tumour, exposing deeper tumour tissue for further treatment. ALA can be given orally and will lead to photosensitisation of target organs in or distant from the alimentary tract similar to that achieved after intravenous administration (Loh et al., unpublished observations). Patients can be given the drug to take just prior to their attendance for treatment, thus minimising the amount of time they need to spend in hospital.

Improved Selectivity

Another factor that may help PDT is to modify drug delivery systems to enhance selectivity. Much work has been done using liposomes as carriers (Jori 1989). With increasing availability of better monoclonal antibodies, a new area of research has been opened up to provide the ultimate precision in drug delivery while the universally cytotoxic property of PDT can be exploited to maximise tumour kill (Popat et al. 1992). Encouraging early clinical results have been reported using this technology for the treatment of gynaecological cancers (Schmidt et al. 1992).

Photodynamic Diagnosis

With the notable exception of Japan, where screening programmes have been in existence for many years, diagnosis of gastric cancers is usually made at a stage too late for curative treatment. In western Europe, although gastroscopy is now a basic investigative tool widely performed, it is disappointing that not many more early gastric cancers are picked up during routine examination. Unless skilled endoscopists are prepared to spend time searching out pre-cancerous lesions, a regime which is economically impractical, little improvement can be expected. Exploitation of the tumour affinity of photosensitisers for diagnostic purposes by looking for increased fluorescence in tumour areas has been attempted with varying results (Kato et al. 1984; Monnier et al. 1990; Zandomeneghi et al. 1988). A major issue is the ethics of subjecting an individual to a prolonged period of photosensitivity for diagnostic purposes, although if this could be done with new photosensitisers like ALA this would be much less of a problem. With improvement in imaging technology and availability of photosensitisers with better tumour affinity, this technique may yet prove to be a valuable tool for gastroenterologists of the future, although it is more likely to be of value for indicating the presence of early neoplastic disease in high-risk patients rather than for mapping the exact distribution of disease.

H. pylori

Yet another area in which PDT might find a role in the future is in treating *H. pylori* (*HP*) infection, as this is localised to areas of the upper gastrointestinal tract that are readily accessible endoscopically. The role of *HP* in the aetiology of gastric malignancy is far from clear, although there have been suggestions of a connection in addition to the more generally accepted link with duodenal ulceration (Moss and Calam 1992). None of the pharmacological eradication regimens has proven entirely satisfactory. We reported in vitro killing of *HP* with PDT using the sensitiser aluminium sulphonated phthalocyanine (Bedwell et al. 1990) under conditions that would be unlikely to effect gastric mucosa. These preliminary findings raised the possibility of using PDT to eradicate *HP*. However, much work needs to be done on photosensitiser and light delivery before in vivo effect can be assessed.

Conclusion

PDT has considerable promise in the management of gastric malignancies, but probably only for the treatment of early disease. It is feasible to treat small areas of neoplastic disease and immediately adjacent normal tissue and be confident that all treated areas will heal safely without risk of perforation. The problem is to know exactly how far the tumour extends, particularly whether there is any lymphatic spread. PDT is only a local treatment, and any part of the tumour not exposed to an adequate light dose will remain viable. Another role may be as a supplement to surgery, to treat small areas of tumour that cannot be removed when the main bulk is removed by surgery. Careful clinical studies with sophisticated imaging to establish the extent of disease spread and to monitor PDT effects will be required to establish the true potential of PDT in the management of gastric malignancy.

References

1. Abulafi AM, Dean R, Allardice JT, Williams NS (1992) Prevention of cutaneous phototoxicity following photodynamic therapy (Abstract). Lasers Med Surg Suppl 4:49
2. Auler H, Banzer G (1942) Untersuchungen über die Rolle der Porphyrine bei geschwulstkranken Menschen und Tieren. Z Krebsforsch 53:65–68
3. Barr H, Chatlani P, Tralau CJ, MacRobert AJ, Boulos PB, Bown Sg (1991) Local eradication of rat colon cancer with photodynamic therapy: correlation of distribution of photosensitiser with biological effects in normal and tumour tissue. Gut 32:517–523
4. Barr H, Krasner N, Boulos PB, Chatlani P, Bown SG (1990) Photodynamic therapy for colorectal cancer: a quantitative pilot study. Br J Surg 77:93–96
5. Bedwell J, Holton J, Vaira D, MacRobert AJ, Bown SG (1991) In vitro killing of Helicobacter pylori with photodynamic therapy. Lancet 335:1287
6. Bedwell J, MacRobert AJ, Phillips D, Bown SG (1992) Fluorescence distribution and photodynamic effect of ALA-induced PPIX in the DMH rat colonic tumour model. Br J Cancer 65:818–824
7. Bugelski PJ, Porter CW, Dougherty TJ (1981) Autoradiographic distribution of hematoporphyrin derivative in normal and tumour tissue of the mouse. Cancer Res 41:4606–4612
8. Chatlani PT, Bedwell J, MacRobert AJ, Bown SG (1992) Distribution and photodynamic effects of AlS_2Pc and AlS_4Pc (di-and tetra- sulphonated aluminium phthalocyanine) in normal and neoplastic colon (Abstract). Lasers Med Sci 7:229
9. Cowled PA, Forbes IJ (1985) Photocytotoxicity in vivo of haematoporphyrin derivative components. Cancer Lett 28:111–118
10. Divaris XG, Kennedy JC, Pottier RH (1990) Phototoxic damage to sebaceous glands and hair follicles of mice after systemic administration of 5-aminolevulinic acid correlates with localised protoporphyrin IX fluorescence. Am J Pathol 136:891–897
11. Dougherty TJ (1990) Photodynamic therapy for the treatment of cancer: current status and advances. In: Kessel D (ed) Photodynamic therapy of neoplastic disease, vol 1. CRC Press, Boca Raton, pp 1–20
12. Figge FHJ, Weiland GS, Manganiello LOJ (1948) Cancer detection and therapy. Affinity of neoplastic, embryonic and traumatized tissues for porphyrins and metalloporphyrins. Proc Soc Exp Biol Med 68:640–641
13. Gomer CJ, Razum NJ (1984) Acute skin response in albino mice following prophyrin photosensitization under oxic and anoxic conditions. Photochem Photobiol 40:435–439
14. Gomer CJ, Rucker N, Murphree AL (1988) Differential cell photosensitivity following porphyrin photodynamic therapy. Cancer Res 48:4539–4542
15. Hayata Y, Kato H, Konaka C et al. (1982) Hematoporphyrin derivative and laser photoradiation in the treatment of lung cancer. Chest 81:269–277
16. Ito Y, Kasugai T (1987) Use of endoscopic laser in gastroenterology. Ann Acad Med Sing 16:290–293
17. Jesionek A, von Tappeiner H (1905) Zur Behandlung der Hautcarcinome mit fluorescierenden Stoffen. Arch Klin Med 82:223
18. Jori G (1989) In vivo transport and pharmacokinetic behaviour of tumour photosensitizers. In: Photosensitizing compounds: their chemistry, biology and clinical use. Wiley, Chichester, pp 78–94
19. Kato H, Aizawa K, Ono J, Konaka C, Kawate N, Yoneyama K, Kinoshita K, Nishimiya K, Sakai H, Noguchi M, Tomono T, Kawasaki S, Tokuda Y, Hayata Y (1984) Clinical measurement of tumor fluorescence using a new diagnostic system with hematoporphyrin derivative, laser photoradiation, and a spectroscope. Lasers Surg Med 4:49–58
20. Kato H, Kawaguchi M, Konoka C, Nishimiya K, Kawate M, Yoneyama K, Kinoshita K, Noguchi M, Ishii M, Shirai M, Hirano T, Aizawa K, Hayata Y (1985) Evaluation of photodynamic therapy in gastric cancer. Lasers Med Sci 1:67–74
21. Kennedy JC, Pottier RH, Pross DC (1990) Photodynamic therapy with endogenous protoporphyrin IX: basic principles and present clinical experience. J Photochem Photobiol B: Biol 6: 143–148

22. Kessel D, Erickson C (1992) Porphyrin photosensitization of multi-drug resistant cell types. Photochem Photobiol 55:397–399
23. Li JH, Guo ZH, Jin ML, Zhao FY, Cai WM, Gao ML, Shu My, Zou J (1990) Photodynamic therapy in the treatment of malignant tumours: an analysis of 540 cases. J Photochem Photobiol B: Biol 6:149–155
24. Lipson RL, Baldes EJ (1960) The photodynamic property of a particular haematoporphyrin derivative. Arch Dermatol 82:508–516
24a. Lipson RL, Baldes EJ, Olsen AM (1961) Haematoporphyrin derivative: a new aid for endoscopic detection of malignant disease. J Thorac Cardiovasc Surg 42:623–629
25. Lipson RL, Baldes EJ, Olsen AM (1964) Further evaluation of the use of haematoporphyrin derivative as a new aid for endoscopic detection of malignant disease. Dis Chest 46:676–679
26. Lipson RL, Baldes EJ, Gray MJ (1967) Haematoporphyrin derivative for the detection and management of cancer. Cancer 20:2255–2257
27. Lipson RL, Baldes EJ, Olsen AM (1961) The use of a derivative of haematoporphyrin in tumour detection. J Natl Cancer Inst 26:1–11
28. Lipson RL, Pratt JH, Baldes EJ (1964) Haematoporphyrin derivative for the detection of cervical cancer. Obstet Gynecol 24:78
29. Loh CS, Bedwell J, MacRobert AJ, Krasner N, Phillips D, Bown SG (1992) Photodynamic therapy of the normal rat stomach: a comparative study between di-sulphonated aluminium phthalocyanine and 5-aminolaevulinic acid. Br J Cancer 66: 452–462
30. MacRobert AJ, Bown SG, Phillips D (1989) What are the ideal photoproperties for a sensitizer? In: Photosensitizing compounds: their chemistry, biology and clinical use. Wiley, Chichester, pp 4–16
31. Malik Z, Djaldetti M (1979) 5-aminolevulinic acid stimulation of porphyrin and hemoglobin synthesis by uninduced Friend erythroleukemic cells. Cell Differ 8:223–233
32. Marriott J (1968) Regulation of porphyrin synthesis. Biochem Soc Sympo 28:61–74
32a. Moan J, Sommer S (1985) Oxygen dependence of the photosensitizing effect of hematoporphyrin derivative in NHIK-3025 cells. Cancer Res 45:1608–1610
33. Moan J, Berg K, Kvam E, Western A, Malik Z, Ruck A, Schneckenburger H (1989) Intracellular localization of photosensitisers. In: Photosensitizing compounds: their chemistry, biology and clinical use. Wiley, Chichester, pp 95–107
34. Monnier Ph, Savary M, Fontoliet Ch, Wagnieres G, Chatelain A, Cornaz P, Depeursinge Ch, van den Bergh H (1990) Photodetection and photodynamic therapy of 'early' squamous cell carcinomas of the pharynx, oesophagus and tracheo-bronchial tree. Lasers Med Sci 5:149–169
35. Moss S, Calam J (1992) Helicobacter pylori and peptic ulcers: the present position. Gut 33:289–292
36. Nelson JS, Liaw LH, Berns MW (1987) Tumor destruction in photodynamic therapy. Photochem Photobiol 46:829–835
37. Patrice T, Foultier MT, Yactayo S, Adam F, Galmiche JP, Douet MC, Le Bodic L (1990) Endoscopic photodynamic therapy with hematoporphyrin derivative for primary treatment of gastrointestinal neoplasms in inoperable patients. Dig Dis Sci 35:545–552
38. Popat S, Vogel J, Wagner U, Biersack J, Krebs D, Schmidt S (1992) Morphological analysis after PDT with antibody-guided phthalocyanines (Abstract). Lasers Med Sci 7:174
39. Potter WR, Mang TS, Dougherty TJ (1987) The theory of photodynamic therapy dosimetry: consequences of photodestruction of sensitiser. Photochem Photobiol 46:97–101
40. Raab O (1900) Über die Wirkung fluorescierender Stoffe auf Infusorien. Z Biol 39:524–546
41. Rassmussen-Taxdal DS, Ward GE, Figge FHJ. (1955) Fluorescence of human lymphatic and cancer tissue following high doses of intravenous hematoporphyrin. Cancer 8:78–81
42. Razum N, Balchum OJ, Profio E, Carstens F (1987) Skin photosensitivity: duration and intensity following intravenous hematoporphyrin derivatives, HpD and DHE. Photochem Photobiol 46:925–928
43. Rimington C (1966) Porphyrin and haem biosynthesis and its control. Acta Med Scand 179(Suppl 445):11–24
44. Roberts WG, Smith KM, McCullough JL, Berns MW (1989) Skin photosensitivity and photodestruction of several potential photodynamic sensitizers. Photochem Photobiol 49:431–438

45. Schmidt S, Wagner U, Popat S, Schultes B, Spaniol S, Biersack J, Krebs D (1992) Clinical results with phthalocyanines (Abstract). Lasers Med Sci 7:204
46. Schwartz SK, Absolon K, Vermund H (1955) Some relationship of porphyrins, x-rays and tumours. Univ Minn Med Bull 27:7–8
47. Sima AAF, Kennedy JC, Balkeslee D, Robertson DM (1981) Experimental porphyric neuropathy: a preliminary report. Can J Neurol Sci 8:105–114
48. Stern SJ, Flock ST, Small S, Thomsen S, Jacques S (1990). Photodynamic therapy with chloroaluminum sulfonated phthalocyanine in the rat window chamber. Am J Surg 160:360–364
49. Svaasand LO (1984) Optical dosimetry for direct and interstitial photoradiation therapy of malignant tumors. In: Doiron DR, Gomer CJ (eds) Porphyrin localisation and treatment of tumors. Liss, New York, pp 91–114
50. Tajiri H, Daikuzono N, Joffe SN, Oguro Y (1987) Photoradiation therapy in early gastrointestinal cancer. Gastrointest Endosc 33:88–90
51. Tralau CJ, Barr H, Sandeman DR, Barton T, Lewin MR, Bown SG (1987) Aluminum sulfonated phthalocyanine distribution in rodent tumours of the colon, brain, and pancreas. Photochem. Photobiol 46:777–781
52. Tralau CJ, Young AR, Walker NPJ, Vernon DI, MacRobert AJ, Brown SB, Bown SG (1989) Mouse skin photosensitivity with dihaematoporphyrin ether (DHE) and sulphonated phthalocyanine (AlSPc): a comparative study. Photochem Photobiol 49:305–312
53. Von Tappeiner H, Jesionek A (1903) Therapeutische Versuche mit fluorescierenden Stoffen. Münch Med Wochenschr 47:2042–2044
54. Von Tappeiner H, Jodlbauer A (1907) Die sensibilisierende Wirkung fluorescierender Substanzen. Gesammelte Untersuchungen über die photodynamische Erscheinung. Vogel, Leipzig
55. Weishaupt KR, Gomer CJ, Dougherty TJ (1976) Identification of singlet oxygen as the cytotoxic agent in photoinactivation of a murine tumor. Cancer Res 36:2326–2329
56. Wolf P, Kerl H (1991) Photodynamic therapy in patients with xeroderma pigmentosum. Lancet 337:1613–1614
57. Zandomeneghi M, Festa C, Angeletti CA, Menconi G, Sicuro T, Cozzani I (1988) Detection of near-infrared porphyrin fluorescence excited in experimental animal tumours by the HeNe laser. Lasers Med Sci 3:99–102

Extended Lymph Node Dissection for Advanced Gastric Cancer and Endoscopic Surgery for Early Gastric Cancer

M. Kitajima, K. Kumai, T. Kubota, Y. Otani, A. Shimada, and A. Oshima

Introduction

Most studies from western countries have not seemed to show a demonstrably increased survival rate with acceptable postoperative morbidity in gastric cancer patients undergoing radical lymphadenectomy [1–3]. The 5-year survival rate of gastric cancer was approximately 20% in most Japanese institutions during the 1950s. According to the national registry of stomach cancer in Japan, the 5-year survival rate of curatively resected gastric cancer improved up to 75% in 1981 [4]. Such remarkable improvement is attributed largely to the system of detecting early gastric cancer by screening tests as well as to the establishment of adjuvant chemotherapy. In more recent studies in Japan, the incidence of early gastric cancer was approximately 40% [5, 6] and this certainly boosted the overall survival curves in gastric cancer patients. In other words, investigation of survival rates according to accurate staging is needed.

The 5-year survival rate of 32.8% for patients with gastric cancer beyond the submucosa remains unsatisfactory [7]. Standardization of prophylactic extended lymphadenectomy could be another possibility for improving the surgical treatment of patients with advanced gastric cancer [8]. In this institution extended radical gastrectomy inclusive of para-aortic lymph nodes for advanced gastric cancer has been performed since 1986. The present study investigates the prognostic significance of para-aortic lymph node dissection in stage III gastric cancer patients, when compared to conventional radical gastrectomy, from 1965 to 1985.

Meanwhile the prognosis of early gastric cancer is fair. Although some western investigators have demonstrated no relationship between survival rate and depth of invasion [9, 10], several Japanese studies showed better outcome of patients with intramucosal gastric cancer [11, 12]. However, gastrectomy is not always the best choice in early gastric cancer patients with poor surgical risk in this study.

Furthermore, small adenocarcinomata existing in the gastric mucosal layer are focused, and the possibility of endoscopic surgery for these early gastric cancers is discussed.

Patients

From 1964 to 1985, 1807 patients with gastric cancer underwent gastric resection in the Department of Surgery, Keio University Hospital. Sixty-four out of the 1807 were treated by extended radical gastrectomy inclusive of para-aortic lymph nodes.

Since 1986, and only in patients with stage III gastric cancer, extended radical gastrectomy including para-aortic lymph node dissection has been performed in 69 out of a total of 522 patients. "Conventional radical gastrectomy" means gastric resection with lymph node dissection along the left gastric artery (LGA), the common hepatic artery (CHA), the celiac artery (CA), the splenic artery (SA), and at the splenic hilus (SH) as well as regional lymph node dissection. "Extended radical gastrectomy" means conventional radical gastrectomy plus lymph node dissection in the hepatoduodenal ligament, at the posterior aspect of the pancreas, and at the root of the mesenterium.

Seven hundred and fifty-seven patients with early gastric cancer underwent gastrectomy from 1964 to 1990. "Early gastric cancer" is defined as a lesion confined to the mucosa or to the submucosa, irrespective of the presence or absence of lymph node metastases [4]. Forty-five patients underwent endoscopic surgery between 1988 and 1990.

Surgical Procedures

The surgical procedure for extended radical lymphadenectomy including para-aortic lymph node dissection in advanced gastric cancer was as follows. After laparotomy was performed by upper median incision, the retroperitoneum was incised from the outer margin of the left colic angle upward to the esophageal hiatus. The lienorenal ligament was cut, and then both the spleen and the pancreas were rotated medially. Lymph nodes surrounding the left renal vessels were dissected. The left adrenal vein was clearly seen (Fig. 1). Then the duodenum was rotated as medially as possible by Kocher's maneuver until the inferior vena cava, left renal vein, and abdominal aorta were visible. The para-aortic lymph nodes were dissected (Fig. 2). After determination of the celiac axis by tracing the trunk of the splenic artery, the nerve plexus and lymph nodes around the celiac axis were dissected. The left gastric artery was then severed at its root.

The entire greater omentum was excised along the transverse colon from the left colic angle to the right end. The left gastroepiploic vessels were severed near the splenic hilus. Lymph nodes around the splenic hilus were dissected. The peritoneum of the anterior leaf of the transverse mesocolon was peeled off towards pancreas. The peritoneum overlying the omental bursa was completely removed with the stomach. The root of the right gastroepiploic artery was severed. The peritoneum of the hepatoduodenal ligament was excised and lymph nodes around the portal vein, common bile duct, and hepatic artery were

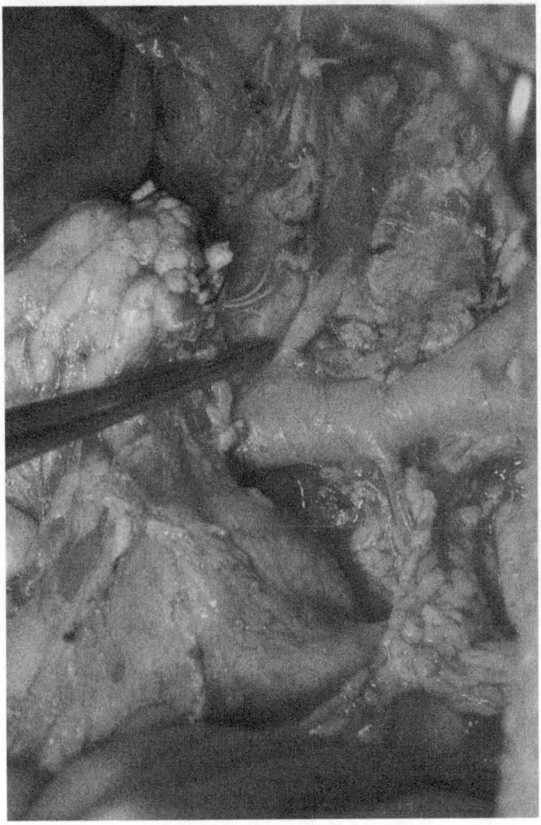

Fig. 1. Lymph node dissection around the left renal vessels

dissected (Fig. 3). The lesser omentum was removed up to the esophageal hiatus. The left gastric vein was severed.

Appropriate gastric resection was selected according to the location of the tumor.

Study Procedure

In accordance with the General Rules for Gastric Cancer Study in Surgery and Pathology in Japan [4], location, gross type, size, serosal invasion, and lymph node metastasis of the tumor were described as surgical findings in all cases. Disseminating peritoneal metastasis and liver metastasis were also described. Gastric cancers were classified into six types based on visual inspection of the mucosal surface of the fresh specimen. Depth of invasion and lymph node metastasis were histopathologically examined using the hematoxylin and eosin staining technique. The cancer stage was classified into four categories based on

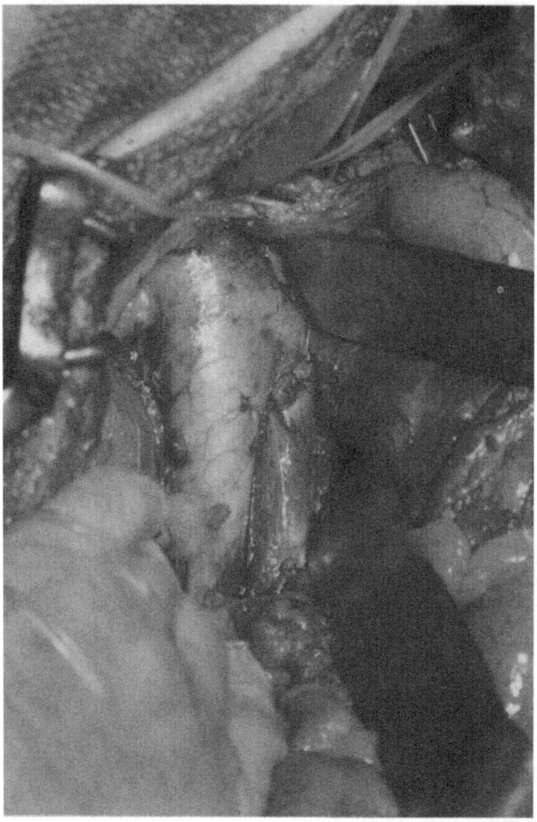

Fig. 2. Para-aortic lymph node dissection

histological findings (Table 1) [4]. PO: no disseminating metastases; P1, P2, P3: disseminating metastases; HO: no liver metastasis; H1, H2, H3: liver metastasis, n(–): no lymph node metastasis; n1(+): regional lymph node metastasis; n2(+): lymph node metastasis along the arteries from celiac axis and at the hilus of spleen; n3(+): lymph node metastasis in the hepatoduodenal ligament, on the posterior aspect of the pancreas, at the root of the mesenterium; n4(+): para-aortic lymph node metastasis.

Para-aortic lymph node metastasis was looked for in 64 cases of randomly performed extended radical gastrectomy.

Two groups of gastric cancer patients at each stage were compared from 1986 to 1990 (group A, $n = 522$) and from 1981 to 1985 (group B, $n = 501$), in order to examine the prognostic significance of extended radical gastrectomy inclusive of para-aortic lymph nodes. Extended radical gastrectomy including para-aortic lymph nodes in group A and conventional radical gastrectomy in group B were performed. Our indications for para-aortic lymph node dissection were defined as serosal invasion or invasion to contiguous structures and lymph node metastasis along the LSA, CHA, CA, SA, or at SH upon gross inspection.

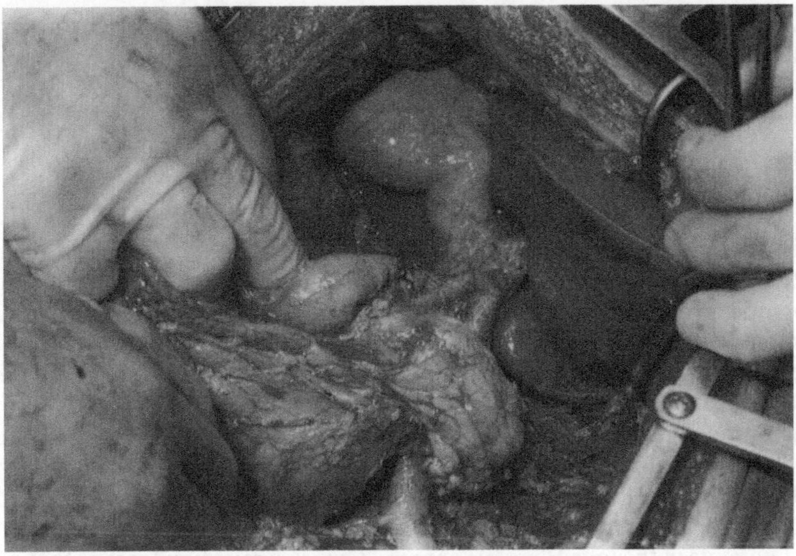

Fig. 3. Lymph node dissection around the portal vein, common bile duct, and hepatic artery

Table 1. Cancer stage based on histologic findings[a]

	Macroscopic or histologic		Histologic	
Stage	Peritoneal metastasis	Liver metastasis	Lymph node metastasis	Depth of invasion
I	P_0	H_0	n(−)	ps(−)
II	P_0	H_0	$n_1(+)$	ssy
III	P_0	H_0	$n_2(+)$	sc
IV	P_1, P_2, P_3	H_1, H_2, H_3	$n_3(+)$, $n_4(+)$	si, sei

[a]See [4], part II, B.4 and Addendum

To investigate the possibility of endoscopic surgery, lymph node metastasis was examined in early gastric cancer cases. Then endoscopic surgery was performed when tumor size was within 2 cm for a protruded lesion or within 1 cm for a depressed lesion, and the histological classification was well differentiated adenocarcinoma. The endoscopic surgical procedure was either endoscopic polypectomy or strip biopsy [13].

Statistics

Survival rate was calculated by cumulative method for each stage, I to IV. When the number of cases was small, survival curves were estimated by life-table analysis using the Kaplan-Meier method [14].

To compare the 5-year survival rates, both the generalized Wilcoxon test and the log rank test were used for evaluations.

Results

Age distribution, surgical procedure, and location of main tumor in each stage of gastric cancer is listed in Table 2. The number of partial resections, including laparoscopic procedure, or endoscopic surgical procedures at stage I and total gastrectomy at stage II increased during the last 5 years of the study. Percentages in stages I and IV also increased during the same 5 years. No other patterns were identified.

The survival rates of patients at each stage from 1964 to 1985 are shown in Fig. 4. The survival rates correspond well to the cancer staging. The curves for stage III and stage IV showed much lower survival rates than the stage I and stage II curves, although conventional radical gastrectomy had been performed in most patients with stage II gastric cancer. "Curative resection" means that all the evident carcinoma, including metastatic nodes, was excised.

Para-aortic lymph node metastasis was found in 4 out of 64 cases, mostly in cases with type 3, corresponding to Borrmann's classification [15], upon gross inspection and with definite serosal invasion or invasion to contiguous structures (Table 3). All four cases with para-aortic lymph node metastasis had more than one metastasis of lymph nodes along LGA, CHA, CA, SA, or at SH. One of four patients is still alive 3 years after extended radical gastrectomy (Fig. 5).

The survival rates at each stage are shown in Fig. 6. There were no significant differences between groups A and B in stages I, II, and IV. Extended radical gastrectomy including para-aortic dissection in stage III gastric cancer improved ($p < 0.05$) the 5-year survival rate compared to that of conventional

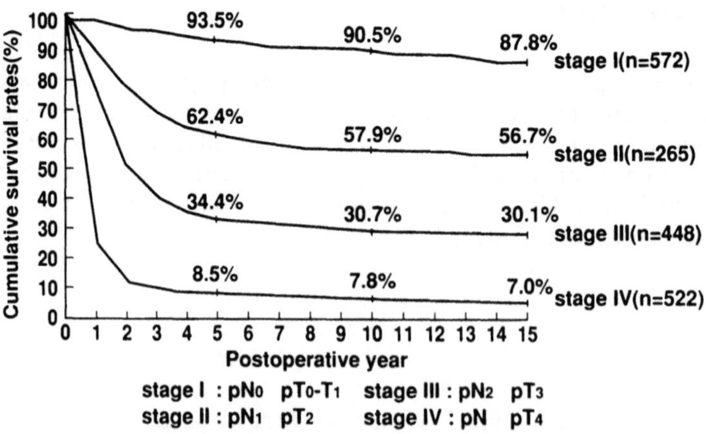

Fig. 4. Cumulative survival curves according to histologic stage

Table 2. Age distribution, location of tumor and surgical method according to stage

Stage		Age (years)	Location of main tumor				Surgical method		
			C upper	M middle	A lower	Entire stomach	Subtotal gastrectomy	Total gastrectomy	Others
Stage I	(1964–1985)	56.9 ± 15.7	84	275	200	3	414	90	55
	(1986–1990)	68.6 ± 12.3	36	106	87	1	135	39	59
Stage II	(1964–1985)	53.9 ± 13.9	27	62	77	3	112	41	18
	(1986–1990)	61.7 ± 12.1	11	18	24	1	28	21	5
Stage III	(1964–1985)	57.2 ± 18.1	86	147	141	10	184	160	42
	(1986–1990)	63.5 ± 12.7	18	42	22	1	32	36	15
Stage IV	(1964–1985)	56.0 ± 14.7	40	38	49	12	37	52	11(41)
	(1986–1990)	60.7 ± 13.7	32	25	39	4	28	42	15(14)

Table 3. Para-aortic lymph node (no. 16) dissection and metastasis

Tumor	Cases with no. 16 dissected		Cases with no. 16 metastasis
Location	C (upper)	10	1
	M (middle)	23	1
	A (lower)	29	2
	Entire stomach	2	0
Gross findings	Type 0	13	0
	1	1	0
	2	10	0
	3	25	3
	4	6	1
	5	9	0
Serosal invasion	S_0	26	0
	S_1	11	1
	S_2	24	1
	S_3	3	2
Depth of invasion (pathology)	m	7	0
	sm	11	2
	pm	10	0
	ss	23	1
	sl	13	1
	si, sei	0	0

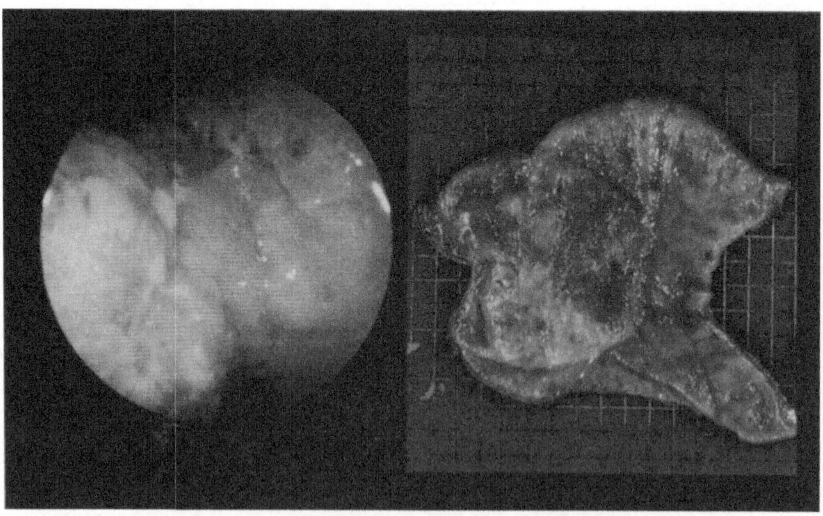

Fig. 5. Endoscopic appearance and surgical specimen from the gastric cancer patient with para-aortic lymph node metastasis who is still alive 3 years after surgery

radical gastrectomy. There were no significant differences in background between the two groups (age distribution, tumor location, surgical procedure, operating time, amount of bleeding and blood transfusion, adjuvant chemotherapy, and so on).

There were significant differences in T3 between groups A and B in regard to survival rate according to depth of cancer invasion by TNM classification (Fig. 7).

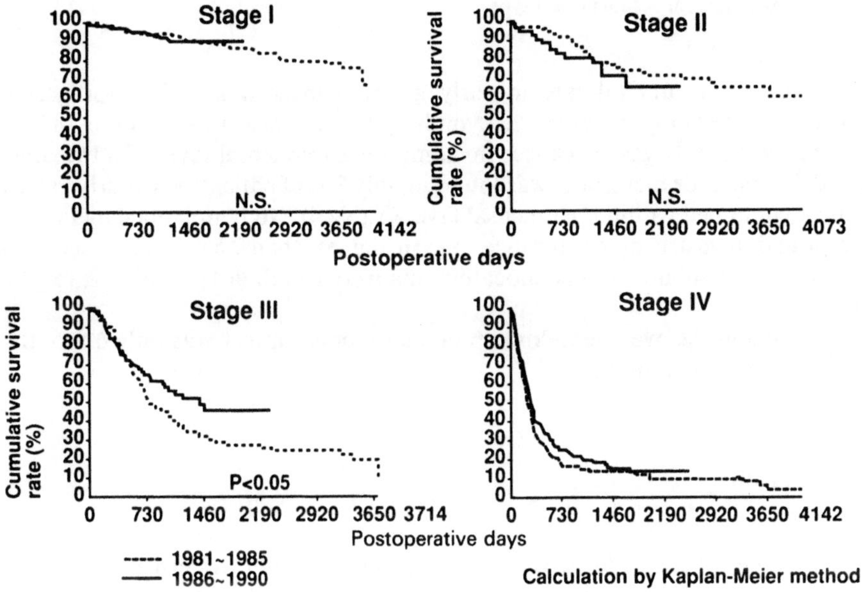

Fig. 6. Cumulative survival curves according to histologic stages

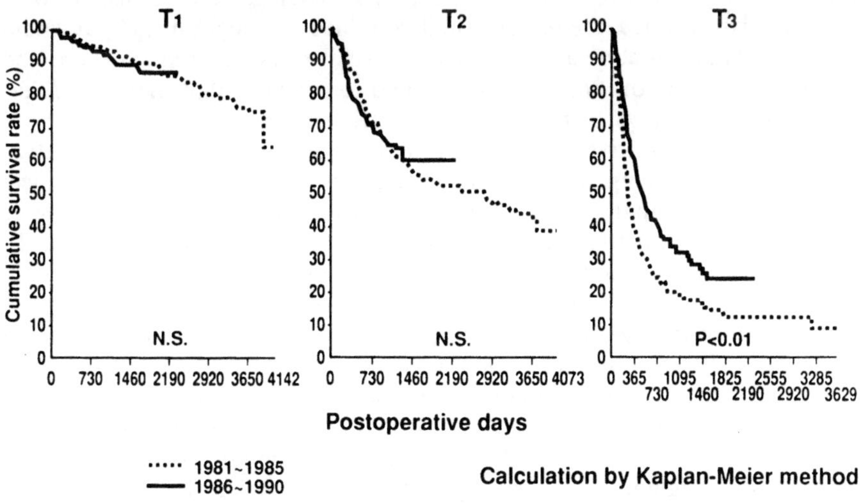

Fig. 7. Cumulative survival curves according to depth of invasion

Table 4. Lymph node metastasis in early gastric cancer

Depth of invasion	No. of cases (%)	n(−)	$n_1(+)$	$n_2(+)$	$n_3(+)$	$n_4(+)$
m	364 (100)	353 (97.0)	8 (2.2)	3 (0.8)	0	0
sm	393 (100)	322 (81.9)	46 (11.7)	20 (5.1)	2 (0.5)	3 (0.8)

m = mucosal type; sm = submucosal type

The 5-year survival rate in early gastric cancer was 85.5%; for gastric mucosal cancer only it was 99%. Lymph node metastasis was found in 18% of patients with early gastric cancer invading the submucosal layer. On the other hand, lymph node metastasis was found in only 3% of patients with early gastric cancer contained within the mucosal layer (Table 4). No lymph node metastasis was found in gastric mucosal cancer measuring less than 2 cm. Recurrence rates of mucosal or submucosal adenocarcinoma were less than 1% and 5%, respectively.

Although the average follow-up of endoscopic surgery was only 6 months, no recurrence was found.

Discussion

The marked difference in survival between Japanese and western studies seems to be attributed to very different pathologic staging systems and aggressiveness of attitude toward eradicating gastric cancer. Most western series potentially "understage" patients relative to the Japanese staging, because usually only perigastric lymph nodes are removed and examined histologically [16]. It would be inappropriate to compare the 5-year survival rates between Japanese and western studies without matching stages and to conclude that there are differences in tumor biology or to give up eradication of gastric cancer.

Despite an aggressive attitude toward resection and lymph node dissection combined with staging accuracy, the prognosis of advanced gastric cancer remains poor in Japan. Extended lymphadenectomy is another challenge to improve the surgical treatment of patients with advanced gastric cancer. To avoid unnecessary deterioration in postoperative morbidity, appropriate indications are needed. The indications for extended radical gastrectomy with para-aortic lymph node dissection reported by several Japanese researchers are similar but slightly different. Our indications are definite serosal invasion or invasion of contiguous structures and lymph node metastasis along LGA, CHA, CA, SA or at SH upon gross inspection, since, in our randomized study, para-aortic lymph node metastasis was found mostly in patients with definite serosal invasion or invasion of contiguous structures. Lymph node metastasis along LGA, CHA, CA, SA or at the splenic hilus was associated with a high incidence of para-aortic lymph node metastasis [17]. Recently, a sternum procedure was indicated for cardiac cancer undertaken with lower esophageal resection and extended lymphadenectomy including para-aortic lymph nodes [18]. By performing extended radical gastrectomy the 5-year survival rate significantly improved from 27.5% with conventional radical gastrectomy to a new figure of 46.0%. This indicates the efficacy of extended radical gastrectomy in advanced cancer. As is always pointed out, this study is not a randomized trial, either. Since there were no significant differences between groups A and B in survival rates for stages I, II, and IV, the effect on survival rate of perioperative care can be neglected. Recent studies from Japan also support our reports [19, 20], although some do not [7].

It is well known that Japan is one of the countries with a high prevalence of gastric cancer. Screening tests have been massively carried out over the last 30 years and resulted in a marked increase in the recorded prevalence of early gastric cancer in Japan, from 1.3% in 1941 through 1945 to 36% in 1965 [21]. The fraction of early gastric cancers among all resected gastric cancers has reached almost 50% during the last 5 years in our institute. The 5-year survival rate in early gastric cancer was 85.5% in this study, which is as good as reported in other studies [22, 23]. Lymph node metastasis was found in only 3% of early gastric cancers localized in the mucosal layer. If cancer localized in the mucosal layer is accurately diagnosed, endoscopic surgery is applicable. Several studies on the accuracy of depth diagnosis using endoscopy or endoscopic ultrasound have been reported [24, 25]. The indications for endoscopic surgery for gastric cancer in our institute seem to be too prudent. However, our results are excellent in spite of the short follow-up. From the point of view of safety, it is not desirable to endoscopically resect a lesion over 2 cm in size.

In conclusion, from 1964 to 1985 the survival rate of patients with stage III gastric cancer was much lower than that of patients with gastric cancer in stage I or II. Since 1986, we have tried extended radical gastrectomy including para-aortic lymph node dissection on stage III gastric cancer patients. The 5-year survival rate after extended radical gastrectomy was better than that after conventional radical gastrectomy.

Endoscopic surgery application is recommended when tumor size is within 2 cm for an elevated lesion or within 1 cm for a depressed lesion and the histologic classification is well-differentiated adenocarcinoma.

Summary

From 1964 to 1985, 1807 patients with gastric cancer underwent gastric resection. The survival rate of gastric cancer patients at stage III (by Japanese classification) is much lower than that of patients at stages I or II, although conventional radical gastrectomy has been performed in most patients with stage III gastric cancer. To improve the survival rate of advanced gastric cancer, extended radical gastrectomy inclusive of para-aortic lymph nodes was performed in 64 cases. Para-aortic lymph node metastasis was found mostly in cases with type 3, corresponding to Borrmann's classification, upon gross inspection and with definite serosal invasion or invasion to contiguous structures. Based on these findings extended radical gastrectomy inclusive of para-aortic lymph nodes has been performed since 1986. Sixty-nine patients with stage III gastric cancer from 1986 to 1990 were compared to 70 patients from 1981 to 1985. Extended radical gastrectomy inclusive of para-aortic lymph nodes for advanced gastric cancer improved the 5-year survival rate compared to that of conventional radical gastrectomy.

From 1964 to 1990, 757 patients with early gastric cancer underwent conventional radical gastrectomy. Among those with early gastric cancer invading to the submucosal layer, lymph node metastasis was found in 18%. On the other hand, in cases of cancer within the mucosal layer, such metastasis was found in only 3%. Endoscopic surgery would be applied when tumor size is less than 2 cm for protruded lesions or less than 1 cm for depressed lesions and the histological classification is well-differentiated adenocarcinoma.

References

1. Gilbertson VA (1969) Results of treatment of stomach cancer: an appraisal of efforts for more extensive surgery and a report of 1,983 cases. Cancer 23:1305–1308
2. Dent DM, Madden MV and Price SK (1988) Randomized comparison of R1 and R2 gastrectomy for gastric carcinoma. Br J Surg 75:110–112
3. Shiu MH, Papacristou DN, Kosloff C et al. (1980) Selection of operative procedure for adenocarcinoma of the mid stomach: twenty years' experience with implications for future treatment strategy. Ann Surg 192:730–737
4. Japanese Research Society for Gastric Cancer (1981) The general rules for the gastric cancer study in surgery and pathology. Jpn J Surg 11:127–139
5. Maruyama K, Gunven P, Okabayashi K et al. (1989) Lymph node metastases of gastric cancer: General pattern in 1931 patients. Ann Surg 210:596–602
6. Kampschoer GHM, Nakajima Y, Van de Verde CJH (1989) Changing patterns in gastric adenocarcinoma. Br J Surg 76:914–916
7. Korenaga D, Moriguchi S, Orita H et al. (1992) Trends in survival rates in Japanese patients with advanced carcinoma of the stomach. Surg Gynecol Obstet 174:387–393
8. Orita K, Sakagami K, Kamikawa Y et al. (1991) Coeliac axis-oriented approach in surgery for advanced gastric cancer. Sem Surg Oncol 7:373–377
9. Bringaze WL III, Chappuis CW, Cohn I Jr et al. (1986) Early gastric cancer: 21-years experience. Ann Surg 204:103–107
10. Carter KJ, Schaffer HA, Ritchie WP Jr (1984) Early gastric cancer. Ann Surg 199:604–608
11. Hioki K, Nakane Y, Yamamoto M (1990) Surgical strategy for early gastric cancer. Br J Surg 77:1330–1334
12. Ichiyoshi Y, Toda T, Minamisono Y et al. (1990) Recurrence in early gastric cancer. Surgery 107:489–495
13. Tada M, Shimada M, Yanai H et al. (1984) A new technique of gastric bipsy (English abstract). Stomach Intestines 19:1107–1116
14. Kaplan EL and Meier A (1958) Nonparametric estimation for incomplete observations. J Am Stat Assoc 53:457–481
15. Borrmann R (1926) Geschwülste des Magens. Heuke FU, Lubarsch O (eds) Handbuch der speziellen pathologischen Anatomie und Histologie, IV/Part 1. Springer, Berlin, pp 864–871
16. Behrns KE, Dalton RR, Jon A van Heerden et al. (1992) Extended lymph node dissection for gastric cancer. Surg Clin North Am 72:433–443

17. Nishi M, Ohta K, Ishihara S et al. (1991) Clinicopathological study about the para-aortic lymph node metastases of gastric cancer. (in Japanese) Shokakigeka 14:165–176
18. Kitajima M and Sohma S (1981) Operation for lower esophageal and cardiac cancer: Sternum splitting procedure. (in Japanese) Herusu Publisher, Tokyo
19. Soga J, Ohyama S, Miyashita K et al. (1988) A statistical evaluation of advancement in gastric cancer surgery with special reference to the significance of lymphadenectomy for cure. World J Surg 12:398–405
20. Maruyama K, Okabayashi K, Kinoshita T (1987) Progress in gastric cancer surgery in Japan and its limits of radicality. World J Surg 11:418–425
21. Muto M, Maki T, Majima S et al. (1968) Improvement in the end-results of surgical treatment of gastric cancer. Surgery 63:229–235
22. Marczell AP, Rosen HR and Hentschel E (1989) Diagnosis and tactical approach to surgery for early gastric carcinoma: a retrospective analysis of the past 16 years in an Austrian General Hospital. Gastroenterol Jpn 24:732–736
23. Itoh H, Oohata Y, Nakamura K et al. (1989) Complete ten-year postgastrectomy follow-up of early gastric cancer. Am J Surg 158:14–16
24. Haruma K, Sumii K, Inoue K et al. (1990) Endoscopic therapy in patients with inoperable early gastric cancer. Am J Gastroenterol 85:522–526
25. Sano T, Okuyama Y, Kobori O et al. (1990) Early gastric cancer: Endoscopic diagnosis of depth of invasion. Dig Dis Sci 35:1340–1344

Stage-Adjusted Chemotherapy of Gastric Cancer

P. PREUSSER, T. BERNS, and H. WILKE

Introduction

Of patients with UICC stage I or II gastric cancer, 50%–80% can be curatively treated by resection [21]. At stage III, 5-year survival is only 15%–20%, and at stage IV (advanced local tumour), patients who survive for 5 years are the exception [8, 12] (Table 1). After "curative" resection of advanced local tumours (stages IIIb, IV), the median overall survival is only 7–15 months [12], while after surgery of limited local tumours that can be resected, but not curatively, and in patients with distant metastases, the median survival is only 4–6 months [2, 10, 14] (Table 2).

In advanced gastric cancer, metastases are found at diagnosis in two-thirds to three-quarters of cases [4, 6, 9, 22–24]. For this reason, locally effective therapy modalities such as surgery and radiation rarely bring satisfactory results in these patients. In such cases, systemic treatment with antineoplastic drugs is a better alternative.

Chemotherapy

Since 1980, various cytostatic drugs have been tested given as single drugs (monotherapy) in disease-oriented phase II trials containing not less than 14 patients who had not undergone previous chemotherapy. In our analysis of these trials, we have only included those in which remissions were defined according to the criteria of the World Health Organisation (WHO) [13, 20].

Few substances induced remission rates of more than 15% (Table 3). The rates of complete remission were higher with cisplatin, doxorubicin and epirubicin than with the other drugs [18].

Since the period of remission induced with single-drug therapy was so short, various combinations of two to four cytostatic drugs were tested in treatment of advanced gastric cancer in both randomised and non-randomised studies [17]. Retrospective analysis of these studies is difficult because of factors like heterogeneity of patient populations with different prognostic factors, and lack of information about extent of disease [1, 3, 5, 7, 11, 15].

Since publication of a prospective, randomised study in which the combinations FAM (5-fluorouracil, doxorubicin, mitomycin C) and FAMTX (5-fluoro-

Table 1. Gastric cancer: 5-year survival after surgery alone

Stage	5-year survival (%)
I	80
II	50–70
III	15–20
IV	0

Table 2. Gastric cancer: median survival after surgery alone

Stage	Resection	Median survival (months)
III	Curative	8–15
IV	Curative	7–8
Locally advanced tumour	Palliative	4–6
Metastases	Palliative	4

uracil, doxorubicin, methotrexate) were compared and a statistically significant advantage of FAMTX shown in regard to remission rate and median overall survival, the combination FAM has ceased to be regarded as the standard chemotherapy regimen for gastric cancer [18]. FAMTX is now the reference treatment with which newer, more effective chemotherapy regimens are to be compared.

Using these newer combinations overall remission rates of 42–47% have been achieved, including 6%–11% complete remissions, with median survival times for all patients of 3–18 months. After these combination therapies, complete remissions were for the first time ever confirmed by pathology departments.

The results after using the ELF combination [etoposide, leucovorin (folinic acid), 5-fluorouracil] are remarkable, as this regimen was only employed in elderly patients (over 65 years) or those who owing to heart disease could not be given combinations containing anthracyclin. Some patients continued to receive pretreatment with carboplatin.

Since the EAP combination (etoposide, doxorubicin, cisplatin) induced serious haematological side effects in a larger percentage of patients than the other combinations, and the results in metastasising gastric cancer were no better than those achieved with the better tolerated ELF regime, EAP is now only used for locally unresectable tumours.

On the basis of the results summarised in Table 4, the FAMTX, ELF and cisplatin/5-fluorouracil combinations are at present undergoing trial in a prospective, randomised and stratified study with the aim of defining a standard chemotherapeutic regime for gastric cancer.

Results of Chemotherapy According to Tumour Stage

There are only a few publications in which results can be analysed separately by disease stage (Tables 3, 4). In metastasised tumours, remission rates of 35%–49% have been induced, together with a median overall survival between 7 and 10 months [18], while in locally unresectable tumours remission rates of 47%–69% have been achieved with a median overall survival of 14–18 months [26]. This means that chemotherapy achieves better results in early-stage disease than in metastasised disease.

Only in more recent studies did patients with locally unresectable tumour undergo thorough clinical and surgical (laparotomy) staging before starting chemotherapy. In three disease-oriented phase II studies, various cytostatic combinations were given preoperatively. After preoperative chemotherapy with methotrexate/5-fluorouracil and cisplatin/5-fluorouracil, complete

Table 3. Chemotherapy of metastasising gastric cancer

Combination	No. of patients	CR *n*	%	CR + PR *n*	%	MS (months)
ELF[a]	59	4	7	27	46	9
FLEP	26	0		9	35	7
EAP	96	8	8	47	49	9
Cisplatin/5-FU	19	2	11	9	47	10
FAMTX	76	5	7	27	36	nr

[a] 41 patients over 65 years old, with or without cardiac risk factors; 18 patients received pretreatment with carboplatin.
CR = complete remission; PR = partial remission; nr = not reported

Table 4. Gastric cancer: results of preoperative chemotherapy in locally advanced disease

Author	Combination	No. of patients	CR *n*	%	CR + PR *n*	%	MS (months)
Verschueren	MTX[a]/5-FU	17		nr	8	47	14
Rorgier et al. [19]	Cisplatin/5-FU	25		nr	14	56	18
Preusser et al.	EAP	35	8	23	24	69	18

[a] middle- to high-dose methotrexate; nr = not reported

tumour resection was possible in more than 50% of patients. Median overall survival times in these studies were 14–18 months or more [16, 19, 26].

EAP was tested in a phase II study in 35 patients with locally advanced, technically unresectable (laparotomy) gastric cancer [26]. With this regimen, 69% remissions were achieved, including 23% complete remissions. After the chemotherapy, resection was possible in 20 of the 35 patients (57%). Six clinically complete and 14 partial remissions were confirmed. The median overall survival was 18 months, and for those who were disease-free after chemotherapy with or without surgery median survival was 24 months. After 3 years, 21% of the patients were alive and free of recurrence.

Although the preoperative studies have included relatively few patients so far, first results seem to suggest that in these disease stages, preoperative chemotherapy allows longer median survival times than are attained through surgery alone. Preoperative chemotherapy ought therefore to be tested in large randomised studies against surgery alone.

Prognostic Factors Relating to Chemotherapy

One thing that is of considerable importance for the planning of therapy is the identification of prognostic factors that allow prediction of the results of chemotherapy. So far, only one study has been published on the subject of prognostic factors for chemotherapy of patients with gastric cancer [11]. The usefulness of the conclusions of many publications is restricted by the fact that, in the analysis of prognostic factors, often chemotherapy programmes are employed that bring about an overall remission rate of no more than 20%, and therefore patient numbers are too low for reliable prognostic factors to be identified.

EAP and ELF are effective chemotherapy programmes for patients with advanced gastric cancer. For this reason, an analysis was carried out to identify prognostic factors for induction of remission and survival rates [25]. The only independent and negative predictive variable for the induction of remission was peritoneal carcinomatosis. Independent predictors for survival were locally advanced tumour versus metastases and male versus female sex. Other relevant factors were, histologically, intestinal versus diffuse type, and patient general condition (WHO criteria) 0 and 1 versus 2 (Table 5).

Table 5. Gastric cancer: prognostic factors for survival (multivariate analysis)

Locally advanced disease versus metastases	$p < 0.0001$
Male versus female sex	$p < 0.008$
Intestinal versus diffuse histological type	$p < 0.08$
General condition WHO grade 0 or 1 versus 2	$p < 0.08$

Summary of Chemotherapy in Gastric Cancer

The treatment of choice in stage I and II gastric cancer is surgery. In these stages, 50%–80% of patients live for 5 years or more after curative resection. When the disease is more extensive, the prognosis is worse.

Because the results of surgery alone in advanced gastric cancer are unsatisfactory, systemic treatment is required in these stages. This is carried out in the form of chemotherapy alone or in combination with surgery. Gastric cancer can be regarded as a chemosensitive tumour, especially on the basis of the published results with new combinations.

Few cytostatics are effective against advanced gastric cancer. The new combinations such as FAMTX, EAP, ELF and cisplatin/5-fluorouracil seem to promise better results. The results obtained with ELF in high-risk patients (age over 65 years, patients with cardiac disease, some with previous antineoplastic treatment) are remarkable.

Only recent studies of perioperative chemotherapy could be included in this analysis, as these used not only clinical but also surgical (laparotomy) staging. Perioperative chemotherapy increased the median survival time above that seen after surgery alone, and for that reason it should undergo further trials.

So far, only one study of prognostic factors for chemotherapy in gastric cancer has been published in which effective chemotherapy programmes were used. The only independent variable for remission was the negative predictive factor of peritoneal carcinomatosis. Independent variables for survival time were locally advanced disease versus metastases and male versus female sex.

These prognostic factors for induction of remission and patient survival are important for retrospective analysis and for the design of new studies. If the search for prognostic factors for chemotherapy is continued, it may in future be possible, by combining relevant factors, to achieve better definition of indications for chemotherapy.

Indications for Chemotherapy

It is not possible to establish a standard chemotherapy protocol for gastric carcinoma at present, because FAMTX, EAP, ELF and cisplatin/5-fluorouracil show comparable antineoplastic activity. Chemotherapy should therefore best be carried out in controlled studies.

In stage I and II tumours chemotherapy is not indicated outside controlled studies. In stages III and IV, when the tumour is unresectable or there are distant metastases, systemic chemotherapy is the main treatment modality.

The decision for chemotherapy can only be made in the light of a knowledge of the efficacy and side effects of the cytostatic drugs and drug combinations that are to be used. Factors prognostic of the induction of remission and survival are important and must be taken into account.

Necessary preconditions for aggressive chemotherapy are: histologically proven advanced gastric carcinoma and/or metastases with measurable diameter according to WHO criteria, patient age 65 years or over, patient's general condition WHO class 2 or below, no previous chemotherapy or radiotherapy, and normal renal, liver, heart and bone marrow function. After two cycles of chemotherapy, careful restaging must be carried out, and if the disease has advanced or the patient's general conditions markedly deteriorated, the chemotherapy should be stopped.

Younger patients with locally advanced, technically unresectable gastric cancer should be treated in controlled studies with intensive chemotherapy using e.g. EAP, so that if objective remission occurs, a second-look operation with resection of the remaining tumours can be carried out (Fig. 1). Because of the high recurrence rate in patients with stage II (30%–50%) and stage III (85%) disease, the combination of effective preoperative chemotherapy followed by resection in these stages should also be tested in controlled studies in the future.

Younger patients in good general condition who have distant metastases (lymph nodes, liver) but no peritoneal carcinomatosis can, according to the present state of knowledge, be treated with FAMTX, ELF or cisplatin/5-fluorouracil (Fig. 1). Patients with peritoneal carcinomatosis should only receive treatment as part of a controlled study, as experience so far is that tested chemotherapy programmes have little effect on this pattern of metastasisation.

For reasons of age or concurrent morbidity, about 60% of all patients with gastric cancer cannot undergo intensive chemotherapy programmes such as with combinations containing cisplatin or doxorubicin. Aggressive chemotherapy is contraindicated in elderly patients because of the increased sensitivity of their organs, and anthracyclins are contraindicated in patients with heart disease. These patients should be treated with better tolerated chemotherapy regimens with fewer undesired side effects, based on 5-fluorouracil/folinic acid, such as the ELF combination, as these cytostatics have no cumulative organ toxicity.

Of particular importance is that in gastric cancer, as in other tumour entities, the efficacy of chemotherapy is dependent on tumour stage. Complete

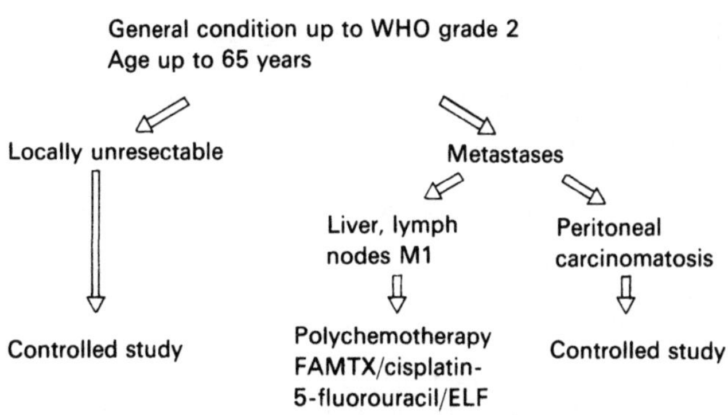

Fig. 1. Flow chart for chemotherapy of gastric carcinoma

and overall remission rates are noticeably higher and median survival noticeably longer in patients with locally advanced disease than in those with distant metastases. In addition, it has recently been shown that technically unresectable tumours can be curatively resected after preoperative chemotherapy has been given.

New developments in the treatment of gastric cancer, such as new chemotherapy programmes, perioperative chemotherapy, and the identification of prognostic factors for chemotherapy could serve as a foundation for stage- and risk-adjusted chemotherapy of this tumour. However, intensive interdisciplinary cooperation will be required if the prognosis of patients with advanced gastric cancer is to be measurably improved.

References

1. Bedikian AY, Chen TT, Khankhanian N, Heilbrun LK, McBride CM, McMurtrey MJ, Bodey GP (1984) The natural history of gastric cancer and prognostic factors influencing survival. J Clin Oncol 2:305–310
2. Bengmark S, Jeppson B (1982) Staging of liver metastases. In: Wess L, Gilberg HA (eds) Liver metastases. G.K. Hall, Boston, pp 268–274
3. Bleiberg H (1985) Prognostic significance of pathological staging in gastrointestinal tumors. Eur J Cancer Clin Oncol 21:655–658
4. Borchard F, Sons HU (1985) Klassifizierung des Magenkarzinoms aus pathologisch-anatomischer Sicht. Therapiewoche 35:161–169
5. Bruckner HW, Stablein DM (1983) Sites of treatment failure: gastrointestinal tumor study group analyses of gastric, pancreatic, colorectal trials. Cancer Treat Rep 2:199–211
6. Clarke JS, Cruze K, El Farra S, Longmire WP (1961) The natural history and results of surgical therapy for carcinoma of the stomach. An analysis of 250 cases. Am J Surg 102:143–149
7. De Lisi V, Cocconi G, Tonato M, Di Costanzo F, Leonardi F, Soldani M (1986) Randomized comparison of 5-FU alone or combined with carmustine, and mitomycin (BAFMi) in the treatment of advanced gastric cancer: a phase III trial of the Italian clinical research group (GOIRC). Cancer Treat Rep 70:481–485
8. Diehl JT, Herrmann RE, Cooperman AM, Hoerr SO (1983) Gastric carcinoma. A ten year review. Ann Surg 198:9–12
9. Dupont JB, Lee JR, Burton GR, Cohn I (1978) Adenocarcinoma of the stomach: review of 147 cases. Cancer 41:941–947
10. Kodama Y, Sugimachi K, Soejima K (1981) Evaluation of extensive lymph node dissection for carcinoma of the stomach. World J Surg 5:241–248
11. Lavin PT, Bruckner HW, Plaxes SC (1982) Studies in prognostic factors relating to chemotherapy for advanced gastric cancer. Cancer 50:2316–2023
12. Meyer H-J, Jähne J, Wilke H (1989) Das organüberschreitende Magenkarzinom. Chir Gastroenterol
13. Miller AB, Hoogstraten B, Staquet M, Winkler A (1981) Reporting results of cancer treatment. Cancer 47:207–214
14. Nekajima T, Harashima S, Hirata M (1978) Prognostic and therapeutic values of peritoneal cytology in gastric cancer. Acta Cytol 22:225–229
15. O'Connell MJ (1985) Current status of chemotherapy for advanced pancreatic and gastric cancer. J Clin Oncol 3:1032–1039
16. Plukker JT, Mulder NH, Verschueren RCJ (1989) Combined chemotherapeutic/surgical approach of locally advanced cancer of the cardia and gastric fundus. EORTC Symposium on Advances in Gastrointestinal Tract Cancer Research and Treatment, Strasbourg, November 1989

17. Preusser P, Achterrath W, Wilke H, Lenaz L, Fink U, Heinicke A, Meyer J, Bünte H (1988) Chemotherapy of gastric cancer. Cancer Treat Rev 15:257–277
18. Preusser P, Wilke H, Achterrath W, Fink U, Stahl M, Lenaz L, Wils J (1992) Chemotherapy of metastatic gastric carcinoma. International Conference on Biology and Treatment of Gastrointestinal Malignancies, Frankfurt, 4–7 February 1992, pp 42–43
19. Rougier P, Mahjoubi M, Oliveira J, Tigaud JM, Lasser P, Droz JP (1989) Treatment of advanced gastric adenocarcinoma (AGC) with 5-FU/platinum combination. EORTC Symposium on Advances in Gastrointestinal Tract Cancer Research and Treatment, Strasbourg, November 1989
20. Scher I, Geller NL, Muggia FM, Rozenczweig M (1987) Clinical evaluation of anticancer treatments: phase II clinical trials. In: Muggia FM, Rozenczweig M (eds) Clinical evaluation of antitumor therapy. Nijhoff, Boston, pp 175–197
21. Speisse B, Hermanek P, Scheibe O, Wagner G (eds) TNM-Atlas. Springer, Berlin Heidelberg New York, pp 90–98
22. Walther HE (1948) Krebsmetastasen. Schwabe, Basel, pp 363–377
23. Warren S (1933) Studies on tumor metastasis. IV. Metastases of cancer of the stomach. N Engl J Med 209:825–828
24. Warwick M (1928) Analysis of one hundred and seventy-six cases of carcinoma of the stomach submitted to autopsy. Ann Surg 88:216–221
25. Wilke H, Preusser P, Fink U, Köhne-Wömpner C, Achterrath W, Stahl M, Meyer H-J, Lenaz L, Freund M, Schmoll H-J (1989) Clinical outcome and prognostic factors in 145 patients with advanced gastric cancer treated with EAP. EORTC Symposium on Advances in Gastrointestinal Tract Cancer Research and Treatment, Strasbourg, November 1989
26. Wilke H, Preusser P, Fink U, Meyer H-J, Stahl M, Seeber S (1992) Neoadjuvant chemotherapy of primarily unresectable gastric cancer. International Conference on Biology and Treatment of Gastrointestinal Malignancies. Frankfurt, 4–7 February 1992, pp 39–40

Subject Index

Springer-Verlag and the Environment

We at Springer-Verlag firmly believe that an international science publisher has a special obligation to the environment, and our corporate policies consistently reflect this conviction.

We also expect our business partners – paper mills, printers, packaging manufacturers, etc. – to commit themselves to using environmentally friendly materials and production processes.

The paper in this book is made from low- or no-chlorine pulp and is acid free, in conformance with international standards for paper permanency.

Batch number: 10583998

Printed by Printforce, the Netherlands